CW01475644

Color Atlas of Otoscopy
From Diagnosis to Surgery

Mario Sanna, M.D.
Professor of Otolaryngology
Department of Head and Neck Surgery
University of Chieti, Chieti, Italy
Gruppo Otologico, Piacenza and Rome, Italy

Alessandra Russo, M.D., Giuseppe De Donato, M.D.
Antonio Caruso, M.D., Abdelkader Taibah, M.D.
Gruppo Otologico, Piacenza and Rome, Italy

with the collaboration of

Essam Saleh, Maurizio Falcioni, Fernando Mancini, Enrico Piccirillo

Foreword by Christian Deguine, M.D.

2nd edition, revised and enlarged

716 illustrations, most in color

Thieme
Stuttgart · New York

Library of Congress Cataloging-in-Publication Data
is available from the publisher

Mario Sanna, M.D.
Professor of Otolaryngology, Head and Neck Surgery
University of Chieti, Chieti, Italy
Gruppo Otologico
Piacenza and Rome, Italy

Alessandra Russo, M.D.
Giuseppe De Donato, M.D.
Antonio Caruso, M.D.
Abdelkader Taibah, M.D.
Maurizio Falcioni, M.D.
Fernando Mancini, M.D.
Enrico Piccirillo, M.D.
Gruppo Otologico
Piacenza and Rome, Italy

Essam Saleh, M.D.
Department of Otolaryngology, Head and Neck Surgery
University of Alexandria, Egypt

© 2002 Georg Thieme Verlag, Rüdigerstraße 14,
D-70469 Stuttgart, Germany
http://www.thieme.de

Thieme New York, 333 Seventh Avenue,
New York, NY 10001, USA
http://www.thieme.com

Typesetting by BEFORE S.r.l., San Benedetto Tr. (AP), Italy

Printed in Germany by Staudigl, Donauwörth

ISBN 3-13-111492-4 GTV
ISBN 1-58890-123-8 TNY   1 2 3 4 5

Foreword

The good fortune of otology resides in the fact that in most cases a diagnosis can be established through careful otoscopic examination: the tympanic membrane is the window to the middle ear.

Otoscopy constitutes the first phase in the examination of the patient. The initiation of the young otologist begins with this basic step. Colleagues of my generation will recall the long months of training which were necessary to understand and identify something in the depths of a narrow, tortuous, and sensitive external canal, often obstructed by physiologic or pathologic secretions. It was difficult to find good textbook illustrations. There were only drawings and lengthy pages of description not worthy of comparison with the unparalleled iconography of Politzer or Toynbee in the last century... Photographs were either absent or, when included, were of such mediocre quality that they were of limited interest. We experienced a feeling of frustration in that era of the electron microscope and of space probes bringing back photos of the earth taken from the moon...

Modern optical systems, in particular the binocular microscope, have permitted an unfettered approach and detailed observation of the tympanic membrane under optimal conditions of lighting and magnification. The addition of observer tubes and video cameras has helped to further familiarize ourselves with the various pathologic conditions. However, the tympanic membrane has long defended itself from photographic intrusion. Inclined in relation to the three spatial planes, and of a diameter of 1 cm (while the normal canal accepts only a 4-mm speculum), it is only through progressive scanning that we view the totality of the surface. Our brain reconstructs the virtual image. Thus, otoscopic photography faces a formidable challenge: to reproduce not what one sees but what one imagines. The solution came with the introduction of the Hopkins optical system, which provides wide-angle capability through a narrow-diameter endoscope, affording an enlarged field of vision and greater depth of field with increased light transmission. The principle is simple; however, utilization of the equipment necessitates a certain degree of experience to obtain quality pictures with regularity. Through my father, to whom I am indebted, I acquired a passion for photography, permitting me to acquire the necessary experience and subsequently to share it. For this reason I feel honored, as friend and colleague, to preface this remarkable volume.

Having perfectly mastered the technical problems, we note with real pleasure that Dr. Sanna and his collaborators offer us more than an "Atlas of Otoscopy," as the title of the volume modestly suggests. It is truly a "Manual of Otology" in that it covers all aspects of inflammatory, infectious, and tumor pathology of the ear, as seen through modifications of the otoscopic image.

The reader, initially attracted by a book of pictures, will be further captivated by a concise text, describing with style and precision the principal pathologic conditions: definition, nature, pathogenesis, and classification accompanied by diagrams. The text indicates as well the complementary examinations indispensable for diagnosis and available therapeutic options. Thus, radiographic images (CT scan, MRI) are juxtaposed with the otoscopic view when deemed appropriate. All pertinent information conforms to the most recently available sources and reflects the consensus of the scientific community.

A particularly interesting and original aspect is presented in the last chapters which deal with the pathology of the skull base: cholesteatoma of the petrous bone, glomus tumors, meningoencephalic herniations—areas in which Dr. Sanna has special experience which he shares with us.

The resident or practitioner desirous of an initiation into otology will find a presentation of auricular pathology which is both general and detailed. Such a structure is thoroughly complementary to the knowledge acquired during his or her medical training. The well-informed otorhinolaryngologist will find an update of the most recent clinical, radiologic, and therapeutic acquisitions in a field which is in constant evolution.

We thank and warmly congratulate the author and his collaborators for this exceptional work which reflects the level of their talent and experience. It clearly represents a significant advance in the field of otology.

Dr. C. Deguine
Lille, France

Preface to the First Edition

Despite advances in diagnostic techniques and imaging modalities, otoscopy remains the cornerstone in the diagnosis of otologic diseases. Every otolaryngologist, pediatrician, or even general practitioner dealing with ear diseases should have a good knowledge of otoscopy.

This atlas is based on 15 years of experience in the Gruppo Otologico in the treatment of otologic and neurotologic disorders. It presents a vast collection of otoscopic views of a variety of lesions that can affect the ear and temporal bone. Many examples are given for each disease so that the reader becomes acquainted with the variable presentations each pathology can have.

While otoscopy alone can establish the diagnosis in some cases, parameters such as history or audiological and neuroradiological evaluation are required in others. An important aspect of this atlas is that it juxtaposes, when appropriate, the clinical picture, radiological diagnosis, and intraoperative findings with the otoscopic findings of the patient. Needless to say, every patient should be considered as a whole and in some particular cases, the otoscopic findings might only be the "tip of the iceberg." Otalgia, otorrhea, and granulations in the external auditory canal are manifestations of otitis externa, but when they persist, particularly in the elderly, they should arouse suspicion of malignancy. Otitis media with effusion can be a simple disease when seen in children, whereas unilateral persistent otitis media with effusion in an adult may be the only sign of a nasopharyngeal carcinoma. A small attic perforation in the presence of facial nerve paralysis and sensorineural hearing loss may be all that is seen in a giant petrous bone cholesteatoma. The manifestation of an aural polyp can vary from a mucosal polyp associated with chronic suppurative otitis media to the much less common but more dangerous glomus jugulare tumor. A small retrotympanic mass may represent an anomalous anatomy such as a high jugular bulb or an aberrant carotid artery. It may also represent frank pathology such as facial nerve neuroma, congenital cholesteatoma, or even en-plaque meningioma.

In each chapter, a surgical summary that lists the different approaches for the management of the pathology dealt with is provided. Throughout the book, emphasis is on how the otoscopic view and the clinical picture may affect the choice of treatment and the surgical technique.

At the end of this atlas, a chapter on postsurgical conditions is presented. The presence of previous surgery poses special difficulties because of the distorted anatomy. Moreover, the otologist should be able to distinguish between what is considered to be normal postsurgical healing and complications that need further intervention.

The authors would like to thank Dr. Clifford Bergman, Medical Editor at Georg Thieme Verlag, for his excellent cooperation and help. Thanks also go to Paolo Piazza, neuroradiologist, for his continuous cooperation and to Maurizio Guida for the illustrations included in the book.

Mario Sanna, M.D.
Alessandra Russo, M.D.
Giuseppe De Donato, M.D.

Preface to the Second Edition

The success of the first edition of *Color Atlas of Oto-scopy* convinced us to update and enlarge it.

In some chapters new otoscopic pictures have been added, as well as intraoperative views, to underline the main features of this book. It is not just a simple color atlas, but also a practical manual in which the surgical indications are presented according to the guidelines of an experienced center.

As some surgical approaches (such as the infratemporal fossa approach type A for class C–D paragangliomas) were only briefly mentioned in the first edition, we added a short description of some of these techniques in this second edition. In this way we aim to give the reader an even more complete idea of the management of these particular pathologies: from otoscopy, through imaging, to the surgical treatment.

With this second edition, our goal is to offer an easy-to-consult book for residents, specialists, and general practitioners.

Drs. Russo, De Donato, and Antonio Caruso, a new young colleague who has been working with us for the past 3 years, helped to accomplish this work with their active and enthusiastic participation.

We would like to thank Dr. Clifford Bergman for his continuous and kind assistance during the preparation of this book.

Mario Sanna, M.D.

Contents

Abbreviations

a	antrum
mfd	middle fossa dura
ss	sigmoid sinus
m	malleus
lsc	lateral semicircular canal
eac	external auditory canal
Ch or CH	cholesteatoma
I	incus
ICA	internal carotid artery

1 Methods of Otoscopy

A preliminary examination is carried out using a head mirror or an otoscope.

For proper otoscopy, the external auditory canal should be cleaned. Few instruments are used for this step, namely, aural speculi of different sizes, a Billeau ear loop, Hartman auricular forceps, and suction tips (Fig. 1.**1**). In cases with a history of recurrent otitis, we prefer to clean the ear visualized with the aid of a microscope (Fig. 1.**2**).

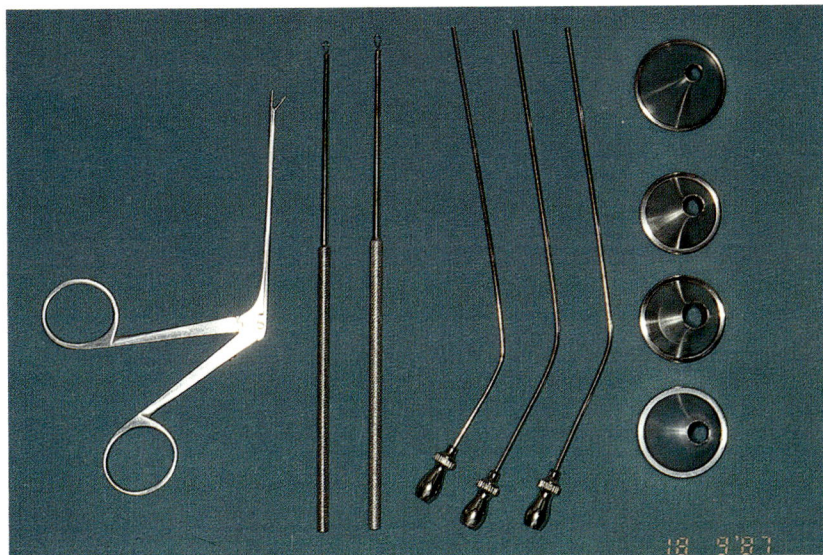

Figure 1.**1**

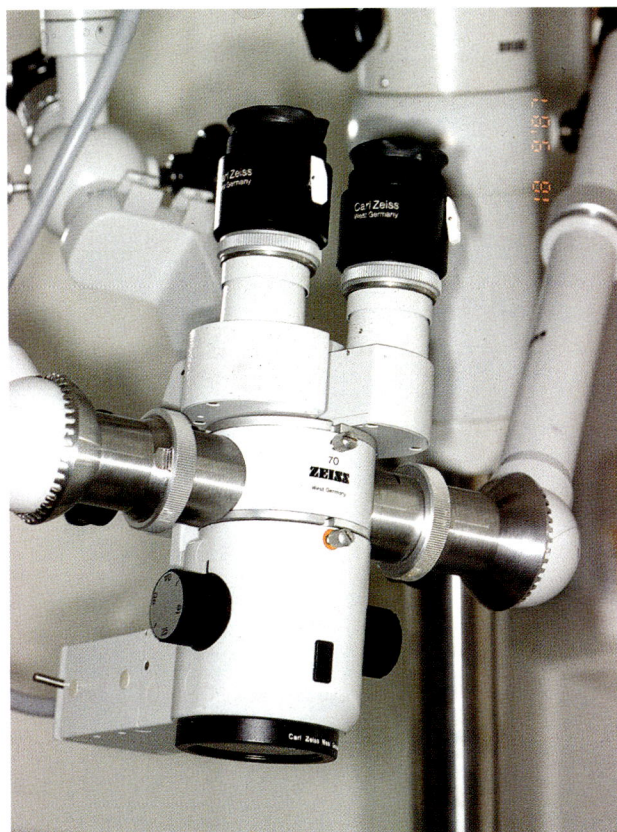

Figure 1.**2**

The use of a rigid 0° 6-cm endoscope (1215AA– Storz, Fig. 1.**3**) connected to a video system enables the patient to see the pathology involving his/her ear (Figs. 1.**4** and 1.**5** show the Endovision Telecam SL 20212001 and the Xenon Light Source 615–Storz). With the help of a video printer connected to the monitor, instant photos of the pathology can be obtained. The rigid 30° endoscope allows evaluation of attic retraction pockets, the extent of which cannot always be determined using the microscope or the 0° endoscope (Fig. 1.**6** shows a series of rigid endoscopes –Storz).

During the last few years, instant photography has also been used in the operating room. A copy of the important steps of the operation is given to the patient while another copy is kept in the patient's chart. The patient is also photographed during the follow-up visit. Thus, for each patient pre-, intra-, and postoperative photographic documentation is obtained.

All the photos in this book were obtained with an Olympus OM 40 camera mounted to the endoscope with a Storz 593-T2 objective. The focus is adjusted to infinity and the diaphragm to 140. We use the TTL-Computer-Flash-Unit Model 600 BA Storz (Fig. 1.**7**). The film used is a Kodak Ektachrome 64T Professional Film (Tungsten).

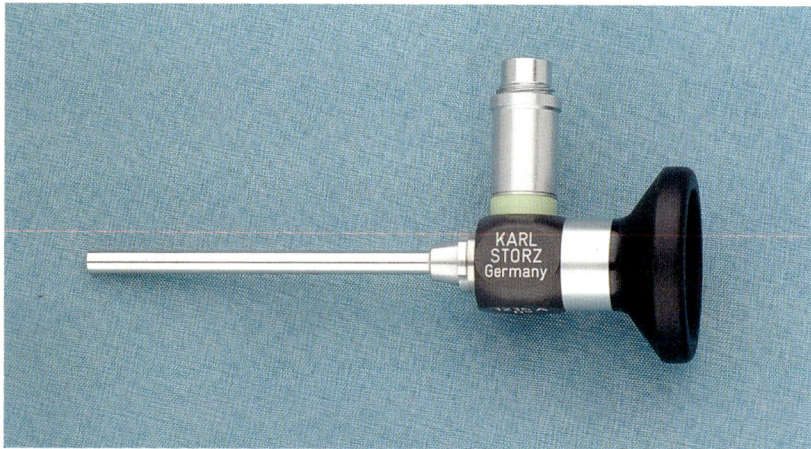

Figure 1.**3**

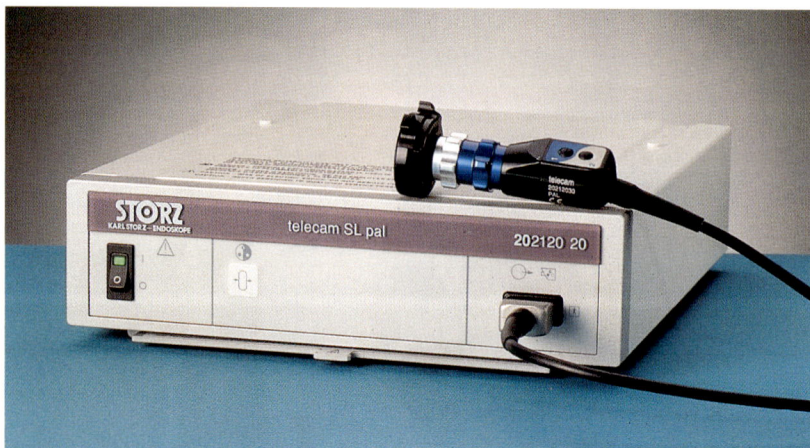

Figure 1.**4**

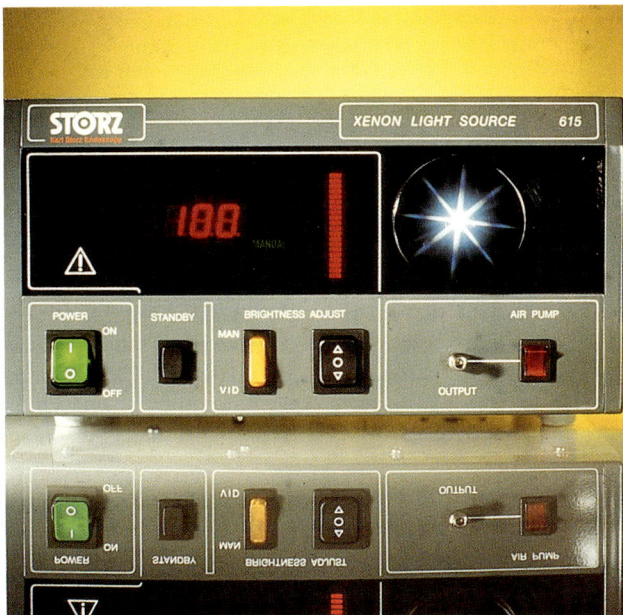

Figure 1.**5**

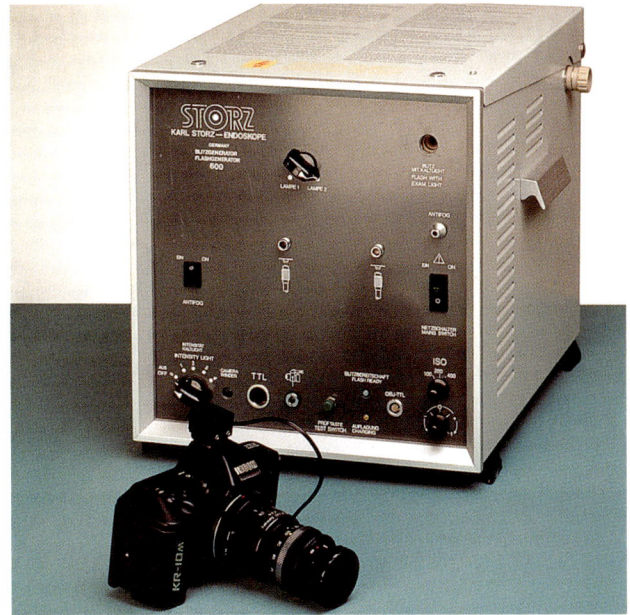

Figure 1.**7**

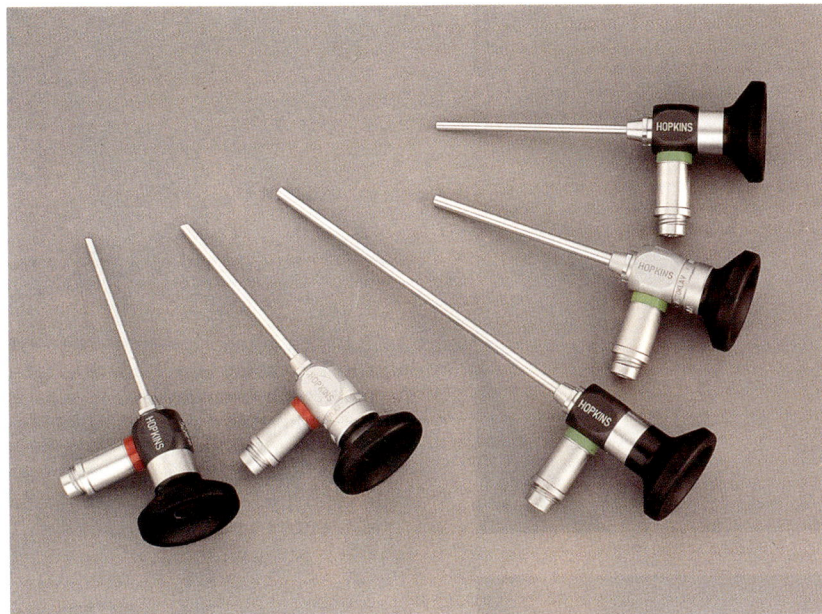

Figure 1.**6**

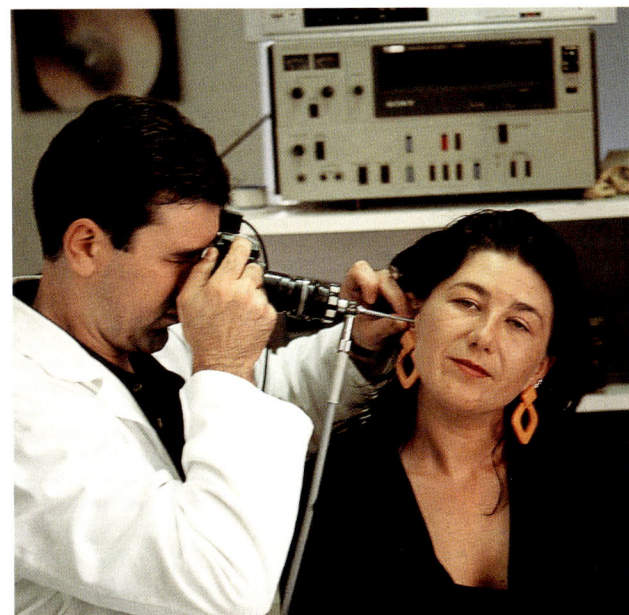

Figure 1.**8**

In all the cases, the examiner sits to the side of the patient whose head is slightly tilted towards the contralateral side. The examiner holds the camera attached to the endoscope with his right hand. With the ring and middle finger of the left hand, the examiner pulls the patient's auricle backwards and outwards to straighten the external auditory canal. The endoscope is advanced over the index finger of the examiner's left hand into the patient's external auditory canal. In this manner, any undue injury to the external auditory canal is prevented (Fig. 1.**8**).

2 The Normal Tympanic Membrane

Anatomy

The tympanic membrane forms the major part of the lateral wall of the middle ear (see Figs. 2.1–2.3). It is thin, resistant, semitransparent, has a pearly gray color, and is cone–like. The apex of the membrane lies at the umbo, which corresponds to the lowest part of the handle of the malleus. Most of the membrane circumference is thickened to form a fibrocartilaginous ring, the tympanic annulus, which sits in a groove in the tympanic bone called the tympanic sulcus. The fibrocartilaginous ring is deficient superiorly. This deficiency is known as

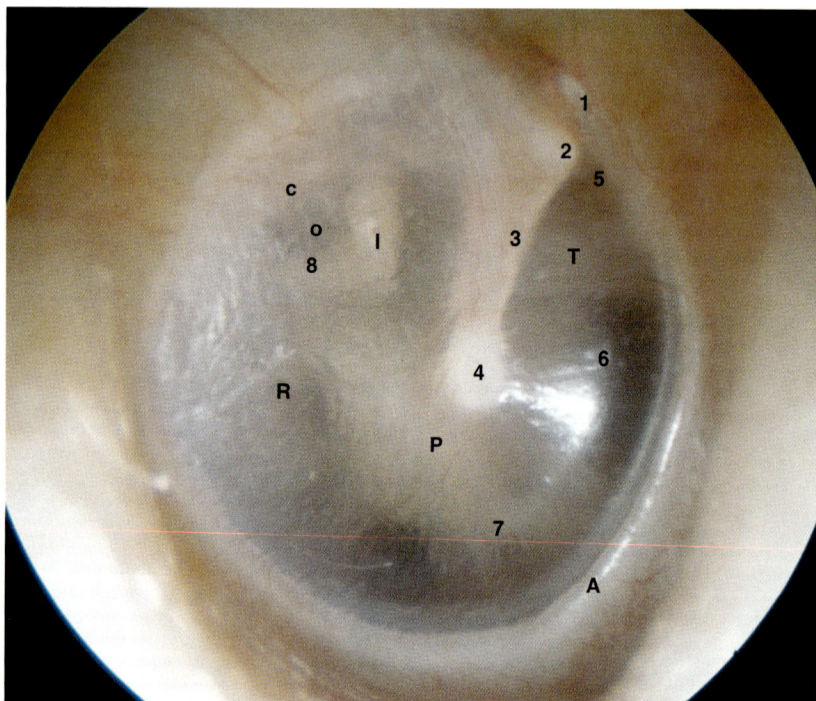

Figure 2.1 Right ear. Normal tympanic membrane. 1 = pars flaccida; 2 = short process of the malleus; 3 = handle of the malleus; 4 = umbo; 5 = supratubal recess; 6 = tubal orifice; 7 = hypotympanic air cells; 8 = stapedius tendon; c = chorda tympani; I = incus; P = promontory; o = oval window; R = round window; T = tensor tympani; A = annulus.

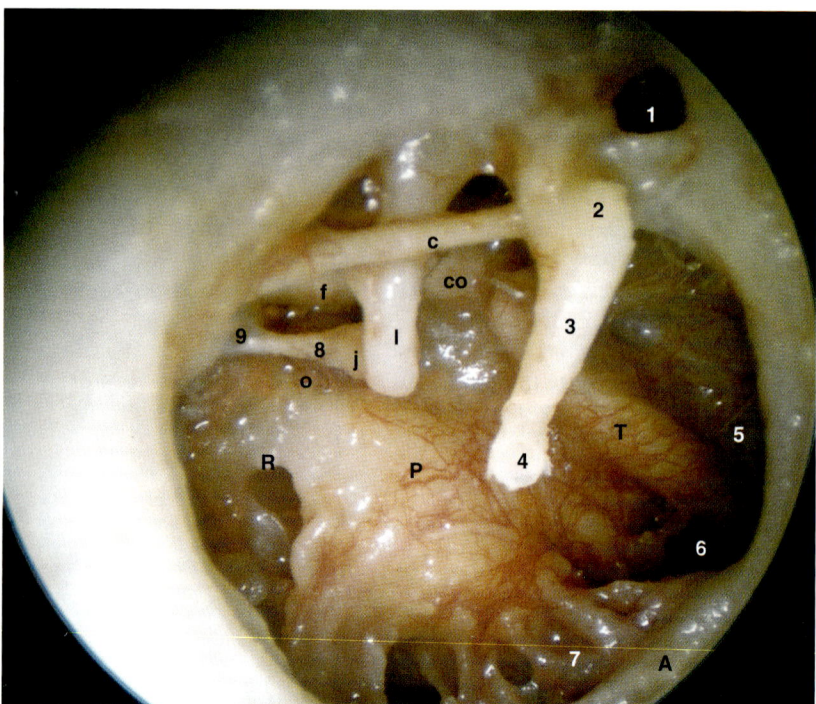

Figure 2.2 Right ear. Structures of the middle ear seen after removal of the tympanic membrane. 9 = pyramidal eminence; co = cochleariform process; f = facial nerve; j = incudostapedial joint. See legend to Figure 2.1 for other numbers and abbreviations.

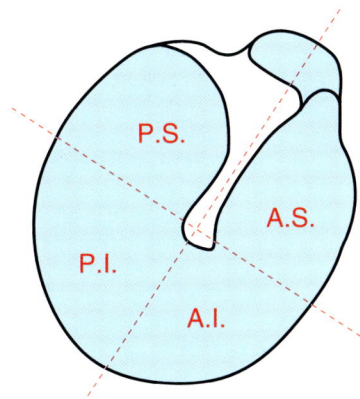

Figure 2.**3** Right ear. Division of the tympanic membrane into four quadrants: A.S. = anterosuperior; A.I. = anteroinferior; P.S. = posterosuperior; P.I. = posteroinferior. This division facilitates the description of different pathologic affections of the tympanic membrane.

the notch of Rivinus. The anterior and posterior malleolar folds extend from the short process of the malleus to the tympanic sulcus, thus forming the inferior limit of the pars flaccida of Shrapnell's membrane. The membrane forms an obtuse angle with the posterior wall of the external auditory canal. It also forms an acute angle with the anterior wall of the canal. It is important to respect this acute angulation in the myringoplasty operation to maintain as much as possible the vibratory mechanism of the tympanic membrane and hence ensure maximum hearing improvement.

The external surface of the tympanic membrane is innervated by the auriculotemporal nerve and the auricular branch of the vagus nerve, whereas the inner surface is supplied by Jacobson's nerve, a branch of the glossopharyngeal nerve.

The blood supply is derived from the deep auricular and anterior tympanic arteries. Both are branches of the maxillary artery.

Histology

The tympanic membrane consists of three layers: an outer epithelial layer continuous with the skin of the external auditory canal, a middle fibrous layer or lamina propria, and an inner mucosal layer continuous with the lining of the tympanic cavity.

The epidermis or outer layer is divided into the stratum corneum, the stratum granulosum, the stratum spinosum, and the stratum basale, which is the deepest layer that rests on the basement membrane.

The lamina propria is characterized by the presence of collagen fibers. In the pars tensa, these fibers are arranged in two basic layers: an outer radial layer that originates from the inferior part of the handle of the malleus and inserts in the annulus, and an inner circular layer that originates primarily from the short process of the malleus. Such a distinct arrangement, however, is absent in the pars flaccida.

The mucosal layer is formed mainly of a simple cuboidal or columnar epithelium. The free surface of the cells possesses numerous microvilli.

Normal Otoscopy

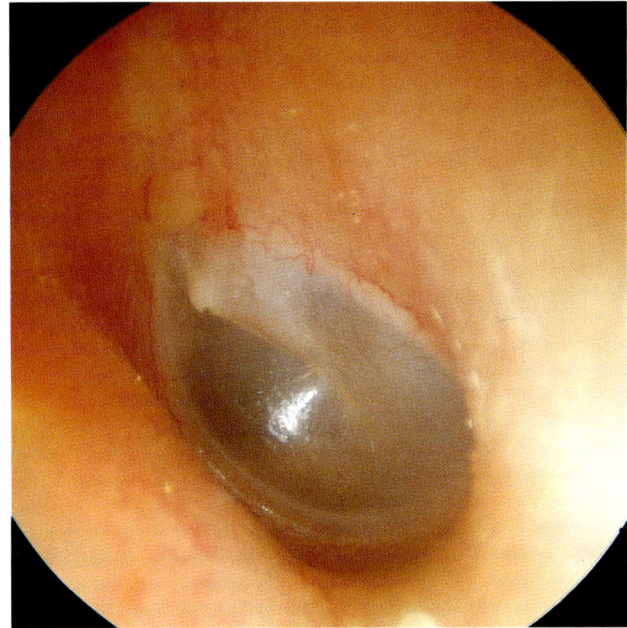

Figure 2.**4** Left ear. Normal tympanic membrane. Note the acute angle formed between the tympanic membrane and the anterior wall of the external auditory canal. The pars tensa with the short process of the handle of the malleus, the umbo, the cone of light, the annulus, and the pars flaccida are seen. Note also the presence of early exostosis in the superior wall of the external auditory canal.

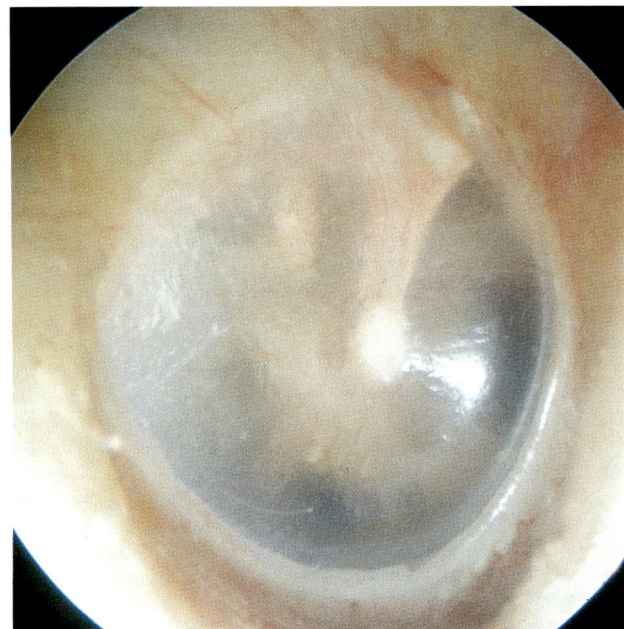

Figure 2.**5** Right ear. Normal tympanic membrane. In this case, the drum is very thin and transparent. The handle and short process of the malleus as well as the umbo and cone of light are well visualized. Through the transparent tympanic membrane, the region of the oval window, the long process of the incus, the posterior arc of the stapes, the incudostapedial joint, the round window, and the promontory can be distinguished. Anteriorly, at the region of the eustachian tube, the tensor tympani canal and the supratubaric recess can be observed.

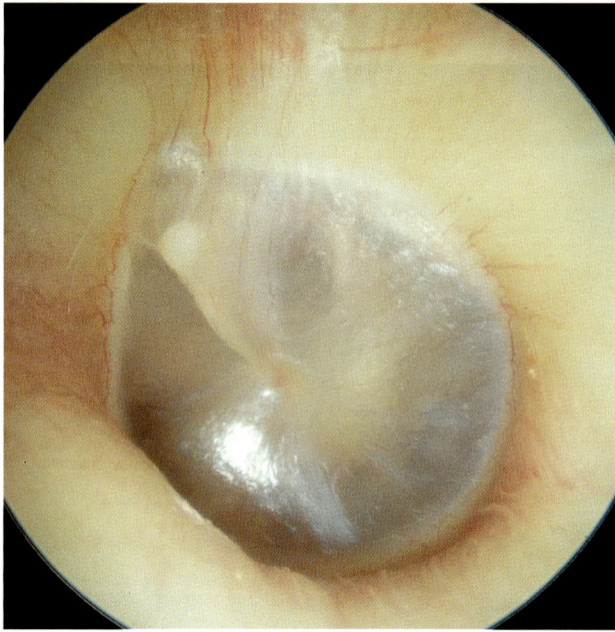

Figure 2.**6**   Left ear. Normal tympanic membrane. The handle of the malleus and cone of light are well visualized through the tympanic membrane; the promontory, the area of the round window, and the air cells in the hypotympanum can be appreciated. The pars flaccida is visualized superior to the short process of the malleus.

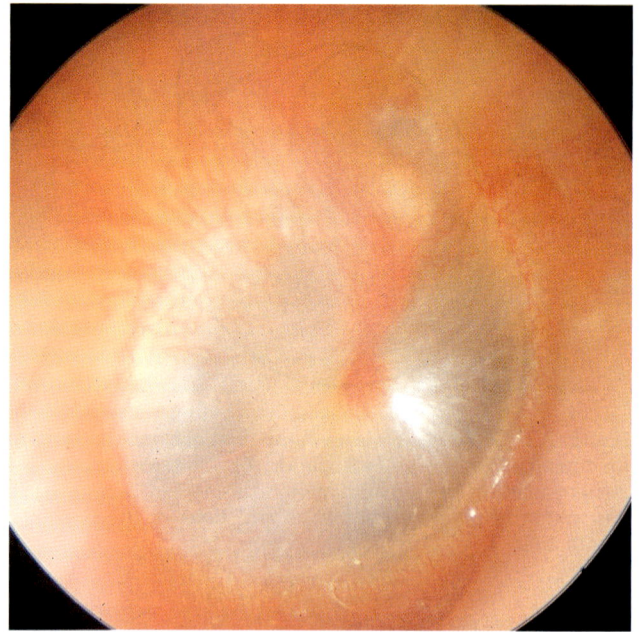

Figure 2.**7**   Right ear. Normal tympanic membrane. The drum, however, is slightly thickened with an accentuated capillary network along the handle of the malleus. The increased thickness of the tympanic membrane obscures all the structures in the middle ear.

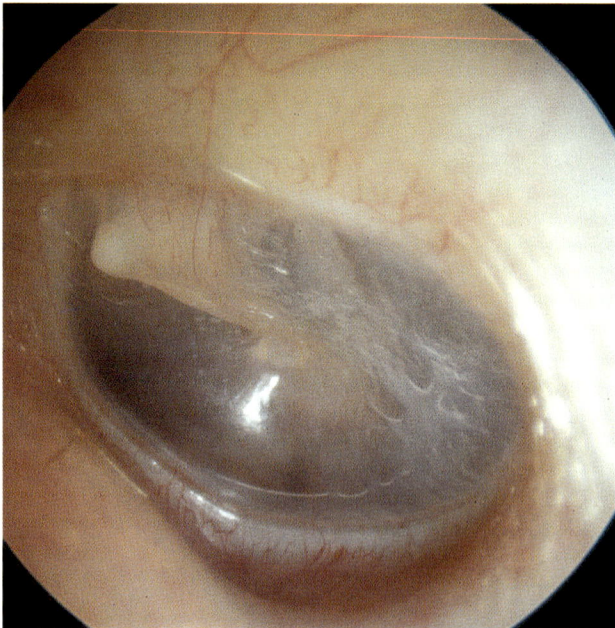

Figure 2.**8**   Left ear. A normal tympanic membrane that is slightly thinned in the anterior quadrant and moderately thickened posteriorly.

3 Diseases Affecting the External Auditory Canal

Exostosis and Osteoma

Exostoses are defined as new bony growths in the osseous portion of the external auditory canal. They are usually multiple, bilateral, and are commonly sessile. They vary in shape, being either round, ovoid, or oblong. The condition is caused by periostitis secondary to exposure to cold water. This explains the high incidence of exostoses among divers and cold-water bathers. Histologically, they are formed from parallel layers of newly-formed bone. It is postulated that the periosteum stimulates an osteogenic reaction with each exposure to cold water, thus causing this stratification.

When exostoses are small they are asymptomatic. Large lesions, however, can occlude the external auditory canal and lead to conductive hearing loss or retention of wax and debris with subsequent otitis externa.

In such cases, and in cases in which a hearing aid is to be fitted, surgical removal of exostoses is indicated. In some cases, surgery is technically difficult and special care is taken to preserve the skin of the external auditory canal. Other structures at risk are the tympanic membrane and ossicular chain medially, the temporomandibular joint anteriorly, and the third segment of the facial nerve posteroinferiorly. A postauricular incision is preferred because it allows good exposure and proper replacement of the skin of the external auditory canal to prevent postoperative scarring and stenosis.

Osteoma is a true benign neoplasm of the bone of the external auditory canal, usually unilateral and pedunculated. Histologically, it can be differentiated from exostosis by the absence of the laminated growth pattern.

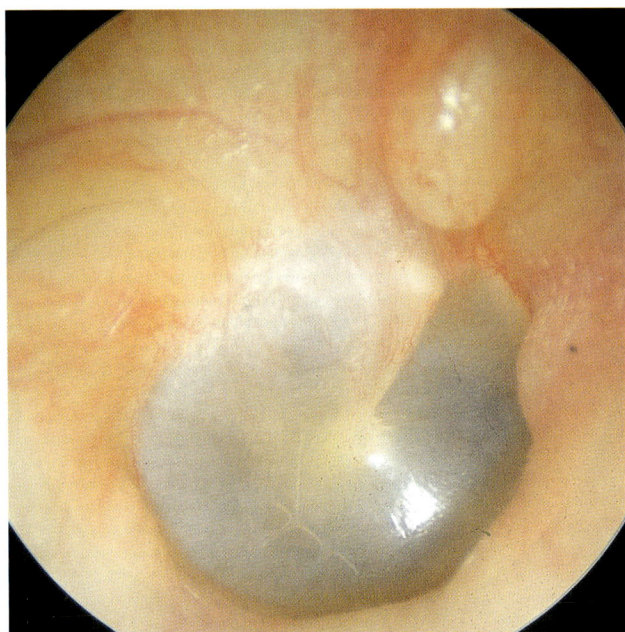

Figure 3.**1**   Right ear. Small exostosis originating from the superior wall of the external auditory canal. Anterosuperiorly, another exostosis is seen in the early phase of formation.

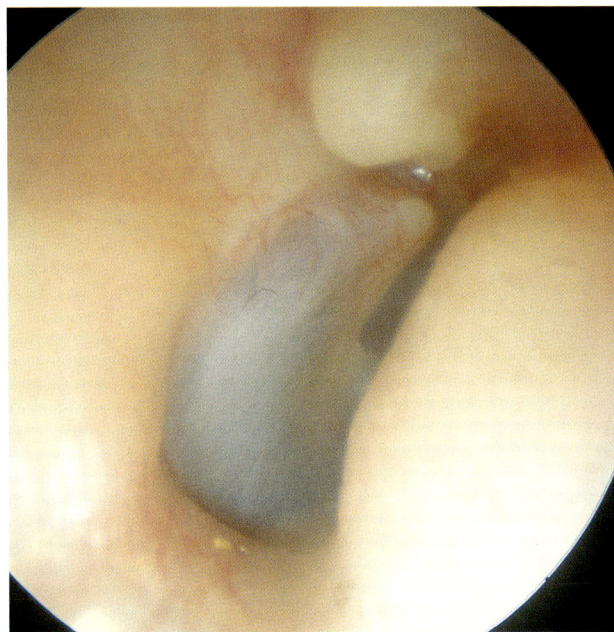

Figure 3.**2**   Right ear. A small asymptomatic exostosis of the superior wall on the external auditory canal is observed. A hump on the anterior wall precludes adequate visualization of the entire tympanic membrane.

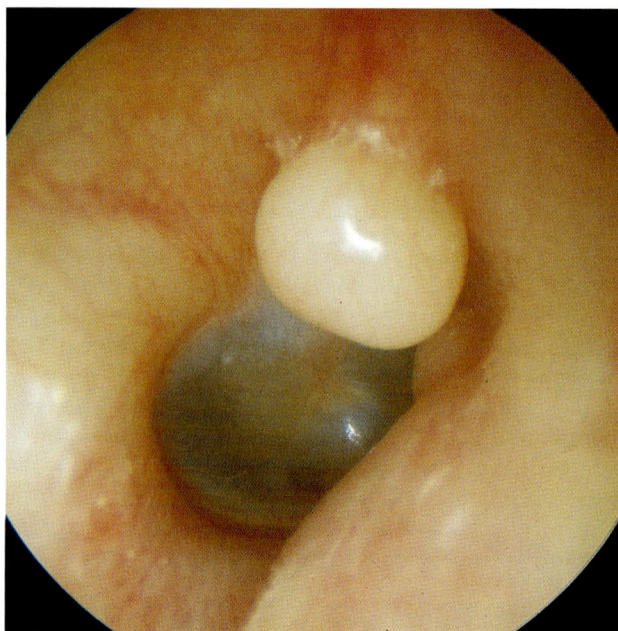

Figure **3.3** Right ear. Osseous neoplasm of the external auditory canal. In this case, given the pedunculated narrow base, an osteoma is a more probable diagnosis. This was confirmed by pathological examination of the removed specimen. Ample bone removal is performed in such cases to avoid recurrence.

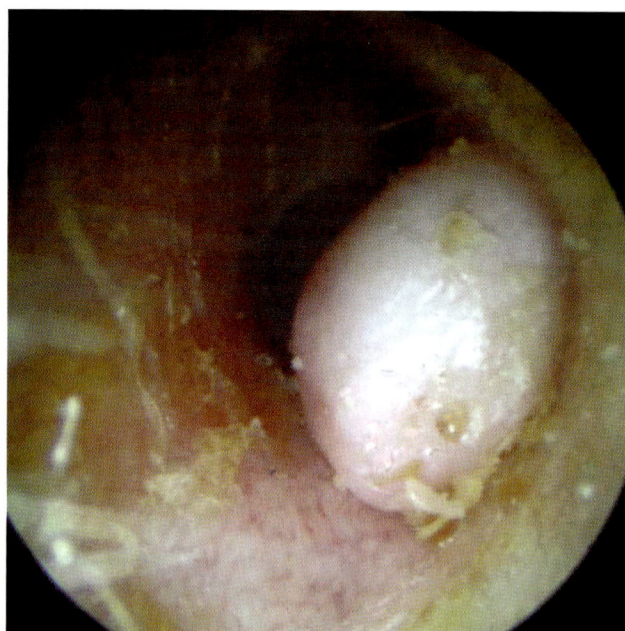

Figure **3.4** Right ear. There is a large osteoma almost totally occluding the lumen of the external auditory canal. The anterior bony canal wall has to be drilled carefully to avoid injuries to the temporomandibular joint.

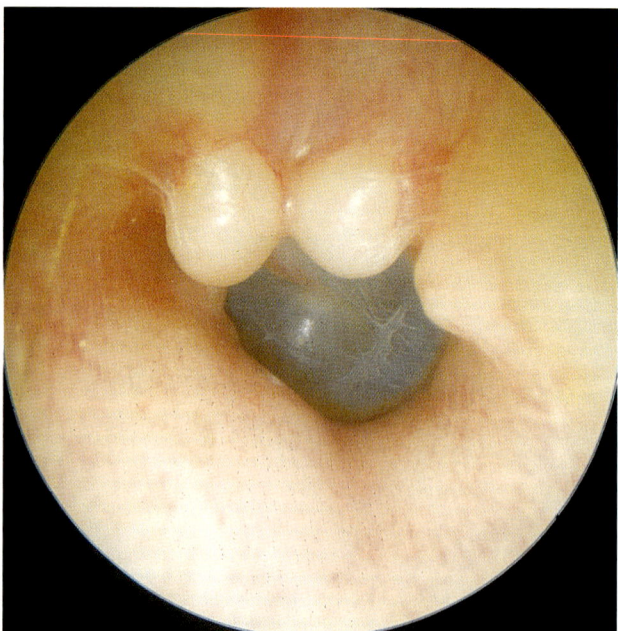

Figure **3.5** Exostosis of the superior wall of the left external auditory canal. The lesion prevents complete visualization of the tympanic membrane.

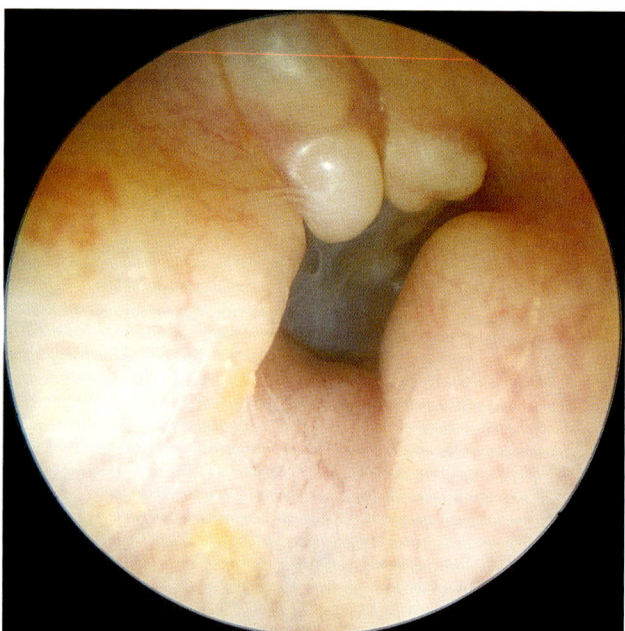

Figure **3.6** Same patient, right ear. Two exostoses are present in the superior wall of the external auditory canal. In addition, the anterosuperior wall shows an additional exostosis. The lesions allow only a limited view of the central part of the tympanic membrane. In this case, regular follow-up and evaluation is necessary because further growth of the lesion could lead to accumulation of debris and cerumen, necessitating surgical intervention.

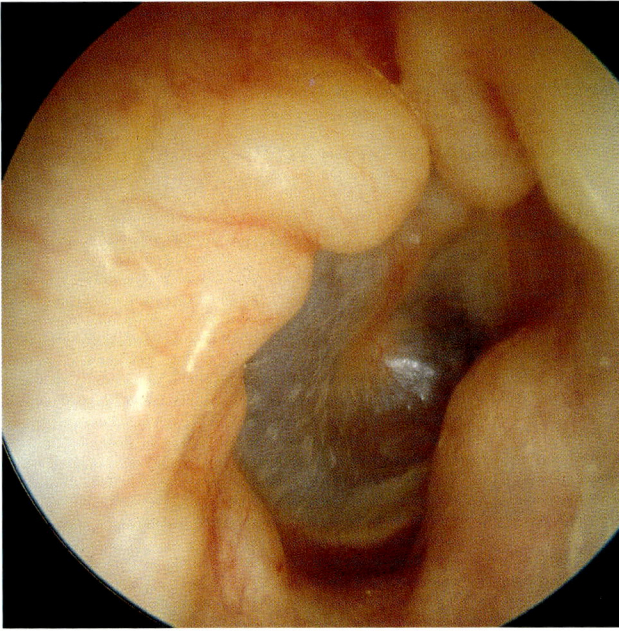

Figure 3.**7**   Right ear. Exostosis of the posterior superior wall of the external auditory canal that precludes visualization of the pars flaccida. A bony hump is also present in the anterior wall of the canal. In this type of case, it is useful to photograph the ear for further follow-up within 1–2 years.

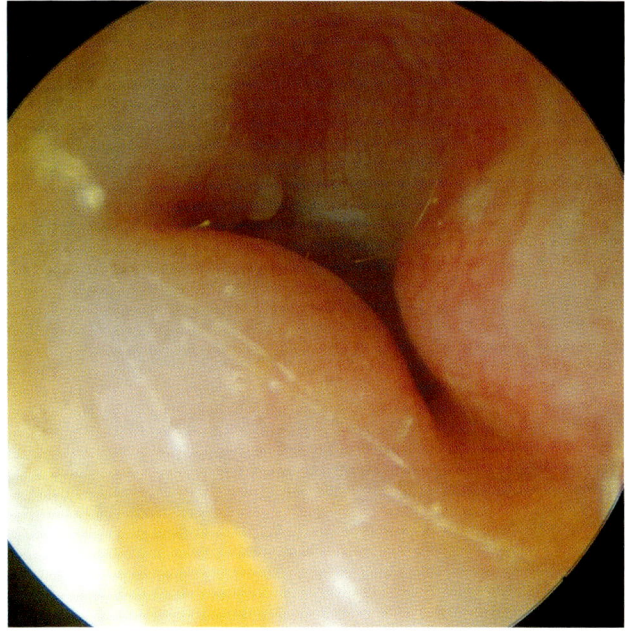

Figure 3.**8a**   Left ear. Obstructing exostosis that causes subtotal occlusion of the external auditory canal. The patient complains of hearing loss and frequent episodes of otitis externa secondary to retention of water and debris inside the canal. A canalplasty under local anesthesia is indicated to restore the size of the external canal.

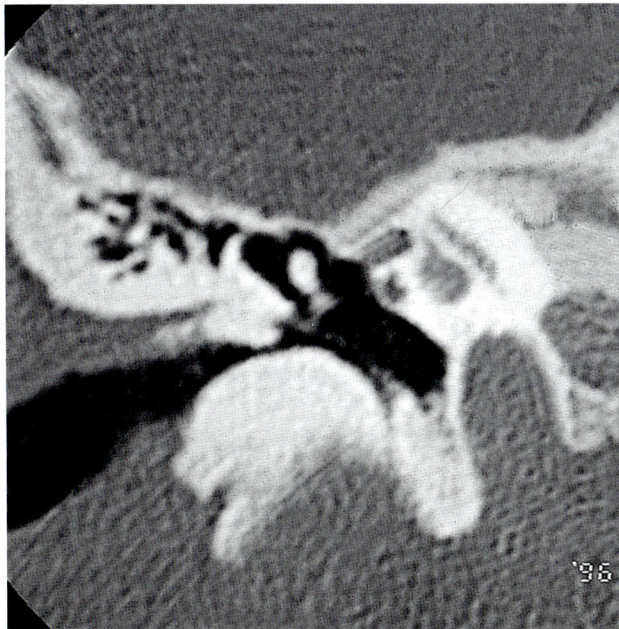

Figure 3.**8b**   Computed tomography (CT) of the same case. The bony external canal is particularly narrowed.

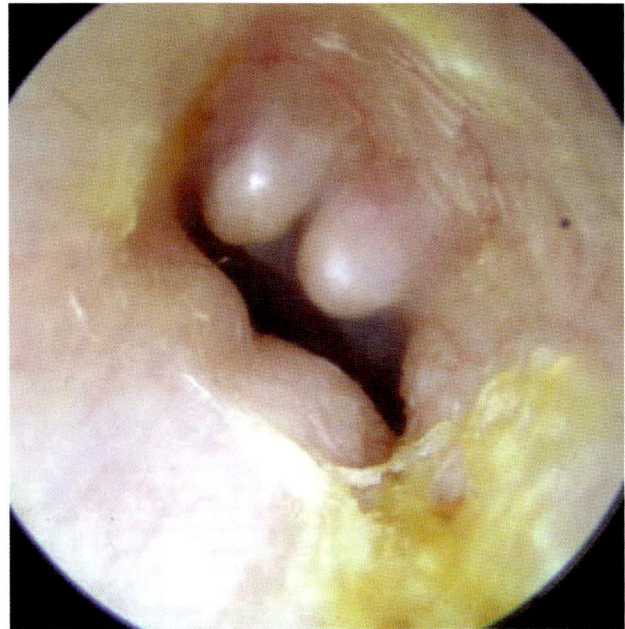

Figure 3.**9**   Left ear. Another case of subtotal occlusion caused by exostosis. Two exostoses are present in the posterosuperior wall, and there is another in the anterior wall of the external auditory canal. In this case, calibration of the ear canal is mandatory to resolve the frequent episodes of otitis externa and conductive hearing loss experienced by the patient.

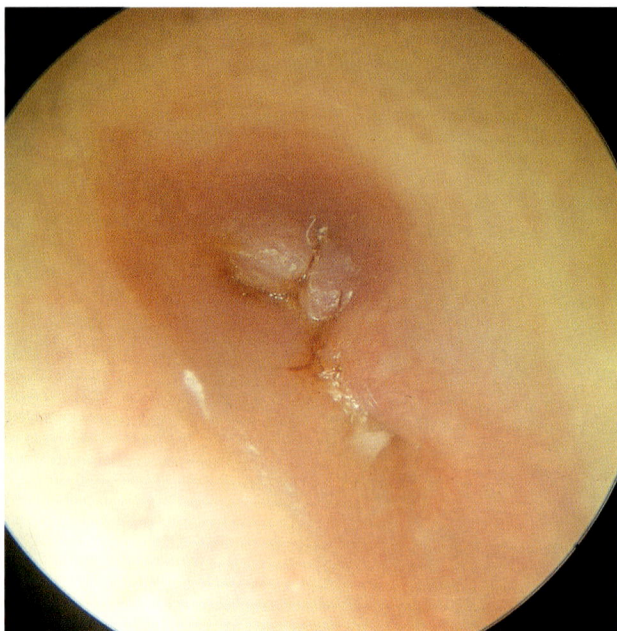

Figure 3.**10**   Obstructing exostosis of the external auditory canal resulting in otitis externa due to accumulation of squamous debris inside the canal. Surgery is essential both to avoid the formation of cholesteatoma and to improve hearing.

Summary

Surgery in cases of exostosis is indicated only in cases with obstructing stenosis with or without hearing loss but with frequent otitis externa due to retention of debris. Surgery can be performed under local anesthesia, preferably using a postauricular incision. This approach allows excellent exposure of the whole meatus, thus minimizing the risk of injury to the tympanic membrane. In addition, it enables the surgeon to preserve the canal skin, thereby avoiding postoperative cicatricial stenosis. After dissecting the posterior limb, the flap is retained by the prongs of the self-retaining retractor. The skin of the anterior wall is incised medial to the tragus and is dissected in a lateral-to-medial direction. While drilling the exostosis, the skin of the canal is protected using an aluminum sheet (the cover of surgical sutures).

Osteoma can be removed by using a curette. In case of recurrence, wide drilling of the bone around its base is also indicated.

Furunculosis

Furunculosis is pustular folliculitis caused by staphylococcal infection of a hair follicle. Infection occurs as a result of microabrasion or of decreased immunity, as in diabetics. It is characterized by severe pain. A tender swelling is seen in the cartilaginous part of the external auditory canal, which may have a central necrotic part.

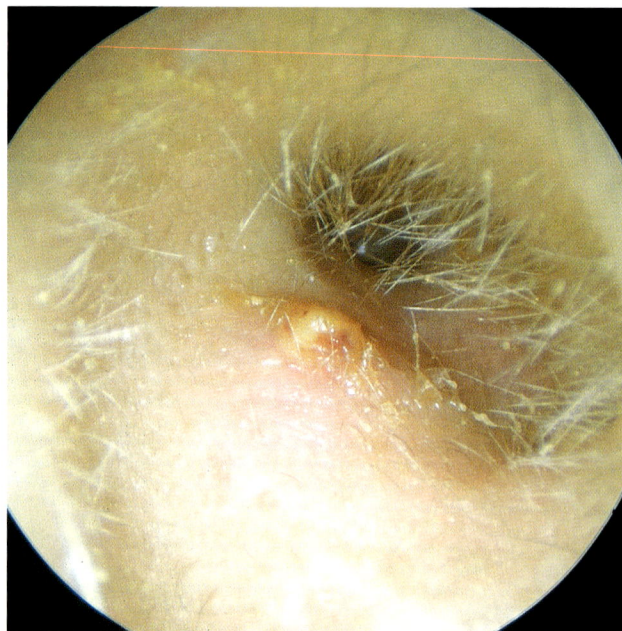

Figure 3.**11**   A furuncle almost totally occluding the meatus. Pain is caused by distention of the richly innervated skin. A central necrotic part is seen.

Myringitis and Meatal Stenosis

Myringitis is an inflammatory process that affects the tympanic membrane. Three forms are recognized: acute myringitis, bullous myringitis, and myringitis granulomatosa.

Acute myringitis is usually seen in association with infection of the external ear (otitis externa) or middle ear (otitis media). It is characterized by hyperemia and thickening of the tympanic membrane, as well as the presence of purulent secretions (Fig. 3.**12**). Therapy consists of administration of general and/or local antibiotics and local steroids.

Bullous myringitis is commonly associated with viral upper respiratory tract infection. It is characterized by the presence of bullae filled with serosanguineous fluid. The bullae are located between the outer and middle layers of the tympanic membrane. The patient complains of otalgia and hearing loss. Therapy consists of antibiotics and steroids (Figs. 3.**13**, 3.**14**).

In granulomatous myringitis, the outer epidermic layer of the tympanic membrane as well as the adjacent skin of the external auditory canal are replaced by granulation tissue. It is generally seen in patients suffering from frequent episodes of otitis externa. In some cases, it may ultimately lead to stenosis of the most medial part of the external auditory canal. It can usually be cured, however, by removing the granulations in the outpatient clinic using the microscope. This is followed by the administration of local steroid drops for nearly 1 month. In refractory cases, however, surgery in the form of canalplasty with free skin graft is necessary.

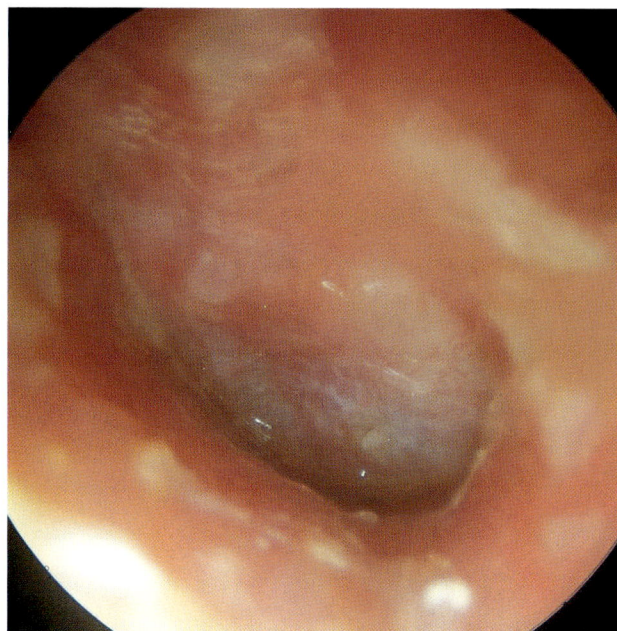

Figure 3.**12**   Left ear. The tympanic membrane is characterized by thickening and hyperemia. In this case, the skin of the external auditory canal is also hyperemic. The tympanic membrane seems lateralized.

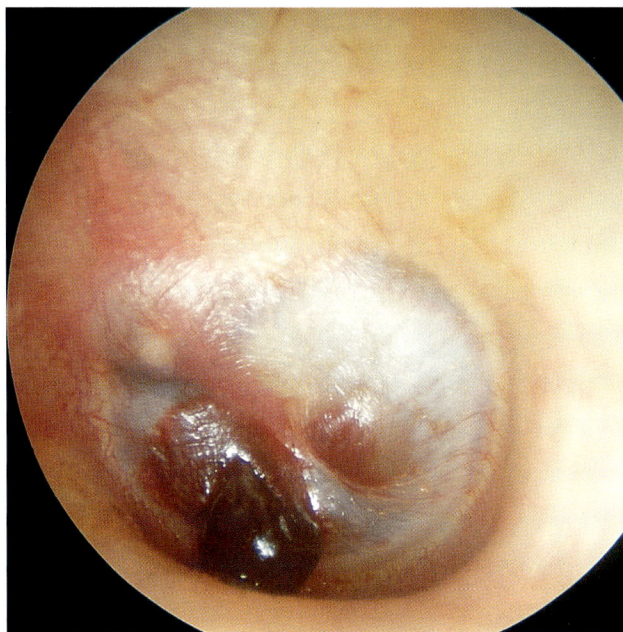

Figure 3.**13**   Left tympanic membrane with a large bulla anterior to the malleus and a smaller one posterior to it.

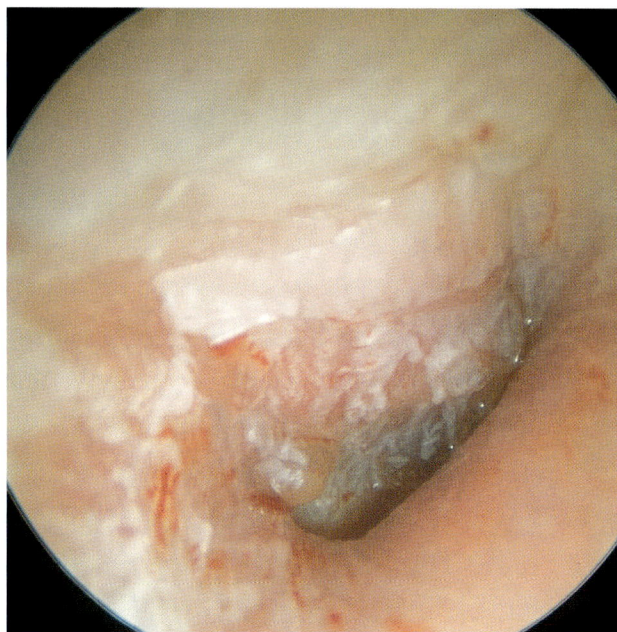

Figure 3.**14**   Right tympanic membrane with a large bulla occupying the entire surface of the membrane. The malleus is not visible.

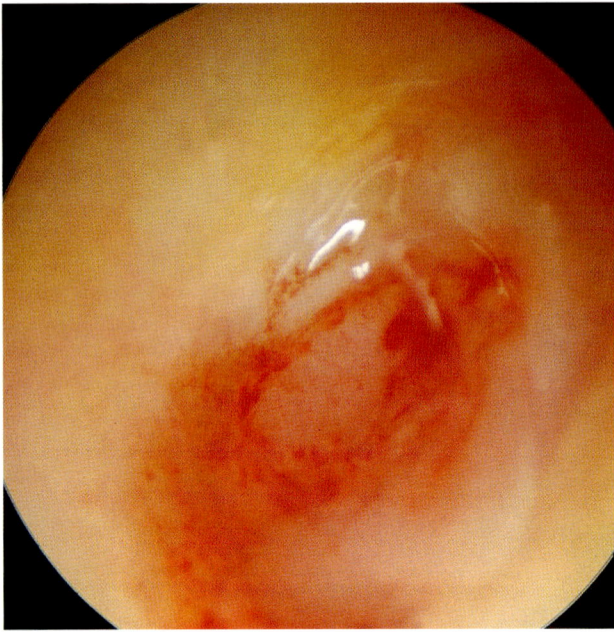

Figure 3.**15** Granulomatous myringitis. The granulomatous tissue has replaced the external skin layer of the tympanic membrane and part of the anterior wall of the external canal. This case was treated by removal of the granulation tissue under local anesthesia in the outpatient clinic. Local steroid drops were then administered for 1 month.

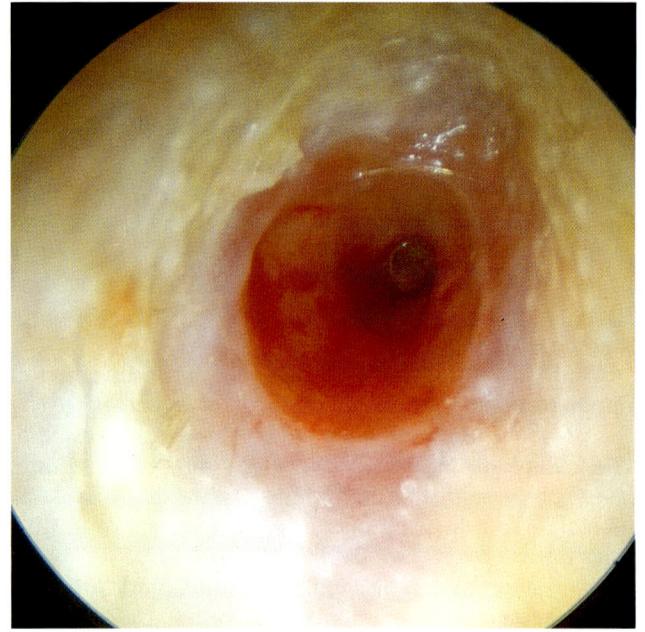

Figure 3.**16** Postinflammatory stenosis of the right external auditory canal of a 68-year-old woman. The patient complained of bilateral continuous otorrhea and hearing loss of 3 years' duration. The otorrhea in the left ear stopped 2 months before presentation. The granulations over the tympanic membrane were removed in the outpatient clinic. A cellophane sheet was inserted into the external auditory canal to avoid the reformation of stenosis. Local steroid drops were administered for 1 month. On follow-up, stenosis was already resolved and the granulation tissue in the external auditory canal was completely replaced by healthy skin.

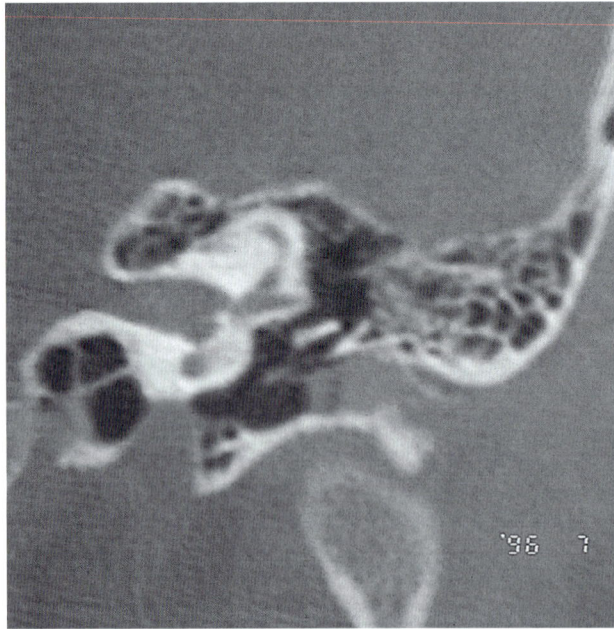

Figure 3.**17** CT of the same case. The bony walls of the external auditory canal are intact. The pathologic skin occupies the lumen of the external auditory canal.

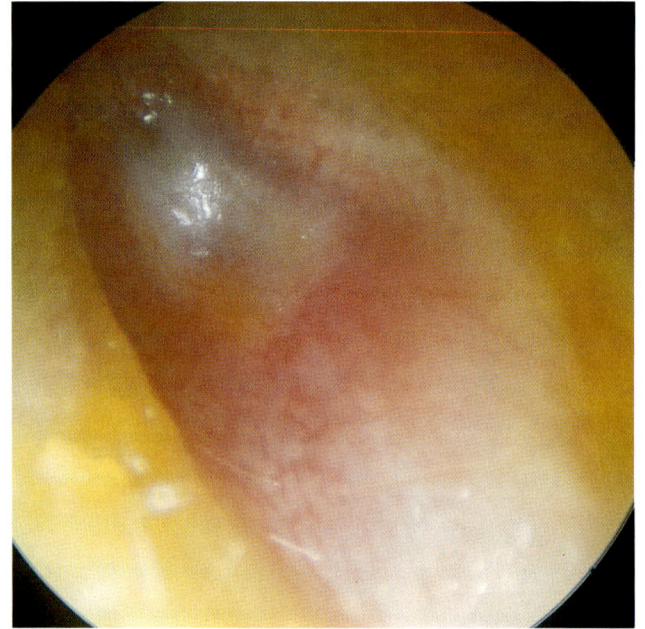

Figure 3.**18** Same patient, left ear (see also CT in Fig. 3.**19**). A canalplasty was performed on this side. After removal of the granulation tissue, myringoplasty and canalplasty were performed.

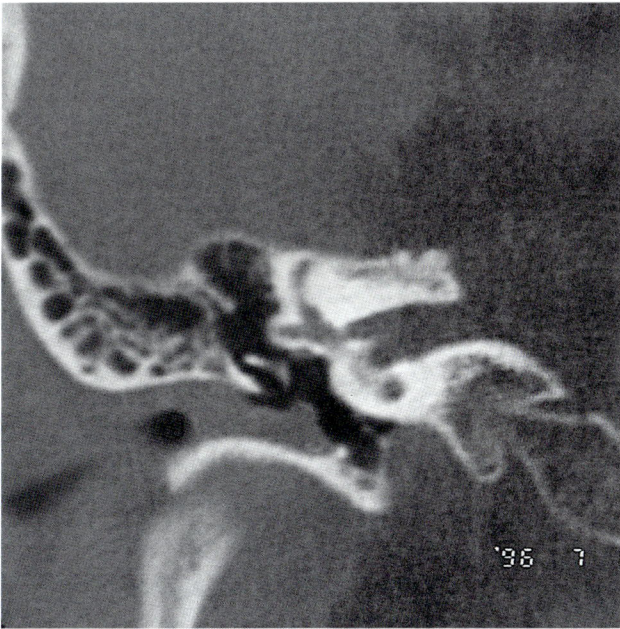

Figure 3.**19**   This CT scan demonstrates a similar lesion on the contralateral side.

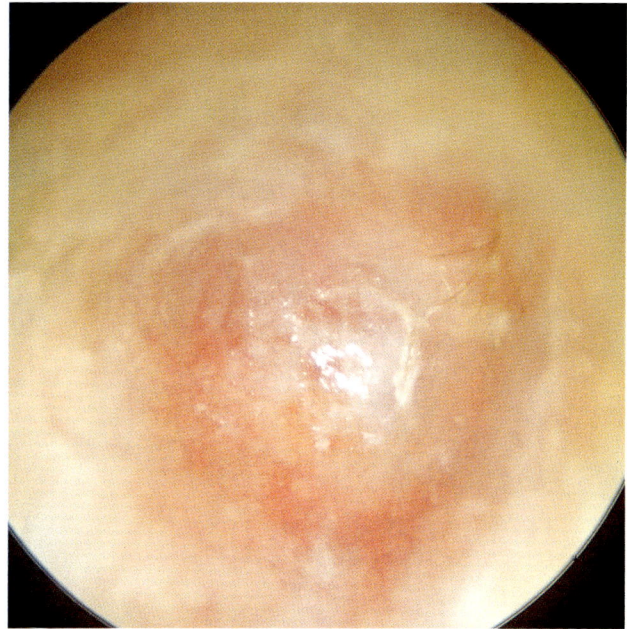

Figure 3.**20**   Right ear. Case similar to that seen in Figure 3.**16**. The patient complained of intermittent otorrhea and hearing loss (see CT scan in Fig. 3.**21**).

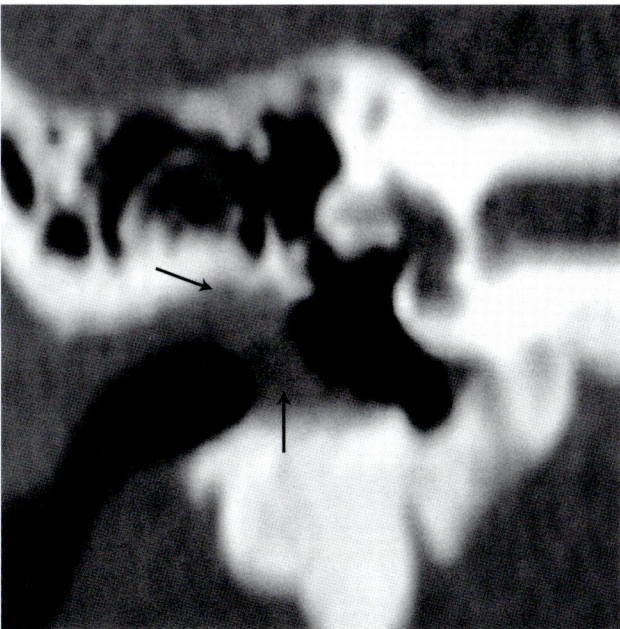

Figure 3.**21**   The CT scan shows thickening of the tympanic membrane and normal bony canal.

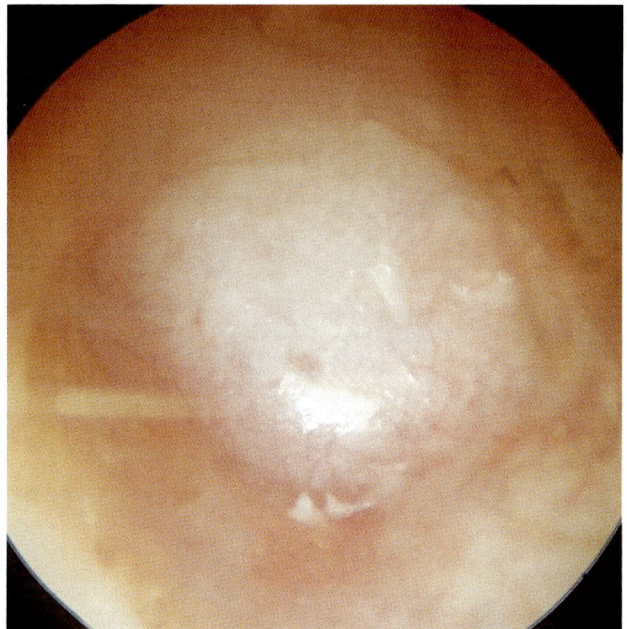

Figure 3.**22**   Same patient, left ear. Two tympanoplasties were previously performed on this ear. Generally, revision surgery is better avoided in patients who have undergone multiple operations and present with canal stenosis associated with lateralization of the tympanic membrane. (For postoperative stenosis of the external auditory canal, see Chapter 14.)

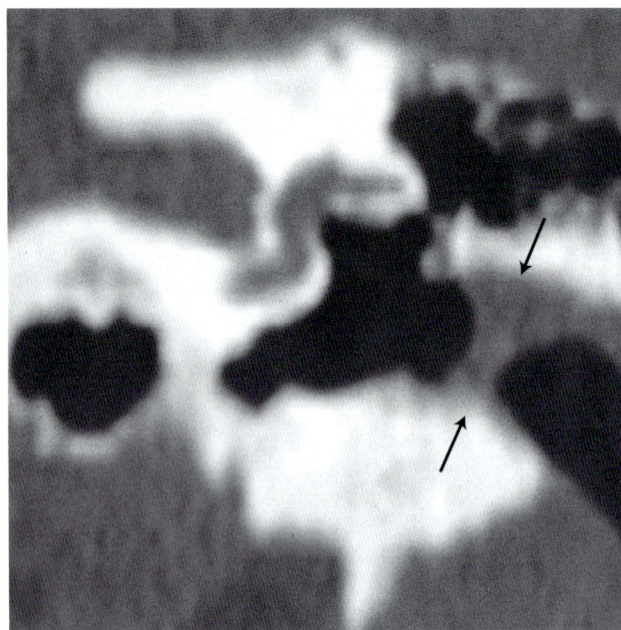

Figure 3.**23** CT scan of the previous case. The tympanic membrane is thickened and lateralized.

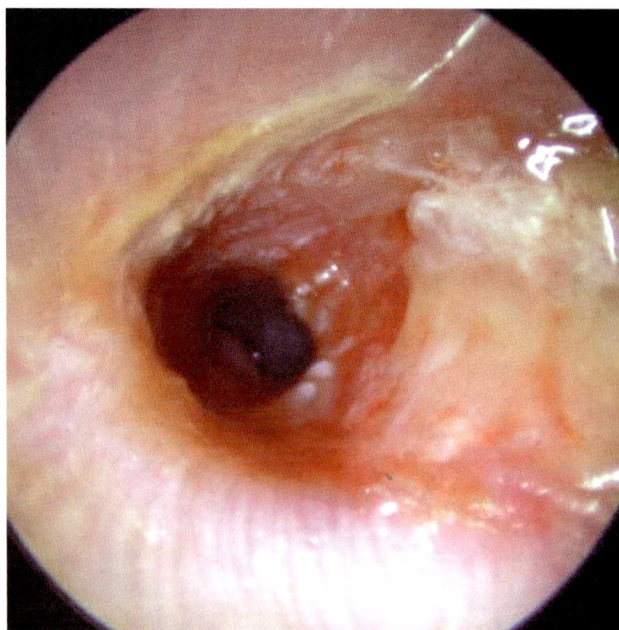

Figure 3.**24a** Left ear. The patient had bilateral postinflammatory external auditory canal stenosis, with bilateral severe conductive hearing loss. In this case, a radical mastoidectomy was performed. At surgery, the tympanic membrane was found to be atelectatic, with an anteroinferior perforation. A granuloma was also removed from the mastoid (cf. Fig. 3.**24b**).

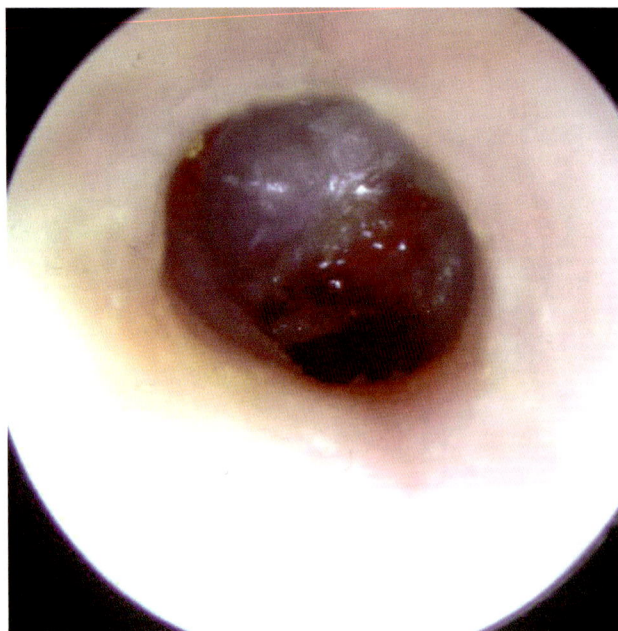

Figure 3.**24b** The right ear in the same patient. A modified radical mastoidectomy was also carried out in this ear. Five months after surgery, this ear developed a postsurgical stenosis. The external auditory canal, the anterior bony canal wall and the tympanic membrane are visible. The attic, facial ridge and residual cavity are obscured by the stenosis. The scar was removed under local anesthesia, and a plastic sheet was inserted for 30 days, with local medication with steroid lotion and boric alcohol being administered.

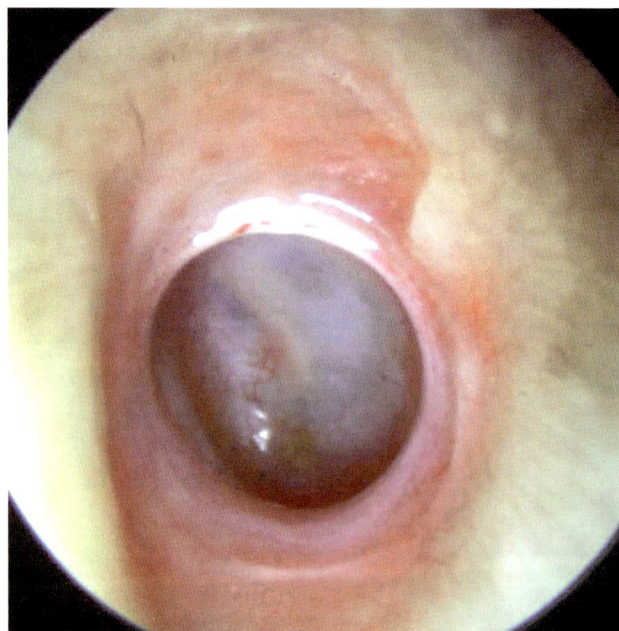

Figure 3.**25** Postinflammatory stenosis in a left ear. The patient had fetid otorrhea. Hearing was normal, and the tympanic membrane was normal. The cicatricial ring was removed and a plastic sheet was inserted to prevent a recurrence of the stenosis.

Summary

Postinflammatory stenosis of the external auditory canal is a difficult pathology to treat. In early cases, in which only granulation tissue is present, it is possible to remove the pathologic tissue (under local anesthesia in the outpatient clinic). This is followed by the insertion of a plastic (polyethylene) sheet to be left in place for about 20 days, during which regular lavage is performed with 2% boric acid in 70% alcohol and local steroid lotions are applied. Surgery is doubtful in well-established cases with excessive cicatricial tissue leading to marked narrowing of the external auditory canal and lateralization of the tympanic membrane (secondary to thickening of the latter). In the majority of cases, restenosis occurs following operative interference. Therefore, it is preferable not to operate in the case of unilateral postinflammatory stenosis. In bilateral cases with marked hearing loss, a hearing aid is prescribed. By contrast, postoperative stenosis has a better prognosis and the results of treatment are more encouraging.

Otomycosis

Otomycosis is more common in tropical and subtropical countries. In the majority of cases, the isolated fungi are of the *Aspergillus (niger, fumigatus, flave-scens, albus)* or the Candida species. Otomycosis is more common in immunocompromised patients and in diabetics. Local factors that favor fungal infections include chronic otorrhea and the presence of epithelial debris. Clinically, the patient complains of otorrhea, itching, and hearing loss. Therapy consists of cleaning the ear to remove all debris and the instillation of local antimycotic preparations as well as lavage with 2% alcohol boric acid drops.

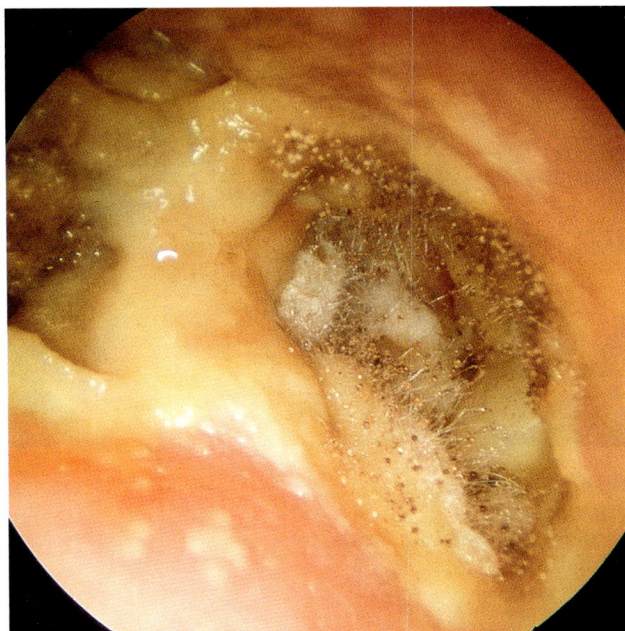

Figure 3.**26** Right ear. Radical mastoid cavity showing cholesteatoma with superimposed fungal infection.

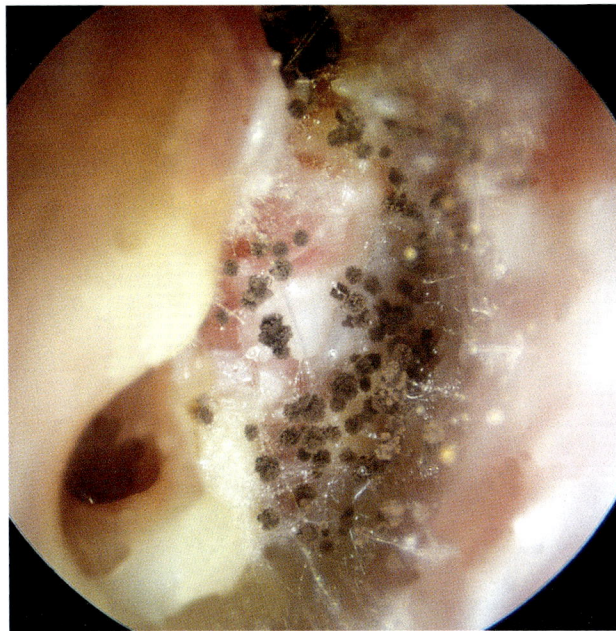

Figure 3.**27** An ear with chronic suppurative otitis media with cholesteatoma showing a superimposed fungal infection. The blackish fungal masses are easily recognized. They should be removed before local antifungal solution is instilled.

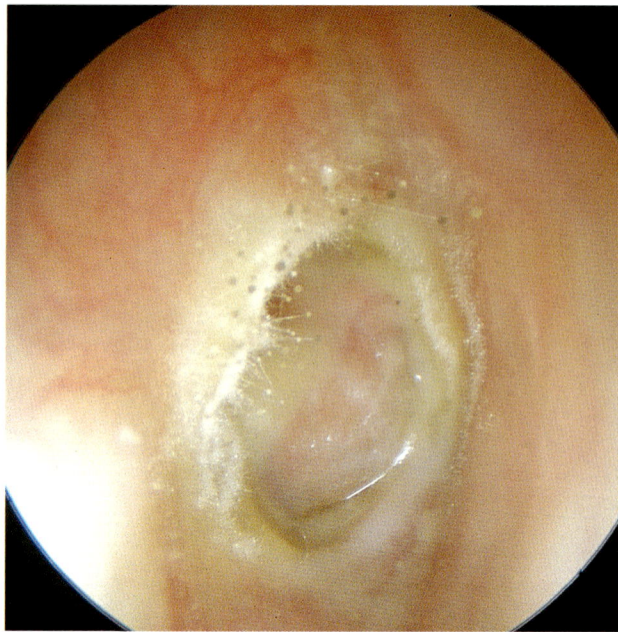

Figure 3.**28**   Another example of otomycosis in a radical mastoid cavity.

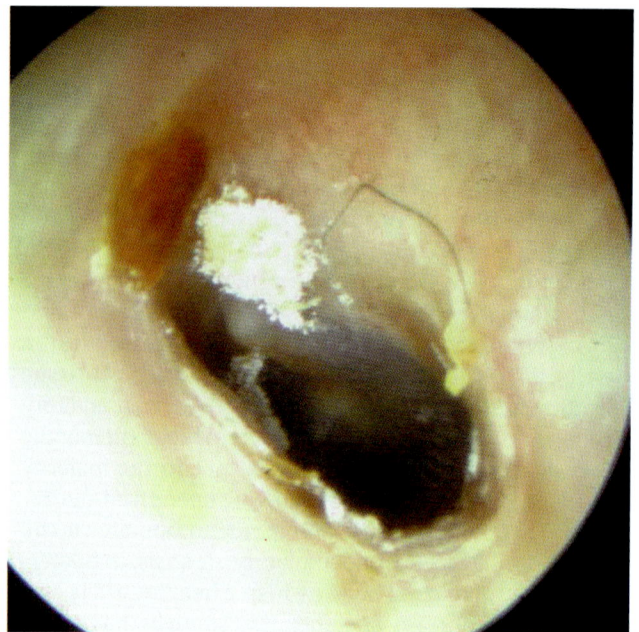

Figure 3.**29**   Another example of otomycosis, in the left ear. There are fungal growths covering the pars flaccida and the skin of the anterior canal wall.

Eczema

Eczema is a dermo-epidermal process of reactive nature resulting from local or general factors. Local factors include allergy, topical medical preparations, or cosmetics, whereas general factors include hepatic or gastrointestinal dysfunction. It manifests by itching, a burning sensation, vesication, and sometimes serous otorrhea. Treatment consists of discontinuing the suspected causative irritant, correction of the systemic disturbances, as well as lavage with boric acid with alcohol and steroid lotion.

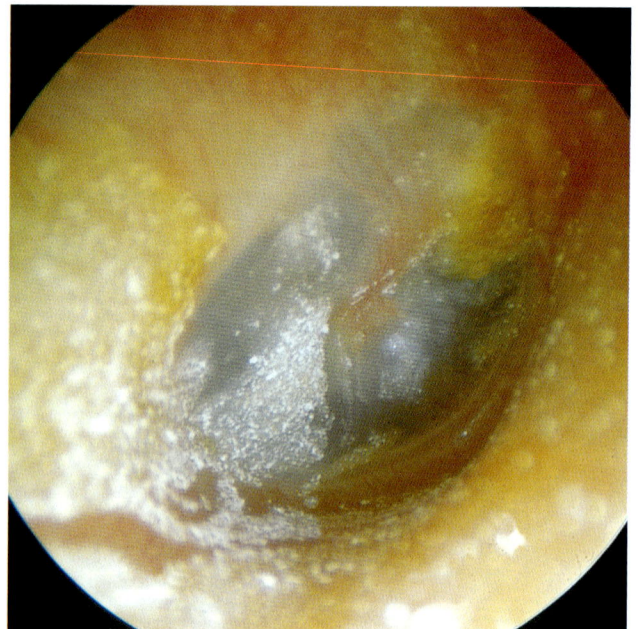

Figure 3.**30**   Right ear. Chronic eczema of the external auditory canal. Squamous debris covering the skin of the external auditory canal can be observed. Successfully treated by the use of local steroid lotion.

Cholesteatoma of the External Auditory Canal

Cholesteatoma of the external auditory canal should be differentiated from keratosis obturans. The latter entails accumulation of desquamated squamous epithelium in the external auditory canal forming an occluding cholesteatoma-like mass. The patient complains of pain and hearing loss. Keratosis obturans is generally bilateral and occurs in young patients, whereas cholesteatoma of the external auditory canal is usually unilateral and occurs in the elderly. In about 50% of patients, keratosis obturans is associated with bronchiectasis and chronic sinusitis. Removal of the mass is sufficient in keratosis obturans. However, in cholesteatoma it may also be necessary to remove the underlying bone followed by reconstruction of the external auditory canal and its skin.

Postoperative (iatrogenic) cholesteatoma of the external auditory canal is generally located at the level of the anterior angle of the tympanic membrane. It usually originates from incorrect repositioning of the skin flaps at the end of the procedure.

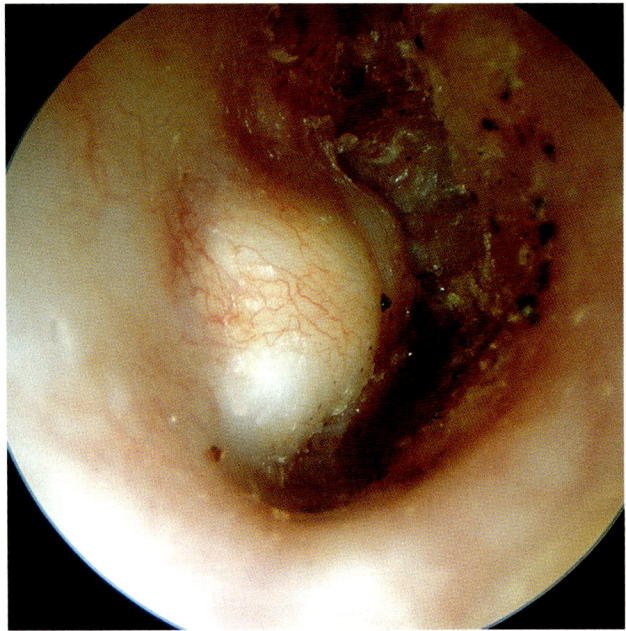

Figure 3.**31**   Cholesteatoma of the external auditory canal, as a result of incorrect repositioning of skin flaps in a previous intact canal wall tympanoplasty. This condition has to be differentiated from exostosis. A probe is used to palpate the mass. If its consistency is tender and soft, cholesteatoma is diagnosed.

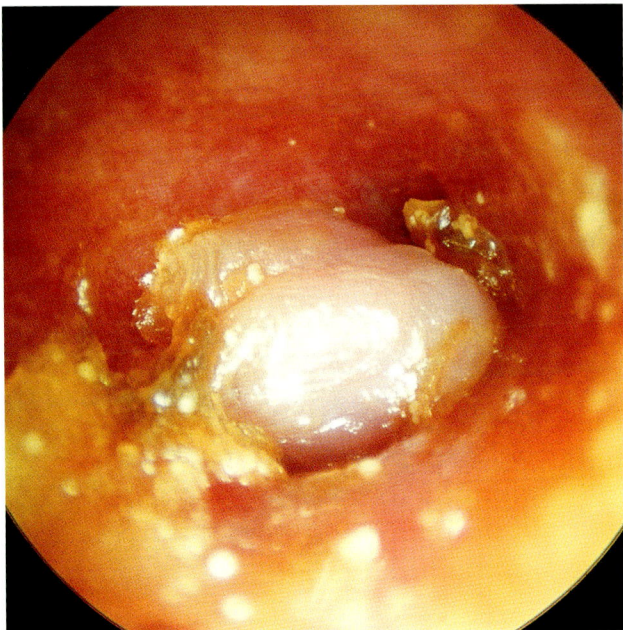

Figure 3.**32**   A case similar to that in Figure 3.**31**. The mass originating from the posterior canal wall inhibits the normal process of epithelial migration towards the outside.

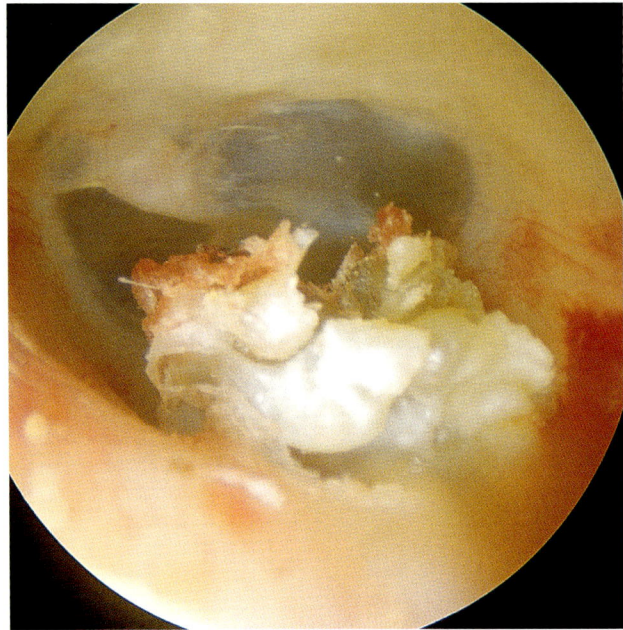

Figure 3.**33**   Cholesteatoma of the inferior wall of the left external auditory canal being removed in the outpatient clinic. In this case, the squamous debris led to erosion of the underlying bone.

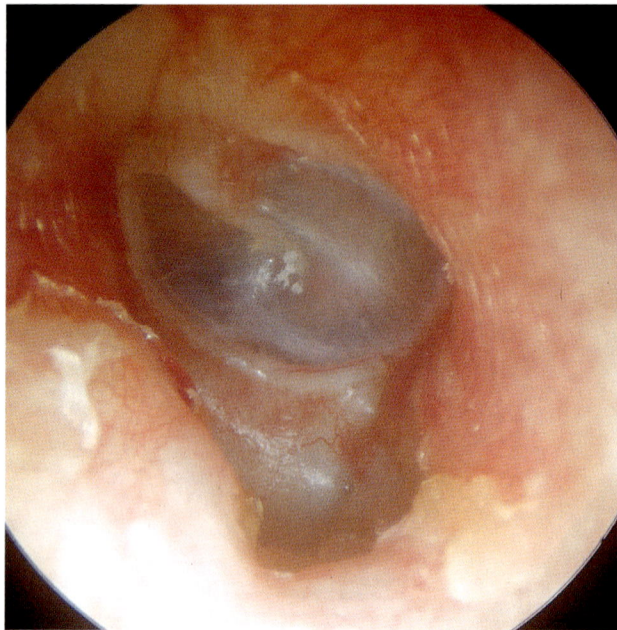

Figure 3.**34**   Same patient, a few months later. Note the bone erosion caused by the cholesteatoma.

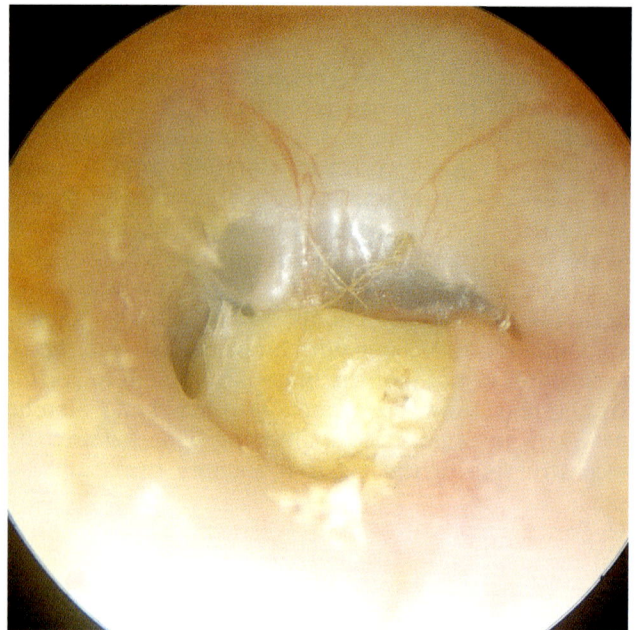

Figure 3.**35**   A case similar to the that in Figure 3.**33**. The cholesteatoma occupies more than half of the external auditory canal and is in contact with the tympanic membrane. The CT scan (Fig. 3.**36**) demonstrates partial erosion of the underlying bone.

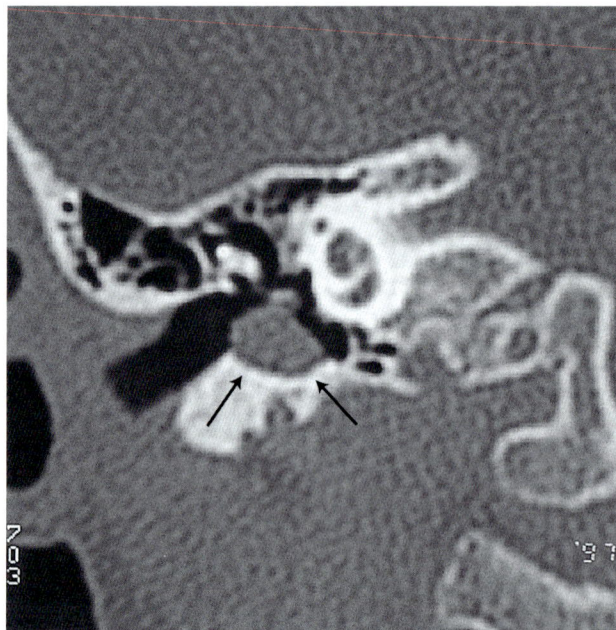

Figure 3.**36**   CT scan of the same case, coronal view. The cholesteatoma is clearly seen in the anteroinferior portion of the external auditory canal, with partial erosion of the underlying bone.

Summary

Postoperative (iatrogenic) cholesteatoma can almost always be removed in the outpatient clinic under local anesthesia using an endomeatal approach. The sac is opened and the cholesteatoma is aspirated. It is advisable to insert a plastic sheet in the external auditory canal for about 3 weeks to prevent the formation of adhesions that could lead to reformation of the cholesteatoma pearl.

Cholesteatoma of the external auditory canal should be surgically removed using a postauricular ap-proach. Wide drilling of the floor of the canal is mandatory to avoid recurrences.

Pathologies Extending to the External Auditory Canal

Some middle ear pathologies can extend into the external auditory canal (e.g., cholesteatomas, glomus tumors, meningiomas, carcinoid tumors, and histiocytosis X). These cases are discussed here to underline the importance of their inclusion in the differential diagnosis of polyps in the external auditory canal. Moreover, taking a biopsy of these polyps in the outpatient clinic without proper radiological study is sometimes hazardous. For a detailed discussion of these pathologies, the reader is referred to the relevant chapters.

Carcinoid Tumors

A carcinoid tumor is an adenomatous neuroendocrinal tumor of ectodermal origin. It has the same histologic and histochemical characteristics as other carcinoid tumors that involve different parts of the body. A carcinoid tumor is suspected whenever an adenomatous tumor of the middle ear has acinic or trabecular histologic features. The diagnosis is confirmed by electron microscopy and immunohistochemistry to demonstrate the presence of serotonin and argyrophilic granules. Surgical removal is indicated. To avoid recurrence, removal of the whole tumor together with the attached ossicular chain is essential.

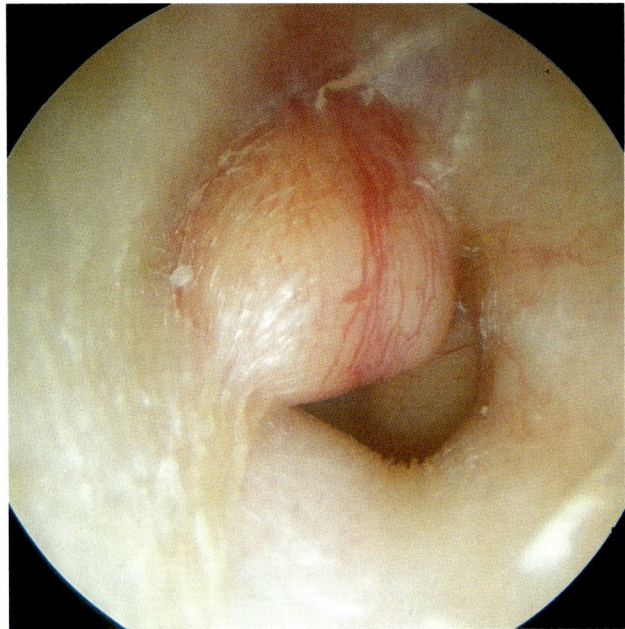

Figure 3.**37** This patient complained of hearing loss in the left ear and otalgia of 3 months' duration. Otoscopy revealed a mass occupying the external auditory canal and originating from its anterosuperior region. The inferior part of the tympanic membrane, which is the only visible part, appears whitish due to the presence of a mass in the middle ear. The audiogram (Fig. 3.**38**) revealed the presence of ipsilateral conductive hearing loss. The tympanogram was type B. CT scan (Figs. 3.**39**, 3.**40**) demonstrated the presence of an iso-intense soft-tissue mass occupying the middle ear and mastoid with extension into the external auditory canal. No erosion of the ossicular chain, nor of the intercellular septa of the mastoid air cells, was noted. Intraoperatively, a glandular-like tissue was found and a frozen section obtained. The biopsy, confirmed by immmunohistochemical and electron-microscopic studies, proved the presence of a carcinoid tumor. A tympanoplasty was performed with total removal of the pathology and the involved malleus and incus.

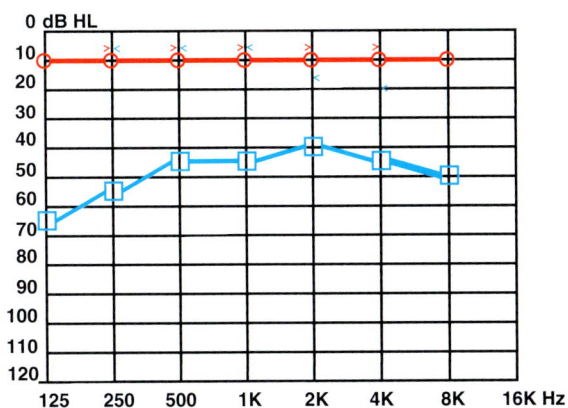

Figure 3.**38** The audiogram shows the presence of significant ipsilateral conductive hearing loss.

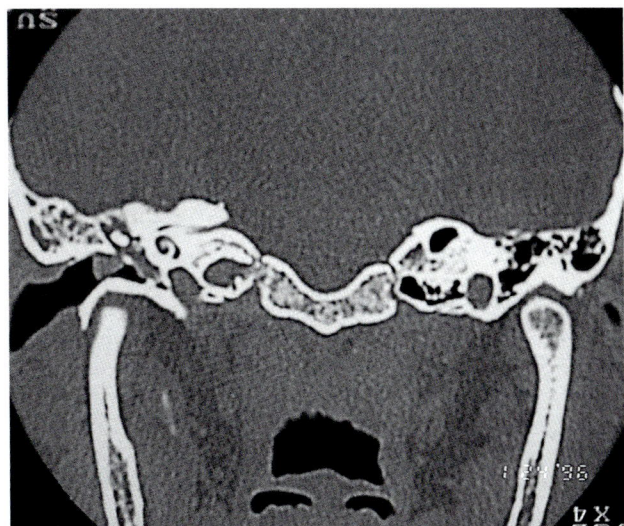

Figure 3.**39** The CT scan demonstrates a soft-tissue mass occupying the middle ear with extrusion through the tympanic membrane.

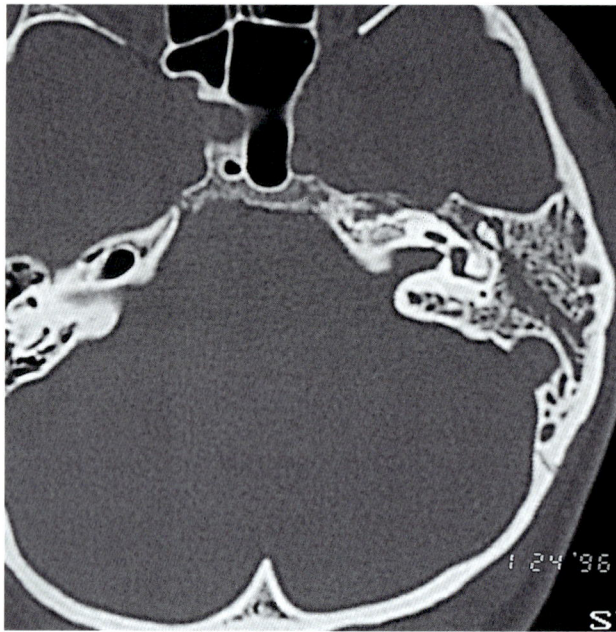

Figure 3.**40** CT scan, axial view. Presence of glue in the mastoid cells without erosion of the intercellular septa.

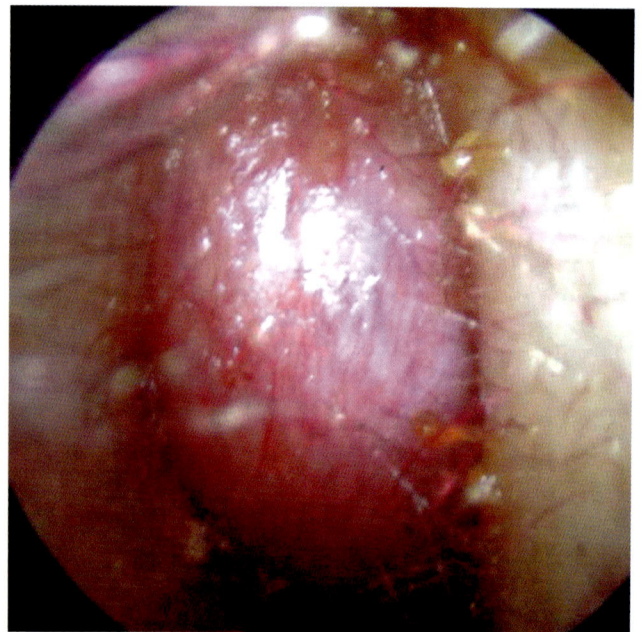

Figure 3.**41** There is a polyp-like mass occupying the external auditory canal. The patient had conductive hearing loss. The CT scan revealed an isointense soft-tissue mass occupying the external auditory canal, the middle ear and the mastoid, without erosion of the ossicular chain or intercellular septa of the mastoid air cells. A frozen section obtained during surgery revealed carcinoid tumor. This diagnosis was later confirmed by immunohistochemistry and electron-microscopy studies. A two-stage tympanoplasty was performed.

Summary

Carcinoid tumors of the middle ear are very rare. They are considered to be a subgroup of adenomatous tumors of the middle ear. Clinically, they manifest as hearing loss, tinnitus, aural fullness, facial nerve paresis, vertigo, and otalgia. These tumors require functional surgery that entails removal of the tympanic membrane and ossicular chain together with the mass. The tympanic membrane is grafted at the same stage, whereas the ossicular chain is reconstructed at a second stage. This strategy ensures that the condition is completely cured.

Histiocytosis X

Histiocytosis X refers to a group of disorders of the reticuloendothelial system characterized by proliferation of cytologically benign histiocytes. The disease can present in three clinical forms, the most benign of which is eosinophilic granuloma, which is usually monostotic. A moderately aggressive form is known as Hand–Schüller–Christian disease. It is characterized by multifocal lesions that are predominantly osteolytic. The most severe form, Letterer–Siwe disease, occurs in children under 3 years of age and presents with diffuse multiorgan involvement. It has a mortality rate of about 40% despite therapy with cytotoxic drugs and corticosteroids. Survivors suffer from diseases such as diabetes insipidus, pulmonary fibrosis, and vertebral column involvement.

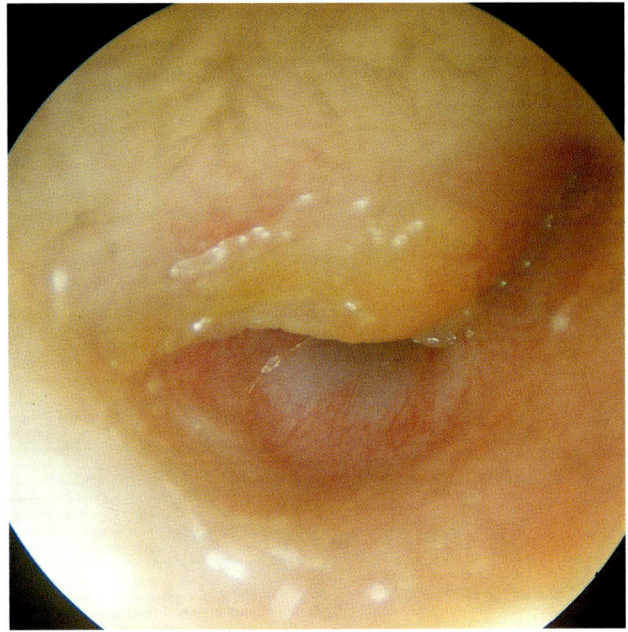

Figure 3.**42** A bulging of the posterosuperior wall of the external auditory canal in a 4-year-old child. A similar picture was also seen in the other ear (see CT scan in Fig. 3.**43**).

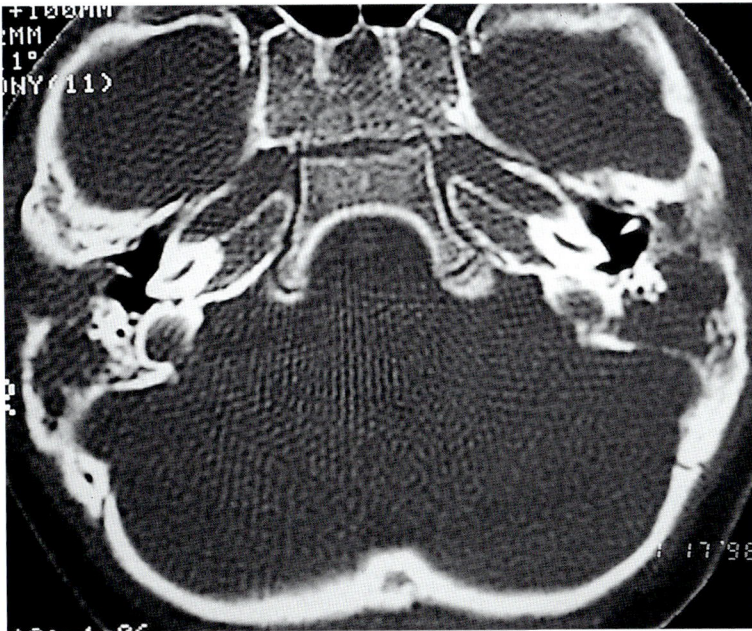

Figure 3.**43** CT scan of the same case as in Figure 3.**42**. The middle ear and mastoid are occupied by an isointense mass. A frozen section obtained during surgery revealed the presence of histiocytosis X. The patient was referred to a specialized center for appropriate staging and therapy with cyto-toxic drugs and corticosteroids.

Other Pathologies

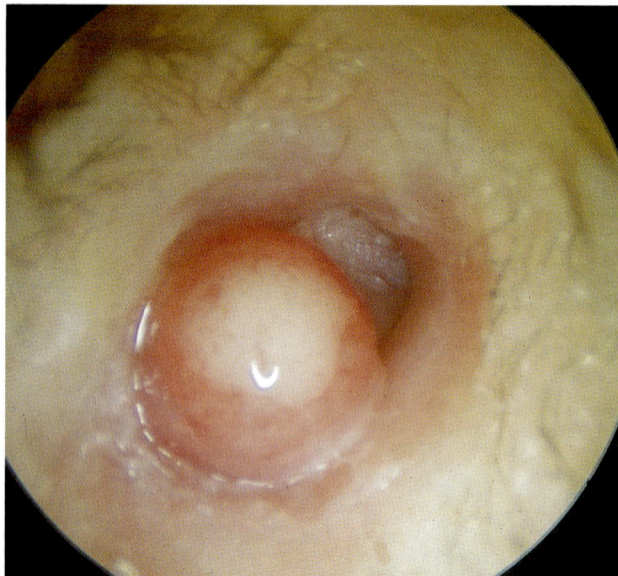

Figure 3.**44** Polyp in the external canal in a child presenting with continuous otorrhea and hearing loss. A CT scan (Fig. 3.**45**) shows the presence of a soft-tissue mass eroding the intercellular septae of the mastoid and the ossicular chain, suggestive of cholesteatoma. This was confirmed during surgery.

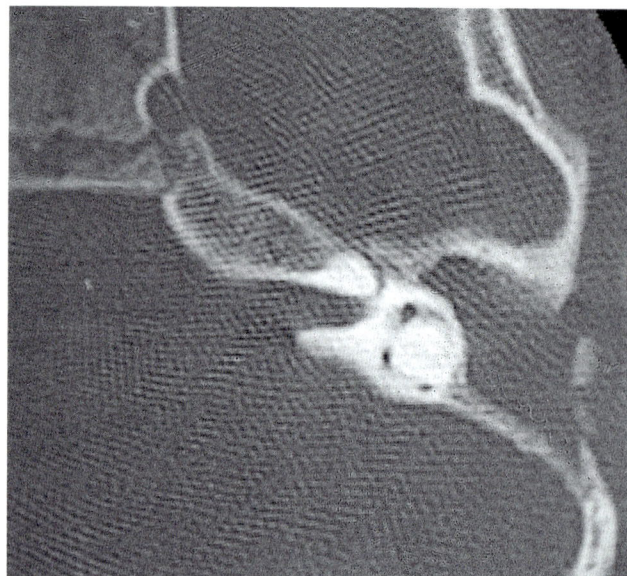

Figure 3.**45** CT scan, axial view. The entire mastoid is occupied by a soft-tissue mass. The intercellular septa of the mastoid and the ossicular chain are absent.

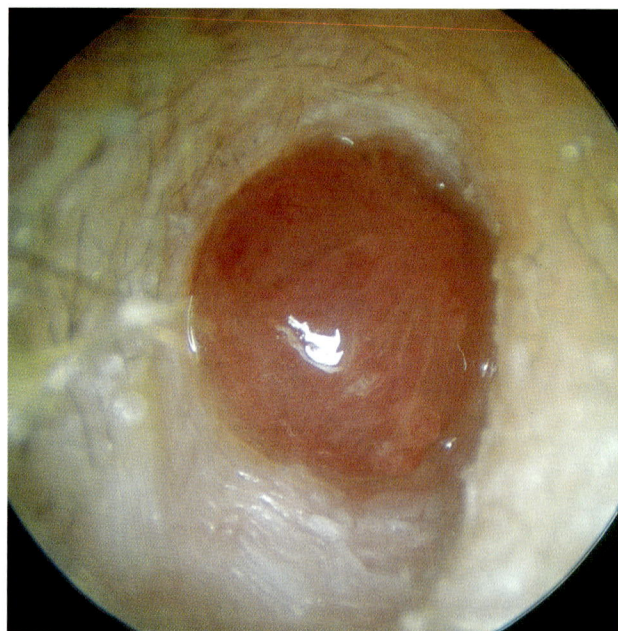

Figure 3.**46** Another example of chronic suppurative otitis media with cholesteatoma that manifests with an aural polyp. Though cholesteatoma presents frequently in this manner, it is absolutely essential to abstain from taking a biopsy of the polyp in the outpatient clinic without performing a CT scan of the temporal bone (see Fig. 3.**47**).

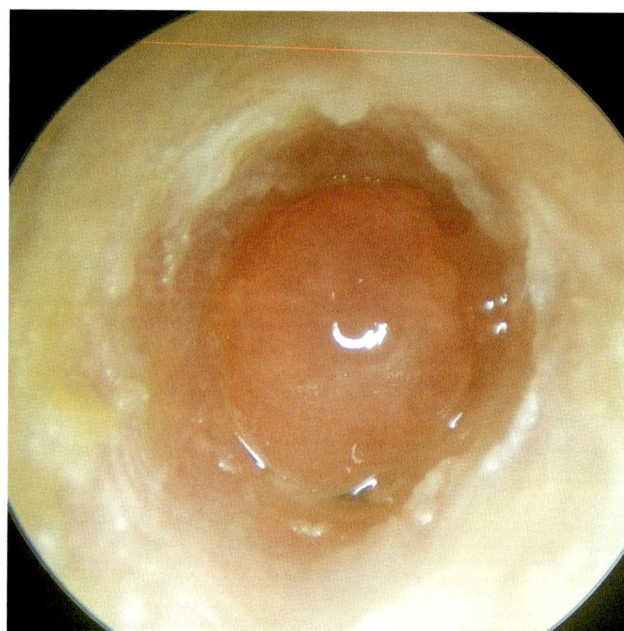

Figure 3.**47** The otoscopic view is very similar to that in Figure 3.**46**. In this case, however, the diagnosis is that of an en-plaque supratentorial meningioma. An outpatient polypectomy in this case might lead to excessive bleeding (see MRI, Figs. 3.**48** and 3.**49**).

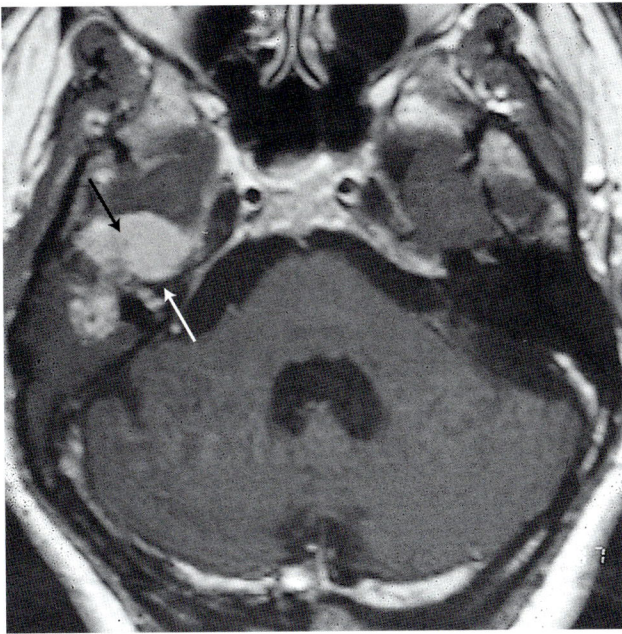

Figure 3.**48** MRI with gadolinium enhancement, axial view. The tumor (arrows) is located in the temporal fossa and reaches the area of the petrous apex and Meckel's cavity.

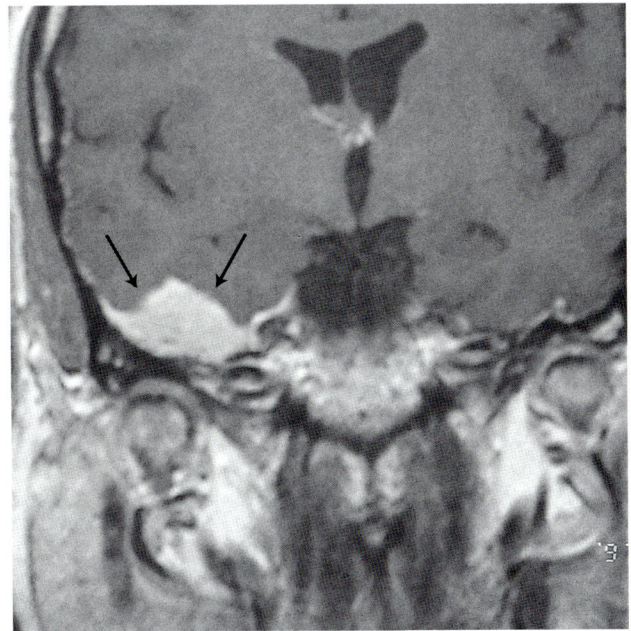

Figure 3.**49** MRI with gadolinium, coronal view. The meningioma displaces the temporal lobe upwards (arrows); pathognomonic tails of the dura are visible.

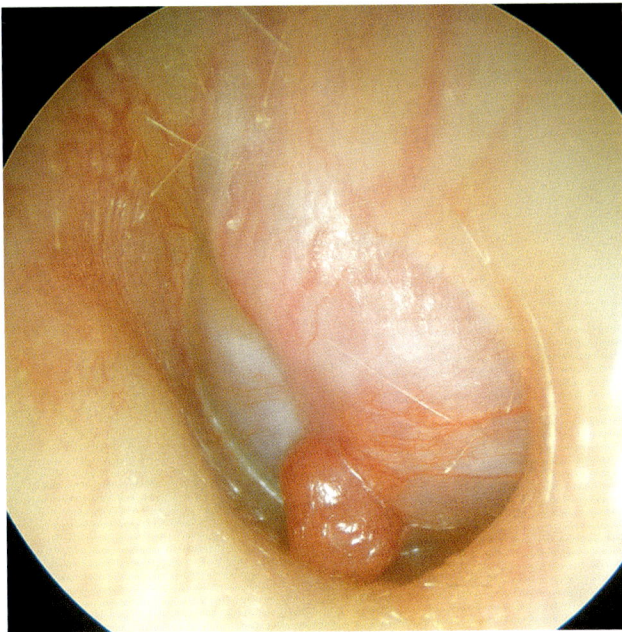

Figure 3.**50** Left ear. Glomus jugulare tumor with extension into the external auditory canal. A biopsy of this lesion might lead to severe and often difficult-to-control hemorrhage.

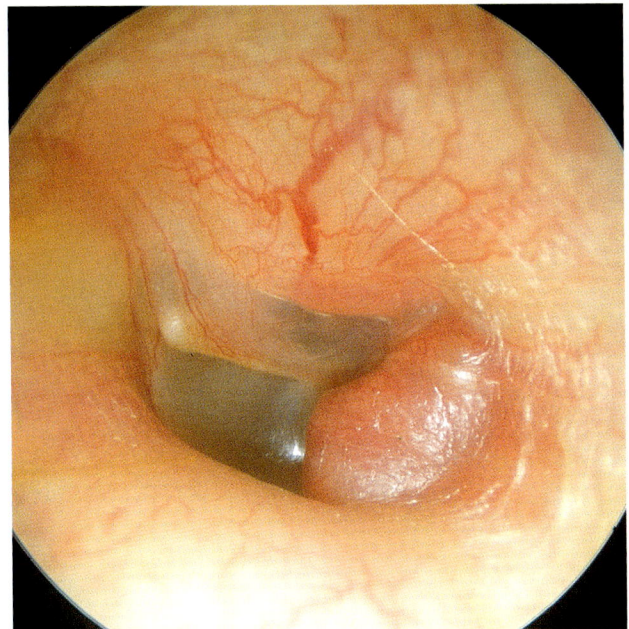

Figure 3.**51** Left ear. Another example of a glomus tumor.

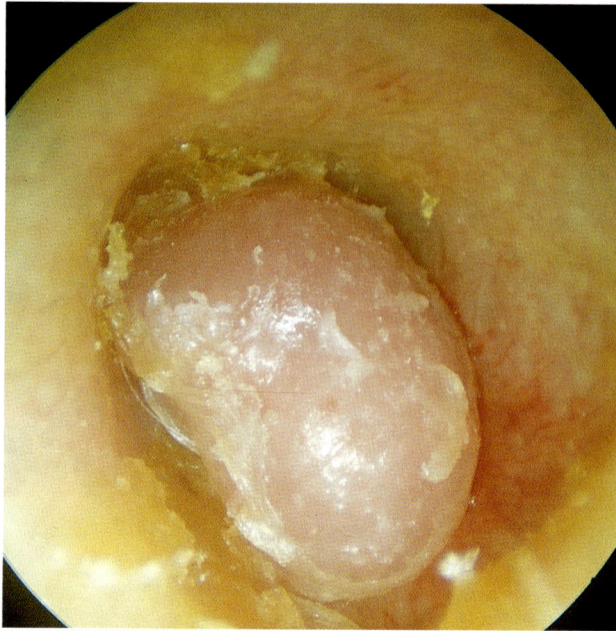

Figure 3.**52** Pulsating neoplasm in the external auditory canal. MRI (Fig. 3.**53**) revealed the presence of a glomus jugulare tumor involving the vertical internal carotid artery.

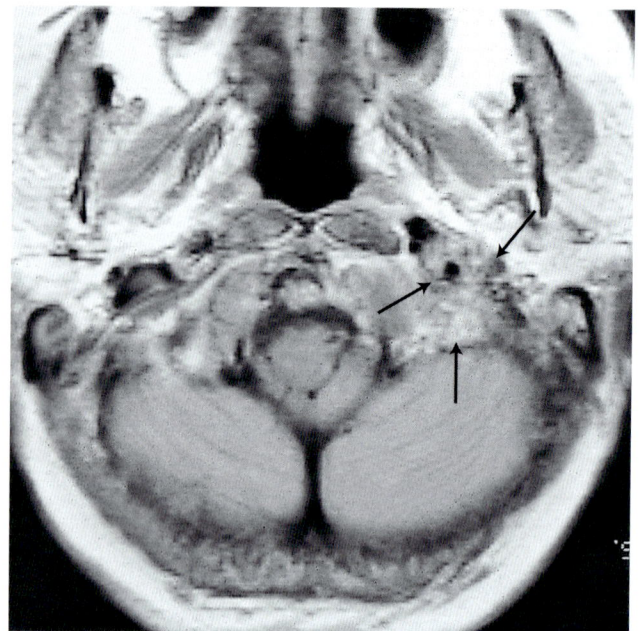

Figure 3.**53** MRI of the same case. A glomus jugulare tumor engulfing the vertical portion of the internal carotid artery is clearly visible.

Necrotizing Otitis Externa (Malignant Otitis)

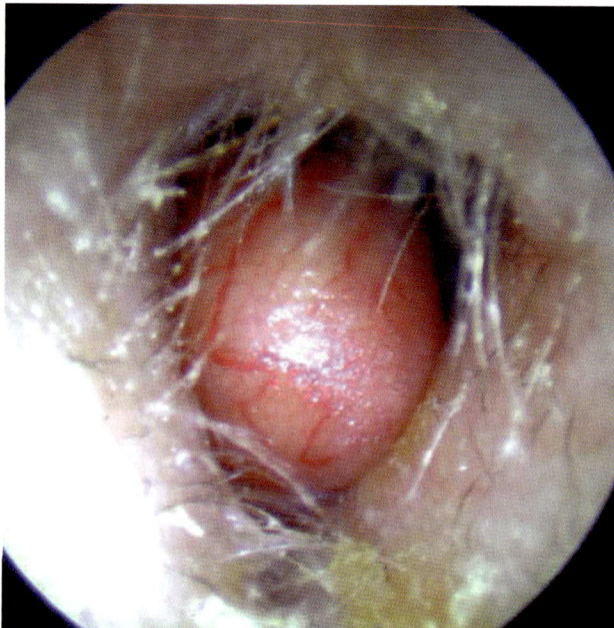

Figure 3.**54** A polyp-like mass is present in the external auditory canal. The patient, who had already undergone two tympanoplasties, complained of pain in the ear. A biopsy excluded neoplastic disease. A scintigraphic examination confirmed the diagnosis of malignant external otitis. The patient was treated with a long course of antibiotic therapy, with final resolution of the pathology.

Temporal Bone Fractures

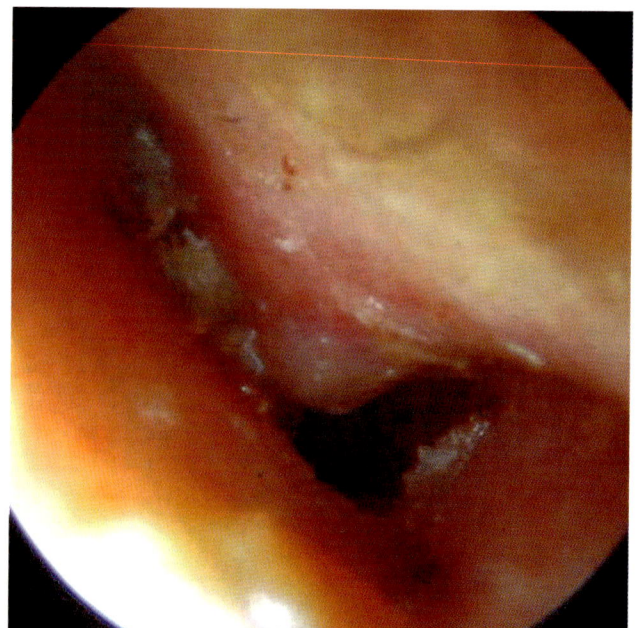

Figure 3.**55** Left ear. Fracture of the anterior bony canal in a patient who had had a car accident. The temporomandibular joint completely occupied the lumen of the EAC. The patient complained of a feeling of fullness and conductive hearing loss.

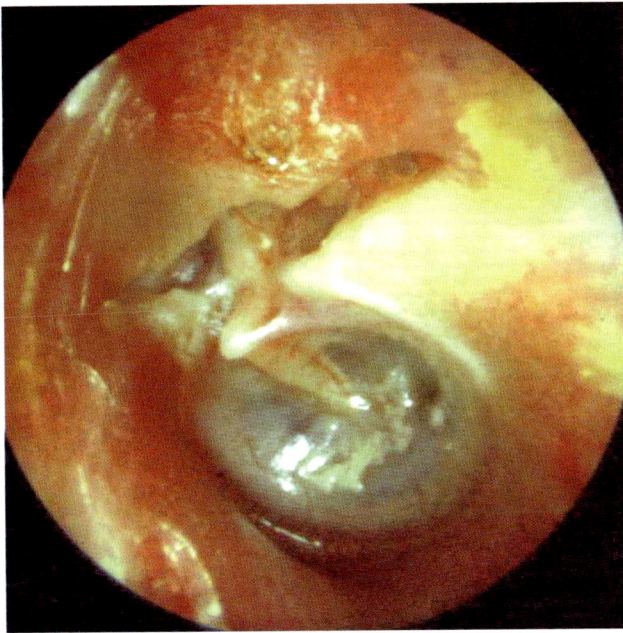

Figure 3.**56** Left ear. Another post-traumatic fracture of the temporal bone. An anteroposterior fissure is seen in the superior canal wall.

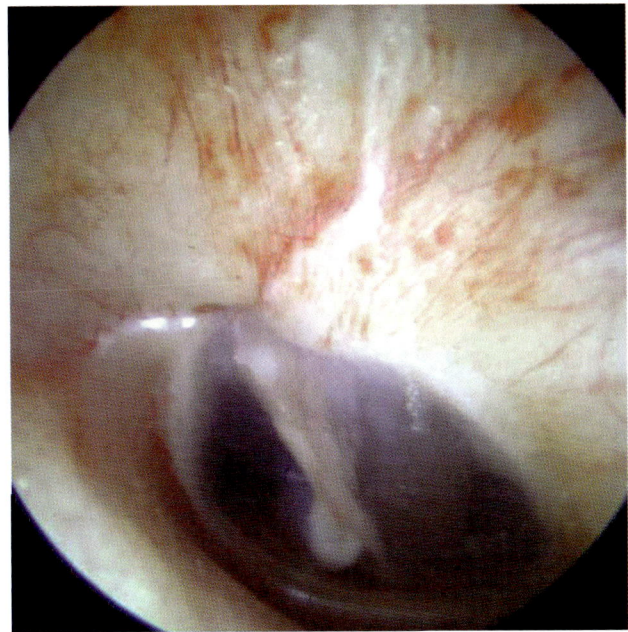

Figure 3.**57** Left ear. A well-established fracture of the temporal bone. The fracture line is located in the superior bony canal wall, with an anteroposterior direction.

Carcinoma of the External Auditory Canal

Basal cell carcinoma is more frequent in the auricle, particularly in subjects with long exposure to the sun. On the other hand, squamous cell carcinoma accounts for about three-quarters of invasive tumors of the external auditory canal and the middle ear. In about 11% of cases, cervical lymph node metastases are present at the time of diagnosis. The most common symptoms include otorrhea, otalgia, hearing loss, facial nerve paralysis, and vertigo. An accurate microscopic examination is important for proper evaluation of the lesion extension. Frequently, an exfoliative lesion is noted, whereas an ulcer is present in other cases. Carcinoma should be suspected when there is a persistent otitis externa characterized by pain and otorrhea that does not resolve adequately with medical treatment. A biopsy of the lesion will clear up any doubts. It is important to perform an accurate examination of the upper deep cervical, postauricular, and parotid lymph nodes (anterior extension of the tumor). The cranial nerves are also evaluated. The facial nerve is the most frequently involved. Involvement of the mandibular nerve indicates tumor extension towards the glenoid fossa. A high-resolution CT scan (bone window) is the most important radiological investigation as it permits the evaluation of bone erosion at the level of the external auditory canal and middle ear. MRI with gadolinium allows evaluation of tumor extension into the soft tissues.

The tumor should be considered to be T3 or T4 if there is infiltration of the posterior or middle cranial fossae, or invasion of the jugular foramen or glenoid fossa. In such cases, whatever the modality of treatment, the prognosis is almost always poor.

Surgery consists of en-bloc removal of the tumor and a trial to include a safety margin of the surrounding healthy tissue in the specimen. Postoperative radiotherapy should be subsequently performed.

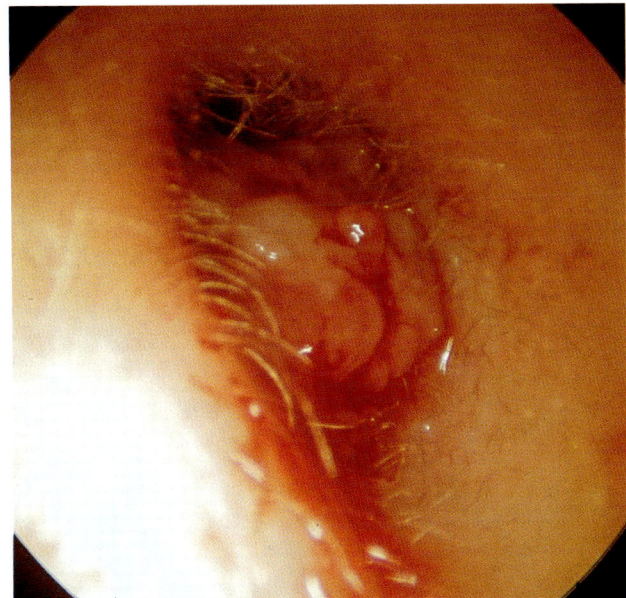

Figure 3.**58** An exfoliative neoplasm that occupies the external auditory canal. The patient complained of otalgia and attacks of bloody otorrhea of 1-month duration. A biopsy was taken and pathologic examination revealed the presence of squamous cell carcinoma. A CT scan (Fig. 3.**59**) demonstrated erosion of the external auditory canal, particularly its anteroinferior wall, without invasion into the glenoid fossa. En-bloc removal of the tumor was performed, together with a superficial parotidectomy. Radiotherapy was performed postoperatively.

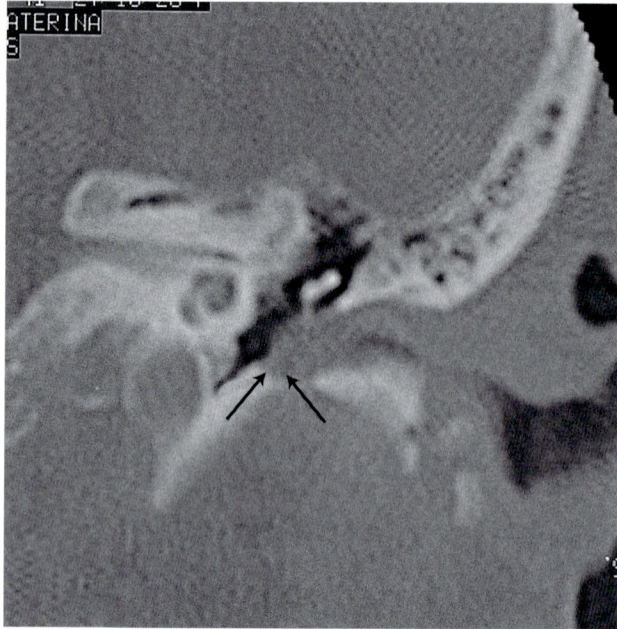

Figure 3.**59**   CT scan demonstrates erosion of the antero-inferior wall of the external auditory canal. The glenoid fossa is not invaded.

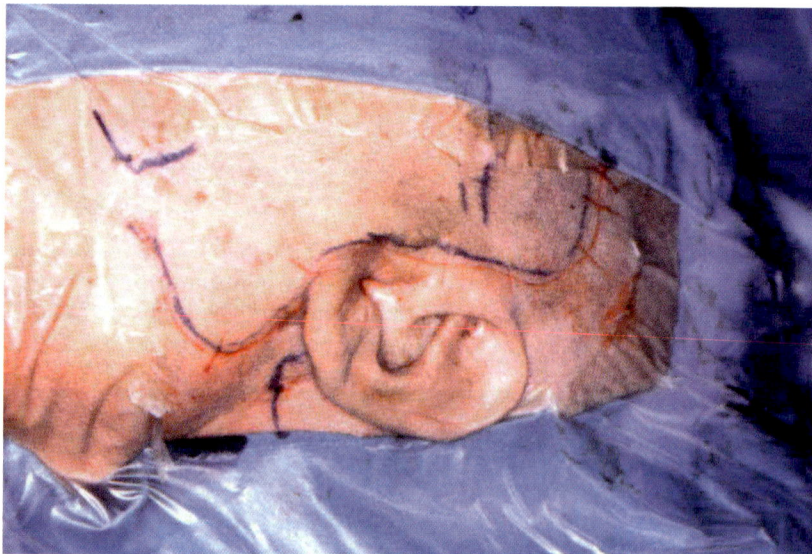

Figure 3.**60a**   Same patient as in Fig. 3.**58**. The preauricular skin incision starts from the parietal region and reaches the submandibular area.

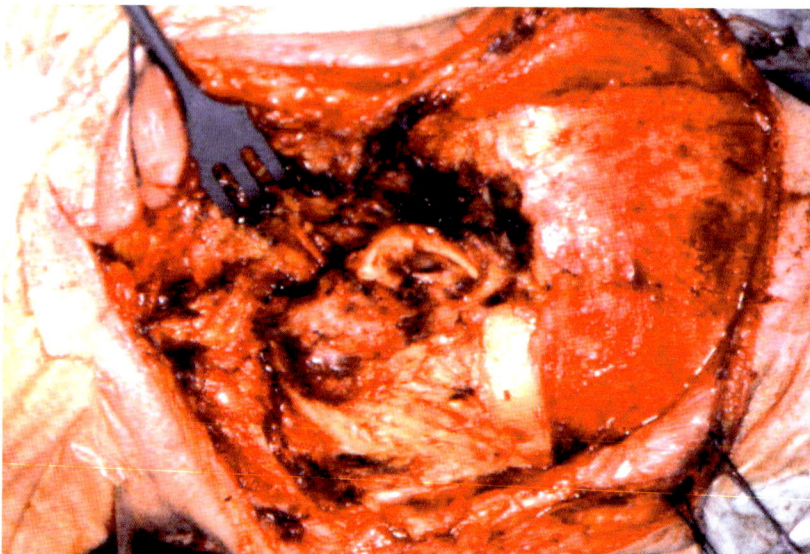

Figure 3.**60b**   The external auditory canal with the cartilage is transected.

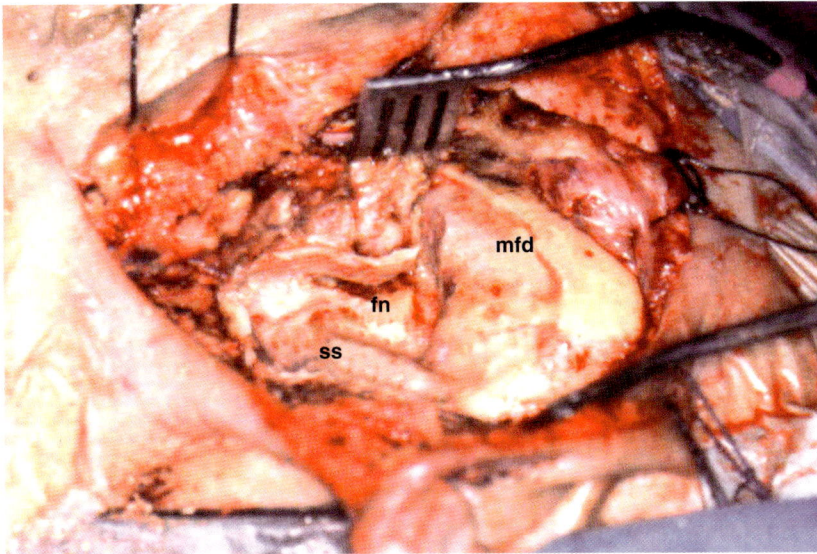

Figure 3.**60c** The external canal skin has been incised laterally. A subtotal petrosectomy has been completed, with middle fossa and sigmoid sinus skeletization and a large posterior tympanotomy.

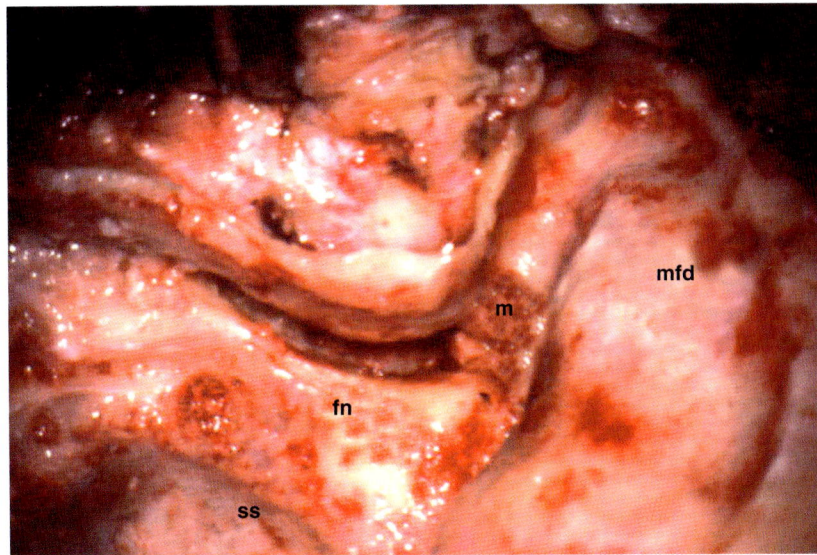

Figure 3.**60d** Higher magnification of the posterior tympanotomy. The third portion of the facial nerve is skeletonized. The incus has been removed, and the malleus is still in place.

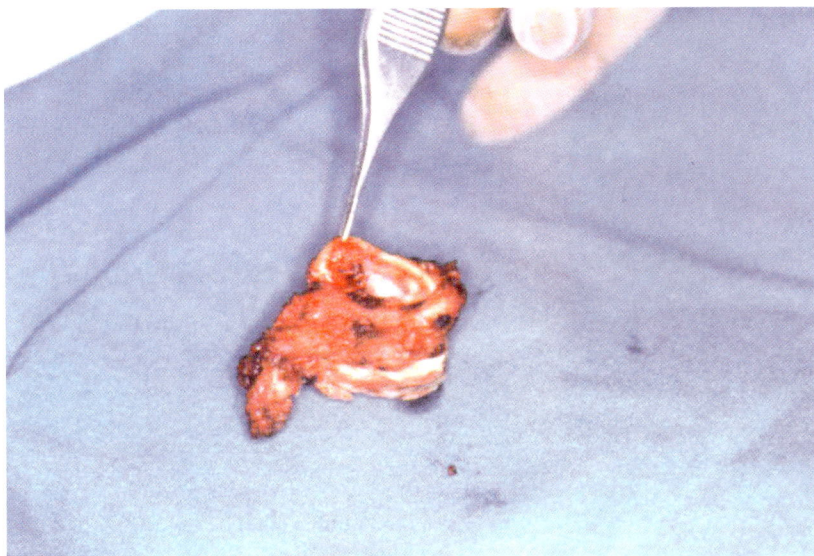

Figure 3.**60e** En bloc removal of the external auditory canal.

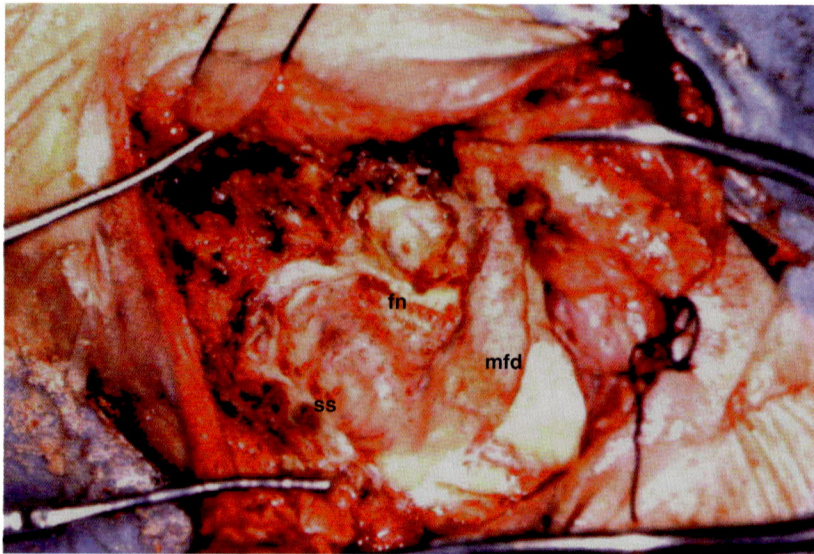

Figure 3.**60f** The external auditory canal has been removed en bloc together with the skin. The facial nerve is identified at the stylomastoid foramen.

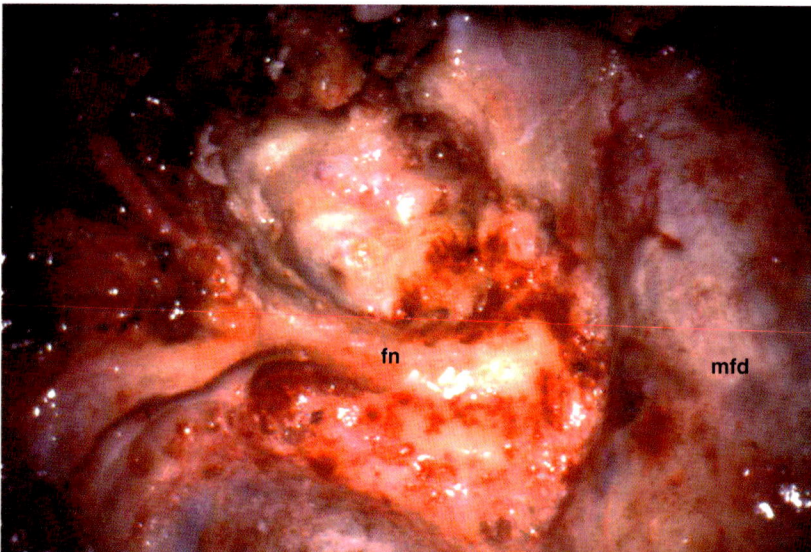

Figure 3.**60g** Higher magnification of the cavity at the end of the procedure. The facial nerve ridge is very low. The extrapetrosal portion of the facial nerve is clearly seen, and the carotid artery is identified.

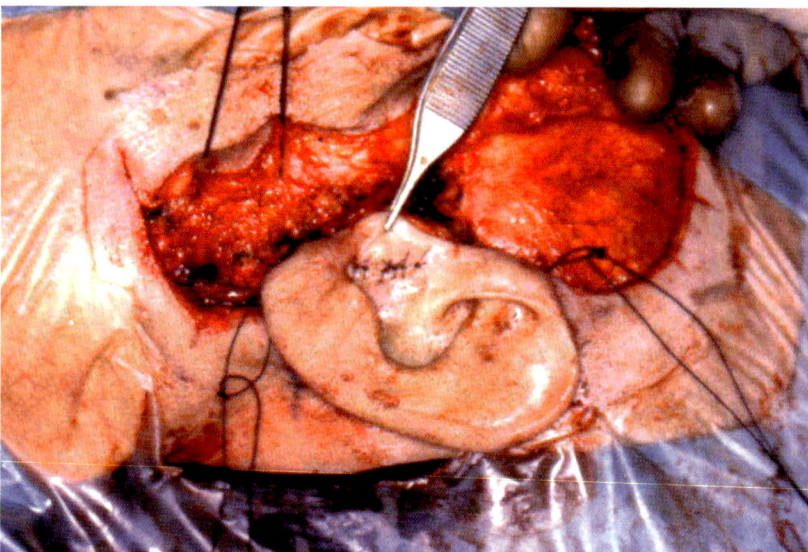

Figure 3.**60h** Blind sac closure of the external auditory canal.

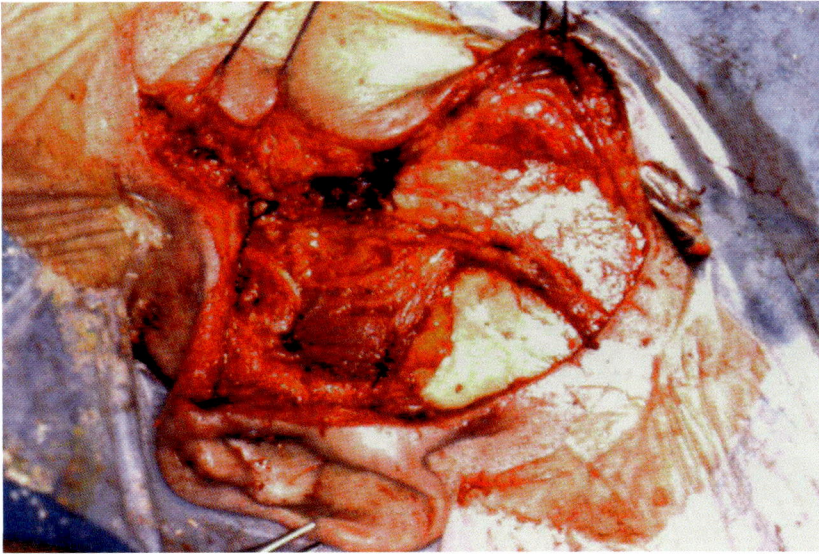

Figure 3.**60i** Closure of the subcutaneous tissue over the fat.

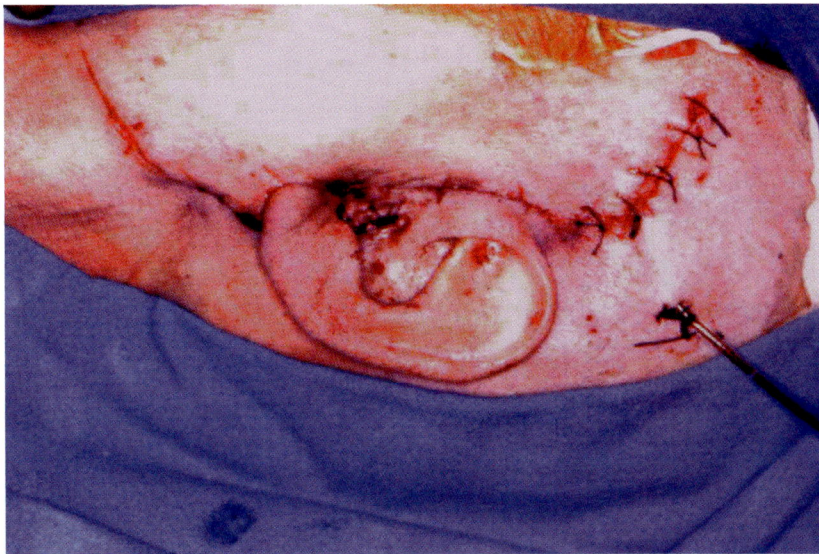

Figure 3.**60j** Skin suture.

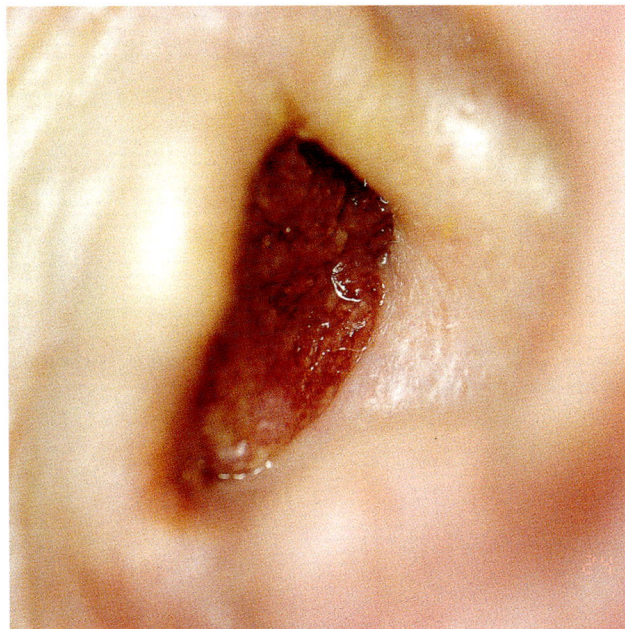

Figure 3.**61** Squamous cell carcinoma protruding through the external auditory canal with extension into the glenoid fossa and infiltration of the middle fossa dura (see CT scan, Fig. 3.**62** and MRI, Fig. 3.**63**). Palliative surgery was performed, followed by radiotherapy.

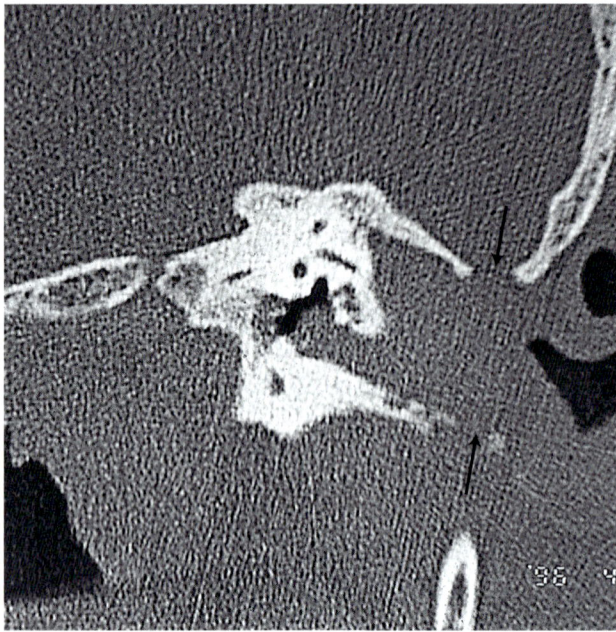

Figure 3.**62**   CT scan. The carcinoma occupies all of the middle ear and the mastoid. The glenoid fossa and the middle fossa plate are eroded.

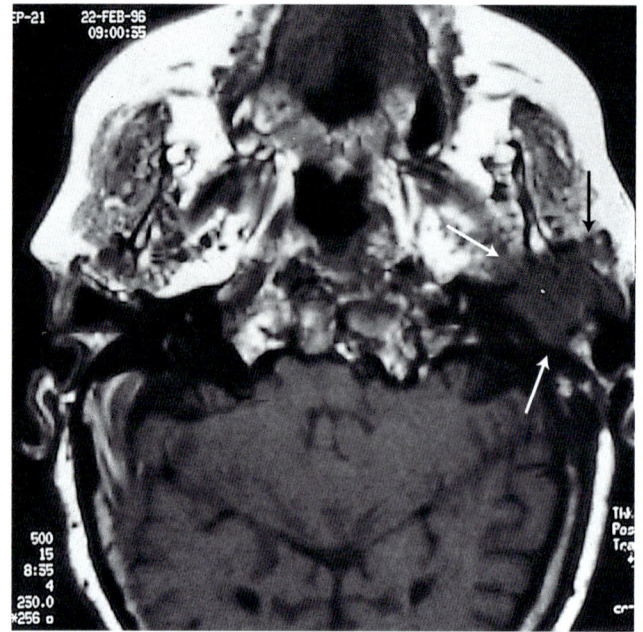

Figure 3.**63**   MRI shows marked anterior extension of the tumor into the infratemporal fossa.

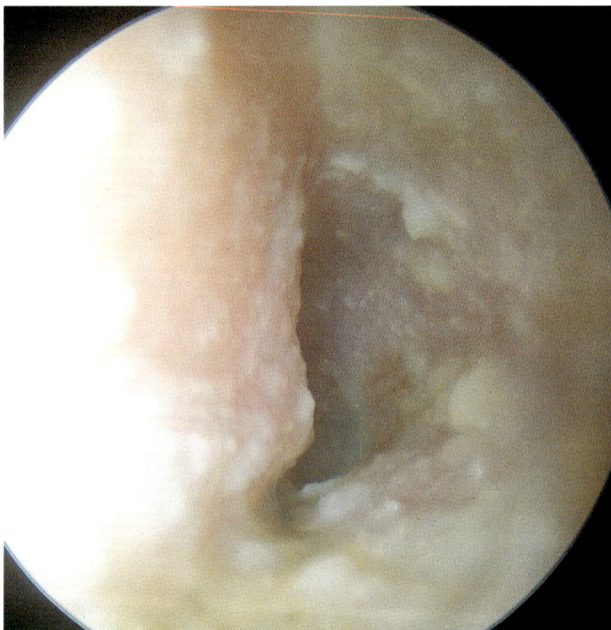

Figure 3.**64**   Squamous cell carcinoma with posterior extension. The mass is infiltrating the skin of the posterior wall of the external auditory canal (see CT scan, Fig. 3.**65**) as a result of which en-bloc resection and subsequent radiotherapy were performed.

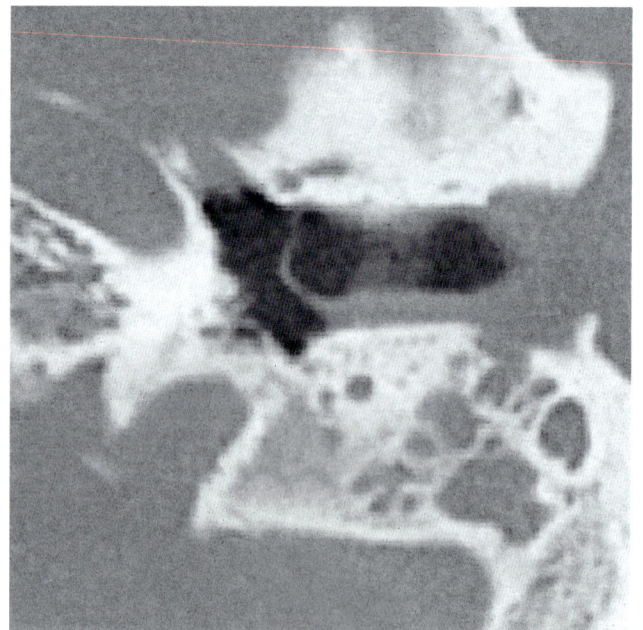

Figure 3.**65**   CT scan, axial view. The tumor has eroded the most lateral portion of the posterior bony wall.

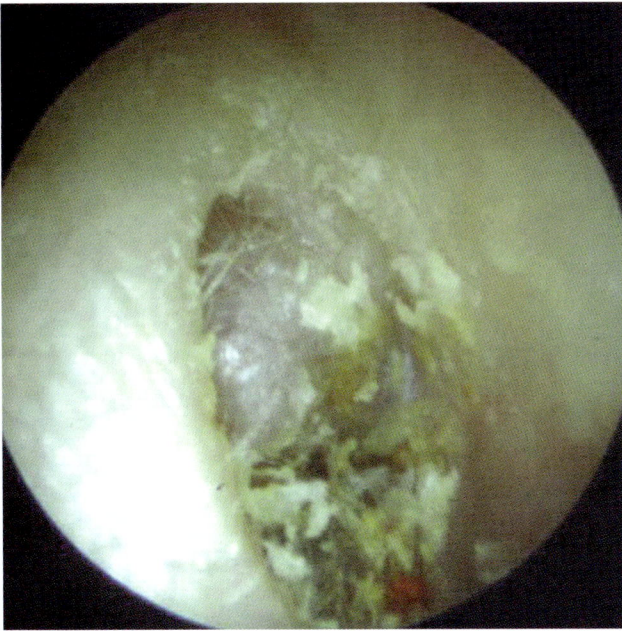

Figure 3.**66a** Right ear. This patient had otalgia, a feeling of fullness and conductive hearing loss. The painful soft mass is protruding from the posterosuperior external auditory canal wall. The histopathological examination after biopsy revealed an adenoid cystic carcinoma (see CT scan in Fig. 3.**66b**).

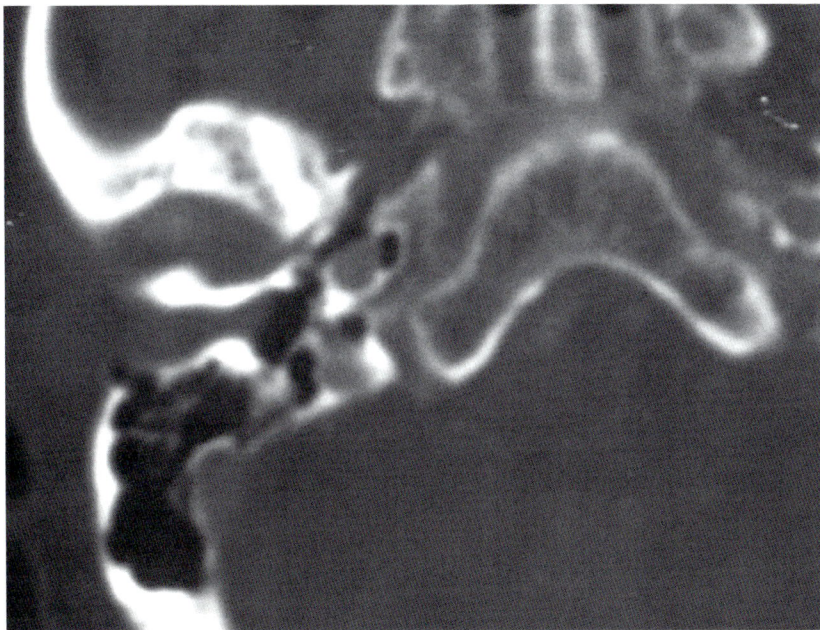

Figure 3.**66b** CT scan of the same patient. This axial view shows the mass (a soft-tissue density) partially occupying the external auditory canal. No erosion of the posterior and anterior bony canal wall is present.

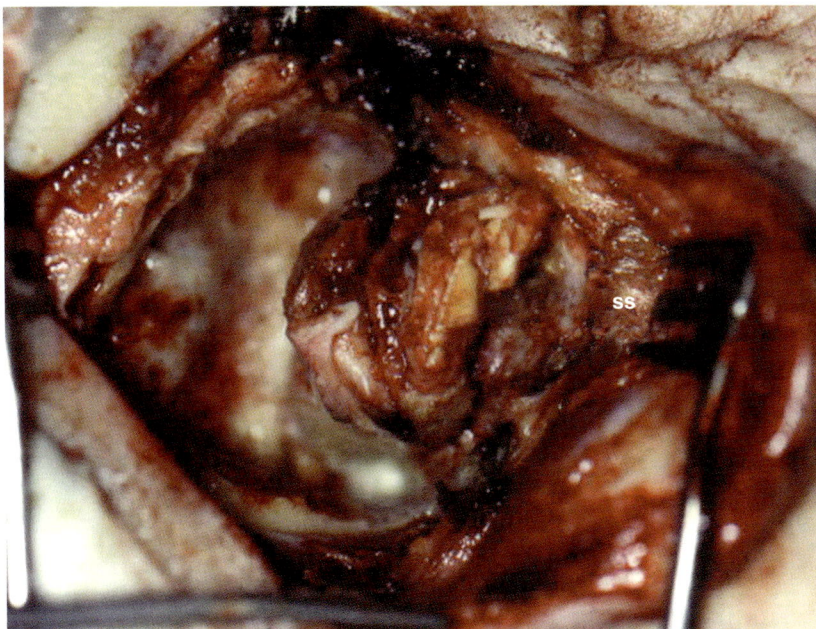

Figure 3.**66c** Intraoperative view of the mass. En-bloc removal of the bony external auditory canal (EAC) was carried out using subtotal petrosectomy, with obliteration of the cavity with abdominal fat and blind sac closure of the the skin of the EAC.

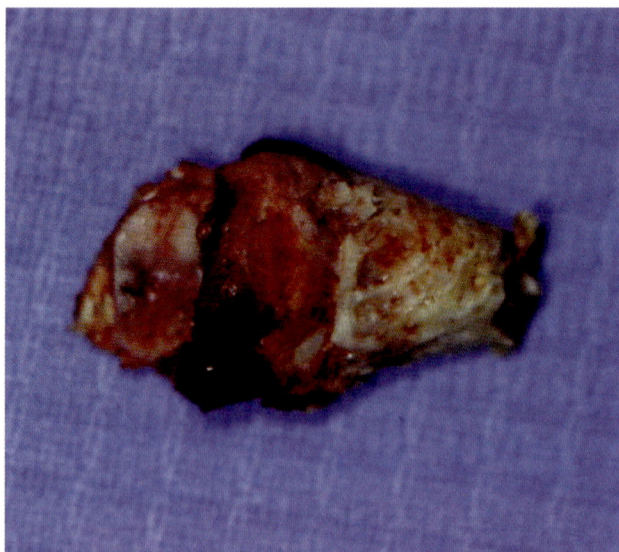

Figure 3.**66d**   The surgical specimen, showing the tumor mass together with the skin, bony wall, malleus and tympanic membrane.

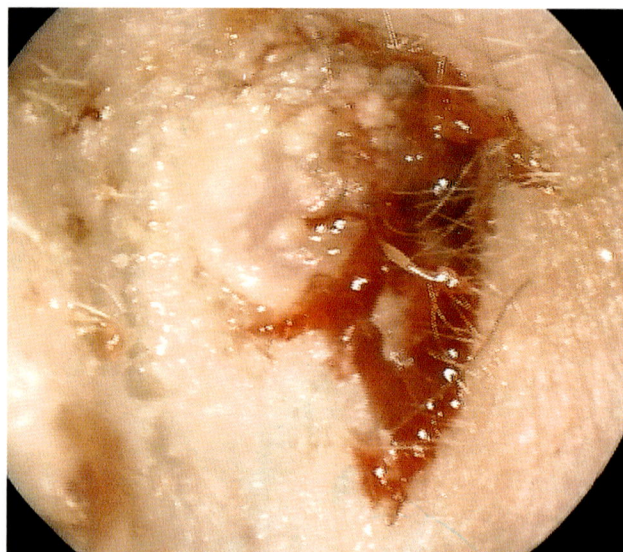

Figure 3.**67a**   Left ear. There is a polypoid mass originating from the anterior wall, occupying the external auditory canal. CT and MRI were carried out (Figs. 3.**67b**, **c**). Pathological examination after biopsy demonstrated a squamous cell carcinoma.

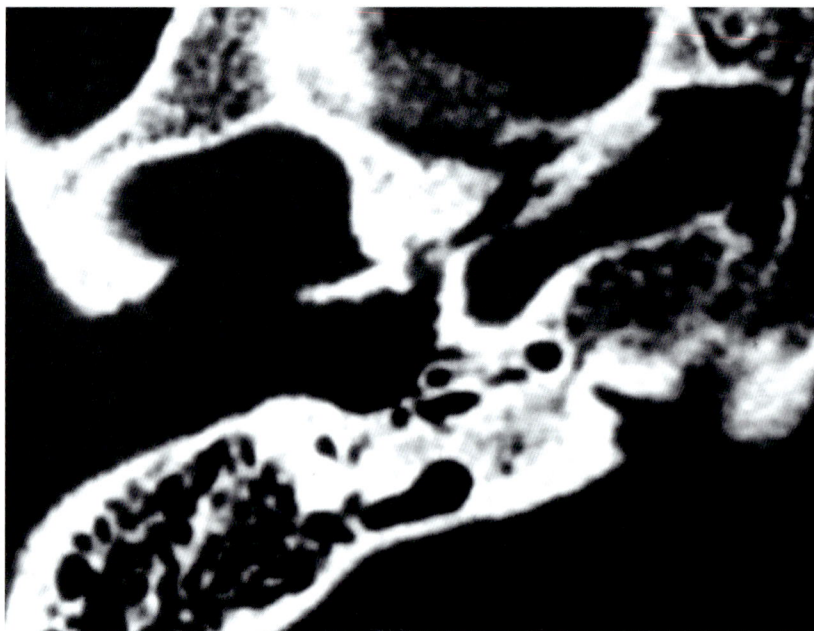

Figure 3.**67b**   The CT scan of the same patient shows a mass occupying the external auditory canal, with erosion of the anterior wall and involvement of the temporomandibular joint. Posteriorly, there is no erosion of the mastoid cortical bone.

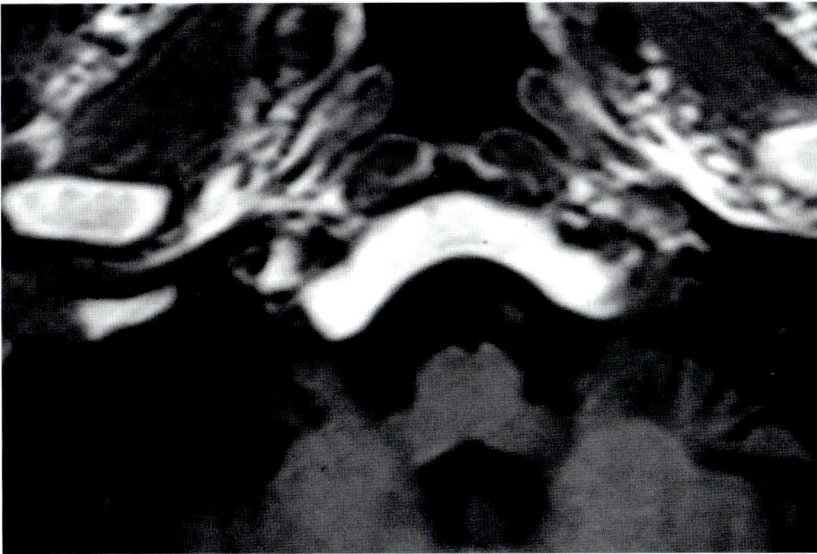

Figure 3.**67c** MRI of the same patient. The mass is spreading anteriorly, invading the glenoid fossa. The preoperative examination was completed with a neck echography which revealed positive unilateral high cervical nodes. A subtotal petrosectomy was associated with a total parotidectomy and a modified radical neck dissection. Radiotherapy was performed postoperatively.

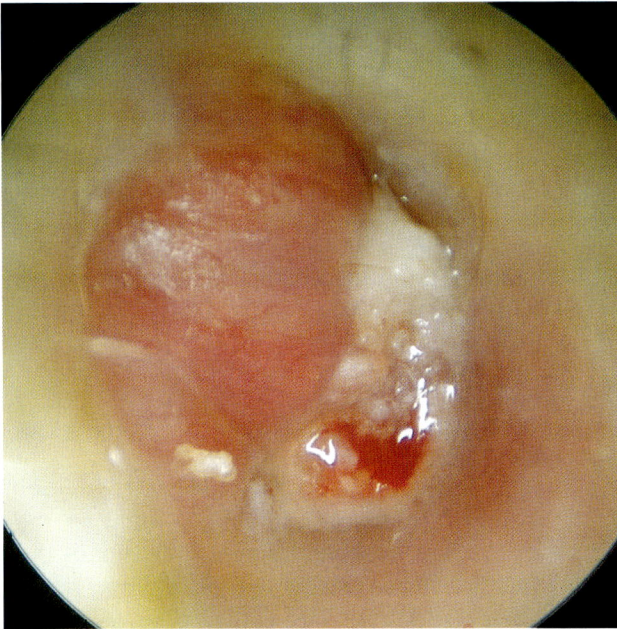

Figure 3.**68** Nasopharyngeal carcinoma extending into the middle ear and external auditory canal. A polypoid massis infiltrating the tympanic membrane and partially filling the external auditory canal (see CT scan, Fig. 3.**69** and MRI, Fig. 3.**70**). The patient was considered inoperable and was referred for radiotherapy.

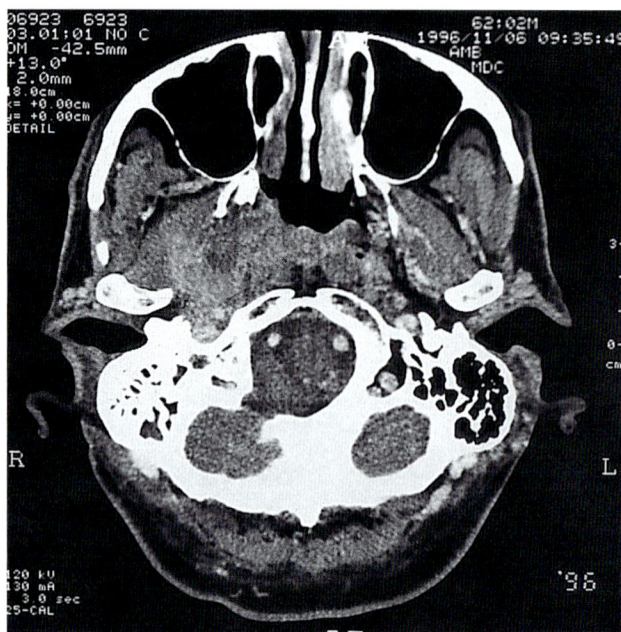

Figure 3.**69** The CT scan demonstrates marked infiltration of the nasopharynx, the pterygoid muscles, and the petrous apex.

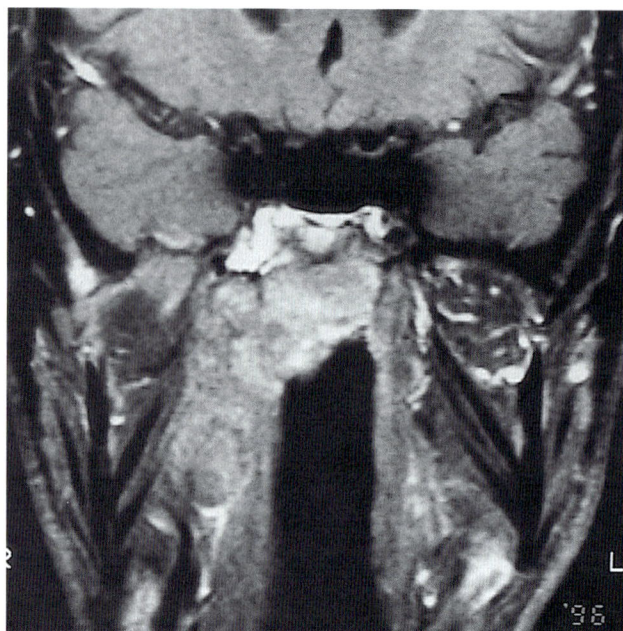

Figure 3.**70** MRI with gadolinium confirms the infiltration.

Summary

A carcinoma arising from the external auditory canal is frequently confused with suppurative otitis. Because of the high incidence of otitis externa and media and because these pathologies are frequently chronic, the diagnosis of carcinoma of the external auditory canal is almost always late. Diagnosis is made by biopsy. A high-resolution CT scan and MRI are necessary for proper evaluation. A high-resolution CT scan determines the osseous erosion caused by the tumor, whereas MRI is superior to CT for the evaluation of soft tissues. MRI shows the presence of dural invasion, intracranial extension, as well as extracranial soft-tissue involvement. Until now there has been no universally accepted system of staging, which is the basis for planning therapy and proper treatment evaluation.

Therapy for carcinoma of the external auditory canal is almost always surgical. Various degrees of resection are utilized according to the extent of the pathology. Very small lesions can be managed by excision biopsy with a safety margin and curettage of the underlying bone.

Lateral en-bloc petrosectomy is the treatment of choice in the majority of carcinomas of the external auditory canal. It entails excision of the external auditory canal (bone and soft tissues), tympanic membrane, and ossicular chain with preservation of the facial nerve. Anteriorly, bone removal extends up to the level of the temporomandibular joint. The cavity can be exteriorized or obliterated with abdominal fat and the external auditory canal closed as a cul-de-sac. When indicated, the resection can include a superficial parotidectomy, resection of the mandibular condyle, and/or neck dissection.

When the tumor has a deeper extension towards the middle ear, en-bloc subtotal resection of the temporal bone is indicated. In such cases, a middle and posterior fossa craniotomy is necessary. Bone removal is performed up to the level of the medial third of the petrous apex and the internal carotid artery. The facial nerve and inner ear are sacrificed.

A more extended procedure is total en-bloc resection of the temporal bone entailing, in addition, the sacrifice of the internal carotid artery, closure of the sigmoid sinus and jugular bulb, and in some cases a total parotidectomy and neck dissection.

4 Secretory Otitis Media (Otitis Media with Effusion)

Secretory otitis media is characterized by the presence of middle ear effusion composed of a transudate/exudate of the mucosa of the middle ear cleft that is formed behind an intact tympanic membrane. Classically, the tympanic membrane is retracted, immobile, dark yellowish or bluish, and thickened. At times, it may be transparent with a hairline (liquid level) or air bubbles visible through it.

The causes are generally: eustachian tube obstruction secondary to mucosal edema due to infection (sinusitis, nasopharyngitis) or allergy; extrinsic pressure on the cartilaginous portion of the eustachian tube due to hyperplasia of glandular or lymphoid tissue or, rarely, due to tumors; malfunction of the tubal muscles, as in children with cleft palate, or malformation of the tube itself, as in Down's syndrome. Other factors that may contribute include: bacteriologic, immunologic, genetic, socioeconomic status, seasonal variation, as well as lack of transmission of specific immunoglobulins in non-breast-fed infants. All these factors cause tubal dysfunction or occlusion, leading to negative middle ear pressure due to oxygen absorption by the mucosa of the middle ear cleft. Normally, the tendency of the tubal walls to collapse at the level of the isthmus can be overcome by an increase in the nasopharyngeal pressure. A negative middle ear pressure up to –25 mm Hg can be thus corrected. On the other hand, with edema of the tubal mucosa, the same increase in the nasopharyngeal pressure cannot overcome a negative middle ear pressure less than –5 mm Hg.

In children, hyperplasia of the adenoid tissue is the most common predisposing factor, and nasopharyngitis is the most frequent cause of secretory otitis media. In adults, the condition is much less common and the presence of persistent unilateral otitis media with effusion can be due to a nasopharyngeal tumor that occludes the tubal opening, or a neoplasm that compresses or infiltrates the tube along its course.

In cases that do not resolve despite proper medical treatment (nasal and systemic decongestants, mucolytics, and antibiotics) or in cases with persistent conductive hearing loss (see Figs. 4.1 and 4.2), the insertion of a ventilation tube is indicated. In children, adenoidectomy is also performed. Surgery aims at alleviating the conductive hearing loss, avoiding the sequelae of otitis media with effusion. Sequelae include recurrent otitis media, tympanosclerosis, adhesive otitis media, retraction pockets with eventual cholesteatoma formation, and in some long-standing cases the formation of cholesterol granuloma (see Chapter 5). In this chapter, some typical cases of otitis media with effusion are shown. For the surgical treatment (myringotomy and ventilation tube insertion), the reader is referred to Chapter 14 on post-surgical conditions.

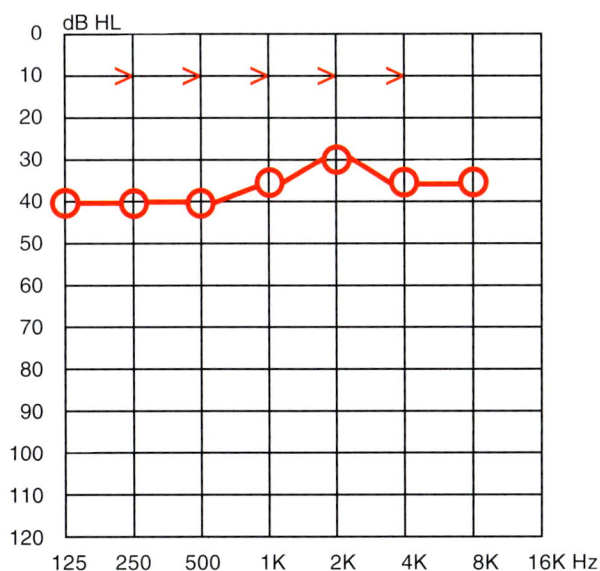

Figure 4.1 Conductive hearing loss. Bone conduction is normal. Air conduction is on an average of 35 dB.

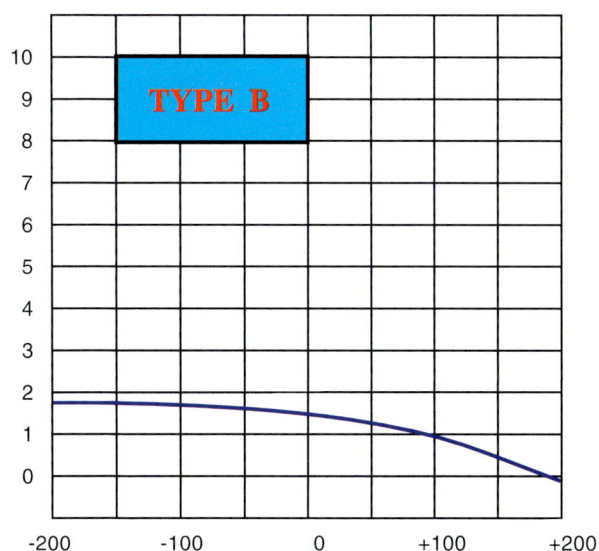

Figure 4.2 Tympanogram type B, typical of middle ear effusion.

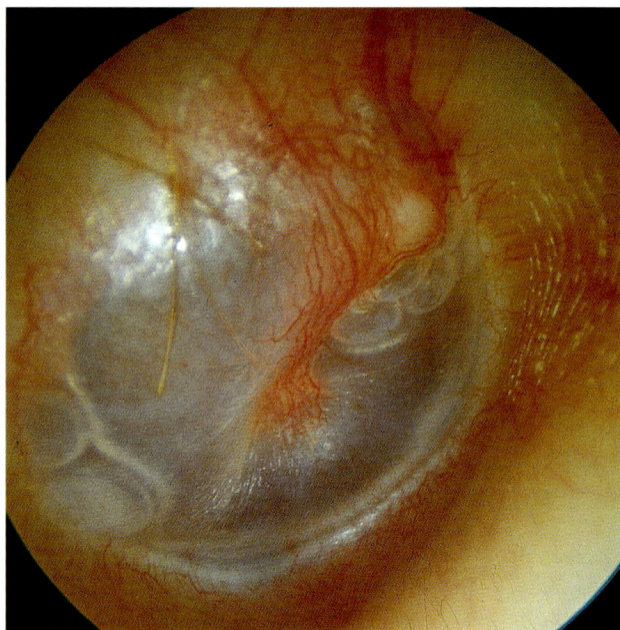

Figure 4.3   Right ear. Secretory otitis media. Air bubbles can be seen anterior to the handle of the malleus and also in the posteroinferior quadrant.

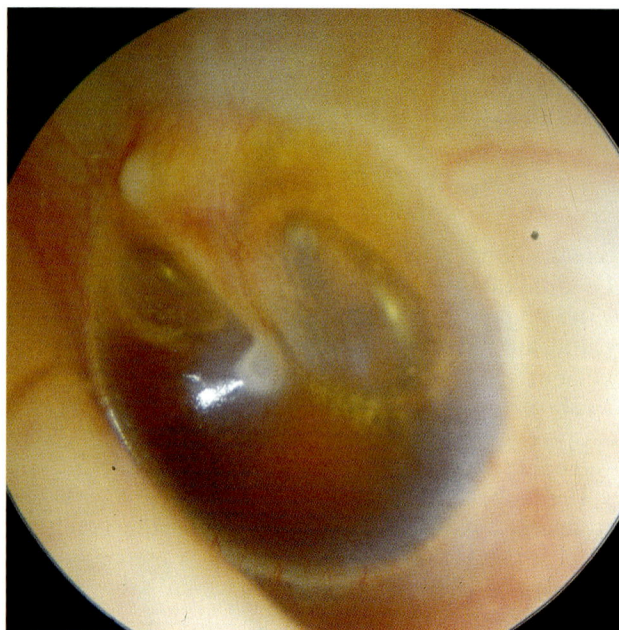

Figure 4.4   Left ear. Secretory otitis media. Middle ear effusion having a reddish color inferiorly and a yellowish color superiorly. In this case, the differential diagnosis includes glomus tympanicum. If doubts still exist after microscopic examination, medical treatment is administered for several weeks and the patient is reexamined.

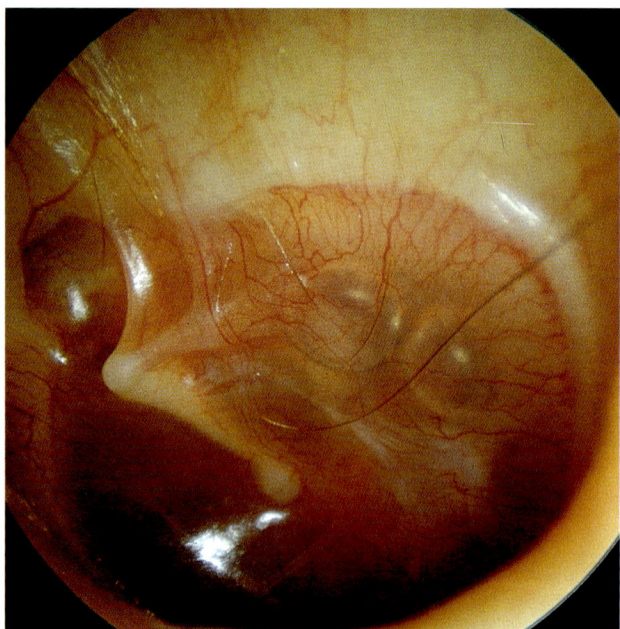

Figure 4.5   Left ear. Secretory otitis media with an apparently dense transudate that gives the tympanic membrane the characteristic dark yellow color. An air-fluid level can be appreciated at the posterosuperior quadrant. The tympanic membrane is diffusely hyperemic. If the condition is not resolved by medical treatment, a ventilation tube should be inserted.

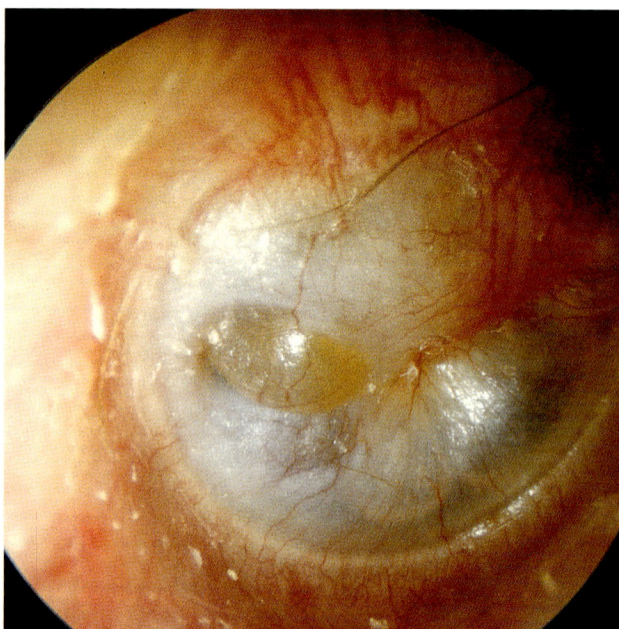

Figure 4.6   Right ear. The presence of glue in the middle ear leads to bulging of the tympanic membrane. In the posterior quadrant, a thinned area of the drum is visualized, through which the yellowish color of the effusion is visible. This area would probably be the site of a future perforation.

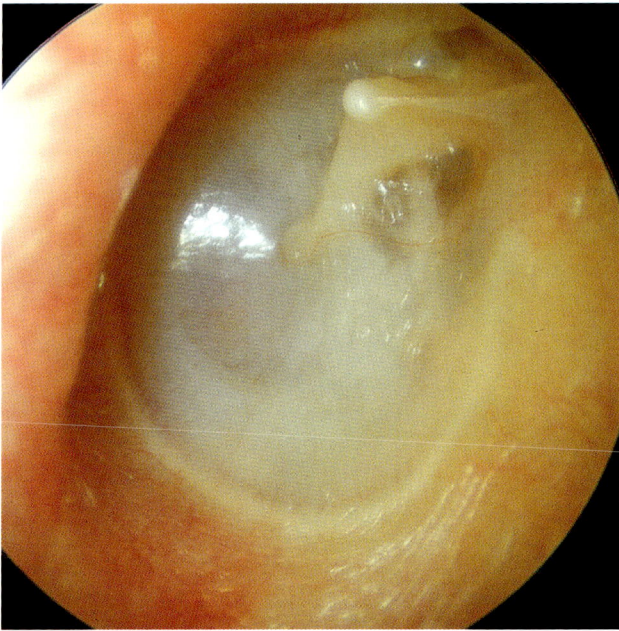

Figure 4.**7** Left ear. Secretory otitis media. The tympanic membrane is thickened. Catarrhal fluid can be seen through the relatively thinner anteroinferior quadrant.

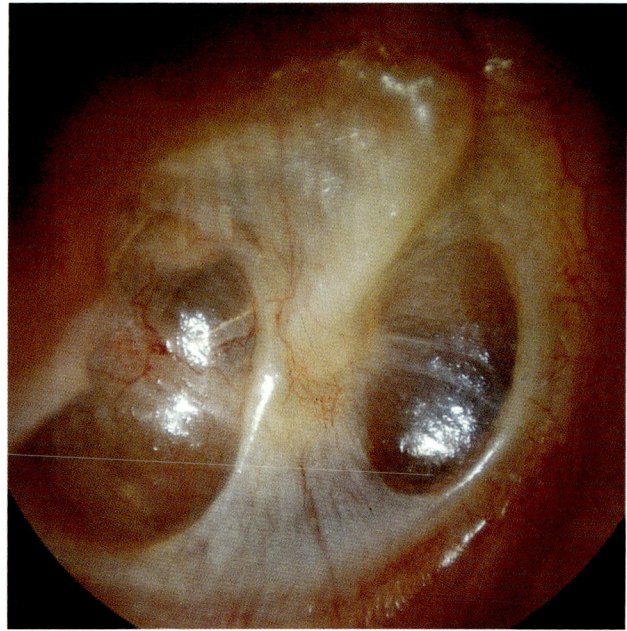

Figure 4.**8** Right ear. Secretory otitis media. The effusion is visible through two thinned areas of the tympanic membrane lying anterior and posterior to the handle of the malleus.

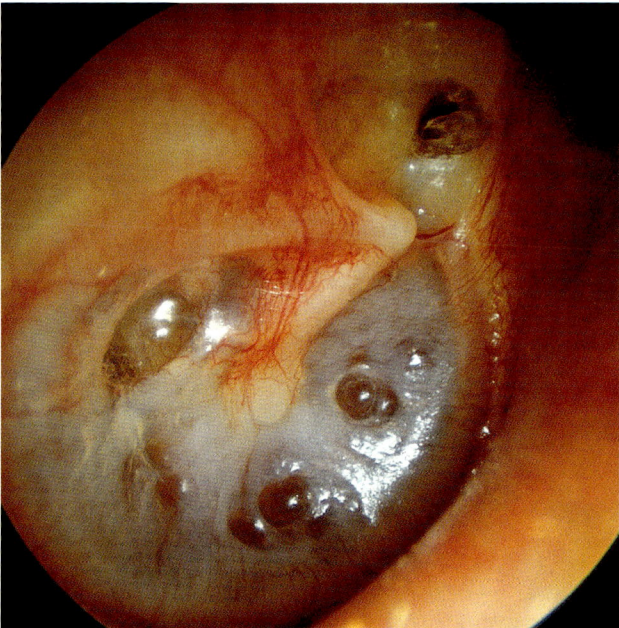

Figure 4.**9** Right ear. Secretory otitis media with tympanosclerosis and epitympanic erosion. The tympanic membrane shows areas of tympanosclerosis alternating with areas of atrophy. Glue is present in the middle ear.

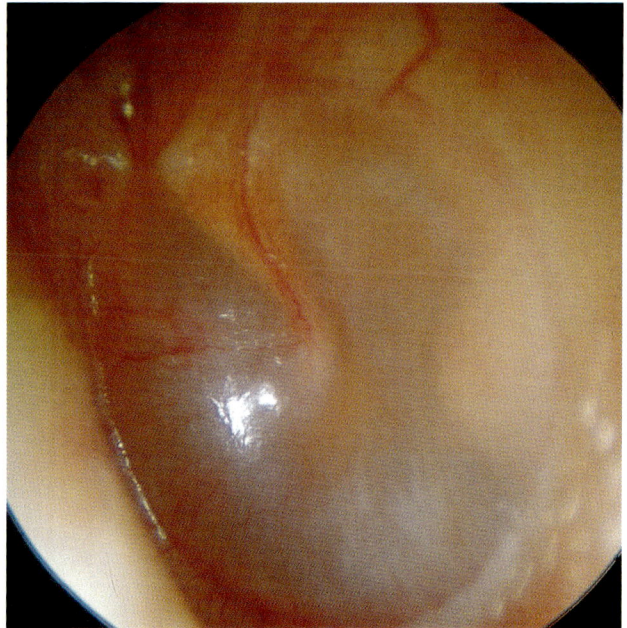

Figure 4.**10** Left ear. Otitis media with effusion and a whitish retrotympanic mass in the posterior quadrant at 3 o'clock can be observed. The presence of congenital cholesteatoma was considered in the differential diagnosis. Exploratory tympanotomy showed only "glue" in the middle ear that was particularly dense in the posterior mesotympanum.

Secretory Otitis Media Secondary to Neoplasms

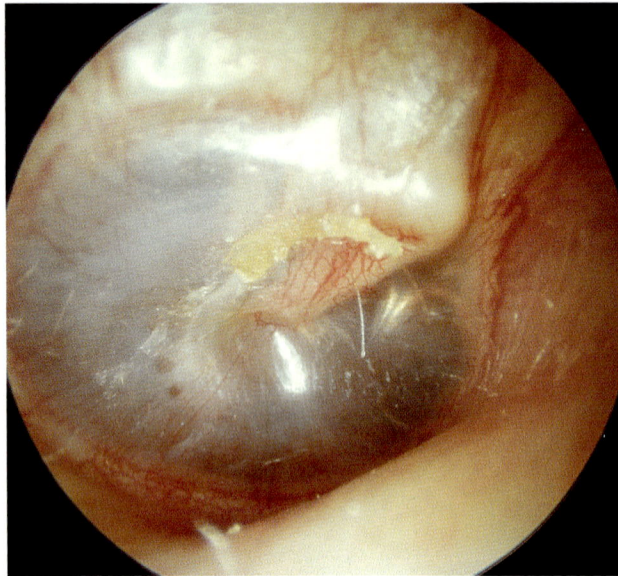

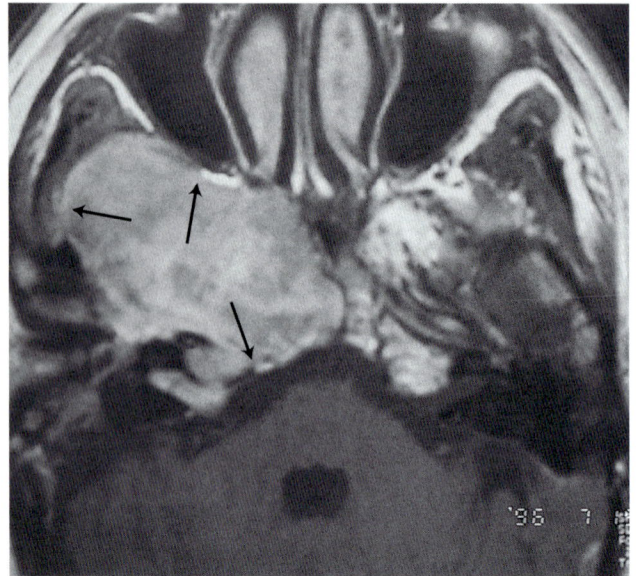

Figure 4.**11**   Right ear. Seromucoid effusion in the middle ear. Air bubbles can be seen in the anterior quadrants of the tympanic membrane. The patient is a 53-year-old woman who presented with a signs of right otitis media with effusion causing conductive hearing loss and ipsilateral paresthesia of the maxillary and mandibular nerves, followed by episodes of trigeminal neuralgia and diplopia in the last few months. Computed tomography (CT) scan and magnetic resonance imaging (MRI) with gadolinium (see following figures) revealed the presence of a

tumor (later proven to be a trigeminal neurinoma) with an intra- and extracranial extension. The tumor compressed the eustachian tube and resulted in the middle ear effusion. Total removal of the tumor was performed in a single-stage operation using an infratemporal type B approach with orbitozygomatic extension (Fig. 4.**14**).

Figure 4.**12**   MRI, axial view, showing the extension of the giant trigeminal neurinoma.

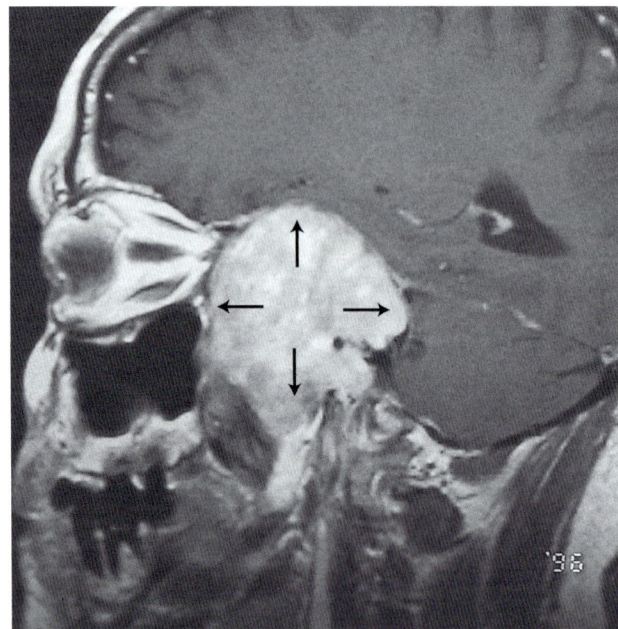

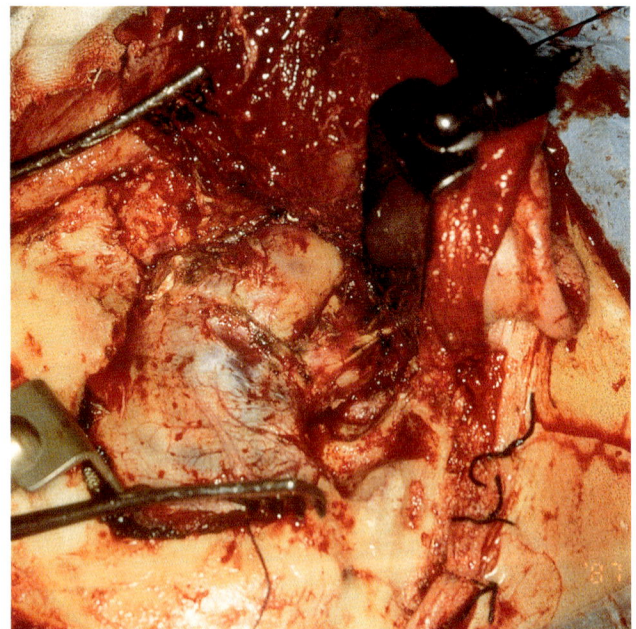

Figure 4.**13**   MRI, sagittal view, confirms the intra- and extracranial extension of the tumor.

Figure 4.**14**   Trigeminal neurinoma removal using an infratemporal type B approach with orbitozygomatic extension.

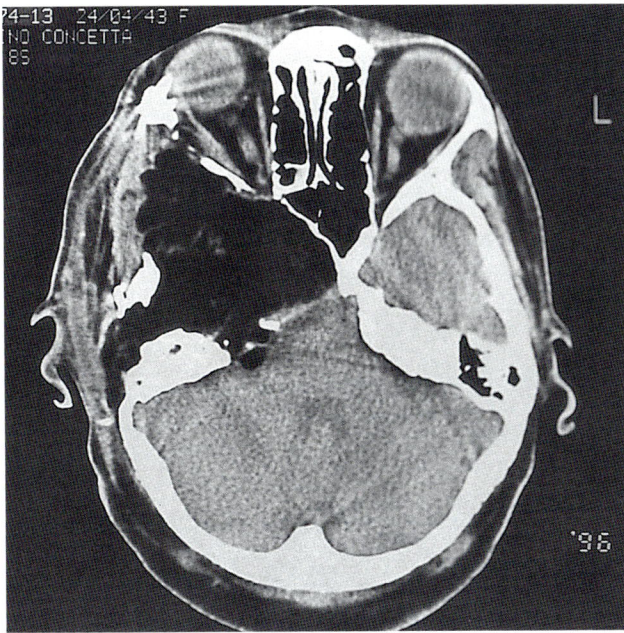

Figure 4.**15** Postoperative CT scan showing total tumor removal.

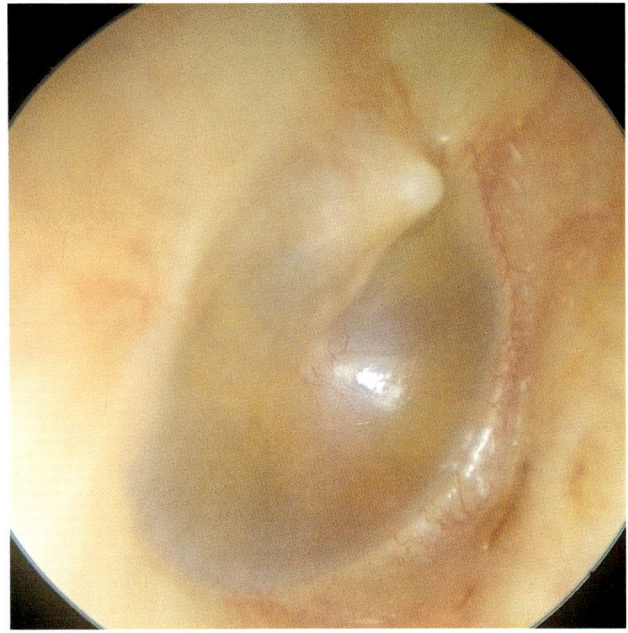

Figure 4.**16** A different case similar to the one in Figure 4.**11**. This 64-year-old woman complained of right nasal obstruction and a sensation of right ear fullness of 1 year's duration. One month before presentation the patient began to suffer from neuralgic pain in the region of the maxillary nerve. The tympanic membrane looks yellowish due to the presence of middle ear effusion (see following figures).

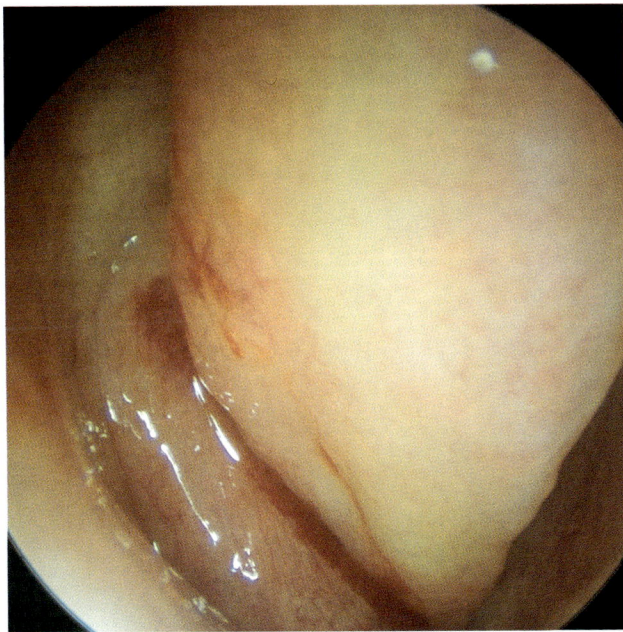

Figure 4.**17** Right nasal cavity, same case. A mass is visualized in the middle meatus. A biopsy proved it to be a neurinoma.

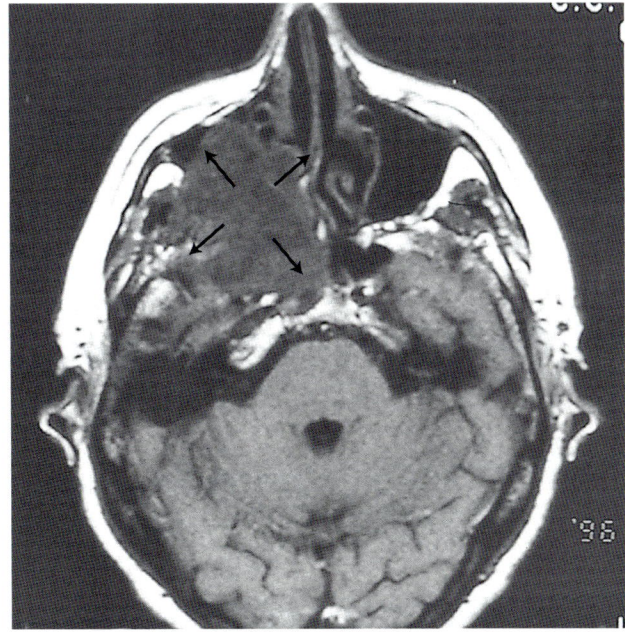

Figure 4.**18** MRI of the same case. A huge trigeminal neurinoma with intra- and extracranial extension can be seen.

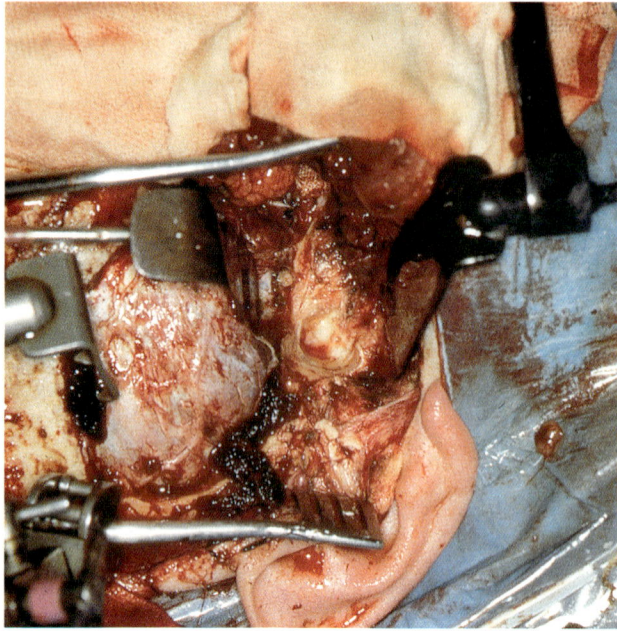

Figure 4.**19**   A single-stage, total removal was accomplished using a preauricular infratemporal subtemporal orbitozygomatic approach.

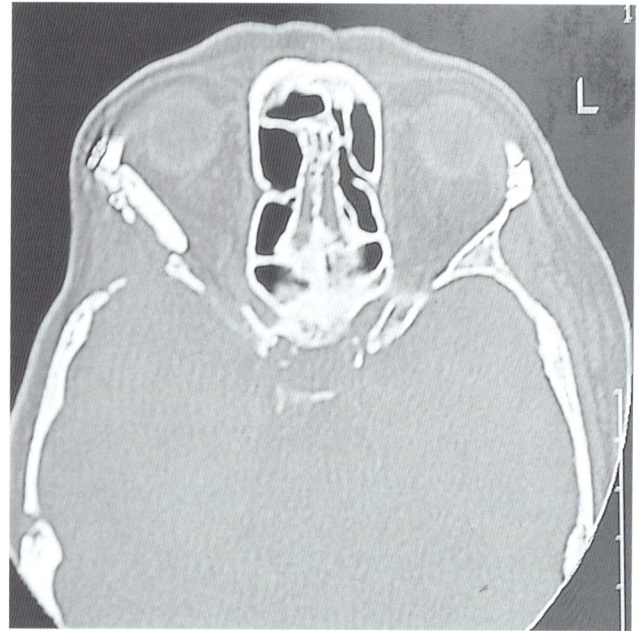

Figure 4.**20**   Postoperative CT scan showing total tumor removal. The floor and the lateral wall of the orbit have been reconstructed.

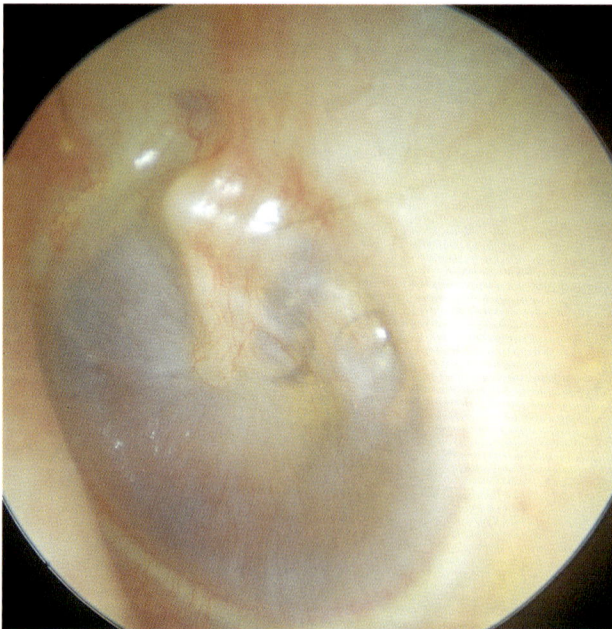

Figure 4.**21**   Left ear. An air–fluid level is seen in a young patient with a juvenile nasopharyngeal angiofibroma.

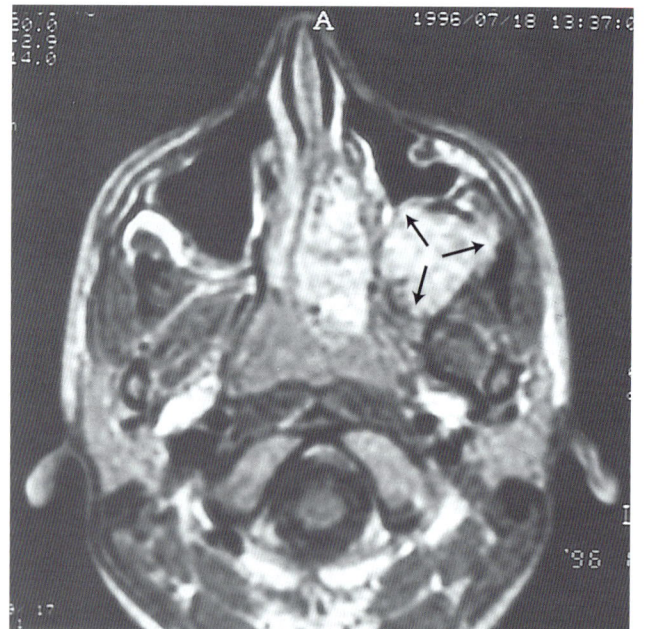

Figure 4.**22**   MRI of the same case. The angiofibroma occupies the nasopharynx, pterygopalatine fossa, and infratemporal fossa on the left side. Removal was accomplished using a Fisch type C infratemporal fossa approach.

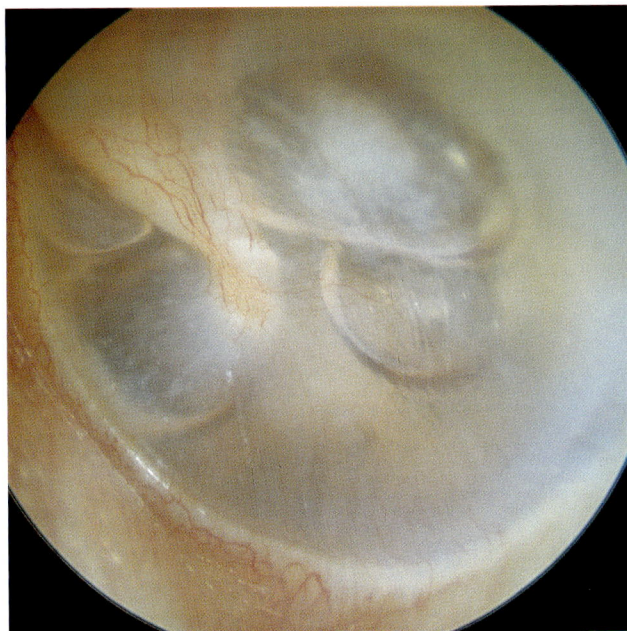

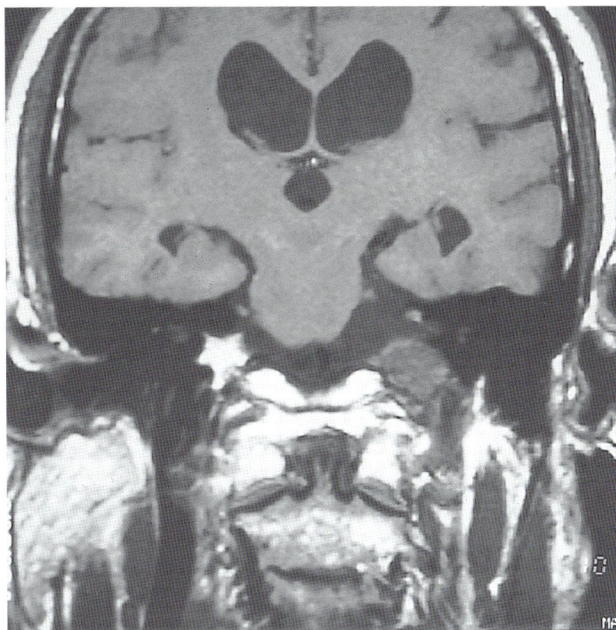

Figure 4.**23** Left ear showing a pulsating air–fluid level in a patient operated 1 year previously to remove a lower cranial nerve neurinoma using a petro-occipital trans-sigmoid approach (POTS) (see preoperative MRI, Fig. 4.**24** and postoperative CT scan, Fig. 4.**25**). The patient complained of a sensation of ear blockage and watery rhinorrhea on leaning forwards. The middle ear is full of cerebrospinal fluid (CSF) passing through open hypotympanic

air cells that communicate with the subarachnoid space. The CSF rhinorrhea was treated by obliterating the eustachian tube and middle ear with the temporalis muscle and by closure of the external auditory canal as a cul-de-sac.

Figure 4.**24** MRI of the same case showing a schwannoma of the lower cranial nerves (T).

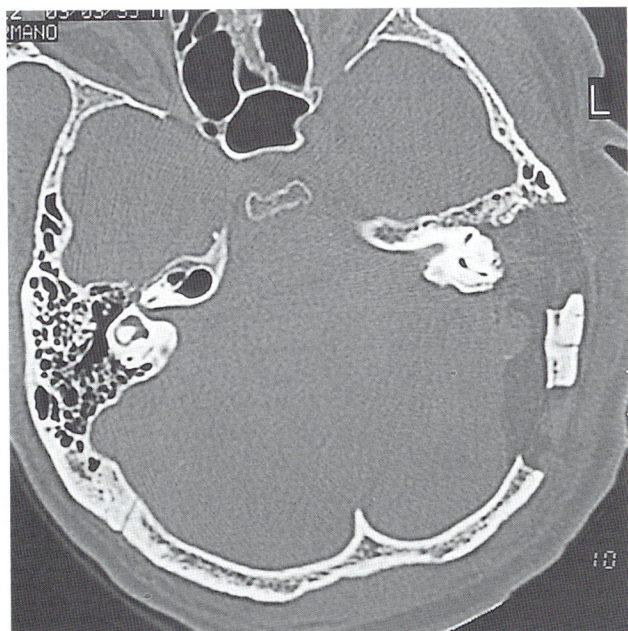

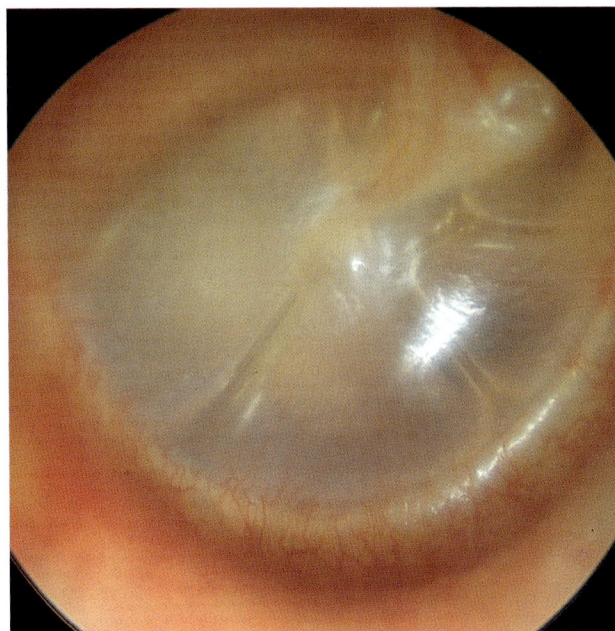

Figure 4.**25** Postoperative CT scan shows the petro-occipital craniotomy and the surgical cavity with preservation of the inner ear.

Figure 4.**26** Right ear. Otitis media with effusion in a 47-year-old female patient who complained of right hearing loss and a sensation of ear fullness of 1 year duration. Nasopharyngeal examination was doubtful. MRI (see Figs. 4.**27** and 4.**28**) demonstrated the presence of a neoplasm at the level of the right Rosen-

müller fossa. A biopsy was performed in this region and revealed the presence of an adenoid cystic carcinoma. The patient was operated on using a type C infratemporal fossa approach and then referred for radiotherapy.

Small nasopharyngeal carcinomas can miss detection on MRI. Therefore, adults with unilateral otitis media with effusion, even with normal radiologic examination, should undergo biopsy of the nasopharynx under local anesthesia.

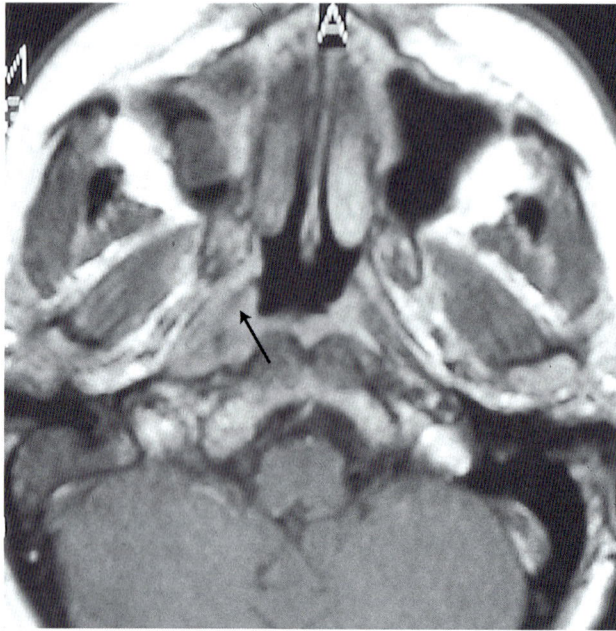

Figure 4.**27** MRI. Small neoplasm at the level of the Rosenmüller fossa (arrow).

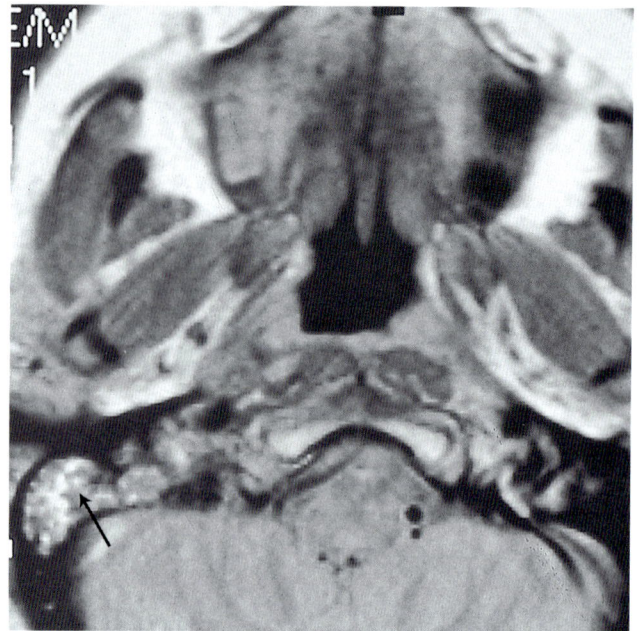

Figure 4.**28** MRI. Effusion in the ipsilateral mastoid is clearly visible (arrow).

Infratemporal Fossa Approach Type C

This is the anterior extension of the type B infratemporal fossa approach. The difference between the two is that in type C the pterygoid process is drilled, providing control of the nasopharynx, the pterygopalatine fossa, and the parasellar area and sphenoid sinus.

Indications

- Tumors of the infratemporal fossa and peritubal areas, such as cylindroma, adenoid cystic carcinoma, etc.
- Persistent or recurrent nasopharyngeal carcinoma after radiotherapy.
- Juvenile nasopharyngeal angiofibroma involving the pterygopalatine and infratemporal fossae.
- Tumors of the infratemporal fossa involving the parasellar area, such as extensive clival chordomas.

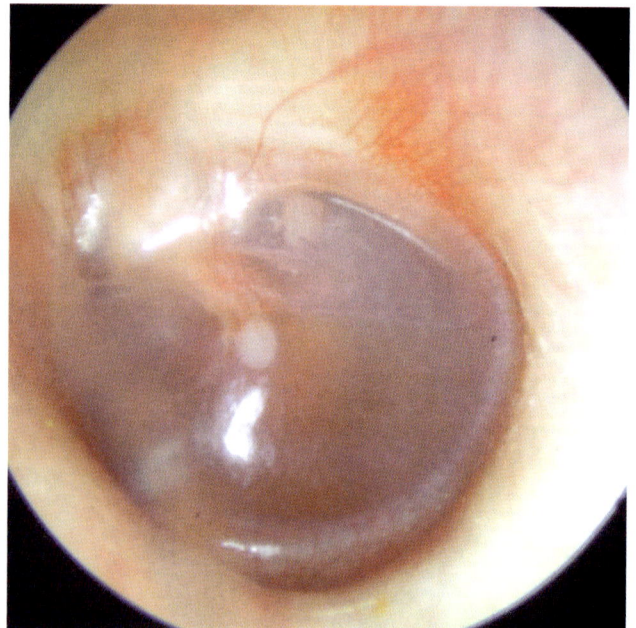

Figure 4.**29a** Left ear. Middle ear effusion is clearly visible. This 14-year-old boy complained nasal obstruction since 3 years, with recurrent epistaxis during the last month and hearing loss. Rhinoscopy showed a soft mass occupying the left nasal fossa.

Surgical Steps

The skin incision is C-shaped, starting above and posterior to the lateral corner of the orbit, extending 3–4 cm behind the postauricular sulcus and ending inferiorly at the angle of the mandible. Cul-de-sac closure of the external auditory canal is carried out and exposure of the extratemporal facial nerve. The best landmark is that the main trunk of the nerve runs along the perpendicular bisection of a line joining the cartilaginous pointer and the mastoid tip. The frontal branch of the nerve is followed until it crosses the zygomatic arch. The skin of the external auditory canal, the tympanic membrane, the incus and the malleus are removed. A subtotal petrosectomy is then performed, with preservation of the labyrinth. The facial nerve is skeletonized.

The temporalis muscle is detached from its bed, to be further reflected anteriorly and inferiorly. The periosteum of the zygomatic arch is elevated, and the arch is transected after two burr holes have been made for refixation at the end of the procedure. The transected arch is reflected inferiorly, together with the temporalis muscle. The vertical segment of the internal carotid artery is identified using a large diamond burr, as described above. Care is taken during this step not to injure the cochlea. The anterior wall of the external auditory canal is then drilled. The capsule of the temporomandibular joint is separated using strong scissors and bipolar coagulation. The articular disk is then removed, exposing the mandibular condyle. The Fisch infratemporal fossa retractor is applied, with inferior displacement of the head of the mandible. The glenoid fossa is drilled. The middle meningeal artery is exposed and cut after bipolar coagulation. The mandibular nerve (cranial nerve V3) is identified and sacrificed. The bony eustachian tube is drilled. The horizontal internal carotid artery is further exposed. The internal carotid artery is retracted anterolaterally, providing sufficient space to drill the petrous apex lying medial to the artery. Drilling of bone inferomedial to the internal carotid artery allows lesions to be removed from the middle clivus. The internal carotid artery is exposed over its vertical and horizontal segments. The bony segment of the eustachian tube is drilled, and the isthmus is identified. Using a septal raspatory, the periosteum of the base of the pterygoid, the greater wing of the sphenoid and the lateral lamina of the pterygoid process are elevated together with the attachment of the lateral pterygoid muscle. The base of the pterygoid is drilled. The vidian nerve, which is formed by the junction of the greater superficial petrosal and the deep petrosal nerve, can be identified. The sphenoid mucosa is also seen. Depending on the type and site of the lesion, the subsequent steps vary.

At the end of the procedure, the temporal muscle is rotated to obliterate the surgical defect, the zygomatic arch is wired into place, and the wound is closed in layers.

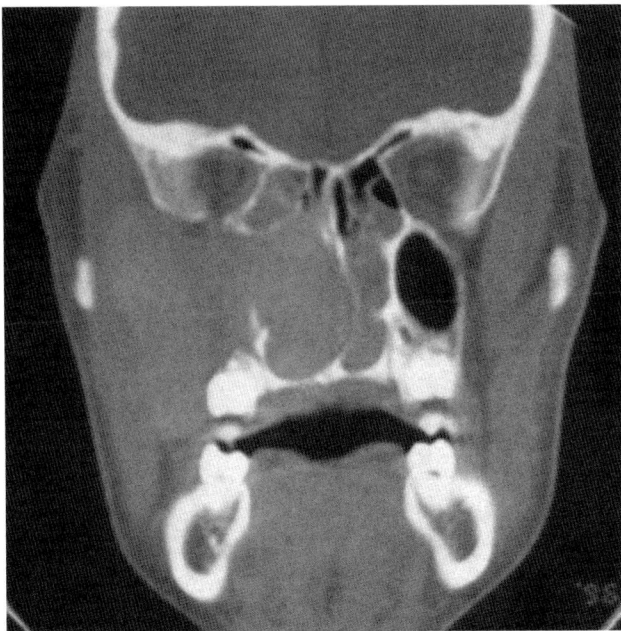

Figure 4.**29b** CT scan, coronal view. The mass occupies the left nasal fossa, the maxillary sinus and the posterior ethmoid, displacing the nasal septum. Retained fluid can be seen in the right nasal fossa.

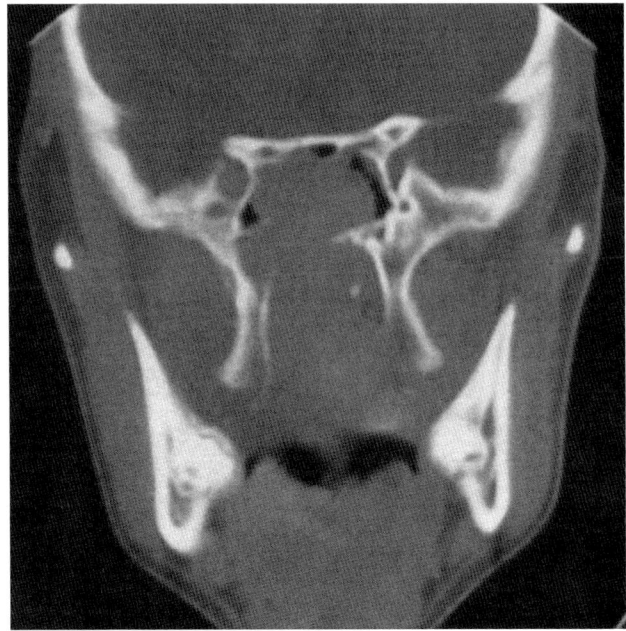

Figure 4.**29c** CT scan, coronal view. The mass occupies the sphenoid sinus and the pterygopalatine fossa.

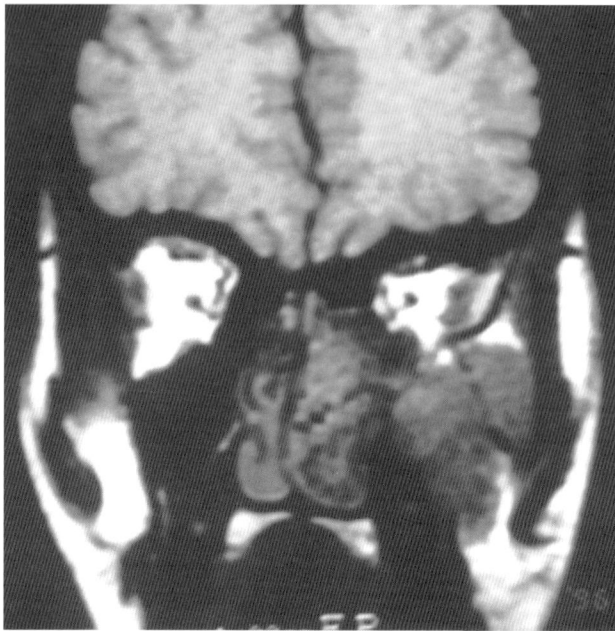

Figure 4.**29d**   MRI, coronal view. The tumor extends from the nasal fossa to the maxillary sinus and posteriorly toward the pterygopalatine fossa.

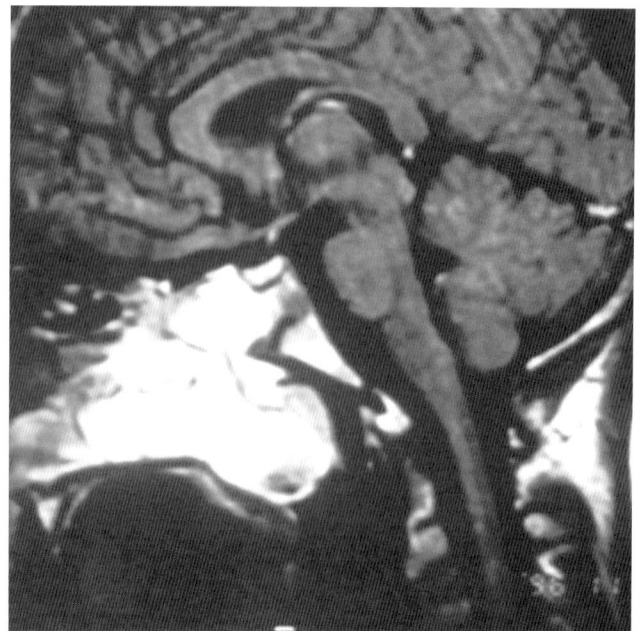

Figure 4.**29e**   MRI, sagittal view. The tumor involves the nasopharynx and the sphenoid sinus and spreads into the left nasal fossa.

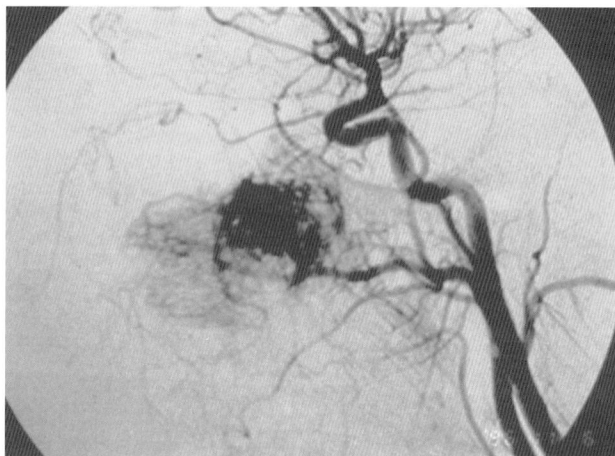

Figure 4.**29f**   Angiography shows that the tumor's vascularization is principally derived from the internal maxillary artery.

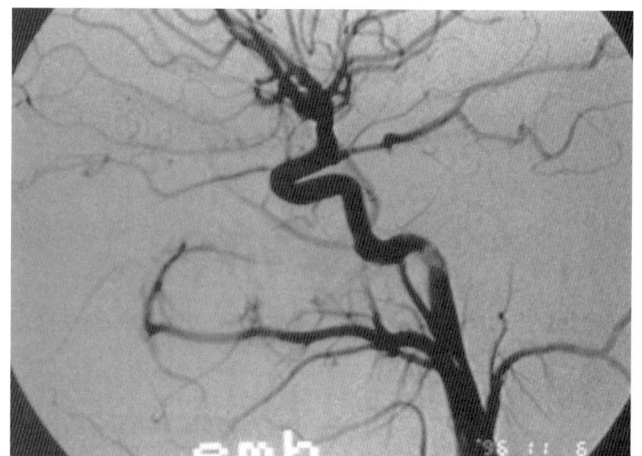

Figure 4.**29g**   Postembolization angiography. The patient underwent surgery 2 days after the embolization.

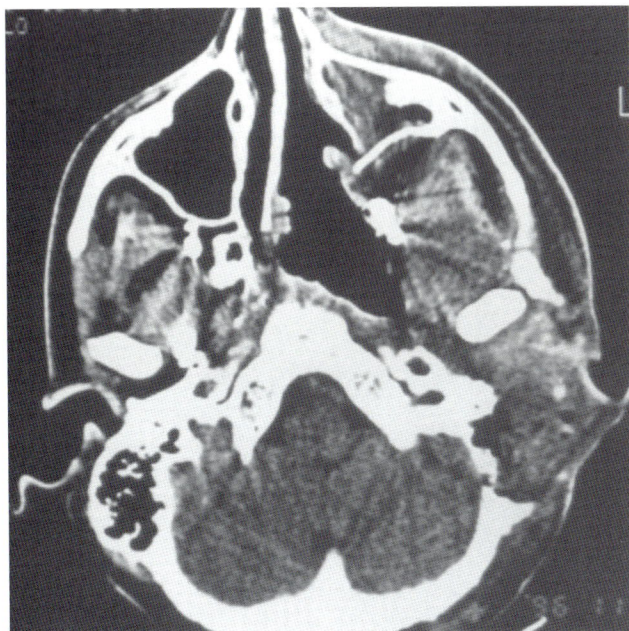

Figure 4.**29h**   Postoperative CT scan, axial view. The tumor was removed using a Fisch infratemporal type C approach.

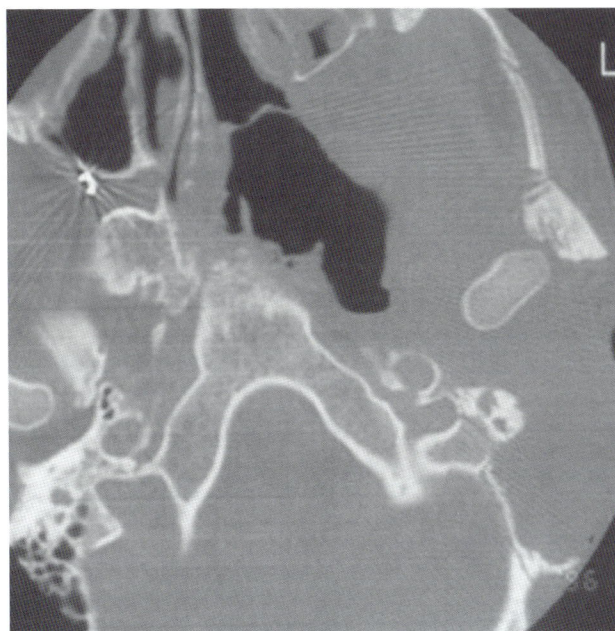

Figure 4.**29i**   High resolution CT scan with bone window, axial view. The pterygopalatine fossa and infratemporal fossa are free of tumor.

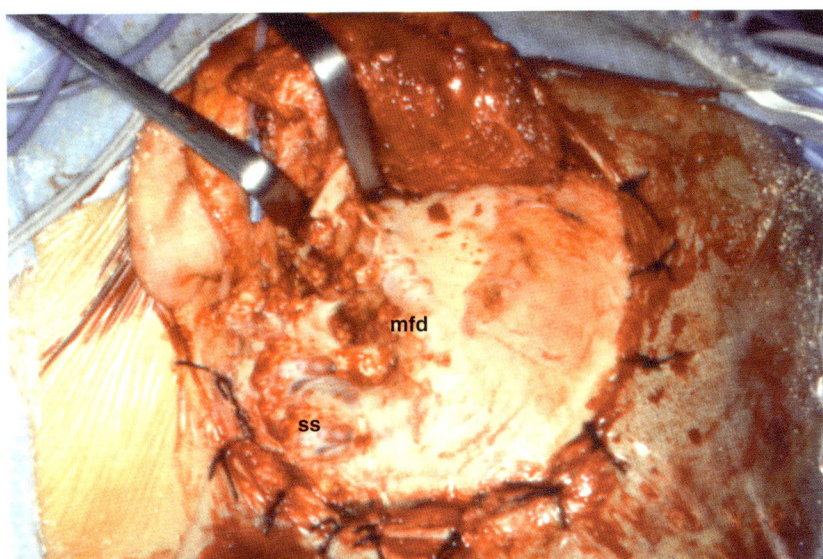

Figure 4.**30a**   Intraoperative view of the same patient as in Fig. 4.**29**, showing the approach. A subtotal petrosectomy was performed. The anterior bony canal wall was removed. The mandibular condyle was displaced inferiorly. The zygomatic arch was temporarily reflected anteriorly, together with the temporalis muscle.

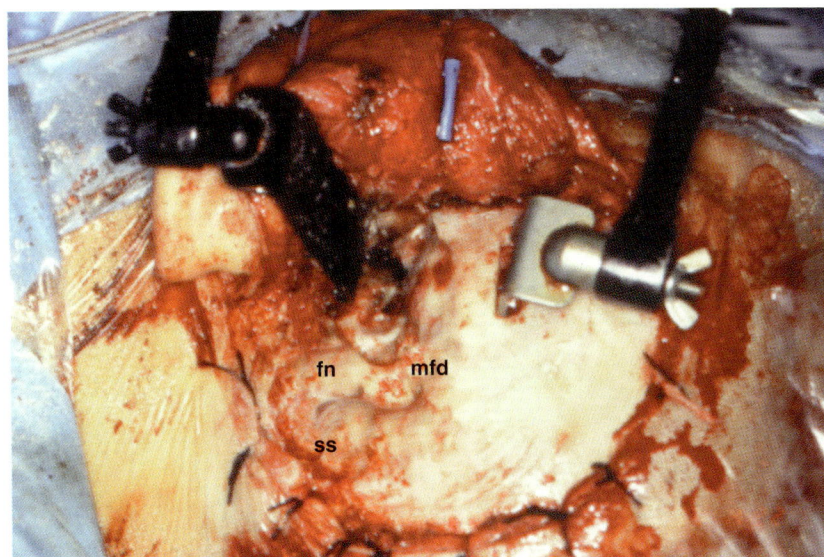

Figure 4.**30b**   An overview of the approach, showing the subcutaneous flap (with the external auditory canal closed as a blind sac) and the temporalis muscle reflected anteriorly. The Fisch retractor is in place, displacing the mandibular condyle inferiorly.

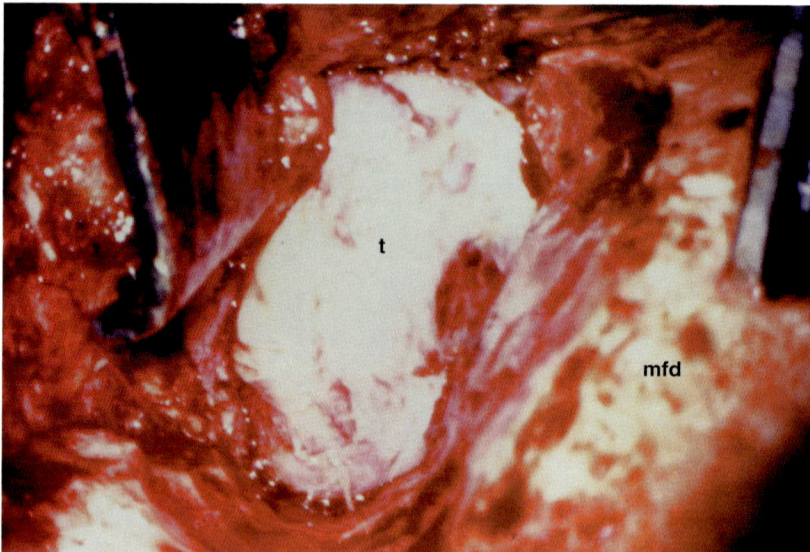

Figure 4.**30c**   Intraoperative view of the tumor (t) reached using the type C infratemporal fossa approach.

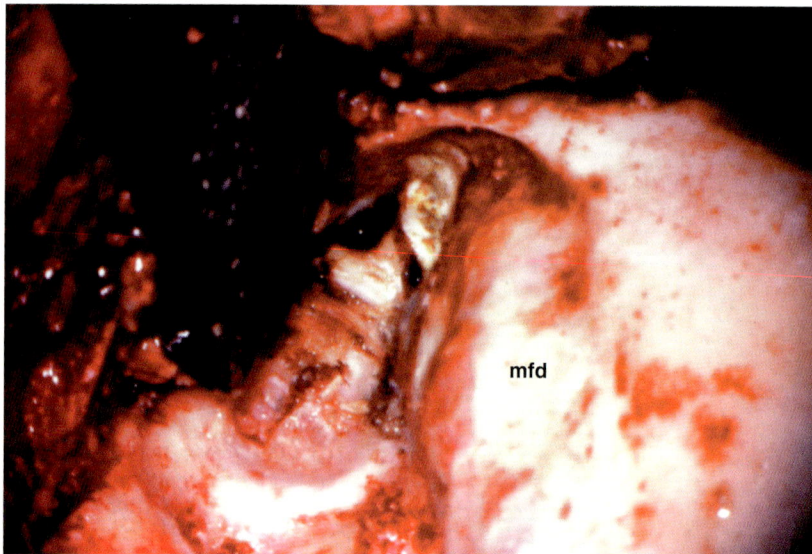

Figure 4.**30d**   The surgical cavity after tumor removal.

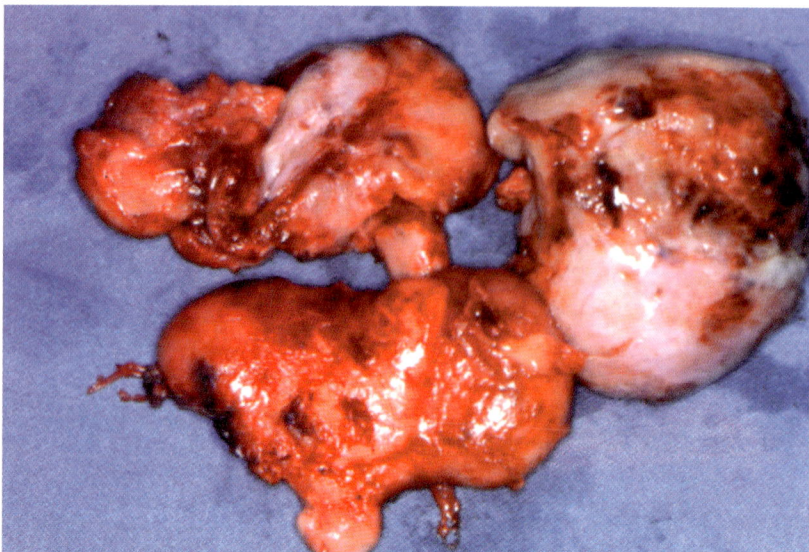

Figure 4.**30e**   Surgical specimen. The tumor mass consists of three blocks.

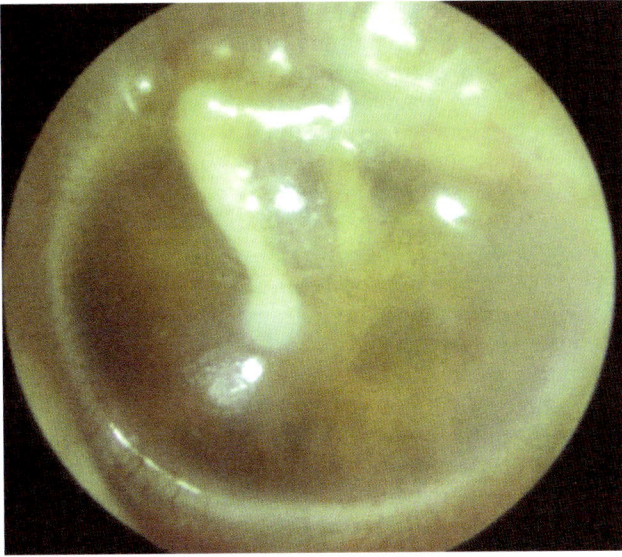

Figure 4.**31a** Left ear. Secretory otitis media. This young patient had already received radiotherapy and chemotherapy treatment 2 years previously for nasopharyngeal carcinoma.

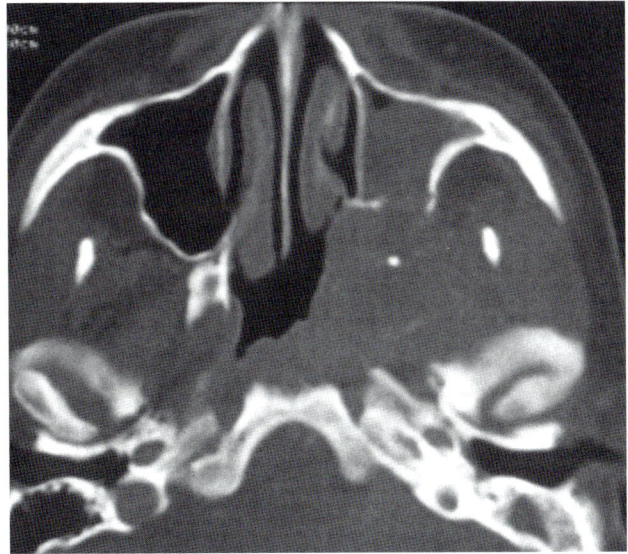

Figure 4.**31b** CT scan, axial view, bone window. In spite of the chemoradiotherapy, there was a recurrence of carcinoma. The tumor involves the pterygopalatine and infratemporal fossa, eroding the posterior wall of the maxillary sinus. The tumor also extends beyond the midline, reaching the contralateral peritubal space.

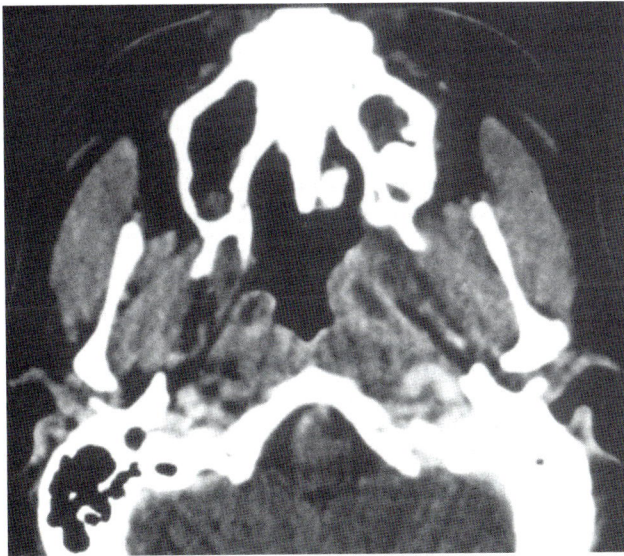

Figure 4.**31c** CT scan, axial view, soft-tissue density. The spreading of the tumor toward the contralateral peritubal space is clearly seen.

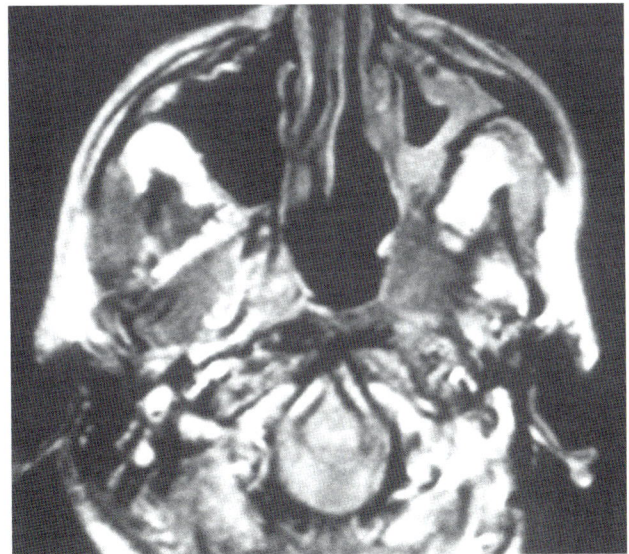

Figure 4.**31d** MRI, 3 years after surgery. The tumor was removed using an extended type C infratemporal fossa approach. The patient is still free of any recurrence after 5 years.

Infratemporal Fossa Approach Type D

This approach is a modification of the type B and type C infratemporal fossa approach, aiming at removal of lesions involving the petrous apex, clivus and cavernous sinus without traversing the middle ear and mastoid.

Indications

- Extradural lesions of the middle or upper clivus, petrous apex, retropharyngeal, parapharyngeal or infratemporal fossa, with or without minimal invasion of the sphenoid sinus–e.g., chordomas, chondrosarcomas, meningiomas and trigeminal neurinomas.
- Intradural or transdural lesions lying ventral to the brain stem, or involving the cavernous sinus, or both–e.g., chordomas, chondrosarcomas and meningiomas.

Surgical Steps

The skin incision is curvilinear, starting at the frontal scalp and extending anterior to the external auditory canal. The skin and soft tissue are elevated. The level of dissection is between the superficial and deep layer of the temporalis fascia. The frontal branch of the facial nerve is thus included in the flap. The periosteum of the zygomatic arch and lateral orbital rim is elevated. More inferiorly, the dissection lies superficial to the masseter fascia, avoiding injury to the facial nerve branches at this level. The main stem of the temporal facial nerve is identified, along with its main branches in the parotid. The temporalis muscle is detached and reflected inferiorly.

Next, a frontotemporal craniotomy is performed. The craniotomy extends anteriorly to just posterior to the lateral orbital rim; superiorly immediately superior to the pterion; and posteriorly behind the mandibular condyle. If necessary, the lateral orbital rim can also be resected.

The zygomatic arch is divided next and reflected inferiorly after two holes have been drilled for refixation, and the condyle of the mandible is retracted inferiorly after its attachments have been cut. The temporal glenoid is drilled. Bone removal extends anteriorly to include the floor of the middle fossa, uncovering the foramen spinosum, through which the middle meningeal artery passes, and the foramen ovale, through which the mandibular nerve passes.

The genu of the internal carotid artery is identified by drilling with a diamond burr at the floor of the eustachian tube.

The artery is followed down to identify its vertical part. The middle meningeal artery is cut after bipolar coagulation. The mandibular nerve is identified. The greater wing of the sphenoid and base of the pterygoid are drilled. This allows exposure of the maxillary nerve at its entrance into the foramen rotundum.

The temporal lobe is slightly retracted, and the middle fossa dura is dissected from the remaining bony floor using a septal raspatory. This fully exposes the maxillary nerve. The gasserian ganglion is also controlled.

The horizontal segment of the internal carotid artery is exposed by drilling anteromedial to the genu of the artery using a diamond burr. The whole intrapetrous internal carotid artery up to the level of the anterior foramen lacerum (superior orbital fissure) can be seen.

The internal carotid artery is elevated from its canal and is retracted laterally, exposing the medially lying petrous apex. Care is taken to elevate the thick periosteal sheath along with the artery in order to protect it, avoiding bleeding from the venous plexus lying in between the two. The petrous apex bone medial to the internal carotid artery is drilled.

With intradural lesions, the dura of the posterior fossa is opened. With lesions extending to the upper clivus, middle fossa, or cavernous sinus, the middle fossa dura is incised. With slight retraction of the temporal lobe, the terminal part of the internal carotid artery is seen before it branches into the anterior cerebral artery and middle cerebral artery. The posterior cerebral artery is seen coursing superior to the oculomotor nerve and the anterolateral surface of the midbrain.

Closure is achieved by suturing the eustachian tube duraplasty using fascia lata, and using a rotation of the temporalis muscle to obliterate the surgical defect. A microvascular latissimus dorsi flap is sometimes needed. The bone flap is returned into place, and the zygomatic arch is wired into place.

Summary

Otitis media with effusion in children is generally bilateral. If it does not resolve despite appropriate medical treatment for a sufficient period, a myringotomy and the insertion of ventilation tubes are indicated. If necessary, adenoidectomy is also performed in the same session.

In all adult cases of unilateral prolonged otitis media with effusion, nasopharyngeal examination is obligatory to exclude nasopharyngeal carcinoma. In these cases it is often advisable to take a biopsy under local anesthesia. Biopsy is still indicated even if the radiologic examination has proved normal. A biopsy should not be attempted, however, during endoscopic examination of the nasopharynx if the mass appears macroscopically vascular. Profuse hemorrhage can occur and may be difficult to control.

5 Cholesterol Granuloma

Cholesterol granuloma is a histologic term used to describe a foreign body, giant cell reaction to cholesterol crystals, and hemosiderin derived from ruptured erythrocytes. Cholesterol granuloma is thought to arise from obstructed drainage and insufficient aeration of cellular compartments of the temporal bone. This leads to reabsorption of air, negative pressure, mucosal edema, and hemorrhage. It can be present in the middle ear, mastoid, or petrous apex. Generally, patients with tympanomastoid cholesterol granuloma have a long history of recurrent otitis media or otitis media with effusion. They also complain of conductive hearing loss, and on otoscopy the tympanic membrane appears bluish in color. In some cases, where granulation tissue is more prevalent, cholesterol granuloma can present as a retrotympanic reddish-brown mass that may cause bulging of the tympanic membrane, thus mimicking a glomus tumor. In these cases, a computed tomography (CT) scan is sufficient to clear up any doubts. A cholesterol granuloma rarely causes bone erosion. On the contrary, bone erosion is characteristic of glomus tumors causing destruction of the jugular hypotympanic septum with an irregular "moth-eaten" contour.

In the initial phases, before cholesterol granuloma is formed, it might be sufficient to insert a ventilation tube, thus preventing further development of the granuloma. When the granuloma has already formed, it is necessary to perform a tympanoplasty with mastoidectomy that opens the intercellular septa, with subsequent aeration of the middle ear and mastoid.

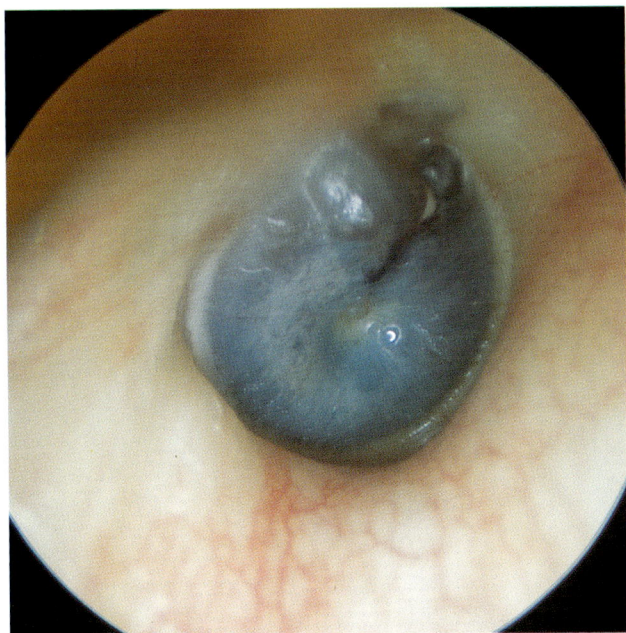

Figure 5.1 Right ear. Typical blue tympanum caused by cholesterol granuloma. The blue color is due to hemosiderin crystals. The granuloma involves not only the middle ear but generally extends into the mastoid air cells.

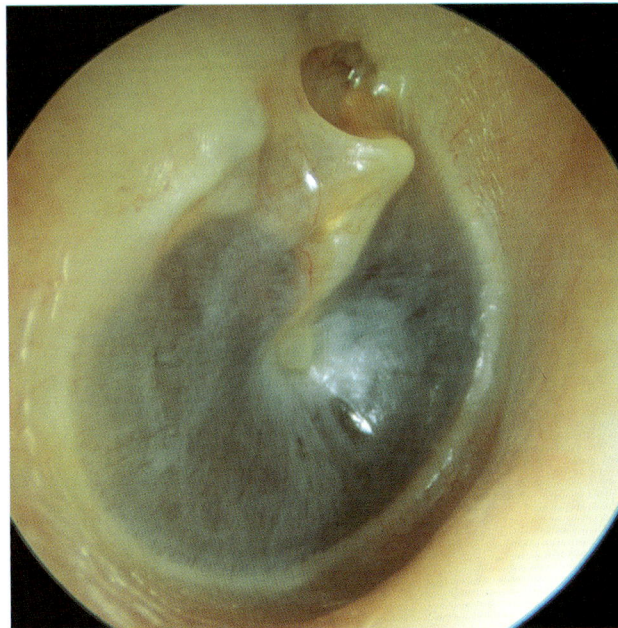

Figure 5.2 Blue tympanum caused by cholesterol granuloma. An epitympanic retraction due to eustachian tube dysfunction is also present.

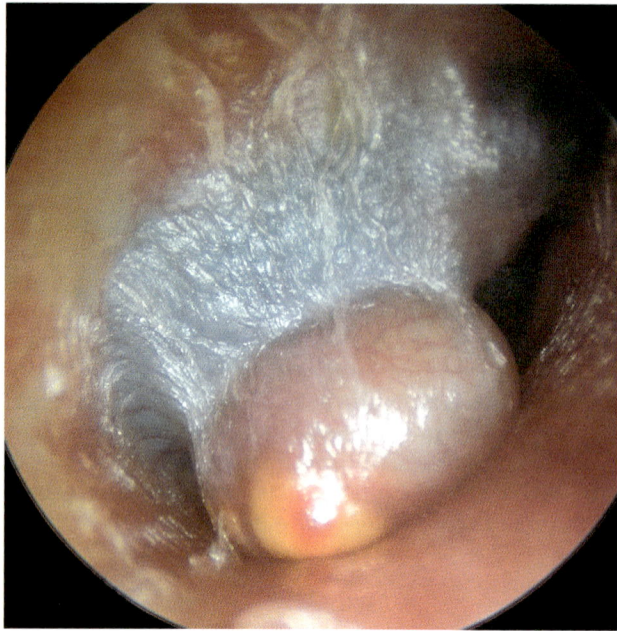

Figure 5.**3** Cholesterol granuloma associated with an inflammatory polyp that leads to bulging of the tympanic membrane.

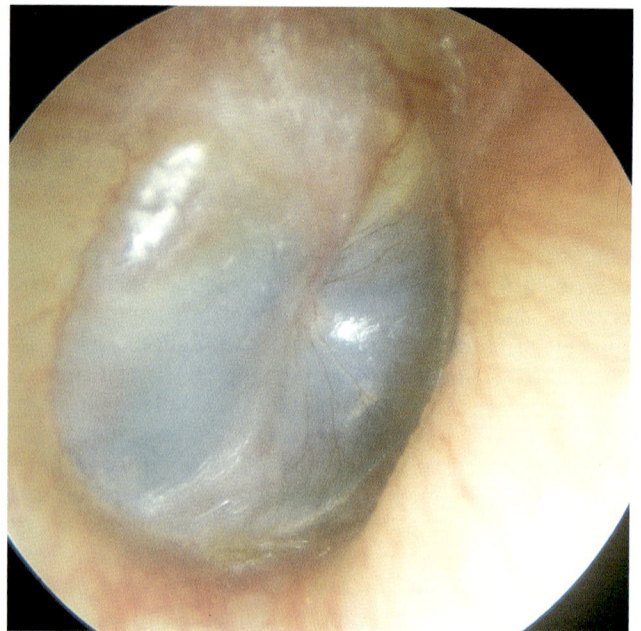

Figure 5.**4** Characteristic blue color of the tympanic membrane caused by a cholesterol granuloma.

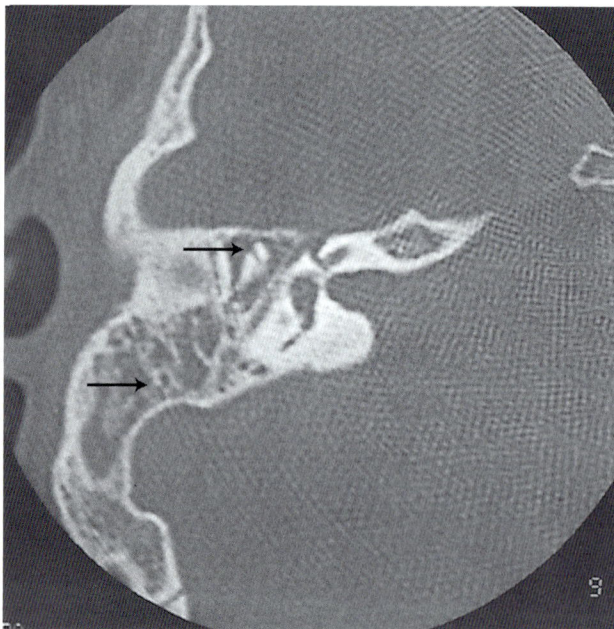

Figure 5.**5** Axial CT of the case shown in Figure 5.**4**. The granuloma and effusion are present in the middle ear and mastoid without causing any bony erosion. The ossicular chain (malleus and incus) is intact and the intercellular septa in the mastoid are preserved.

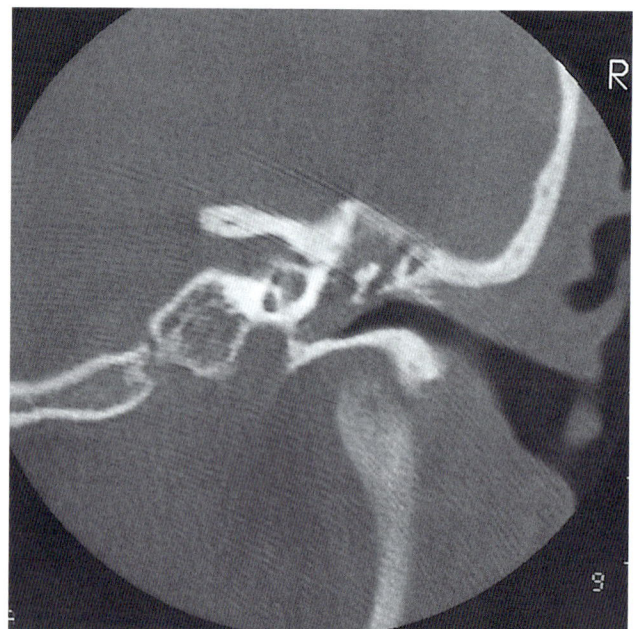

Figure 5.**6** Coronal CT scan of the same patient.

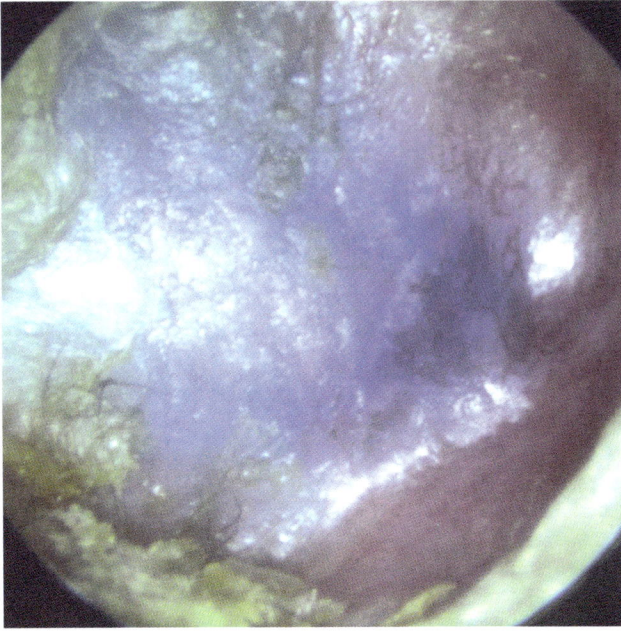

Figure 5.**7**   Characteristic blue color of the tympanic membrane, with lateralization, caused by cholesterol granuloma (open tympanoplasty).

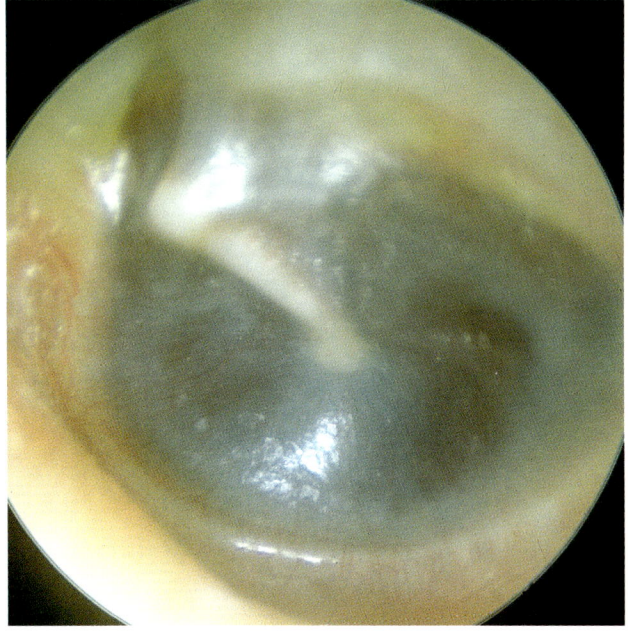

Figure 5.**8**   Left ear. A 17-year-old male patient complained of conductive hearing loss of 1 year's duration accompanied by left nasal obstruction. Otoscopy revealed the presence of a left cholesterol granuloma. Rhinoscopy showed the presence of a nasopharyngeal swelling that extended into the left nasal cavity. The swelling was suggestive of a juvenile nasopharyngeal angiofibroma.

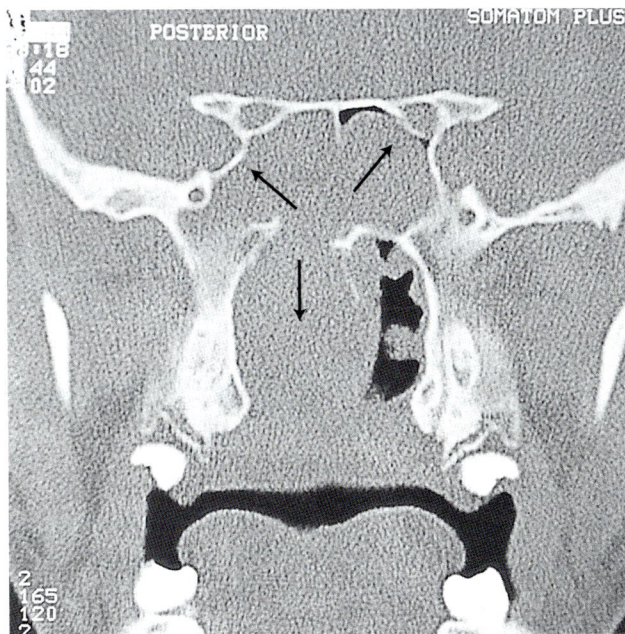

Figure 5.**9**   CT, coronal view. Involvement of the nasopharynx and the sphenoidal sinus.

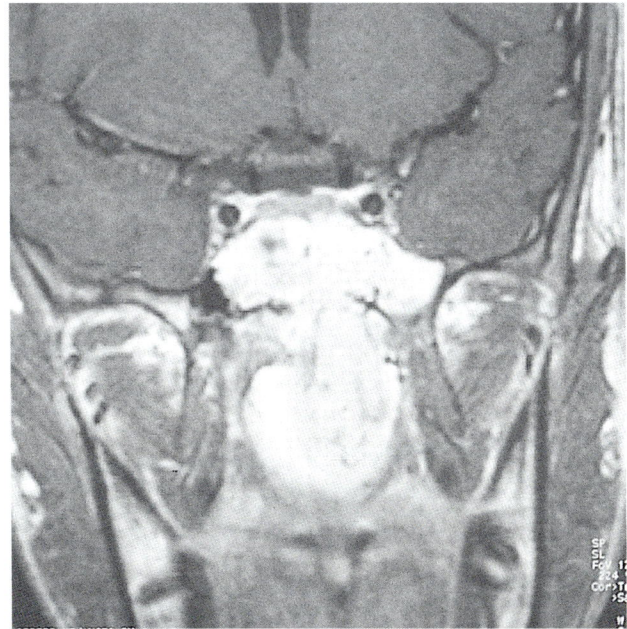

Figure 5.**10**   Magnetic resonance imaging (MRI) of the same case, coronal view, showing the extension of the angiofibroma.

Figure 5.**11**   MRI of the same case, sagittal view, showing the extension of the tumor from the ethmoid to the rhinopharynx pushing the soft palate.

Figure 5.**12**   MRI of the same case, axial view. Involvement of the middle ear and mastoid by the cholesterol granuloma can be observed.

Figure 5.**13**   The angiofibroma was removed, after being embolized, using a midfacial degloving approach.

Figure 5.**14**   Postoperative CT (1 year) confirming the total tumor removal.

6 Atelectasis, Adhesive Otitis Media

Adhesive otitis media is characterized by complete or partial adhesions between the thin retracted and atrophic pars tensa and the medial wall of the middle ear. Necrosis of the long process of the incus or the stapes suprastructure can also occur, with a resultant natural myringostapedopexy. It should be differentiated from atelectasis and from simple drum retraction, in which the tympanic membrane is mobile with the Valsalva or Toynbee maneuvers.

Sadè (1979) distinguished five grades of atelectasis (Fig. 6.1): grade I is characterized by a mild retraction of the tympanic membrane; in grade II the retracted tympanic membrane comes in contact with the incus or the stapes; in grade III the tympanic membrane touches the promontory; grade IV is adhesive otitis media; and in grade V there is a spontaneous perforation of the atelectatic ear drum with otorrhea and polyp formation.

Nakano (1993) proposed two types of adhesive otitis: type A, in which the retracted and atrophic tympanic membrane adheres completely to the promontory, and type B, in which retraction and adhesion affect mainly the posterior part of the tympanic membrane, usually without retraction of its anterior half.

Histologically, the tympanic membrane is atrophic due to thinning or even absence of the lamina propria. It can be hypothesized that the negative middle ear pressure caused by eustachian tube dysfunction or persistent secretory otitis media leads to atrophy of the elastic fibers of the pars tensa. An occasional episode of acute suppurative otitis media might form adhesions between the mucosa of the promontory and the retracted tympanic membrane.

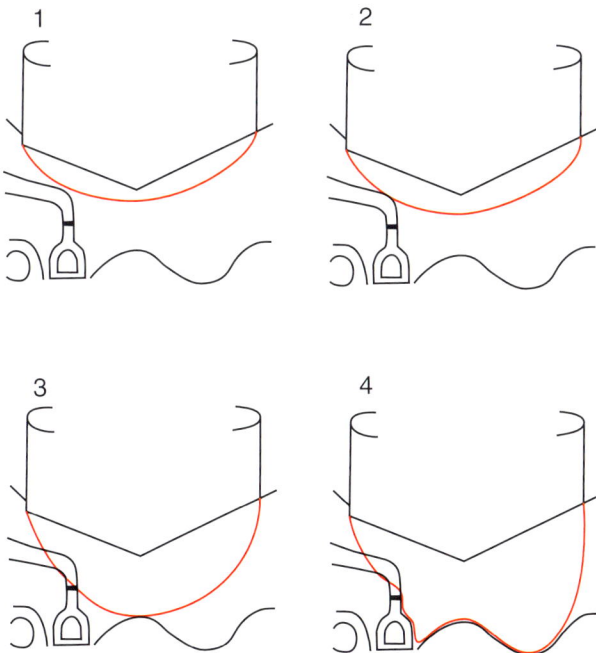

Figure 6.1 Sadè classification of atelectasis (modified) (see text).

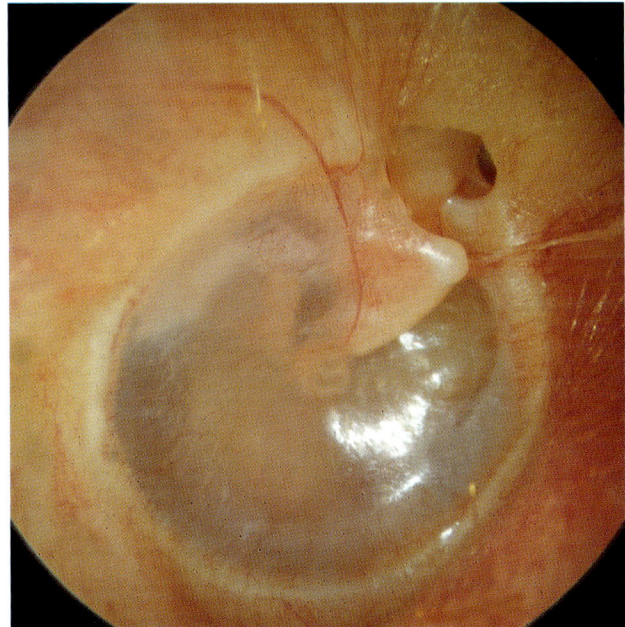

Figure 6.2 Right ear. Sadè grade I atelectasis. The tympanic membrane is retracted but does not come into contact with the middle ear structures. A mild retraction of the pars flaccida, through which the head of the malleus is visible, is also noted. The base of the retraction pocket is under control, with no sign of cholesteatoma. It is also possible in this case to assume that the drum is mobile on Valsalva or Toynbee maneuvers. This patient presented with very mild conductive hearing loss and a normal tympanogram (type A) (see Figs. 6.3 and 6.4).

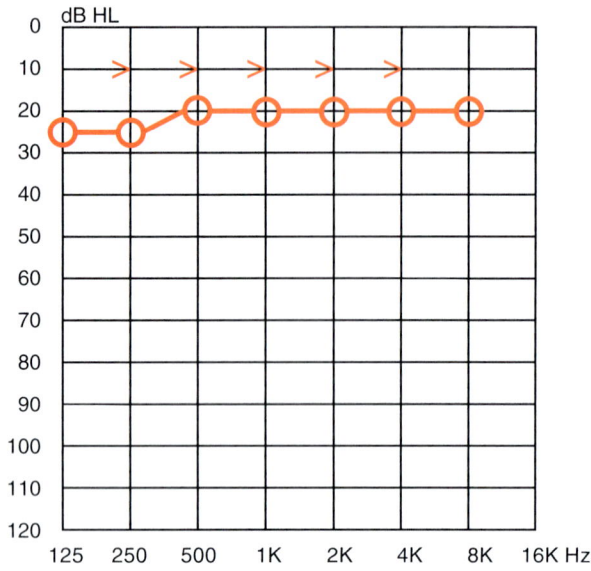

Figure **6.3**   Audiogram of the same case. Mild conductive hearing loss.

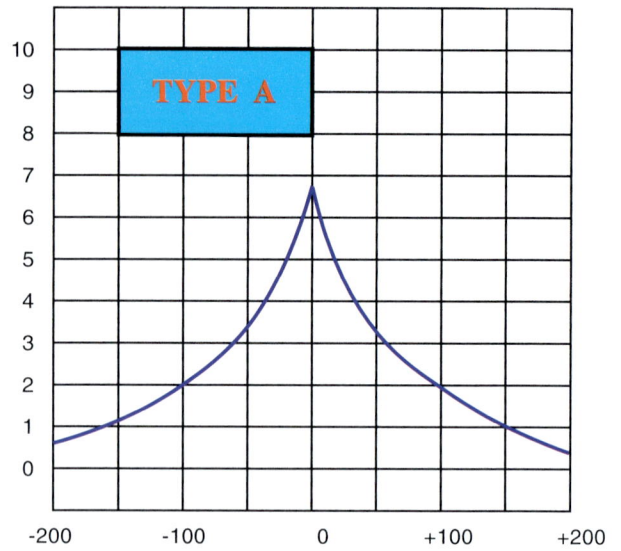

Figure **6.4**   Tympanogram of the same case. Normal or type A.

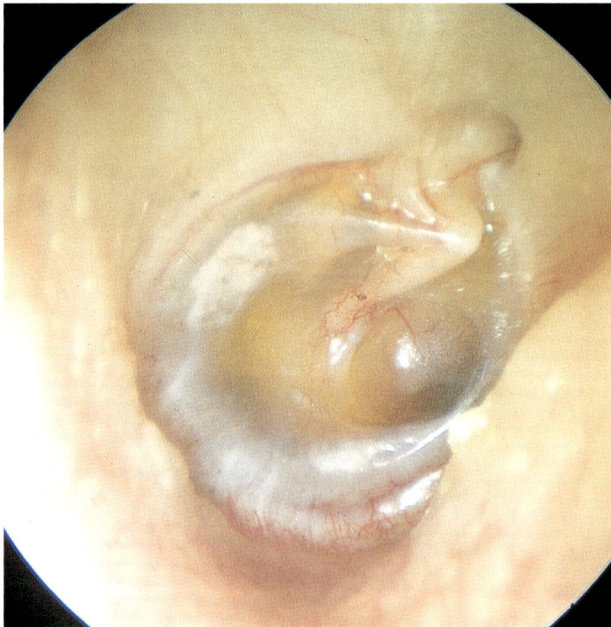

Figure **6.5**   Right ear. Grade I atelectasis with the malleus slightly medialized. An epitympanic retraction pocket is also seen. Middle ear effusion with yellowish color can be appreciated. Pure tone audiogram revealed a 40-dB conductive hearing loss (Fig. 6.**6**), whereas the tympanogram was type B, i.e., typical of middle ear effusion (Fig. 6.**7**). In this case, the insertion of a ventilation tube is indicated to avoid further retraction of the tympanic membrane, to aerate the middle ear, and to improve hearing.

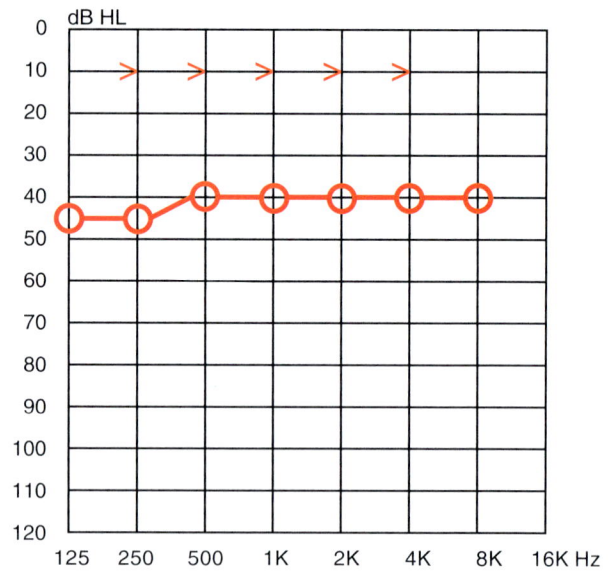

Figure **6.6**   Audiogram of the same case, showing a 40-dB conductive hearing loss.

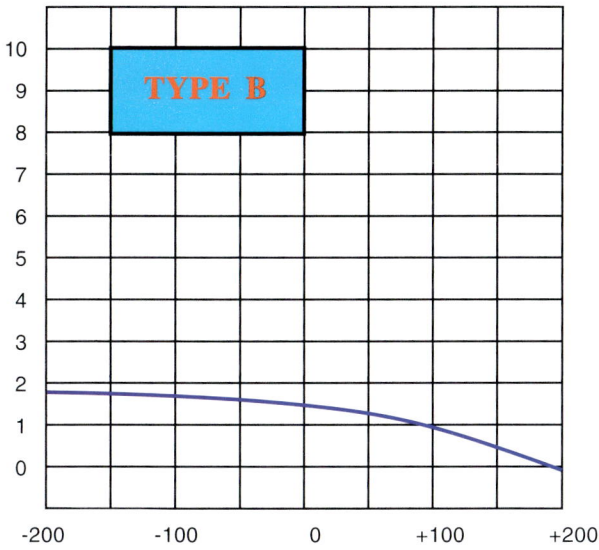

Figure 6.**7** Type B tympanogram of the same case, typical of middle ear effusion.

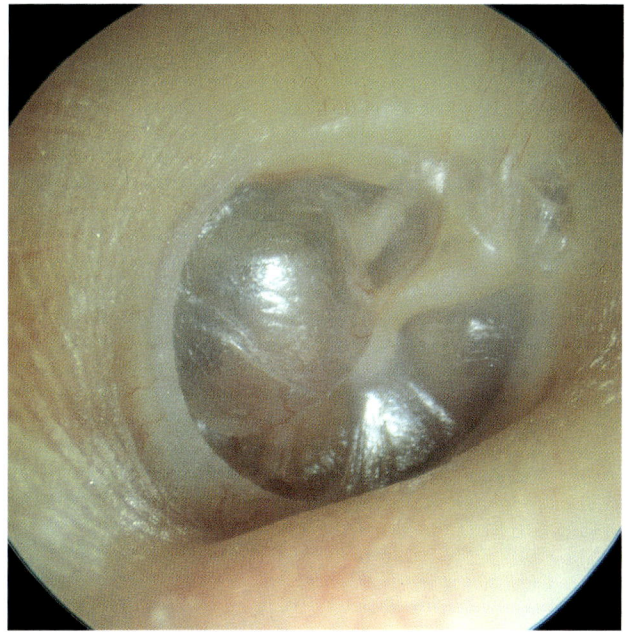

Figure 6.**8** Right ear. Grade I atelectasis. The tympanic membrane is markedly thinned due to partial resorption of the lamina propria. The incus is seen in transparency. Pure tone audiogram is normal (Fig. 6.**9**), whereas the tympanogram has a very high compliance (Fig. 6.**10**). As the tympanic membrane is mobile with the Valsalva maneuver, insertion of a ventilation tube is not indicated.

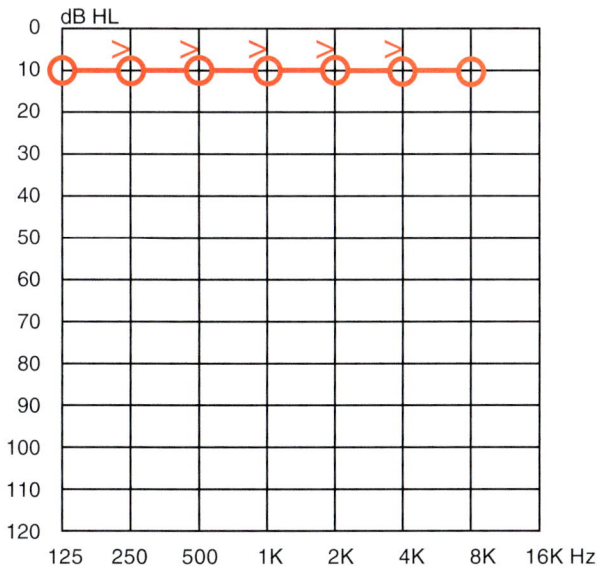

Figure 6.**9** Audiogram of the same case.

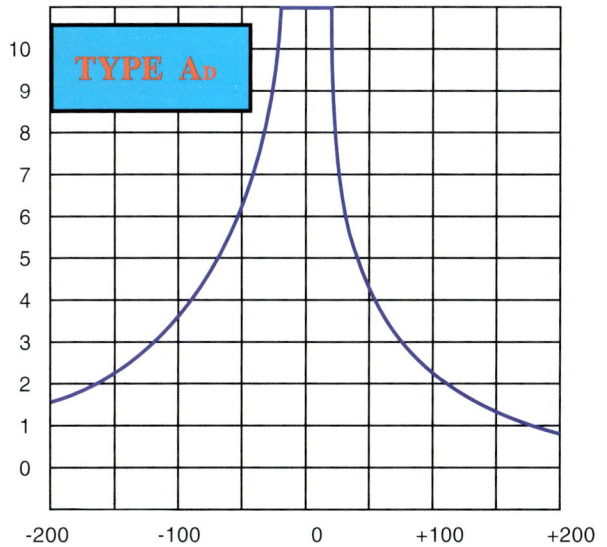

Figure 6.**10** Tympanogram of the same case, type Ad according to the classification of Liden-Jerger, 1976.

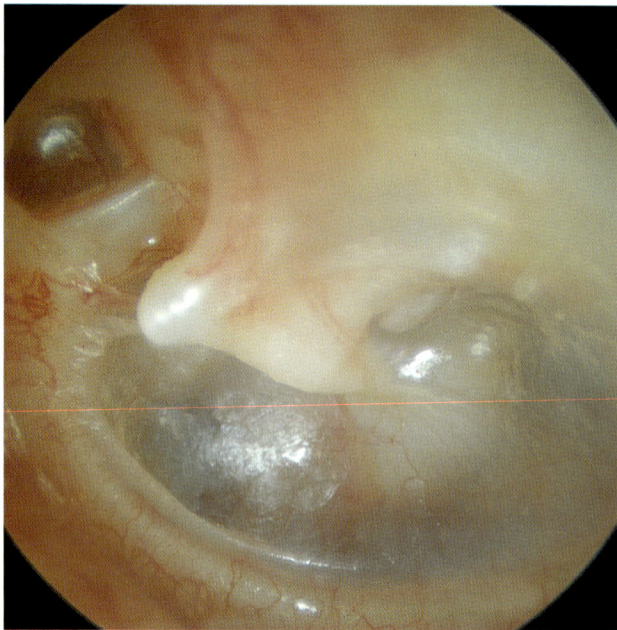

Figure 6.**11**   Left ear. Grade II atelectasis with marked epitympanic retraction. The tympanic membrane touches the incus. The malleus is medialized. Air–fluid levels are seen in the anteroinferior quadrant. The insertion of a ventilation tube is necessary to restore normal conditions.

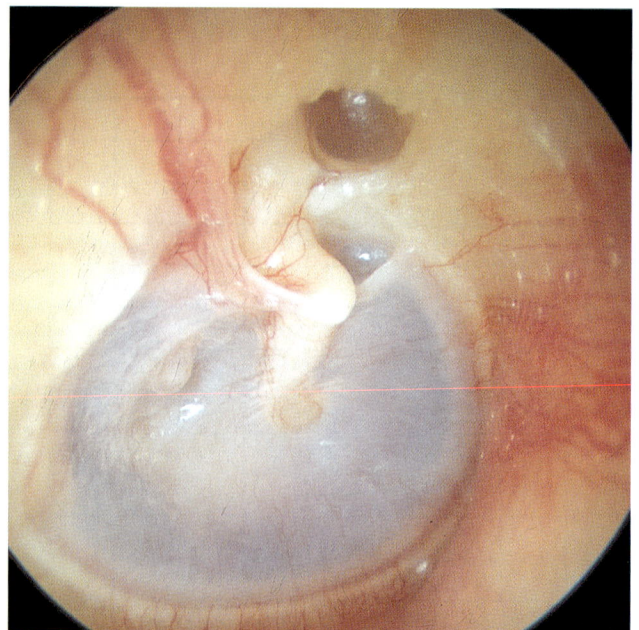

Figure 6.**12**   Right ear. Grade II atelectasis. A condition similar to the previous case, but with the onset of thickening of the tympanic membrane.

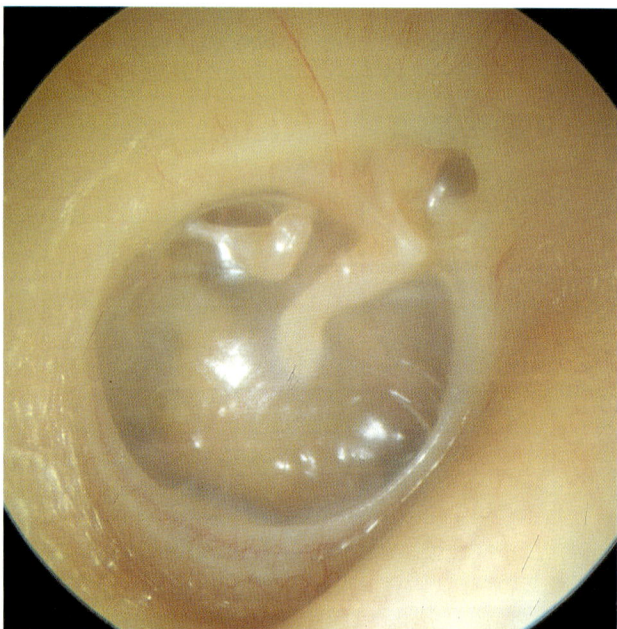

Figure 6.**13**   Right ear. Grade II atelectasis. The tympanic membrane is very thin due to absence of the fibrous layer. The membrane adheres to the incudostapedial joint and the tensor tympani tendon. Insertion of a ventilation tube is indicated.

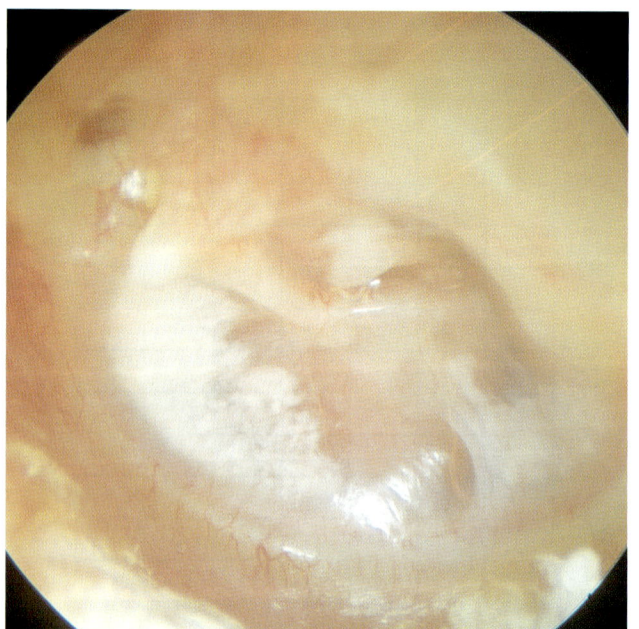

Figure 6.**14**   Left ear. Grade III atelectasis. The tympanic membrane is touching the promontory and the incus. An air–fluid level and a tympanosclerotic plaque can be seen in the anterior quadrant.

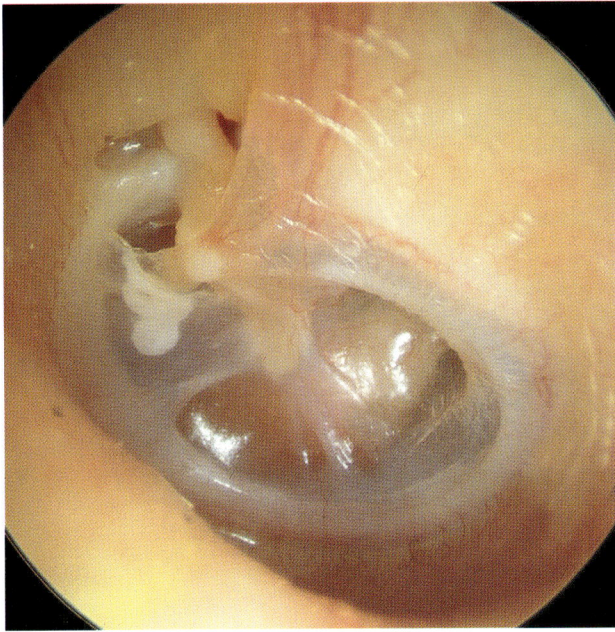

Figure 6.**15**   Left ear. Grade III atelectasis. The thin and atrophic tympanic membrane is in contact with the promontory. Middle ear effusion is seen. A tympanosclerotic plaque is present in the anterosuperior quadrant. The head of the malleus is visible through an epitympanic retraction pocket. The insertion of a ventilation tube is indicated.

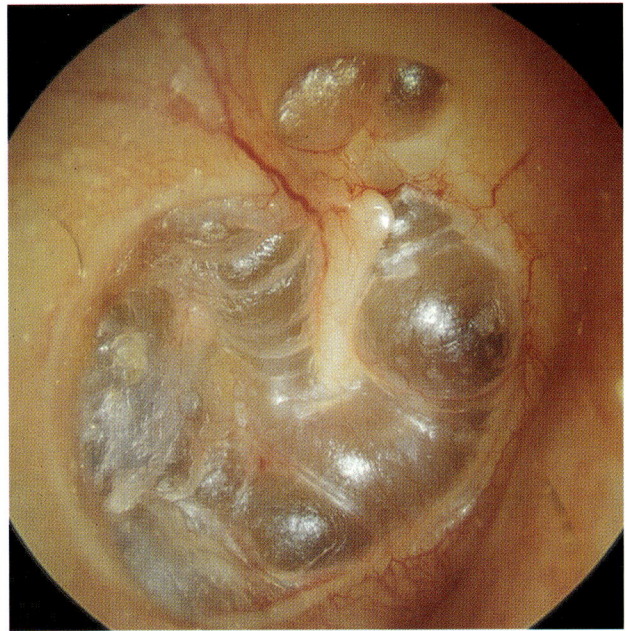

Figure 6.**16**   Right ear. Adhesive otitis media or grade IV atelectasis associated with a mild epitympanic retraction pocket. The thin and atrophic tympanic membrane completely covers the promontory. The tympanic membrane retraction has caused erosion of the long process of the incus, with a subsequent spontaneous myringostapedopexy. As the patient has no hearing loss, surgery is not indicated.

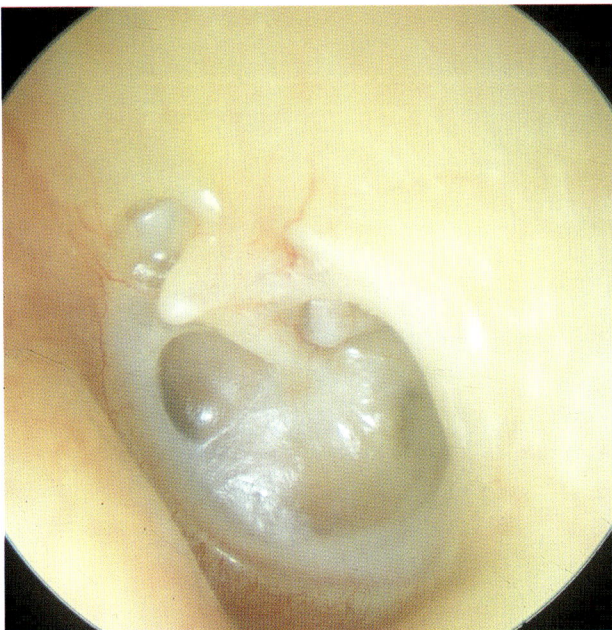

Figure 6.**17**   Left ear. Grade IV atelectasis. The malleus is medialized and adherent to the promontory. The tympanic membrane is atrophic. The epidermal layer of the membrane is adherent to the incudostapedial joint, the promontory, and the round window. A retraction pocket corresponding to the eustachian tube orifice is also seen. Middle ear effusion is present. Insertion of a ventilation tube is indicated.

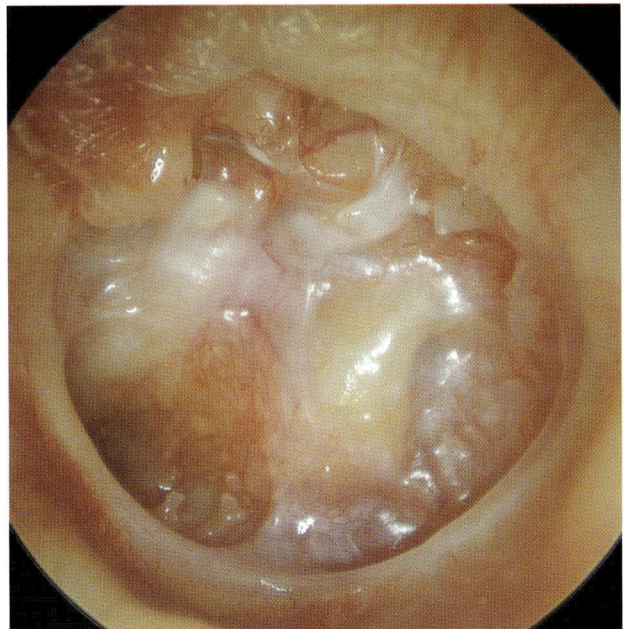

Figure 6.**18**   Left ear. Adhesive otitis media. This case represents the long-term sequela of persistent secretory otitis media with chronic eustachian tube dysfunction. The fibrous and mucosal layers of the tympanic membrane have been resorbed, whereas the epidermal layer is completely adherent to the medial wall of the middle ear. The promontory, round and oval windows, as well as residues of the ossicular chain are all visible. The handle of the malleus is completely medialized and partially eroded. The long process of the incus is eroded, whereas the stapes suprastructure is completely absent. As the patient is not suffering from otorrhea, surgery is not advised.

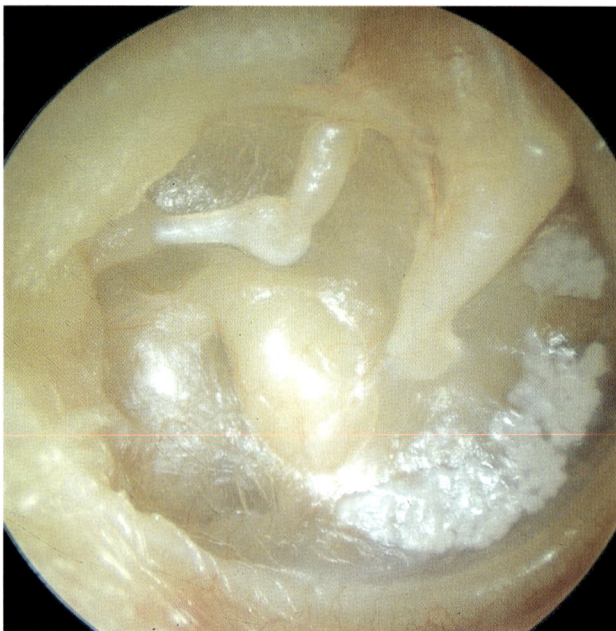

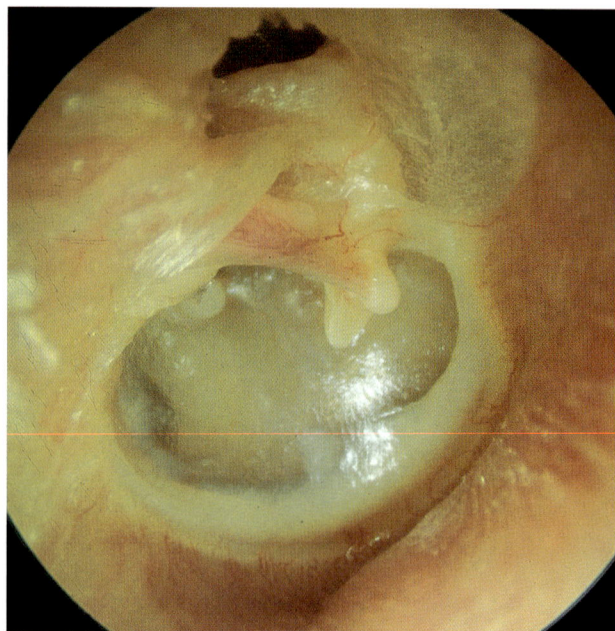

Figure **6.19** Right ear. The thin and atrophic tympanic membrane adheres to the promontory, incudostapedial joint, pyramidal process, and stapedius tendon. The long process of the incus is partially eroded. Calcifications are present in the anterior quadrants. As hearing is normal, surgery is not indicated.

Figure **6.20** Right ear. Atelectasis associated with marked epitympanic erosion through which the head of the malleus and body of the incus are seen covered with epithelial squamae. The

tympanic membrane is thin and transparent due to absence of the fibrous layer. The handle of the malleus is amputated. The long process of the incus is eroded, and a natural myringostapedopexy is seen. The promontory, round window, head of the stapes, and oval window can be seen through the thin tympanic membrane. Despite the attic epithelialization, a true cholesteatoma has not yet formed. Regular follow-up of such patients is vital. Should the disease progress with cholesteatoma formation, surgery in the form of an open tympanoplasty is indicated.

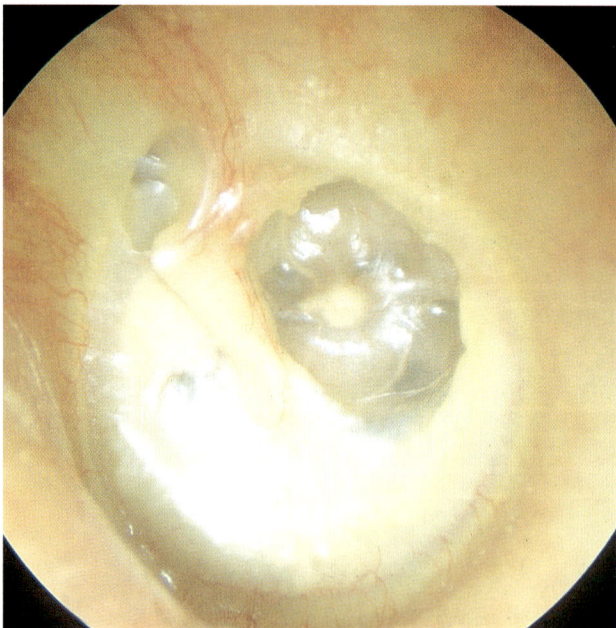

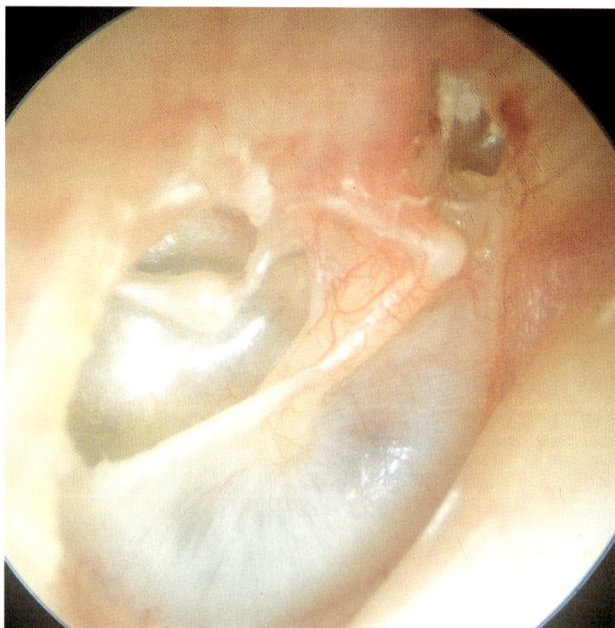

Figure **6.21** Left ear. Posterior retraction pocket. The tympanic membrane remains adherent to the stapes head even after Valsalva maneuver (myringostapedopexy). The remaining part of the tympanic membrane is thick and shows tympanosclerosis. Audiometry revealed normal hearing. Patients with myringostapedopexy generally have good hearing; therefore, surgery is not indicated except if conductive hearing loss develops and/or a posterior retraction pocket is associated with frequent otorrhea. Surgery varies from simple myringoplasty (when the tympanic membrane needs reinforcement) to tympanoplasty (in which the ossicular chain is eroded and needs ossiculoplasty).

Figure **6.22** Right ear. The tympanic membrane, being adherent to the long process of the incus, caused erosion of the latter with subsequent conductive hearing loss (see Fig. 6.**23**). The second portion of the facial nerve is seen superior to the oval window. The head of the stapes and the stapedius tendon are also visible. Tympanoplastic surgery was performed in this patient. The tympanic membrane was reinforced and the incus interposed between the handle of the malleus and the stapes.

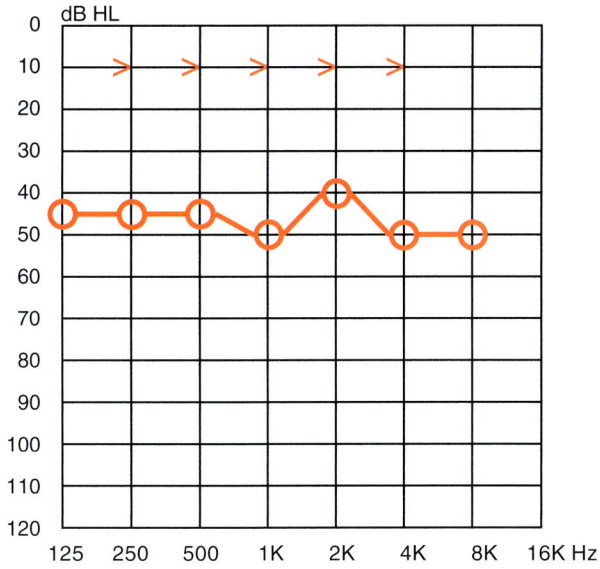

Figure 6.**23** Audiogram in the same case showing conductive hearing loss.

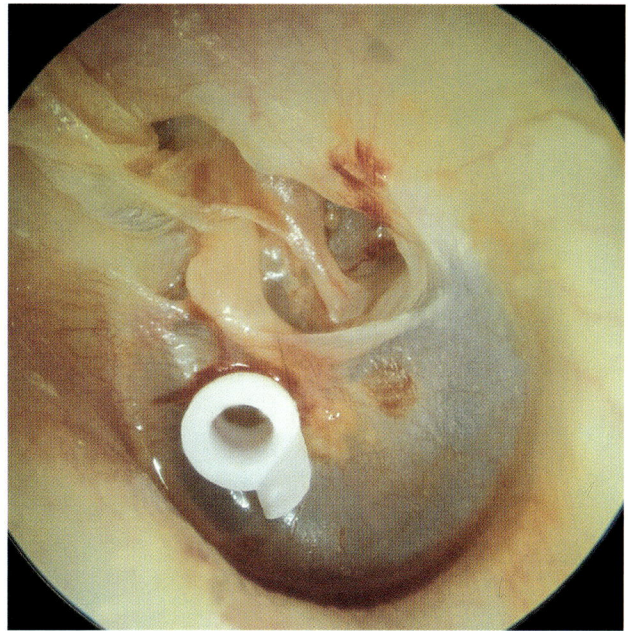

Figure 6.**24** Left ear. Meso- and epitympanic retraction pockets that adhere to the head of the malleus, the partially eroded long process of the incus, and the incudostapedial joint. A ventilation tube has been inserted in the anterior quadrant to avoid further retraction that might lead to cholesteatoma.

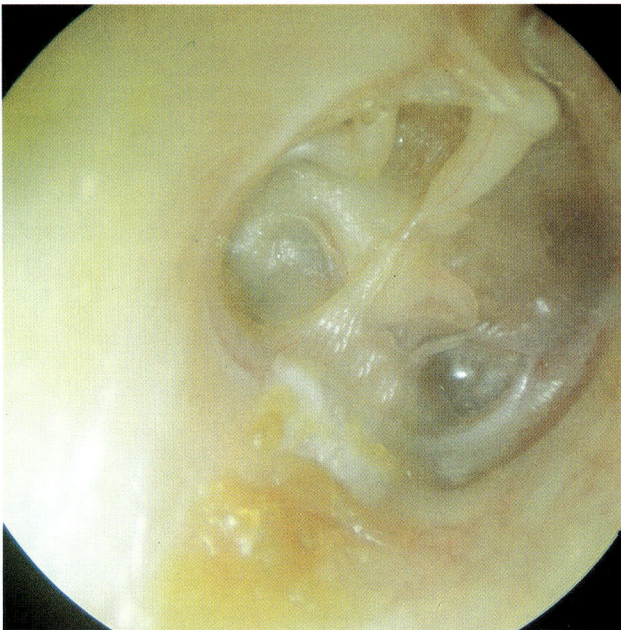

Figure 6.**25** Right ear. Grade IV atelectasis. All of the middle ear structures can be seen in transparency. Starting from the malleus and moving in a clockwise direction, we can distinguish the tubal opening, the hypotympanum, the promontory, the round window, the stapedius tendon, and the incudo-stapedial joint.

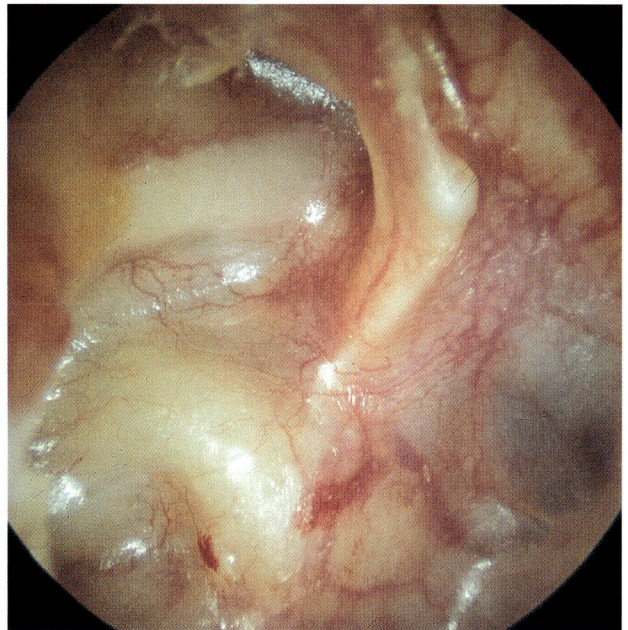

Figure 6.**26** Right ear. Large mesotympanic retraction pocket that caused erosion of the incus and stapes suprastructure. The second portion of the facial nerve passing superior to the oval window, the promontory, and the round window can all be seen in transparency. In patients with good social hearing and no otorrhea, surgery is not indicated.

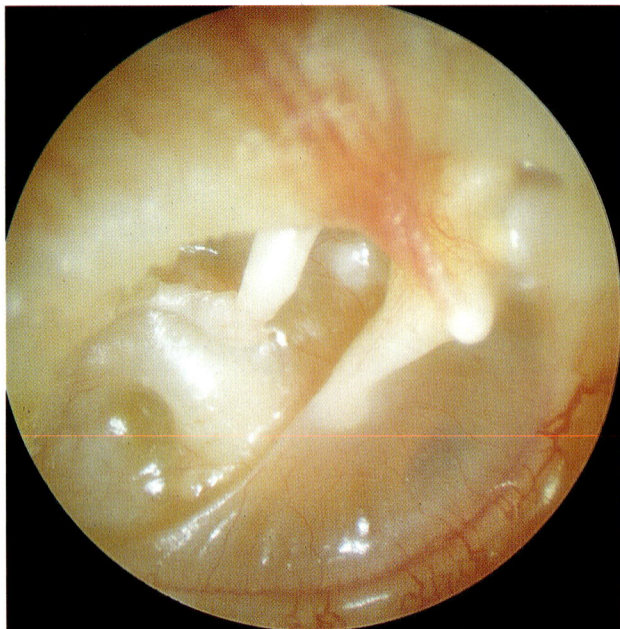

Figure 6.**27**   Right ear. Posterior retraction pocket. The tympanic membrane adheres to the promontory, the round window, the partially eroded long process of the incus, the head of the stapes, and the stapedius tendon. The processus cochleariformis is clearly visible between the malleus and the long process of the incus. Middle ear effusion can be observed anterior to the malleus and in the region of the oval window. In this case, ventilation tube insertion is indicated in an attempt to prevent further erosion of the ossicular chain and the formation of mesotympanic cholesteatoma.

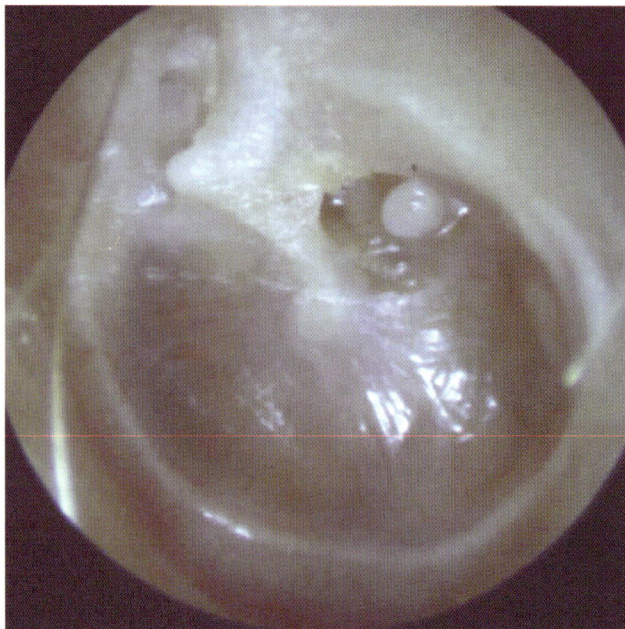

Figure 6.**28**   Left ear. Grade II atelectasis with erosion of the long process of the incus, and adhesion of the tympanic membrane to the head of the stapes. The whole of the tympanic membrane is very thin. Audiometry showed that the patient had good hearing. In this case, surgery is not indicated.

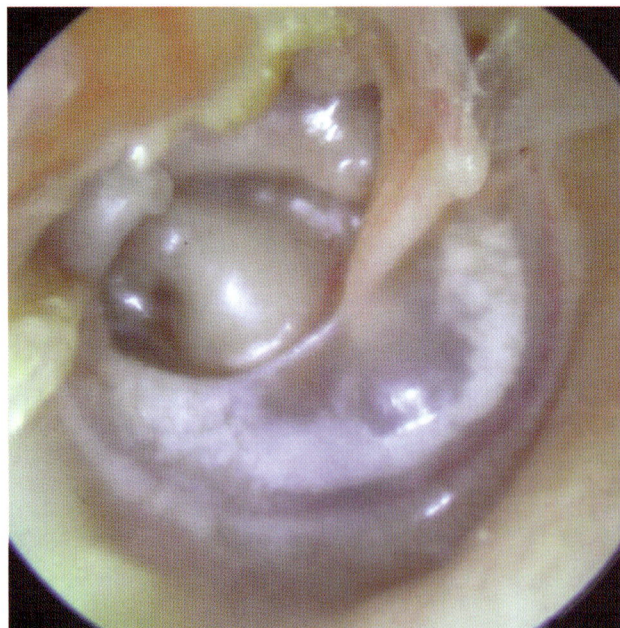

Figure 6.**29**   Right ear. Large posterior retraction pocket. The long process of the incus and stapes superstructure are absent. The round window, oval window, promontory, cochlear process and secondary portion of the facial nerve are clearly visible in transparency.

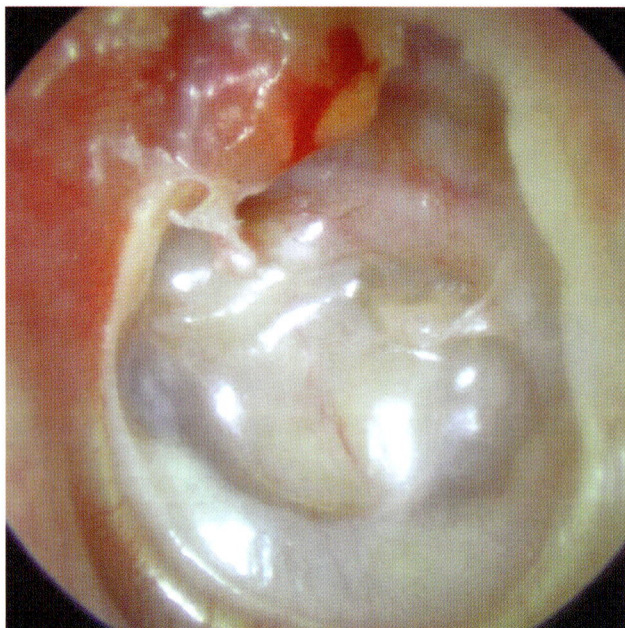

Figure 6.**30**   Left ear. A grade IV atelectatic ear. The epidermal layer of the tympanic membrane is completely adherent to the medial wall of the middle ear. The residues of the ossicular chain are visible. The stapes superstructure is partially eroded but still present. The patient had otorrhea. In this case surgery is indicated.

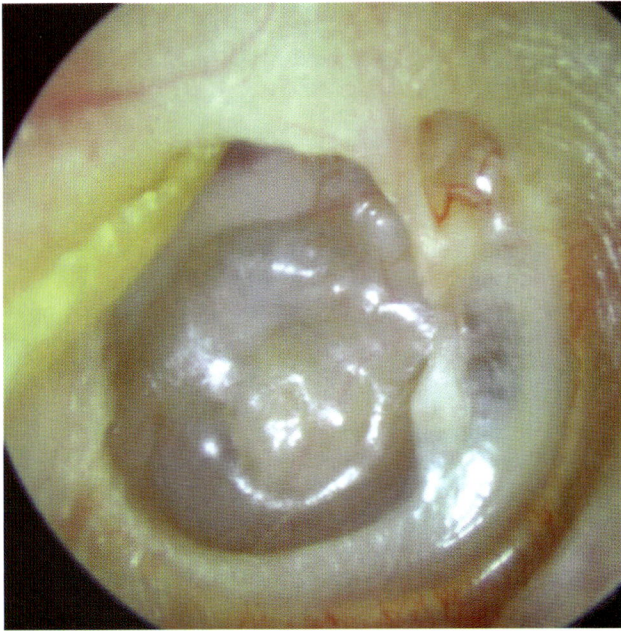

Figure 6.**31** Right ear. Grade IV atelectasis. The long process of the incus, the head of the malleus, and stapes superstructure are absent. The second portion of the facial nerve can be seen, as well as the round and oval windows. The patient had otorrhea. Surgery is indicated, with reconstruction of the tympanic membrane using tragal perichondrium and cartilage.

Summary

In grade I, II, and III atelectasis, a long-term ventilation tube is usually inserted to prevent further retraction of the tympanic membrane. However, in cases with marked conductive hearing loss that denotes erosion of the incus or the superstructure of the stapes, ossiculoplasty is performed after extraction and sculpturing of the eroded incus or using a homologous incus. A large disk of tragal cartilage is used to reinforce the tympanic membrane.

Indications for surgery in adhesive otitis media include cases with tympanic membrane perforation (grade V according to Sadè 1979), with or without polyps, granulation or otorrhea, those cases with a large infected retraction pocket causing frequent otorrhea, or those with conductive hearing loss due to ossicular chain erosion. In all these cases a tympanoplasty is performed using a postauricular incision. A disk of tragal cartilage is used with the perichondrium adherent to its lateral surface. If the handle of the malleus is present, it is incorporated into the cartilaginous disk after a triangular defect has been created to accomodate it. This technique has the advantage of preventing retraction and adhesions between the tympanic membrane and the promontory. At the same time, it enables repair of the tympanic membrane perforation with the tragal perichondrium.

It can be concluded that there is no single treatment for the atelectatic ear. The milder the degree of atelectasis, the more conservative the treatment is. It should be noted, however, that in the long term conservative treatment (e.g., ventilation tube) has not been found to modify the further evolution of atelectasis. As atelectasis results from eustachian tube dysfunction, the ideal solution would be correction of this defect. At present, there is no acceptable "functional" surgery for the eustachian tube. Individual treatment should be administered according to the consequences of this dysfunction in each case. Such a strategy, however, requires a flexible approach and versatile surgical techniques.

7 Non-Cholesteatomatous Chronic Otitis Media

The difference between acute and chronic otitis media is not the duration of the disease but rather the anatomo-pathological characteristics. Untreated acute otitis media persisting for months is still a process that tends essentially to return to normality. On the other hand, a chronic otitis, even if the ear stops discharging, has anatomopathological sequelae of clinical importance.

The most commonly encountered forms are active chronic suppurative otitis media, characterized by otorrhea, and inactive chronic suppurative otitis media, in which the ear is dry. Naturally, the active form may become quiescent either spontaneously or following treatment. The ear becomes dry and the condition is designated inactive. A dry perforation, however, may be infected, leading to ear discharge. In this latter case, the mucosa may be hyperplastic and thick due to interstitial edema, fibrosis, or cellular infiltration. In some cases, polyps are formed which may be large enough to occupy the external auditory canal. In other cases, persistence of suppuration can lead to ulceration of the mucosa, formation of granulation tissue, and even bone resorption. The anatomical sequelae of chronic otitis media vary. They may be in the form of a simple central tympanic membrane perforation, erosion of the ossicular chain, or formation of tympanosclerosis. Both the active and inactive forms cause functional alterations such as conductive or mixed hearing loss (very rarely sensorineural). The absence of squamous epithelium in the middle ear has led to the designation of this form as a "safe type" of otitis media. This is to distinguish it from cholesteatoma, which is considered "unsafe" due to the potential complications that may arise from the presence of keratinized squamous epithelium in the middle ear.

General Characteristics of Tympanic Membrane Perforations

Tympanic membrane perforations are usually present at the pars tensa. Pars flaccida perforations are generally associated with epitympanic cholesteatoma.

If a tympanic membrane perforation does not heal spontaneously, the epithelial and mucosal layers creep and meet along the borders of the perforation. This pathological communication between the middle and external ear can be considered a true "air fistula." In the presence of a tympanic membrane perforation, the patient is subject to recurrent infections and ear discharge.

Whenever tympanic membrane perforations are diagnosed, the following three assessments must be carried out: 1) At the level of the perforation the site, size, and state of the remainder of the tympanic membrane around the perforation should be determined. 2) At the level of the middle ear, the state of the mucosa, the con-

dition of the ossicular chain (if possible), and the presence or absence of epithelialization should be evaluated. 3) The otoscopic examination has to be complemented with pure tone audiometry to obtain a better understanding of the ossicular chain (possible erosion of the incus, fixity of the chain).

Pars tensa perforations can be either central or marginal. Marginal perforations lie at the periphery of the tympanic membrane with absence of the fibrous annulus. Marginal perforations are considered "unsafe" because the skin of the external auditory canal, in the absence of the annulus, can easily advance towards the middle ear, giving rise to cholesteatoma.

Otoscopic examination can often define the junction between the skin and mucosa at the borders of the tympanic membrane perforation. At this junction the squamous epithelium has a "velvety" appearance. The presence of a red de-epithelialized ring along the perforation rim indicates the evagination of the mucosa towards the external surface of the tympanic membrane residue. However, invagination of the skin towards the inner surface of the tympanic membrane residue is more difficult to diagnose. This inward skin migration is favored by the atrophy of the mucosa which occurs as a result of the perforation. At the time of myringoplasty, freshening of the edge of the perforation not only promotes the attachment of the graft but also greatly reduces the risk of leaving entrapped skin on the undersurface of the drum, which may lead to iatrogenic cholesteatoma.

Conductive hearing loss caused by tympanic membrane perforation has two main causes: 1) Reduction of the tympanic membrane surface area on which the acoustic pressure exerts its action. 2) Reduction of the vibratory movements of the cochlear fluids, because sound reaches both windows at nearly the same time without the dampening and phase-changing effect of the intact tympanic membrane.

The site of the perforation cannot be correlated to a particular audiometric pattern. However, it is generally observed that hearing loss occurs more in the low frequencies and that for perforations of the same size, hearing loss occurs more in posterior perforations than in anterior ones.

The majority of posttraumatic and postotitic perforations heal spontaneously. When large portions of the tympanic membrane are lost or when chronic or recurrent infections occur, the perforation may become permanent. In these cases, the tympanic membrane must be repaired (myringoplasty) to restore the normal physiology of the ear.

Posterior Perforations

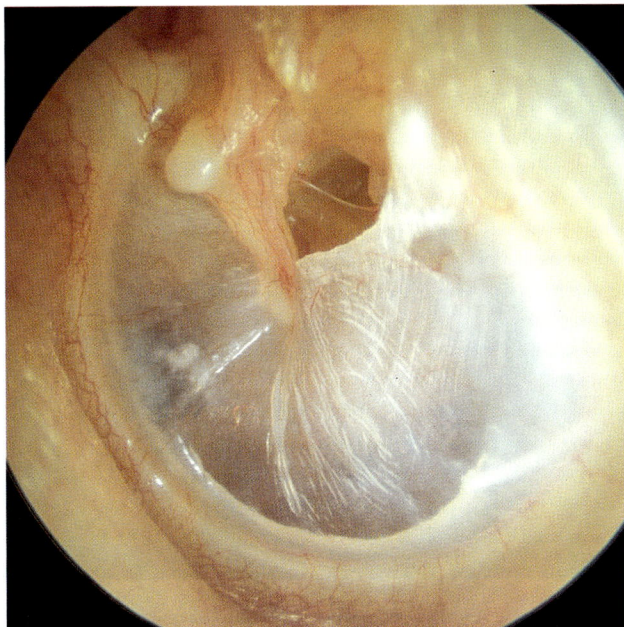

Figure 7.**1**   Left ear. The tympanic membrane is very thin due to atrophy of the fibrous layer. A posterosuperior marginal perforation is seen. This perforation is risky because the skin of the external auditory canal can easily advance into the middle ear, forming a cholesteatoma. In this case, a myringoplasty using an endomeatal approach is indicated.

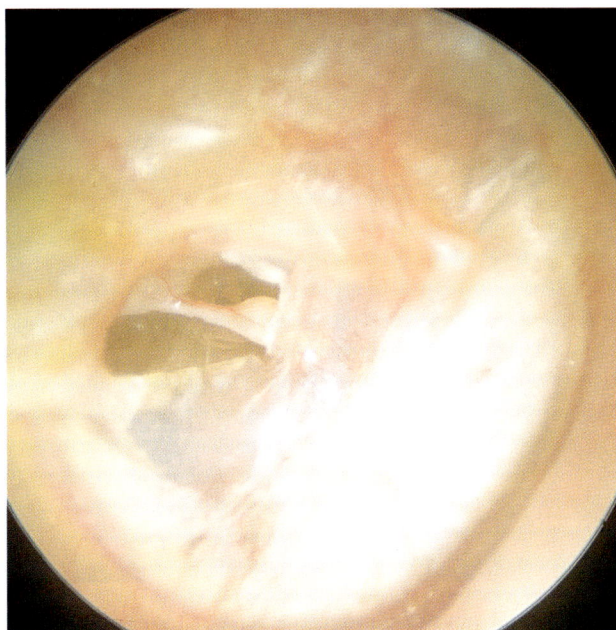

Figure 7.**2**   Right ear. Marginal posterosuperior perforation through which the intact incudostapedial joint, the stapedius tendon, and the pyramidal process can be seen.

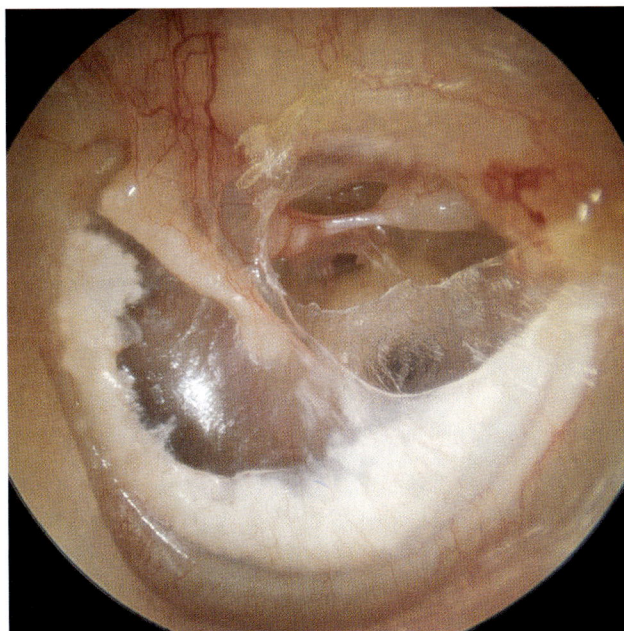

Figure 7.**3** Left ear. Perforation of the posterosuperior quadrant of the tympanic membrane. Visualized through the perforation are the incudostapedial joint, the stapes, the stapedius tendon, the pyramidal process, the promontory, and the round window. The residue of the tympanic membrane is very thin due to absence of the fibrous layer. Tympanosclerosis can be seen in the marginal part of the drum residue. From the surgical point of view, posterior perforations are the easiest to repair, especially when partial reconstruction of the tympanic membrane is all that is required. When the residue of the tympanic membrane is transformed into a rigid tympanosclerotic plaque, it is advisable to remove it, conserving the epidermal layer to be laid over the graft.

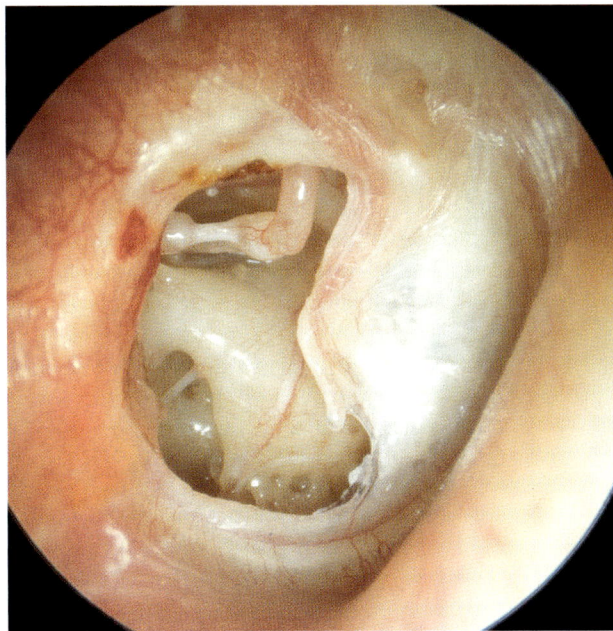

Figure 7.**4**   Right ear. Large perforation of the posterior quadrants. Normal middle ear mucosa. The incudostapedial joint is intact. The oval window with the annular ligament surrounding the footplate can be seen. The pyramidal eminence, the stapedius tendon, the round window, and Jacobson's nerve running on the promontory are also visible. The remaining anterior quadrants of the tympanic membrane are tympanosclerotic and rigid, blocking the mobility of the malleus.

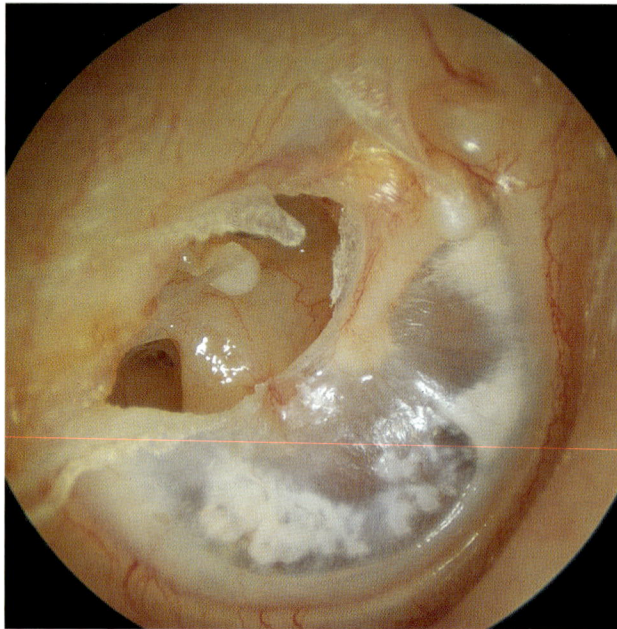

Figure 7.**5**   Right ear. Presence of chronic otitis media. Dry perforation of the posterior quadrants of the tympanic membrane, through which the head of the stapes and the round window are visible. The long process of the incus is necrosed. The middle ear mucosa is normal. The tympanic membrane residue shows tympanosclerosis with alternating areas of calcification and areas of thinned membrane due to atrophy of the fibrous layer. The operation, performed through a post-auricular incision, will also include the reconstruction of the ossicular chain using the autologous incus.

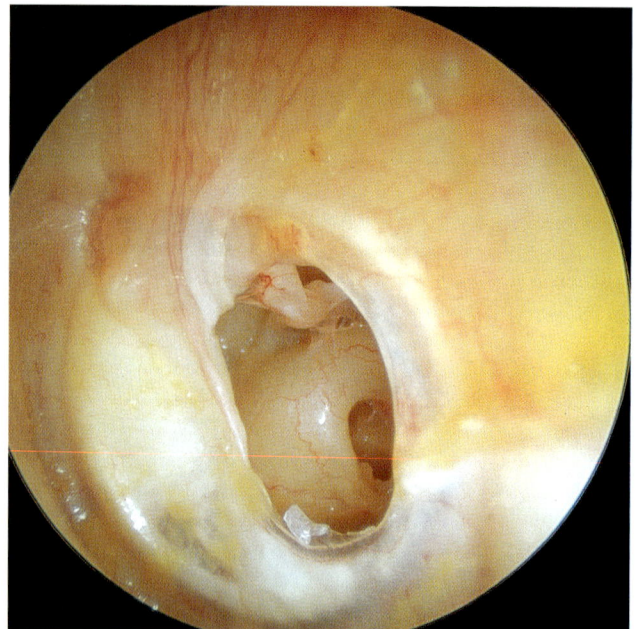

Figure 7.**6**   Left ear. Posterior nonmarginal perforation. The incudostapedial joint, the promontory, and the round window are all discernible.

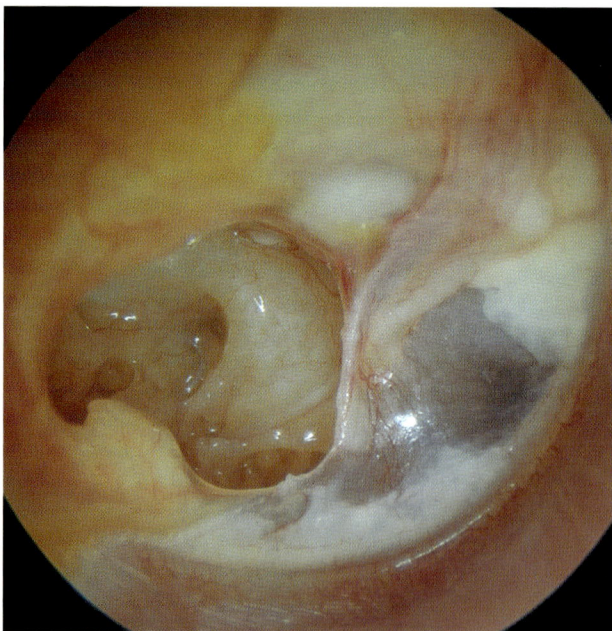

Figure 7.**7**   Right ear. Presence of simple chronic otitis media; a posteroinferior drum perforation. The middle ear mucosa is normal. The round window and Jacobson's nerve running on the promontory are seen. The incus can also be appreciated posterior to a retromalleolar tympanosclerotic plaque. The tympanic membrane residue shows areas of atrophy alternating with areas of tympanosclerosis.

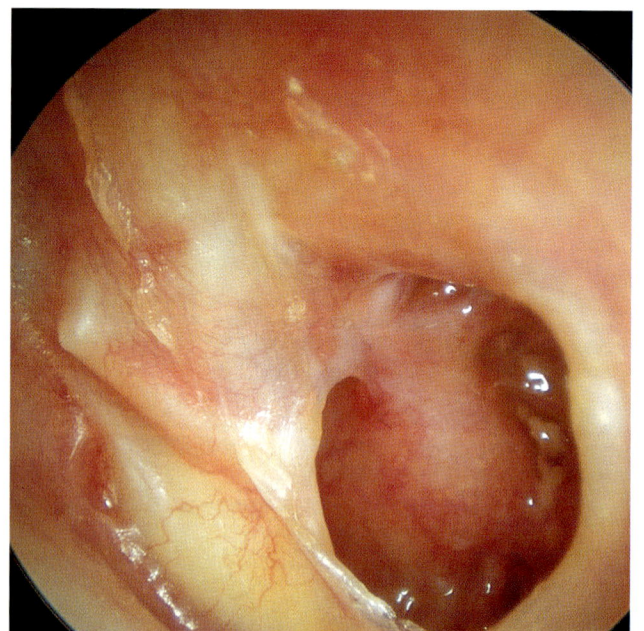

Figure 7.**8**   Left ear. Perforation of the posterior quadrants of the tympanic membrane. The skin advances along the posterosuperior border of the perforation towards the incudo-stapedial joint. The middle ear mucosa appears hypertrophic. Mucoid discharge is also present. A tympanosclerotic plaque can be seen in the residue of the tympanic membrane.

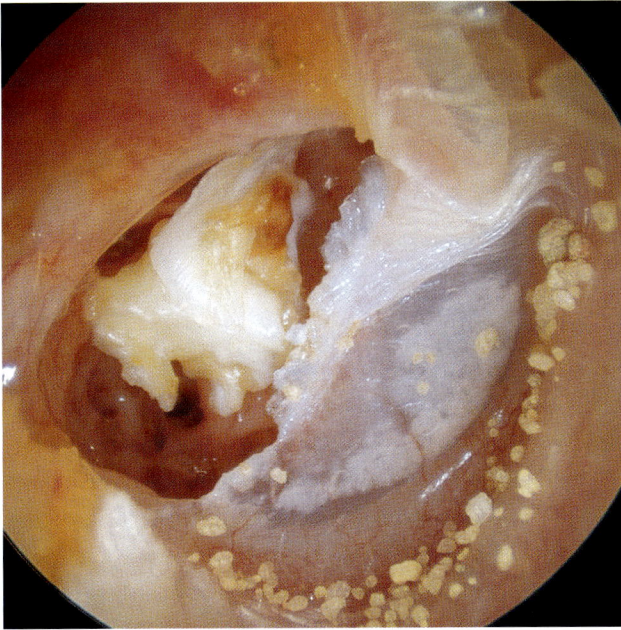

Figure 7.**9**   Right ear. Marked posterior marginal perforation, through which the skin penetrates into the middle ear. The ossicular chain is not identifiable.

Anterior Perforations

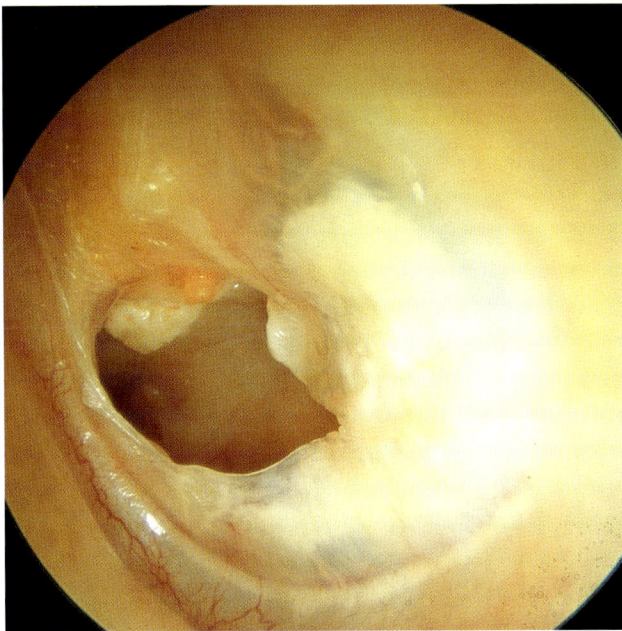

Figure 7.**10**   Left ear. Anterior perforation of the tympanic membrane, through which the tubal orifice is visible. A white mass is present behind the anterosuperior margin of the perforation. This mass can be either a cholesteatoma or a tympanosclerotic plaque. The consistency of the mass can be tested using an instrument under the microscope; the cholesteatoma is soft and will break, whereas tympanosclerosis is generally hard.

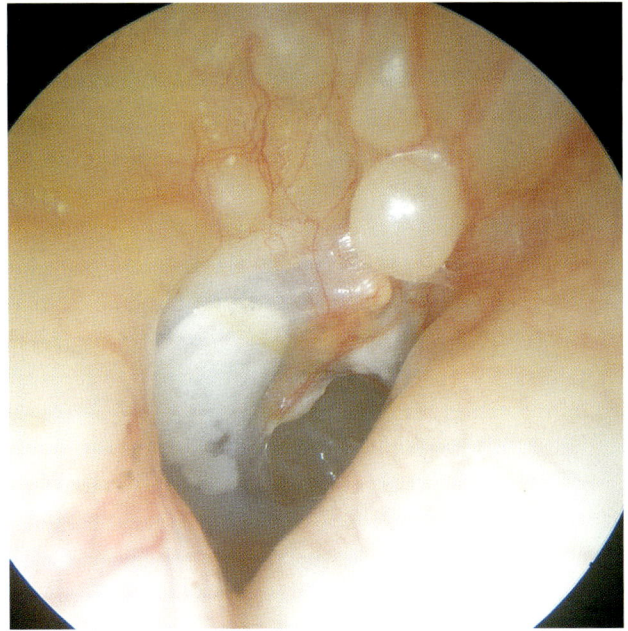

Figure 7.**11**   Right ear. Anterior perforation in a patient with anterior and posterior humps of the external auditory canal as well as exostosis of the superior canal wall. In this case, canalplasty should be performed at the same time as myringoplasty.

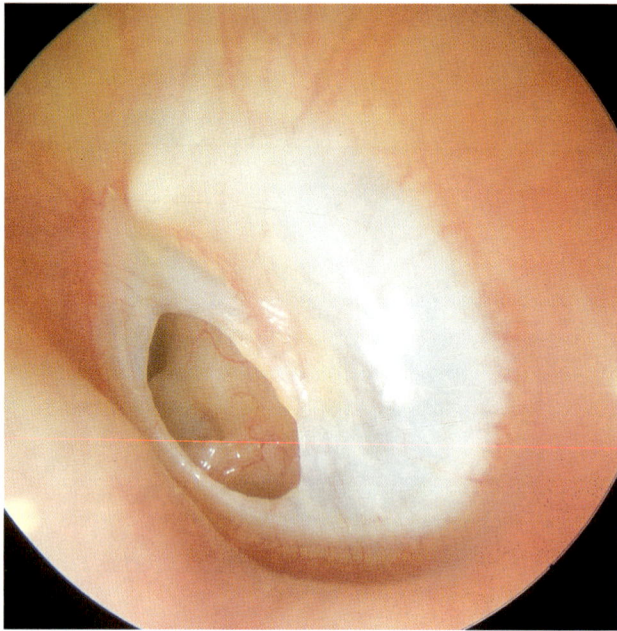

Figure 7.**12**   Left ear. Dry anteroinferior perforation. The middle ear mucosa is normal. The tympanic membrane residue shows tympanosclerosis, giving it a white appearance. The tubal orifice can be seen from the anterior margin of the perforation.

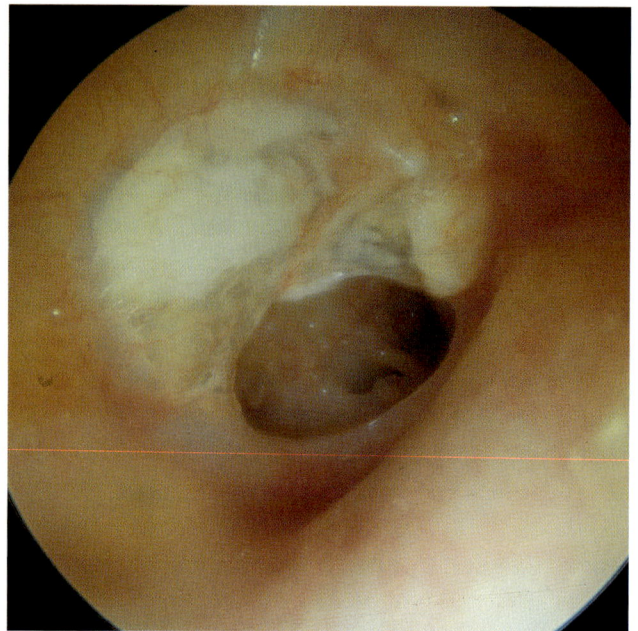

Figure 7.**13**   Right ear. Anteroinferior perforation. The posterior and anterior residues of the tympanic membrane show tympanosclerosis. The anteroinferior residue of the drum is de-epithelialized. The tubal orifice is also visible.

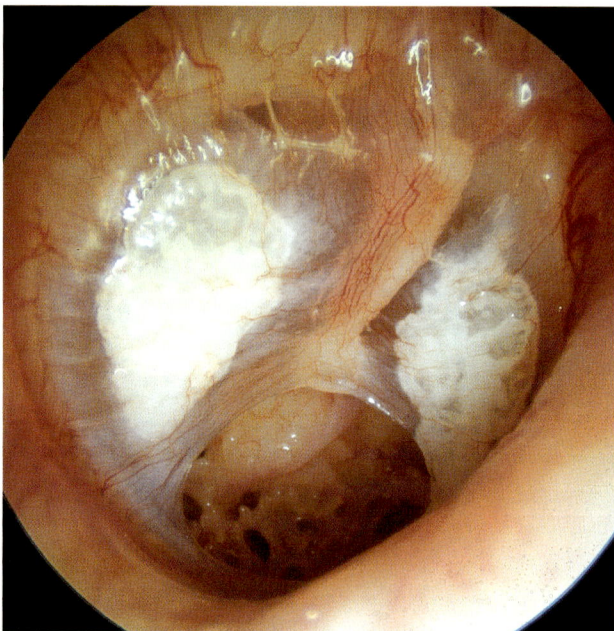

Figure 7.**14**   Right ear. Anteroinferior perforation. Two tympanosclerotic plaques are observed: one anteromalleolar and the other retromalleolar. The middle ear mucosa is normal. The hypotympanic air cells are seen through the perforation.

Subtotal and Total Perforations

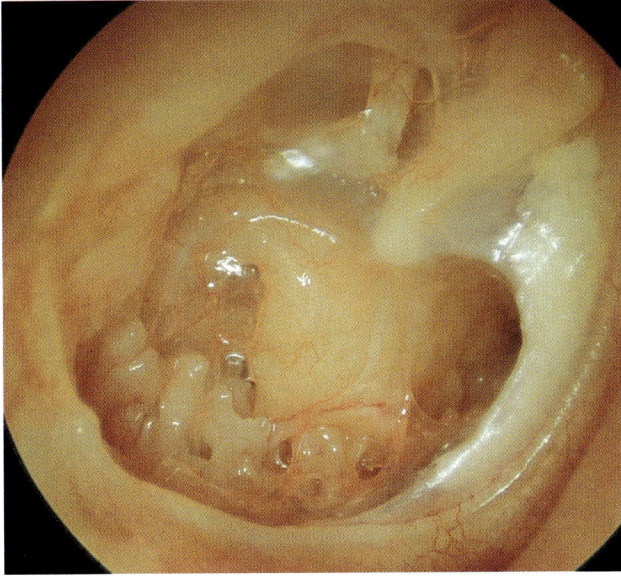

Figure 7.**15** Right ear. Large tympanic membrane perforation. The tubal orifice, the hypotympanic air cells, the promontory, the round and oval windows, and the intact stapes can be viewed. An onset of necrosis of the incus can be distinguished.

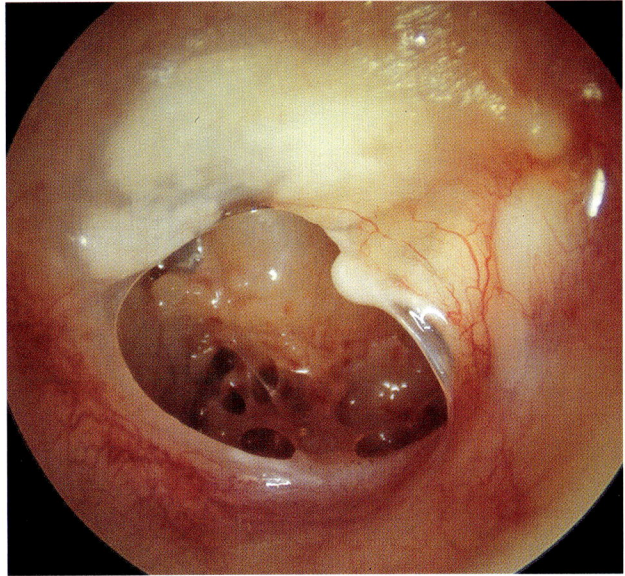

Figure 7.**16** Right ear. Perforation of the inferior quadrants of the tympanic membrane. All the tympanic membrane residue shows dense tympanosclerosis. Removal of these sclerotic plaques during myringoplasty assures an adequate vascularity to the graft, and thus a high success rate for the operation.

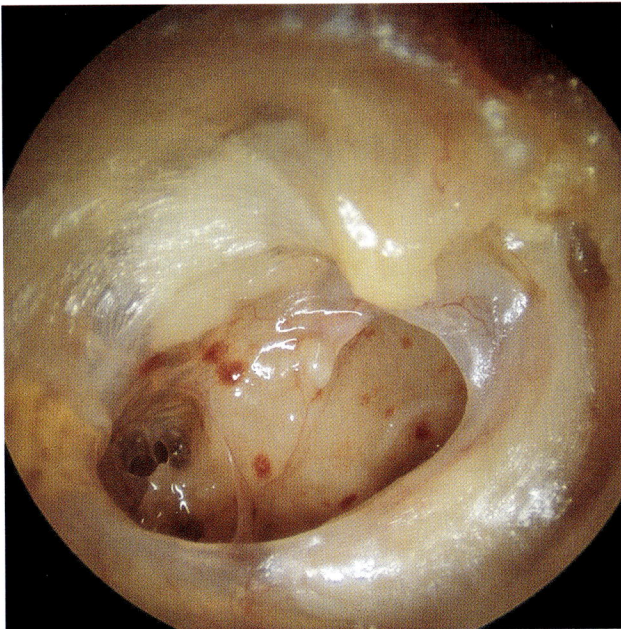

Figure 7.**17** Right ear. Similar case. The promontory and the round window are visible. A tympanosclerotic plaque that engulfs the ossicular chain is seen at the level of the posterosuperior border of the perforation.

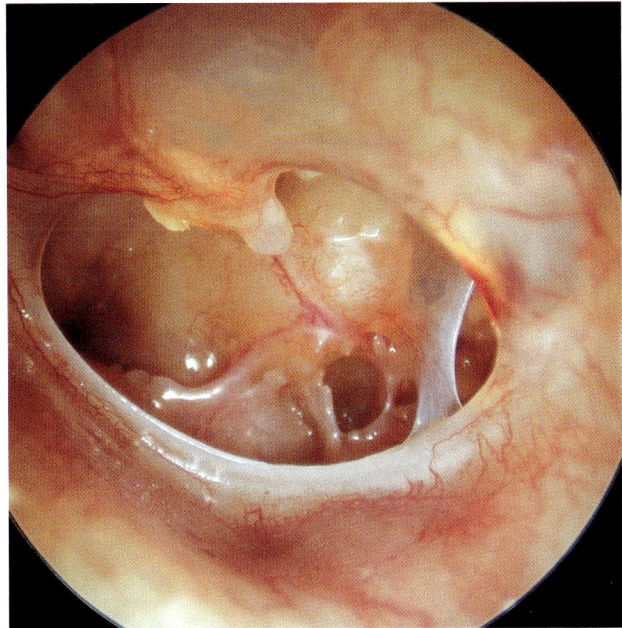

Figure 7.**18** Left ear. Subtotal perforation. The annulus as well as a fibrous rim are visualized along the inferior border of the perforation. The handle of the malleus is medialized. The tubal orifice, the hypotympanic air cells covered with mucosa, Jacobson's nerve on the promontory, and the long process of the incus are visible. The residue of the tympanic membrane is thickened. In cases in which only a small anterior residue of the tympanic membrane is found, an overlay technique in which the graft is put over the annulus is used, thus preventing detachment of the anterior part of the graft leading to reperforation.

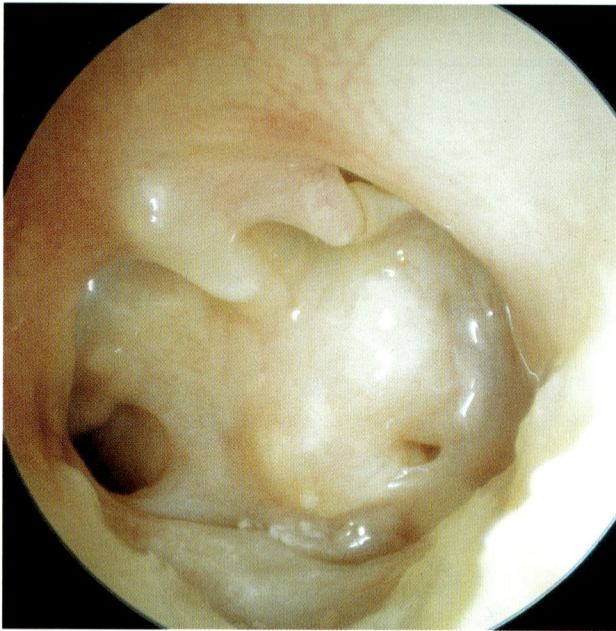

Figure 7.**19**   Left ear. Total perforation of the tympanic membrane through which evolving tympanosclerotic plaques are visible. The stapes and the stapedius tendon are visible. The long process of the incus is partially eroded. The handle of the malleus is medialized and adherent to the promontory. The tubal orifice and the hypotympanic air cells are also noted.

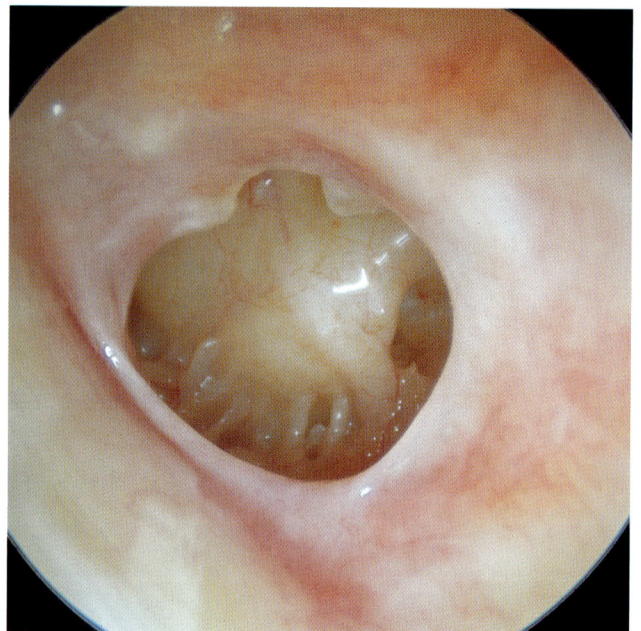

Figure 7.**20**   Left ear. Subtotal perforation of the tym- panic membrane. The middle ear mucosa is normal. The tympanic membrane residue is de-epithelialized. The incudo-stapedial joint, the medialized handle of the malleus, and the hypotympanic air cells are visible.

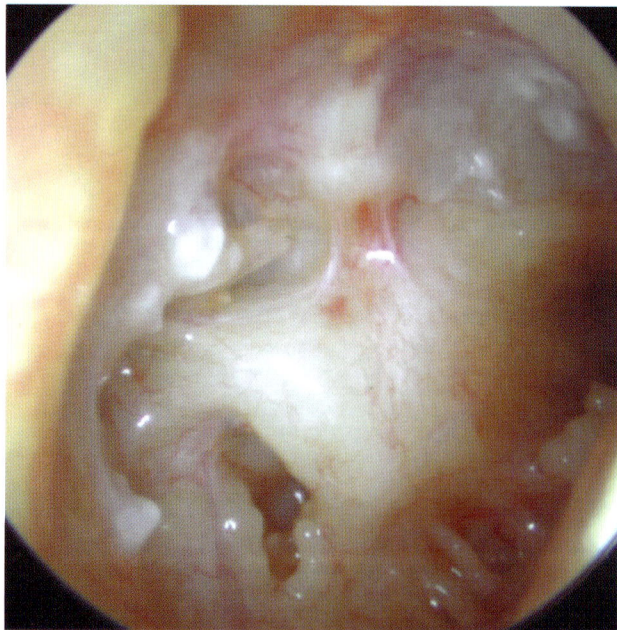

Figure 7.**21**   Right ear. Total perforation, with absence of the annulus. The mucosa of the middle ear is normal. The malleus and incus are absent. The stapes superstructure is present. The round window is clearly seen, as well as the hypotympanic cells and eustachian tube.

Posttraumatic Perforations

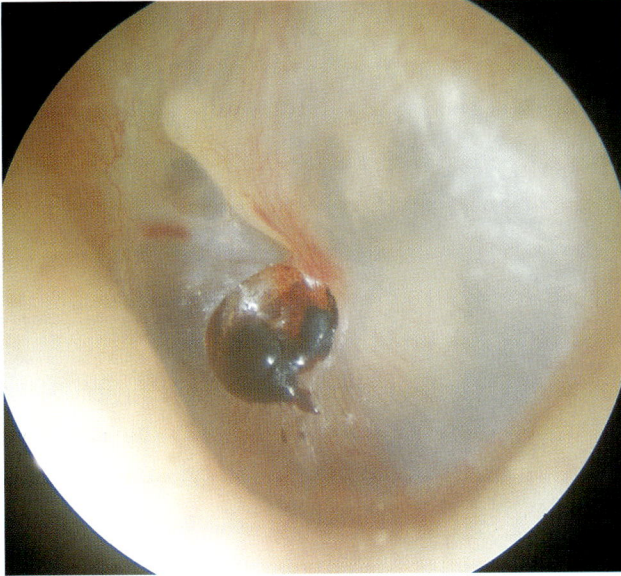

Figure 7.**22** Left ear. Posttraumatic perforation of the tympanic membrane in the region of the cone of light. The blood clot over the perforation has not been removed. This clot helps to guide spontaneous healing of the drum.

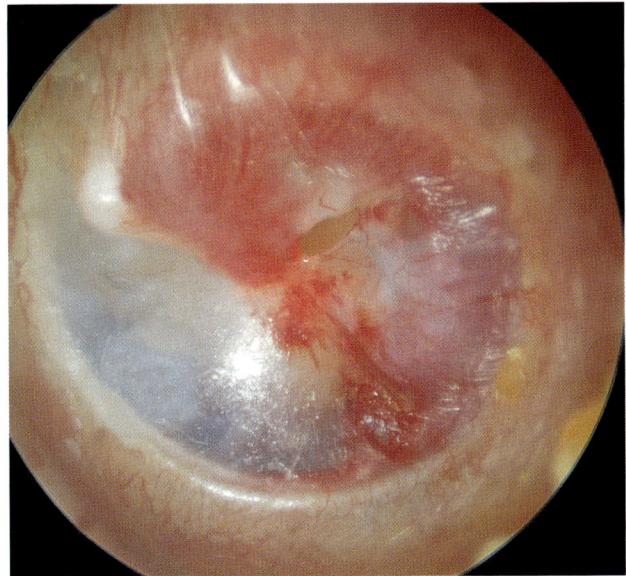

Figure 7.**23** Left ear. Posttraumatic perforation in the postero-superior quadrant. The characteristic radial tear, running in the same direction as the fibers of the tympanic membrane, is apparent. Hemorrhagic points separating the epidermal layer from the fibrous layer are visible. These tiny hemorrhages are typical of posttraumatic perforations. This type of tympanic membrane perforation has a very high incidence of spontaneous healing.

Summary

The presence of a tympanic membrane perforation that does not heal spontaneously, as in chronic otitis media, represents an anatomical and functional defect that needs surgical correction in the majority of cases.

Myringoplasty is indicated in cases with and without otorrhea, with a small or a large air–bone gap, and with no age limit. It is contraindicated when the tympanic membrane perforation is present in the only hearing ear.

Myringoplasty is generally performed using a post-auricular incision under local anesthesia–except for children, in whom general anesthesia is used. The tympanic membrane is repaired by an autologous temporalis fascia graft. We prefer the underlay technique in the majority of cases because it gives better results both anatomically and functionally. The overlay technique is used in selected cases when the anterior residue of the tympanic membrane is pathologic or absent. When properly performed, the overlay technique gives optimal results in these cases. Canalplasty is done whenever bony humps of the external canal are present that limit control of the perforation borders. If reperforation occurs after myringoplasty (in about 5% of cases), a revision operation is indicated after a few months. The results of the first and second operations in terms of graft take and reperforation are generally comparable.

Perforations Complicated or Associated with Other Pathologies

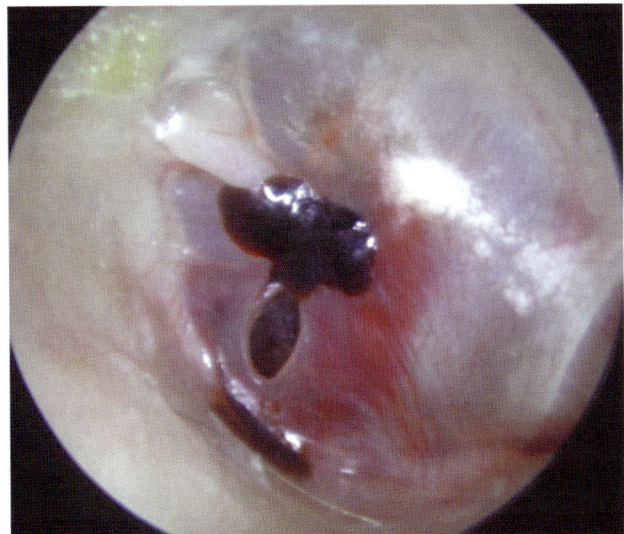

Figure 7.**24** Left ear. Posttraumatic perforation of the tympanic membrane, anterior to the handle of the malleus. A blood clot has not been removed. Generally, posttraumatic perforations heal spontaneously.

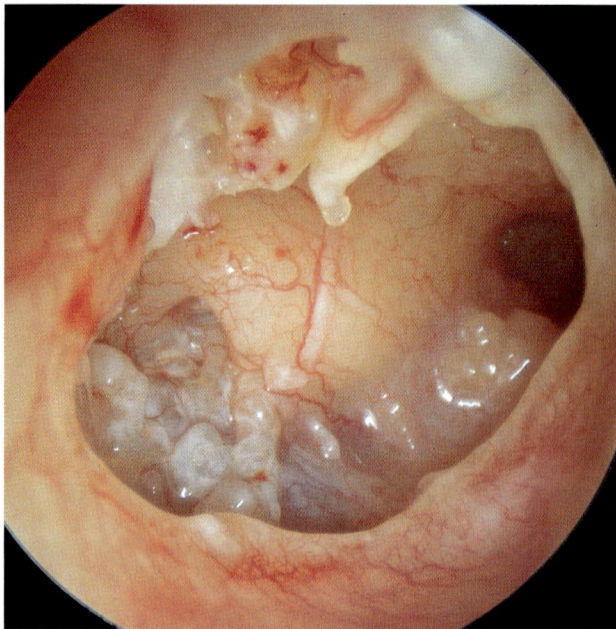

Figure 7.**25**   Right ear. Total perforation. Epidermization is present in the regions of the mesotympanum and the ossicular chain. The round window, hypotympanic air cells with thickened mucosa, Jacobson's nerve running on the promontory, and the tubal orifice are well visualized. This case is an example of chronic otitis media complicated by the presence of skin in the middle ear. Tympanoplasty should be staged. In the first stage, the skin is removed without traumatizing the ossicular chain, and the tympanic membrane is reconstructed. In the second stage, the middle ear is checked for any residual skin, and the ossicular chain is reconstructed.

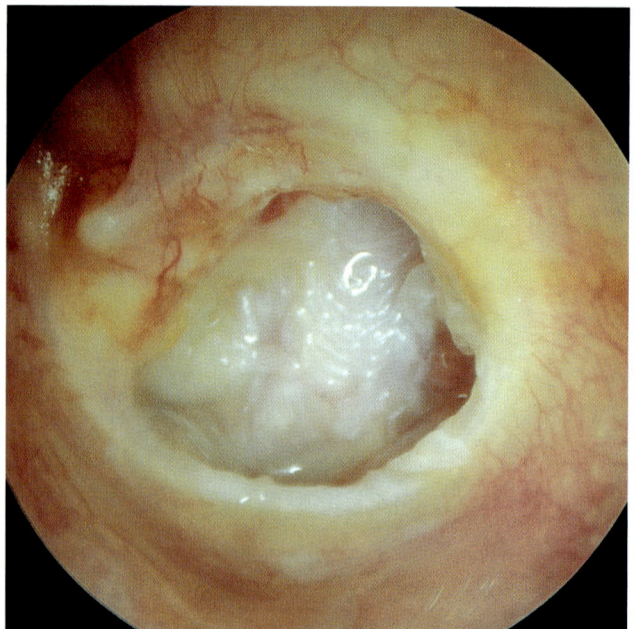

Figure 7.**26**   Left ear. Large perforation with diffuse epidermization of the middle ear associated with purulent otorrhea. In these cases, even if the ossicular chain proves intact, mastoid exploration should be done. A second stage is performed 1 year after the first operation to check for any skin residues.

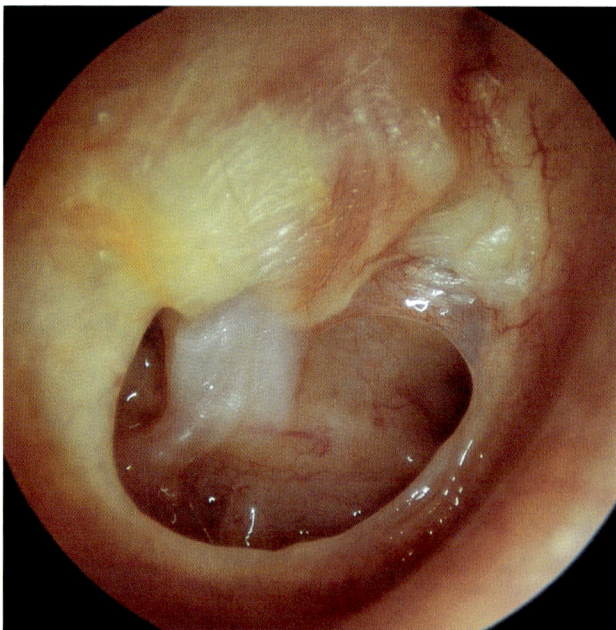

Figure 7.**27**   Right ear. Perforation of the inferior quadrants of the tympanic membrane, the residues of which show tympanosclerosis. Epidermization is evident over the promontory. Since epidermization is limited in this case, a single-stage tympanoplasty can be performed.

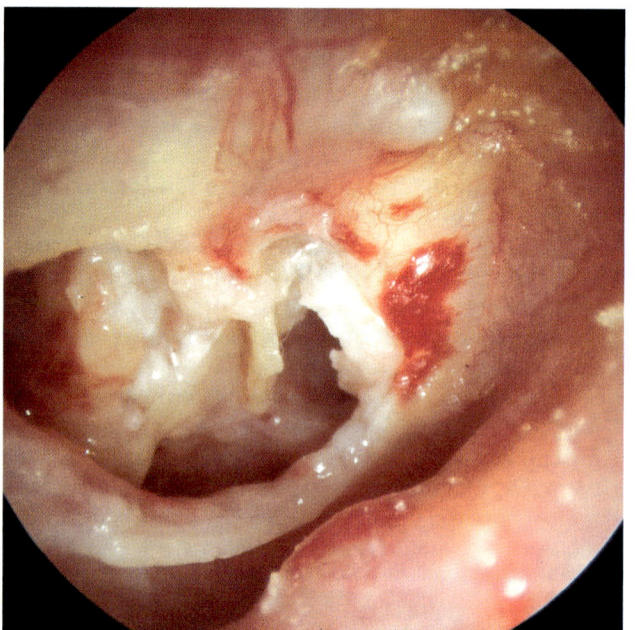

Figure 7.**28**   Right ear. Another example of chronic otitis media complicated with diffuse epidermization of the middle ear. Surgery follows the same rules as for cholesteatoma.

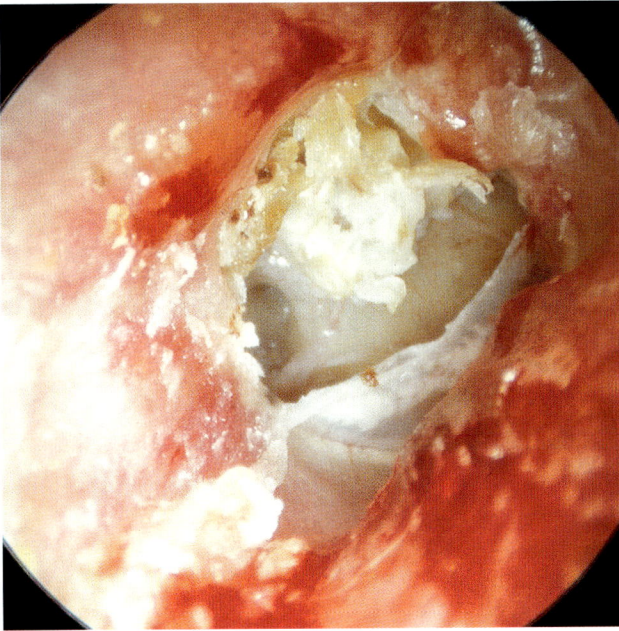

Figure 7.29 Right ear. Large tympanic membrane perforation. The anterior drum residue shows tympanosclerosis. The ossicular chain is difficult to identify because of the presence of epidermization at this level. The round window is visible. A staged tympanoplasty is also indicated in this case.

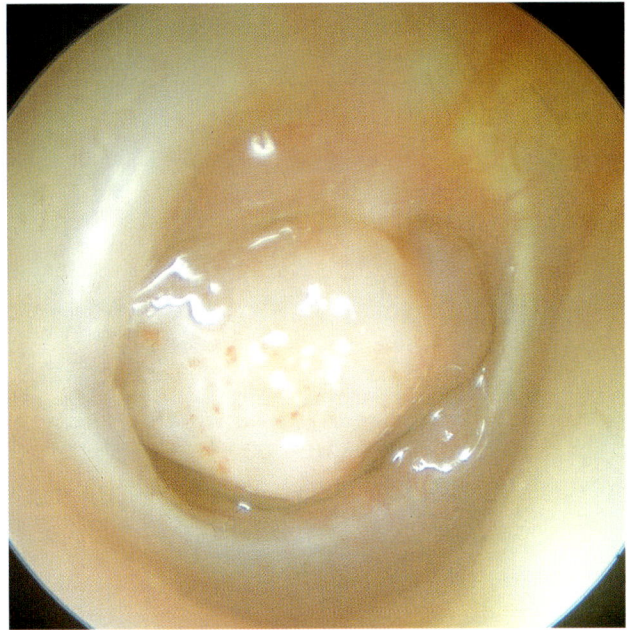

Figure 7.30 Right ear. Granulomatous otitis media. A roundish mass fills the middle ear. Serous otorrhea is present.

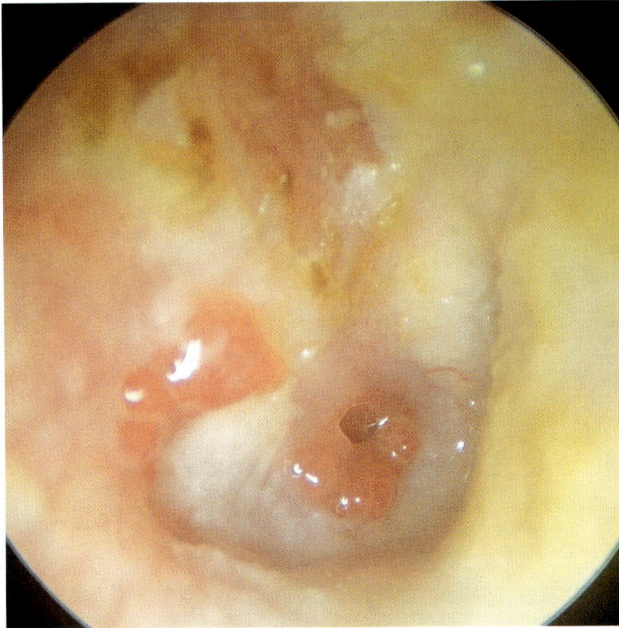

Figure 7.31 Right ear. Small perforation of the inferior quadrants of the tympanic membrane, with eversion of the mucosa onto the outer layer of the membrane. Tympanosclerosis, both antero- and posteromalleolar, can be observed.

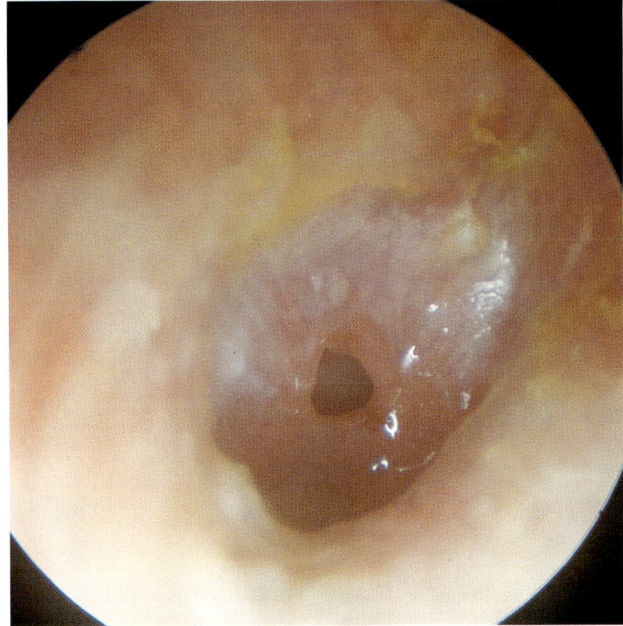

Figure 7.32 Right ear. Case similar to that in Figure 7.31. The mucosa has replaced the epithelial layer. Ear discharge is also present. During myringoplasty, curettage of the everted mucosa is necessary until the fibrous layer of the tympanic membrane is reached.

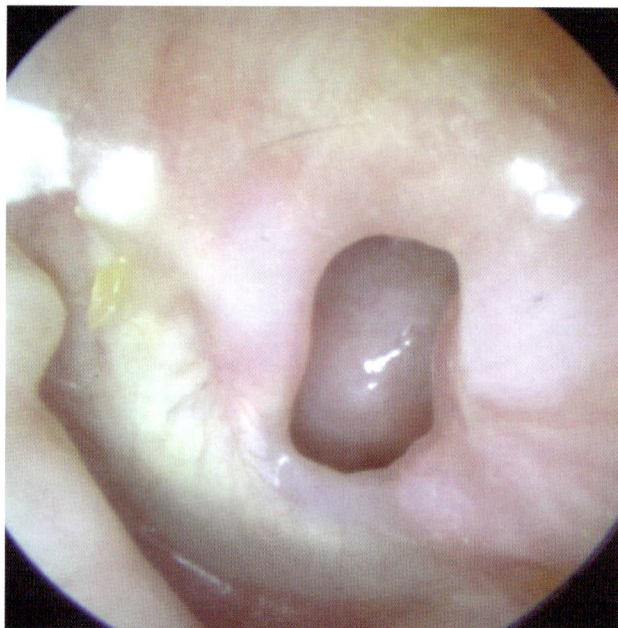

Figure 7.**33**   Left ear. Central perforation. The patient complained of otorrhea. Surgery is indicated. The thicker, disepithelialized part of the tympanic membrane must be removed before reconstruction.

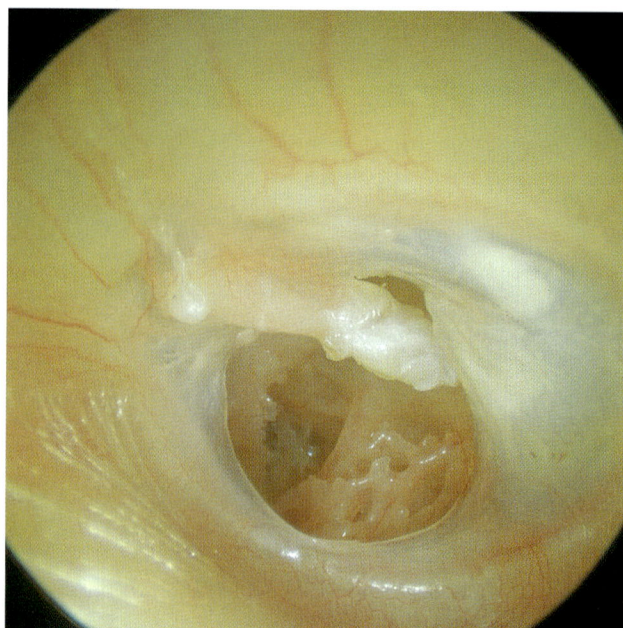

Figure 7.**34**   Left ear. Perforation of the anterior quadrants. Skin envelopes the handle of the malleus. During myringoplasty, curettage of the skin is necessary before reconstruction.

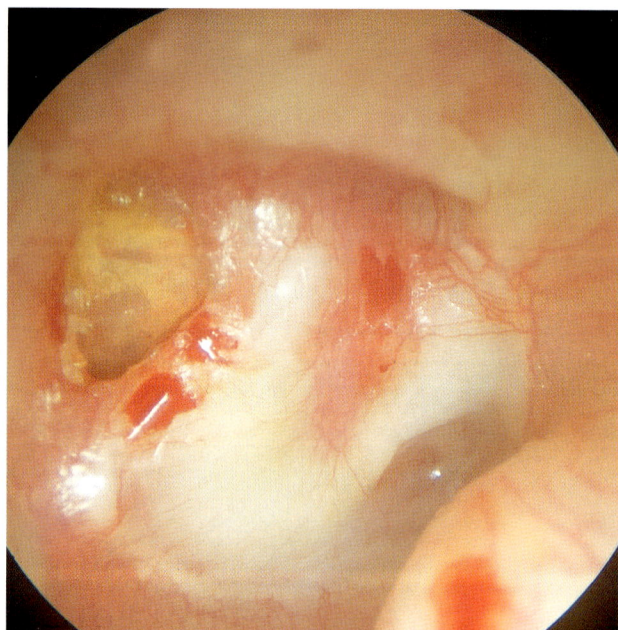

Figure 7.**35**   Right ear. Posterior perforation. The residues of the tympanic membrane appear whitish and bulging. During surgery, the middle ear was occupied by granulomatous tissue that proved to be tuberculosis (TB) on histopathological examination. This patient had a past history of pulmonary TB. Tuberculous otitis media should be suspected in cases of pulmonary TB presenting with otorrhea.

Tympanosclerosis

Tympanosclerosis is characterized by fibroblastic invasion of the submucosal spaces of the middle ear followed by thickening, hyalinization, and fusion of collagen fibers into a homogenous mass with calcium deposits and phosphate crystals. Though the pathogenesis is not yet clear, it seems that chronic otitis media is a predisposing factor. Two distinct forms are recognized:

Tympanosclerosis with intact tympanic membrane. This is characterized by calcareous plaques (chalk patches) in the fibrous layer of the tympanic membrane. The antero- and posteromalleolar regions are usually involved. The periannular region of the inferior quadrants is also affected, forming a horseshoe pattern. The pars tensa is rigid, thick, and loses its elasticity, assuming a whitish aspect. Atrophic and thinned areas can also occur. Infrequently, in very advanced cases, the tympanosclerotic plaques occupy all the middle ear spaces, attic, and aditus and completely block the ossicular chain. The tympanic membrane in these cases is very thick or even replaced by the plaques.

Tympanosclerosis associated with tympanic membrane perforation. The perforation is frequently central or subtotale, and the annulus, infiltrated by calcium deposits, is well visualized. Frequently, submucous nodular deposits are encountered in the middle ear. Ossicular fixation or erosion due to devitalization as a result of loss of blood supply can also occur. The middle ear mucosa is very thin, with reduced vascularity. In some cases, tympanosclerotic plaques are seen extruding from the mucosa to present as white middle ear masses.

Tympanosclerosis Associated with Perforation

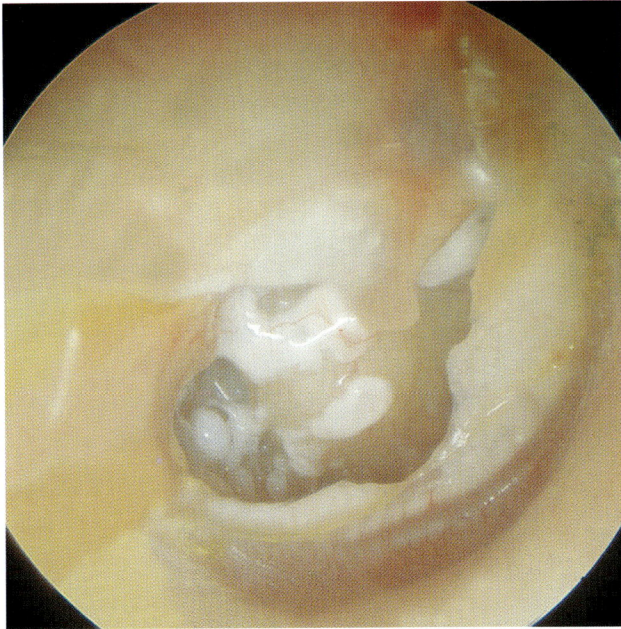

Figure 7.**36**   Right ear. Tympanosclerosis associated with perforation. The tympanic membrane residues and the middle ear (promontory and hypotympanum) show the characteristic plaques. The malleus is blocked by tympanosclerosis.

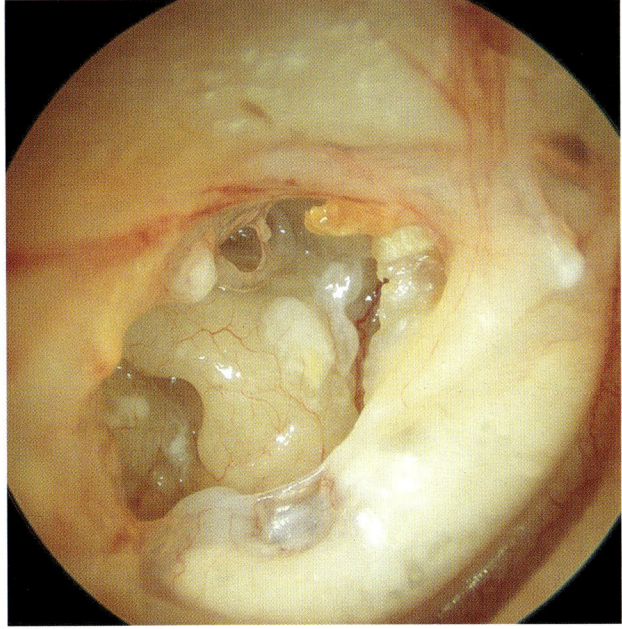

Figure 7.**37**   Right ear. Tympanosclerosis with perforation. A large tympanosclerotic plaque is noted in the anterior residue of the tympanic membrane. The middle ear is also involved. The promontory, oval window, stapes footplate, and round window can be appreciated.

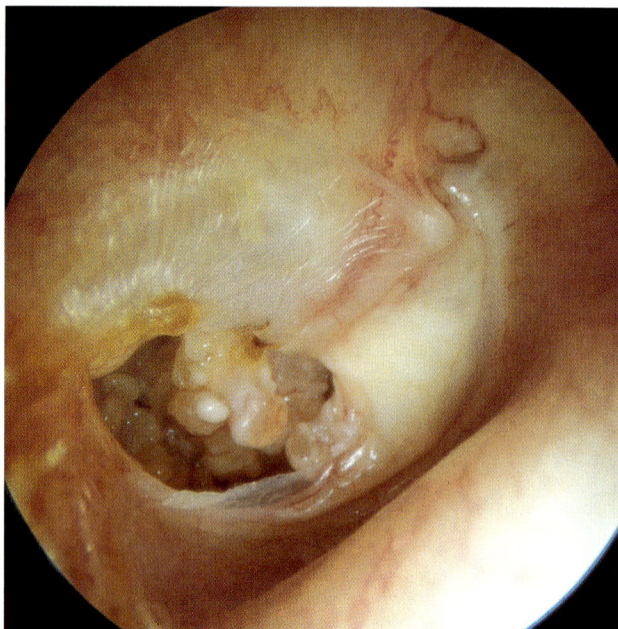

Figure 7.**38**   Right ear. Perforations of the inferior quadrants with tympanosclerosis involving the residues of the tympanic membrane and the middle ear.

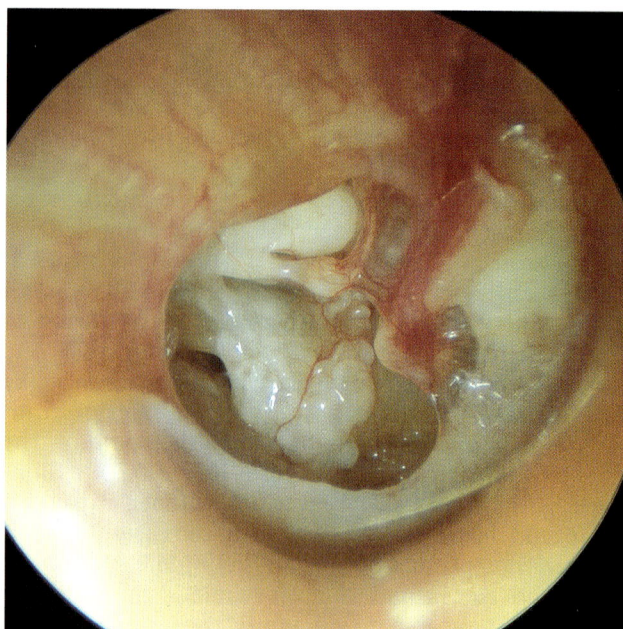

Figure 7.**39**   Right ear. Tympanosclerosis with perforation. The tympanosclerotic process involves the anterior residues of the tympanic membrane and the mucosa of the promontory reaching to the posterior mesotympanum. At this level, ossification of the stapedius tendon is seen. The tympanic segment of the fallopian canal is covered by a sclerotic plaque. The long process of the incus is eroded.

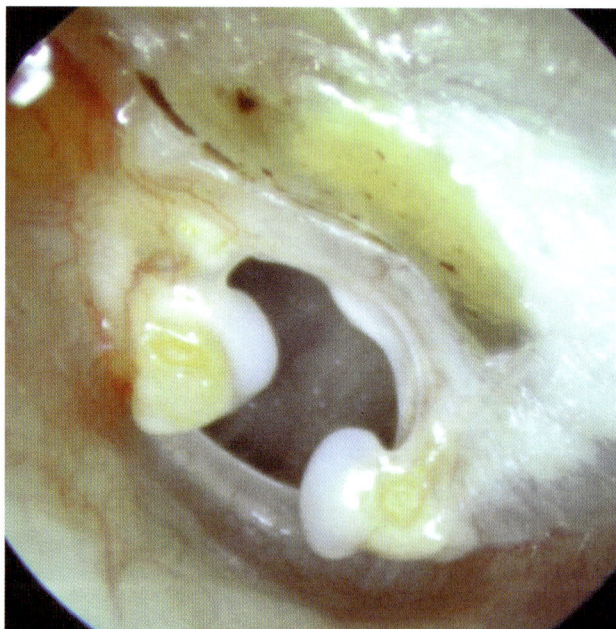

Figure 7.**40**   Left ear. An anterior dry perforation, with tympanosclerosis in the residual tympanic membrane, is visible.

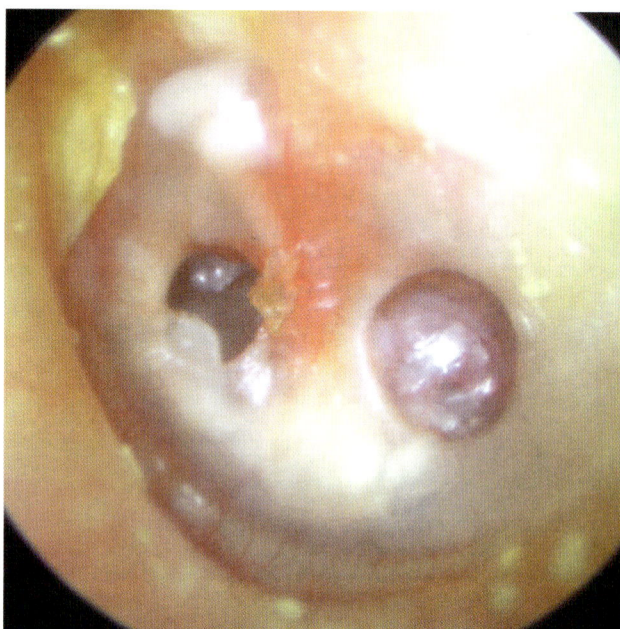

Figure 7.**41**   Left ear. Tympanosclerotic appearance of the tympanic membrane, with an anteromalleolar perforation and posteromalleolar inflammatory polyp.

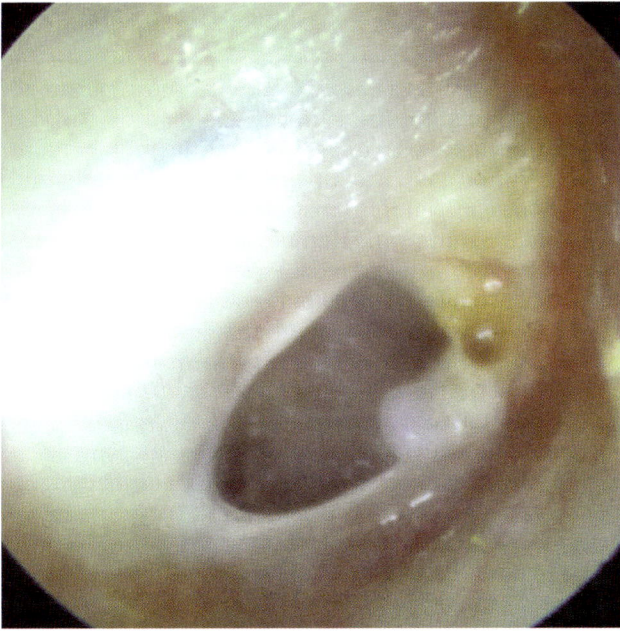

Figure 7.**42** Right ear. An anteroinferior perforation is present. The middle ear mucosa is normal. The residual tympanic membrane shows thick tympanosclerosis.

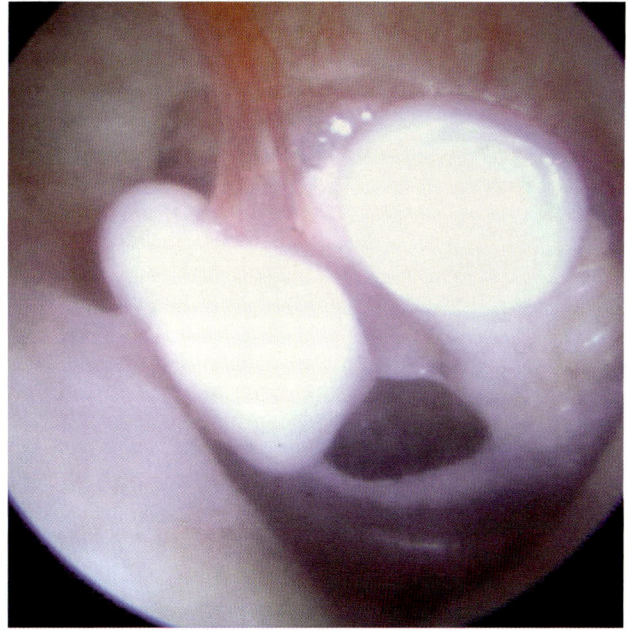

Figure 7.**43** Left ear. Central inferior perforation. Two white tympanosclerotic plaques are present anteriorly and posteriorly to the malleus.

Tympanosclerosis with Intact Tympanic Membrane

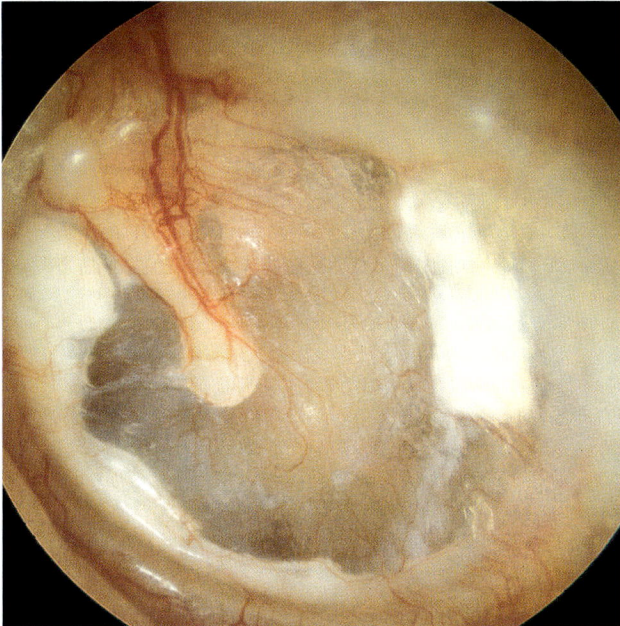

Figure 7.**44** Left ear. Tympanosclerosis and intact drum. The majority of the tympanic membrane is thinned due to atrophy of the fibrous layer. Two tympanosclerotic plaques are present near the anterior and posterior margins.

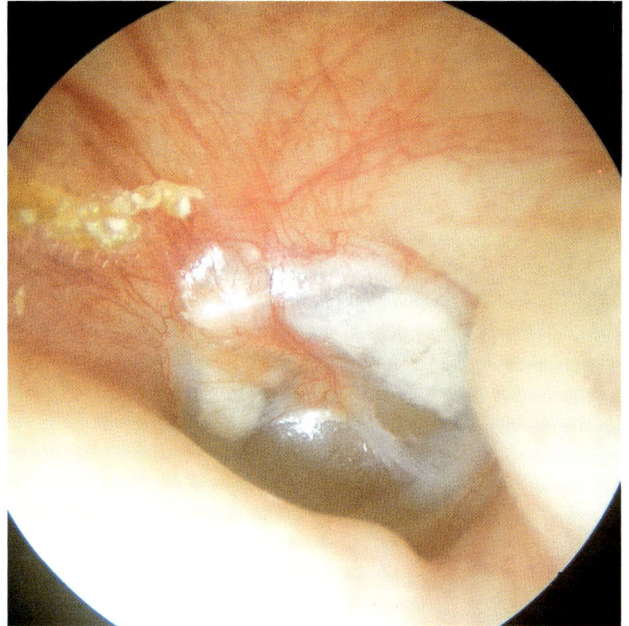

Figure 7.**45** Left ear. The intact tympanic membrane shows tympanosclerotic plaques lying both anterior and posterior to the malleus that alternate with areas of atrophy (in the inferior quadrants).

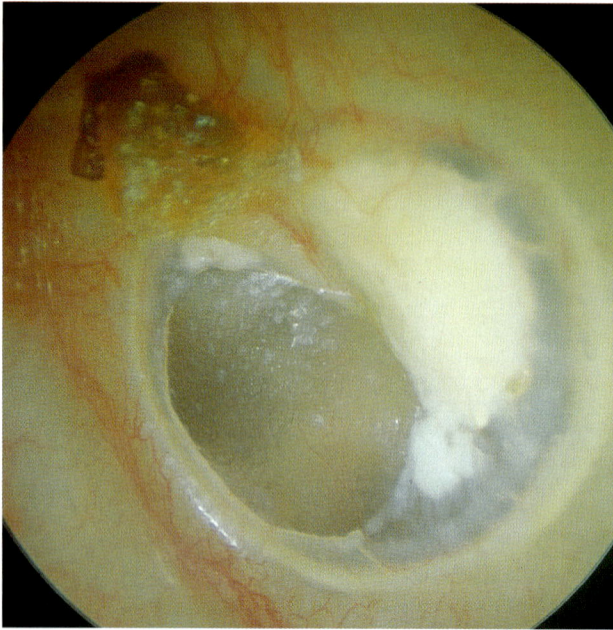

Figure 7.**46**   Left ear. Tympanosclerosis with intact drum. A large plaque is visible in the posterior quadrants of the tympanic membrane. The anterior quadrants are thinned and atrophic, allowing visualization of the tubal orifice.

Summary

Chronic otitis media associated with tympanosclerosis represents a more complex anatomopathological entity. In cases with intact tympanic membrane, surgery is indicated in the presence of a significant air–bone gap, signifying ossicular chain involvement. Should erosion or fixation of the ossicles be found, ossiculoplasty is performed. Fixation of the stapes is an indication for stapedotomy.

In cases associated with tympanic membrane perforation, it is often possible to perform a single-stage reconstruction in which myringoplasty is performed with or without ossiculoplasty. A fixed stapes, however, is an indication for staging, where myringoplasty is performed first, followed by a second-stage stapedotomy after a few months. In all suspected cases, the patient should be informed preoperatively of the possibility of staging surgery.

In a small percentage of cases of chronic otitis media with tympanosclerosis, a good postoperative functional level can deteriorate with time due to refixation of the ossicular chain, with a consequent air–bone gap. In such cases, after achieving closure of the tympanic membrane, a hearing aid is recommended.

8 Chronic Suppurative Otitis Media with Cholesteatoma

Cholesteatoma is an epidermal inclusion cyst localized in the middle ear, whose capsule and matrix is formed from stratified squamous epithelium. The desquamating debris includes pearly white lamellae of keratin that accumulate concentrically, forming the cholesteatomatous mass.

The term *cholesteatoma* is actually a misnomer. It is derived from the Greek "chole" or bile, "steatos" or fat, and "oma" or tumor. There is no relation between cholesteatoma and bile or fat. The suffix "oma" (tumor), however, is more appropriate because cholesteatoma can be considered an epidermal inclusion cyst.

Cholesteatoma can be divided into congenital (middle ear or petrous bone) and acquired (middle ear or petrous bone). Congenital cholesteatoma is derived from entrapped ectodermal cellular debris during embryonic development. When it involves the middle ear, it appears as a whitish retrotympanic mass that may be localized either anterior or posterior to the malleus (see Chapter 9). When it involves the petrous part of the temporal bone, it is termed *congenital petrous bone cholesteatoma* and in the majority of cases it is localized in the petrous apex (see Chapter 10). In this chapter we will deal exclusively with cholesteatoma involving the middle ear. Petrous bone cholesteatoma is dealt with in a later chapter.

Acquired cholesteatoma of the middle ear can be caused by invasion of the skin of the external auditory canal into the middle ear through a marginal perforation. It can also originate from a epitympanic retraction pocket that becomes so deep that keratin debris can no longer be expelled, leading to its accumulation and subsequent cholesteatoma formation. Such retraction pockets can remain asymptomatic until they become infected, resulting in otorrhea and hearing loss. In other cases, the only symptom might be progressive hearing loss due to erosion of the ossicular chain by the developing cholesteatoma.

Because it is not always easy to establish a clear distinction between epitympanic or posterosuperior retraction pockets and cholesteatoma, we prefer to follow up these patients with otomicroscopy and endoscopy. In cases in which the retraction pocket becomes deep, giving rise to a cholesteatoma, a tympanoplasty is indicated. Because of the early stage of the disease, surgery can be done in a single stage.

Fetid otorrhea and hearing loss are the main complaints in cholesteatoma. In addition, complicated cases can manifest with vertigo and/or facial nerve paralysis. Vertigo occurs as a result of labyrinthine fistula, which is most commonly located in the lateral semicircular canal. Facial paralysis can be caused by pressure of the cholesteatoma sac or neuritis.

In rare cases, the cholesteatoma can invade the labyrinth, cochlea, posterior and middle fossa durae, the internal auditory canal, and the petrous apex, forming a petrous bone cholesteatoma (see Chapter 10).

Treatment of cholesteatoma is exclusively surgical. Early this century, radical mastoidectomy, a destructive procedure for the middle ear, was performed with the only goal being eradication of infection to save the ear.

In the early 1950s, the concept of tympanoplasty was introduced. Tympanoplasty was aimed at eradication of infection as well as reconstruction of the tympano-ossicular system. Today, two types of tympanoplasty are employed: closed tympanoplasty, in which the posterior canal wall is preserved, and open tympanoplasty, in which the posterior canal wall is drilled. Both techniques, when performed appropriately and with the proper indications, can produce excellent results in terms of eradication of cholesteatoma and restoration of hearing. In children, the closed technique is preferred, performed in two stages, in the majority of cases due to cildren's highly cellular mastoids and in an attempt to preserve the anatomy of the ear as much as possible. In adults, particularly in epitympanic cholesteatoma with marked erosion of the scutum, in cases with sclerotic mastoids, or when middle ear atelectasis is present, an open tympanoplasty is performed (see also Chapter 14).

Epitympanic Retraction Pocket

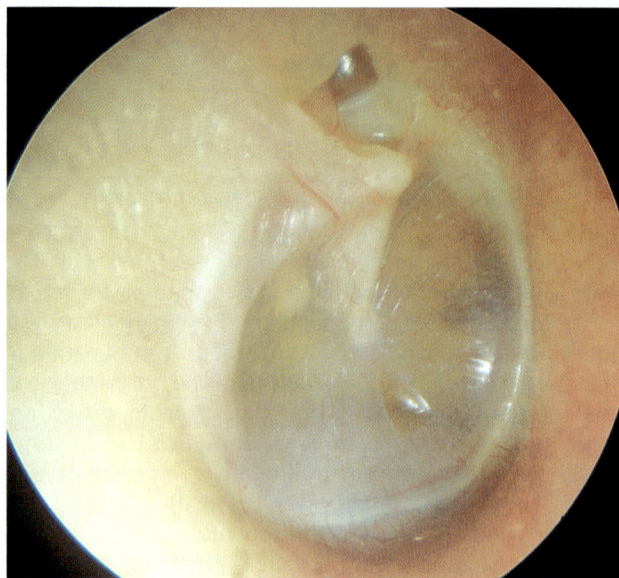

Figure 8.**1** Right ear. Early epitympanic retraction pocket. The tympanic membrane shows grade I atelectasis. Middle ear effusion with characteristic yellowish coloration of the drum is seen. In the anterosuperior quadrant, the tubal orifice is visible in transparency, whereas the long process of the incus is evident in the posterosuperior quadrant. In the area of the cone of light, an atrophic part of the tympanic membrane due to a previous myringotomy can be appreciated.

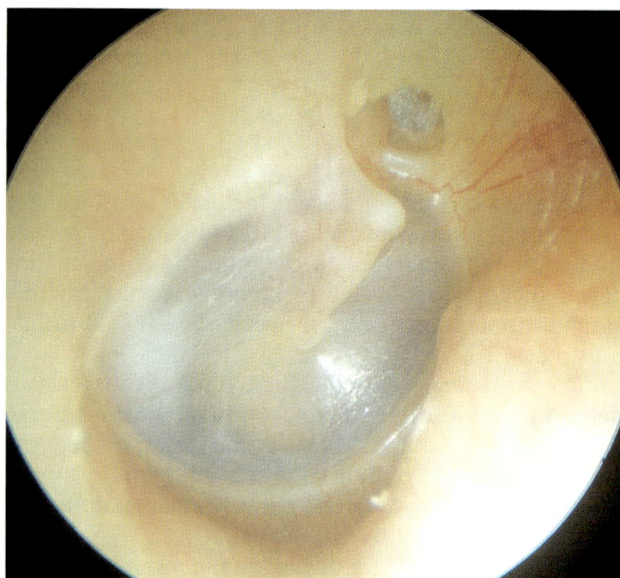

Figure 8.**2** Right ear. Epitympanic retraction pocket with the onset of tympanosclerosis of the pars tensa of the tympanic membrane.

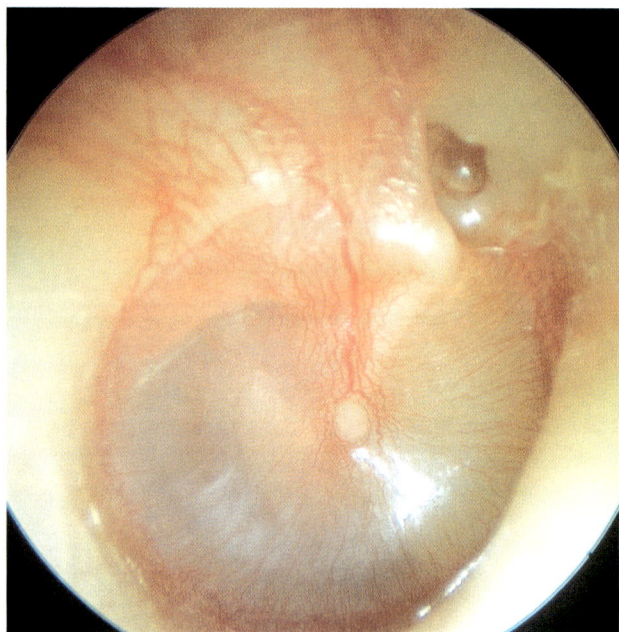

Figure 8.**3** Right ear, similar case. The anterior quadrants of the pars tensa are retracted and thickened.

Figure 8.**4** Right ear. A large controllable epitympanic retraction pocket with erosion of the scutum. The head of the malleus is seen. Middle ear effusion gives the tympanic membrane the characteristic yellowish coloration. To prevent progression of the retraction pocket and the formation of adhesions, myringotomy, ventilation tube insertion, and regular follow-up are indicated. These cases frequently represent the transition from a

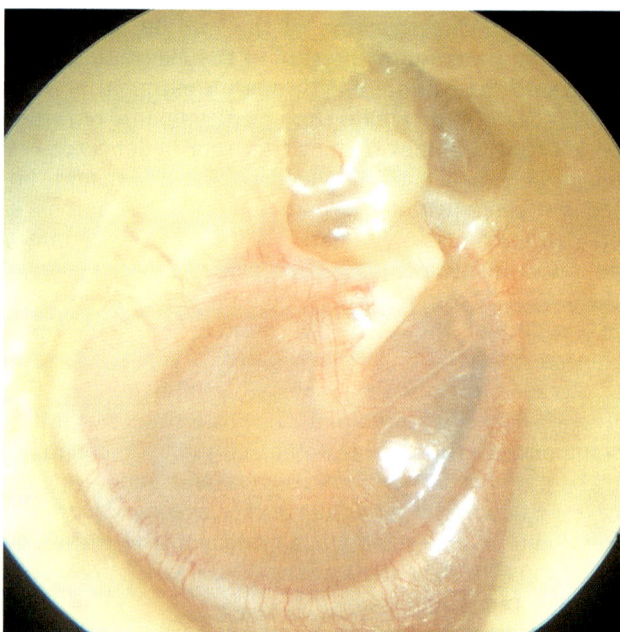

simple retraction pocket to an initial attic cholesteatoma. The distinction between the two is sometimes difficult. In suspected cases, a high-resolution computed tomography (CT) scan (bone window) is beneficial for better evaluation of the extension of the retraction pocket. In cases where the condition remains stable with regular follow-up and where hearing is normal, no surgery is required. If the pocket extends deeper, giving rise to a frank cholesteatoma, surgery is indicated. If hearing is normal, an open tympanoplasty (modified Bondy technique) is performed in a single stage.

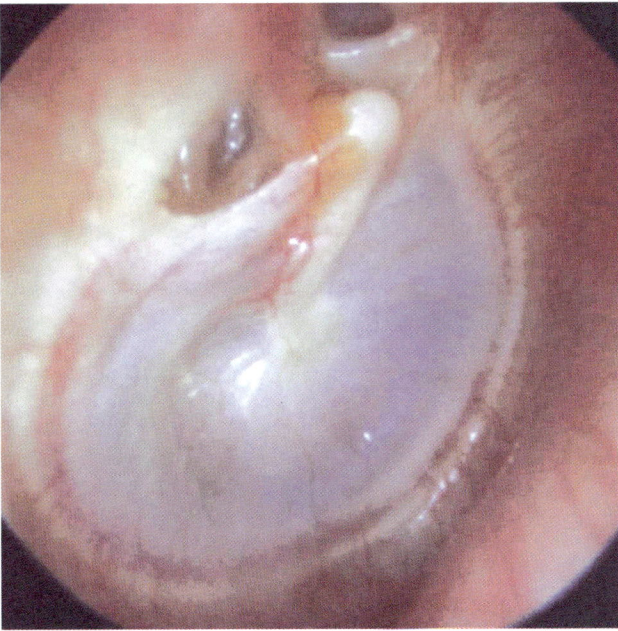

Figure 8.**5**   Right ear. An epitympanic and postmalleolar retraction pocket that can be monitored endoscopically. The pars tensa is thick, with some slide retraction. In this case, surgery is not indicated, but regular endoscopic follow-up examinations are necessary.

Epitympanic Cholesteatoma

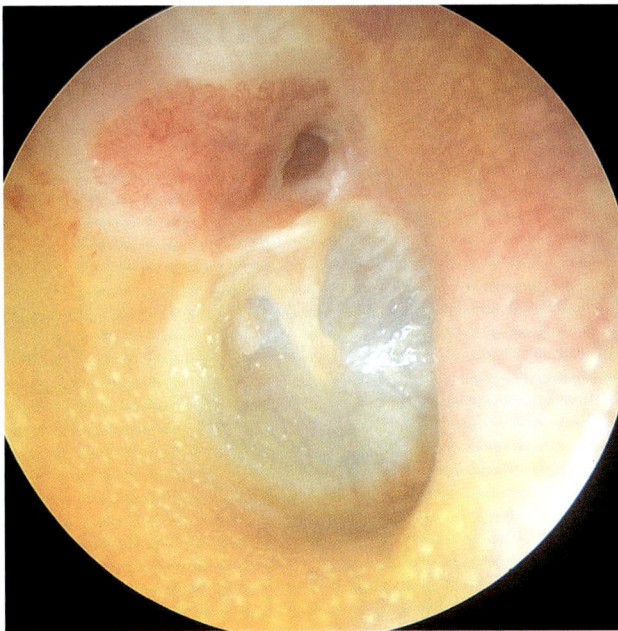

Figure 8.**6**   Right ear. Epitympanic erosion with cholesteatoma. The patient complained of fetid otorrhea and attacks of bloody ear discharge of several years' duration. Inflammatory tissue is seen surrounding the area of epitympanic erosion. As preoperative hearing was nearly normal (see audiogram, Fig. 8.**7**), a single-stage open tympanoplasty in the form of a modified Bondy technique was performed. This technique allows eradication of the cholesteatoma and also conserves hearing (for the modified Bondy technique, see Chapter 13).

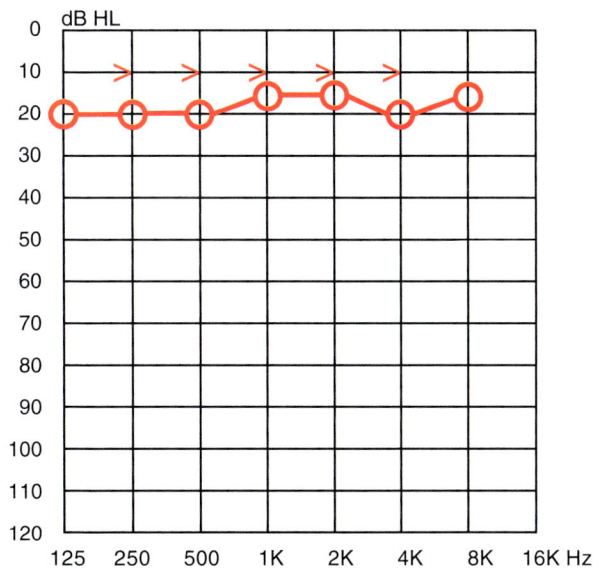

Figure 8.**7**   Audiometry of the case described in Figure 8.**6**. Normal preoperative hearing.

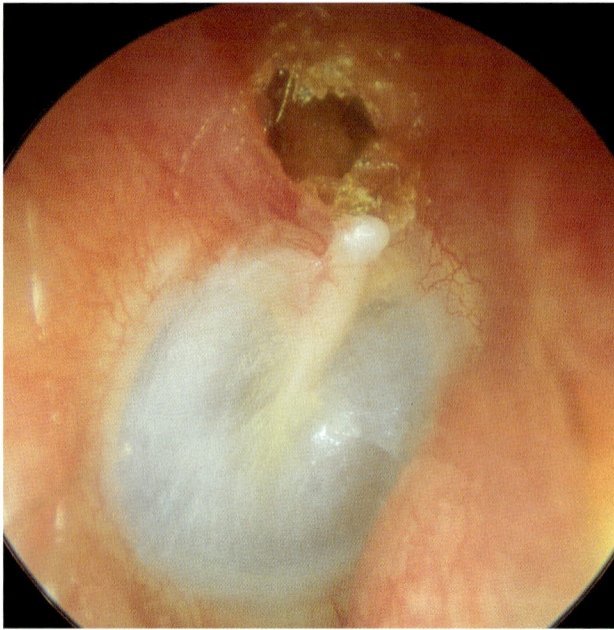

Figure 8.**8**   Right ear. Epitympanic erosion with cholesteatoma. The tympanic membrane is completely tympanosclerotic. The patient did not complain of otorrhea (dry cholesteatoma).

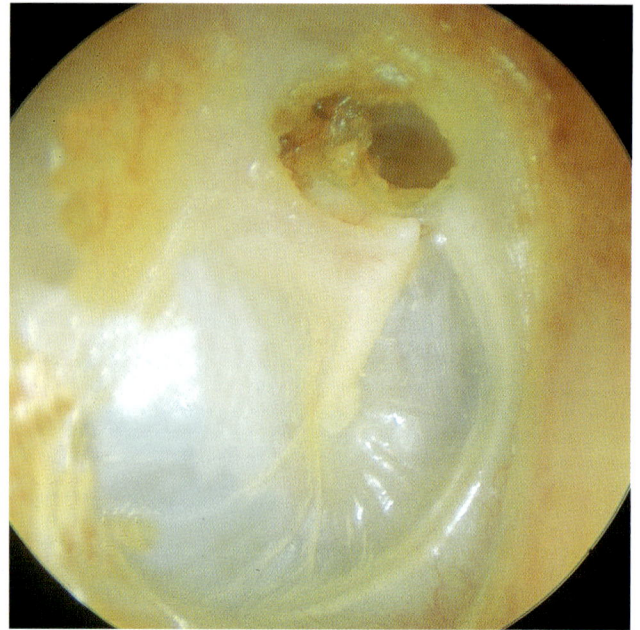

Figure 8.**9**   Right ear. Epitympanic erosion with cholesteatomatous squamae. The patient did not complain of otorrhea. The pars tensa is intact. Intraoperatively, the cholesteatoma was found to have partially eroded the head of the malleus and the short process of the incus. The ossicular chain, however, maintained its continuity. A modified Bondy technique was performed and the normal preoperative hearing was conserved.

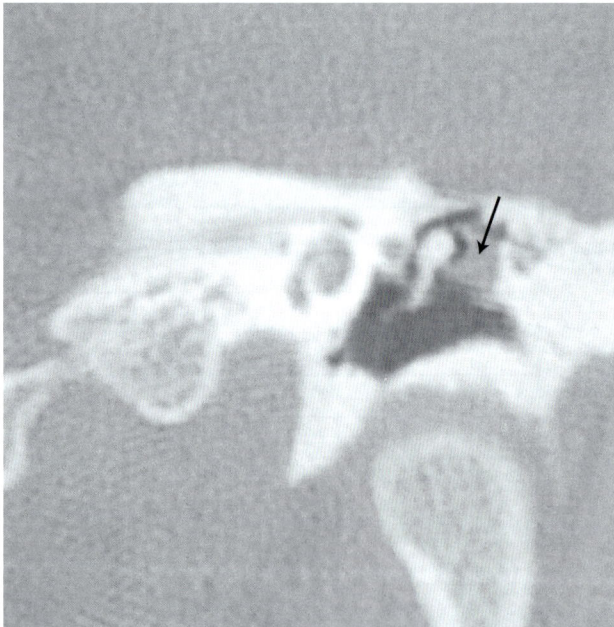

Figure 8.**10**   CT of the previous case, coronal view. The cholesteatoma is located in the epitympanic area. The middle ear is free.

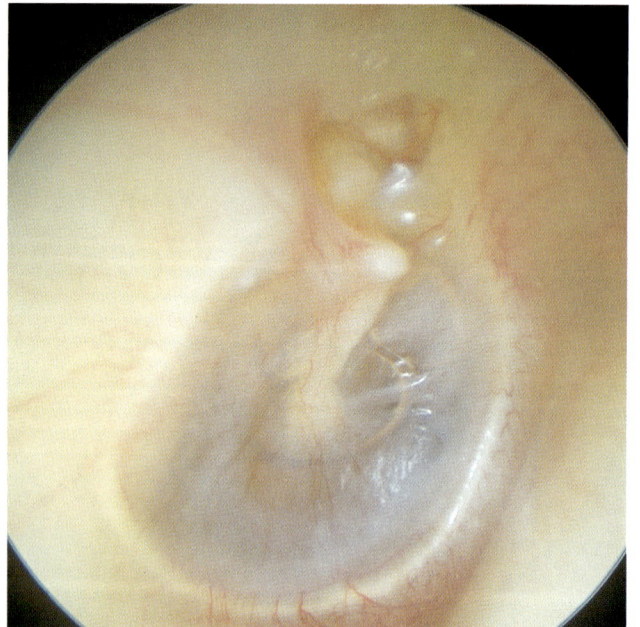

Figure 8.**11**   Right ear of a 46-year-old patient suffering from bilateral cholesteatoma. An epitympanic erosion with cholesteatoma and middle ear effusion showing an air–fluid level can be seen. CT scan (Fig. 8.**13**) demonstrates choles-teatoma extension into the mastoid. Intraoperatively, a fistula of the lateral semicircular canal was encountered, as well as erosion of the incus. A single-stage open tympanoplasty was performed with autologous incus interposition between the handle of the malleus and the head of the stapes. In patients with bilateral cholesteatoma, an open technique is preferred.

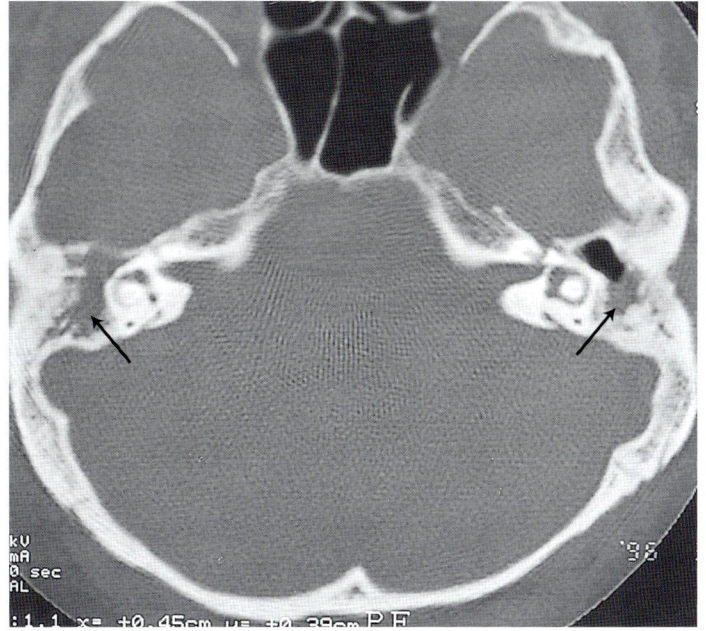

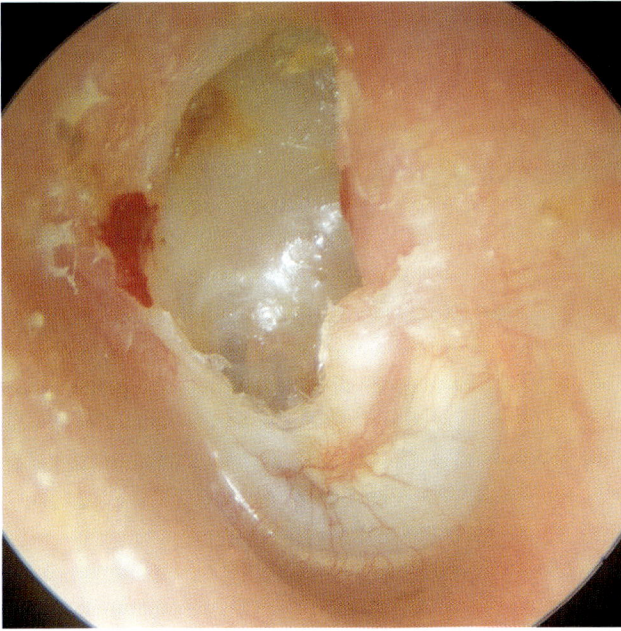

Figure 8.**12**   Left ear of the same patient. Cholesteatoma with marked erosion of the scutum and epidermization of the attic and mesotympanum. The cholesteatoma debris was partially cleaned. The residual pars tensa shows tympanosclerosis. Intraoperatively, the ossicular chain was absent. The otoscopic view of the left ear is apparently more advanced than the right ear. This, however, was not the case intraoperatively since the marked epitympanic erosion shown here allowed self-cleaning of the cholesteatoma debris (see CT scan, Fig. 8.**13**). Because of the total destruction of the ossicular chain, a second stage was programmed for functional reconstruction.

Figure 8.**13**   CT of the previous case showing cholesteatoma extension in the mastoid in the right ear and self-cleaning of the cholesteatoma debris in the left ear.

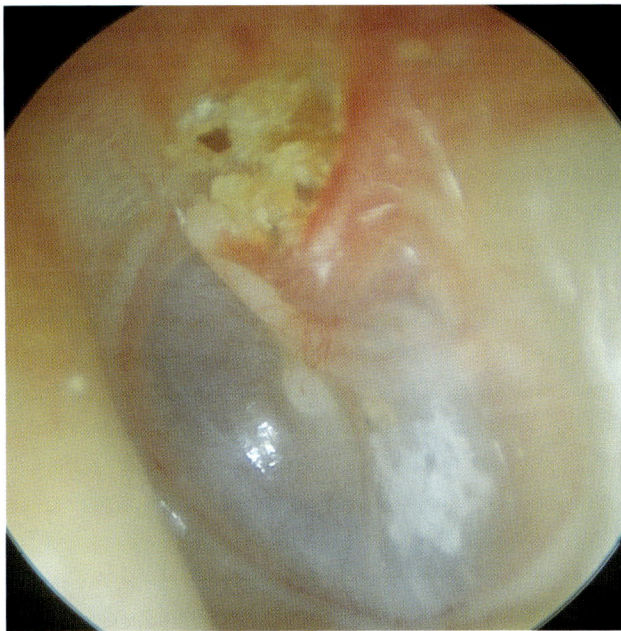

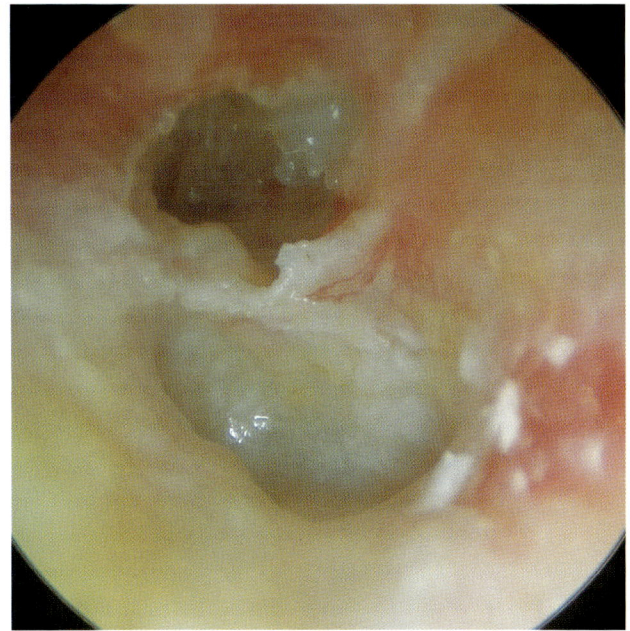

Figure 8.**14** Left ear. Small epitympanic erosion with cholesteatoma. The skin surrounding the erosion is hyperemic and everted.

Figure 8.**15** Left ear. Large epitympanic erosion with cholesteatoma and fetid otorrhea. The head of the malleus and body of the incus are eroded.

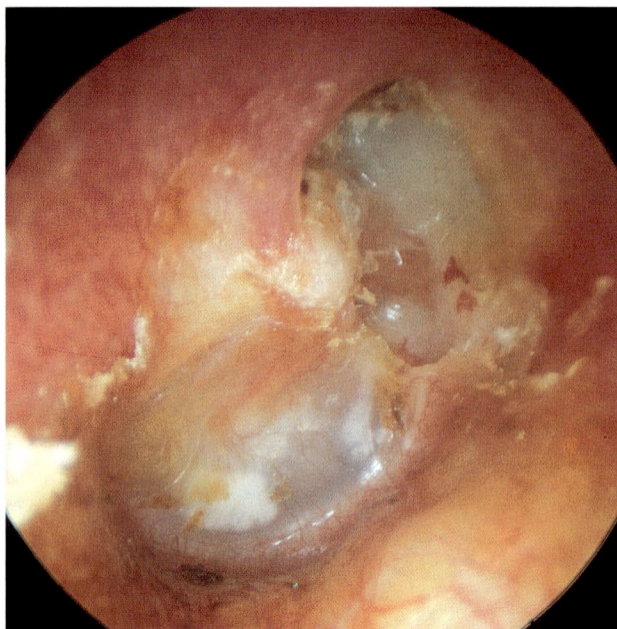

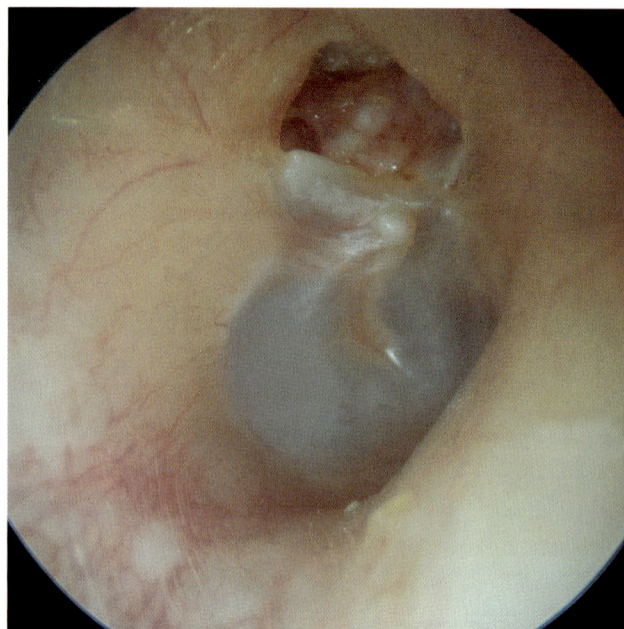

Figure 8.16 Right ear. Large epitympanic erosion with cholesteatoma. This 18-year-old patient did not have otorrhea. Ipsilateral hearing was normal, whereas the contralateral side showed severe sensorineural hearing loss secondary to a previous surgery of radical mastoidectomy. Given the intact ossicular chain, an open tympanoplasty (modified Bondy technique) was performed. According to our strategy, cholesteatoma in the only hearing ear is one of the absolute indications for performing an open technique. The reason is that this technique, if properly per-formed, ensures complete eradication of the pathology and bet-ter long-term follow-up, thus minimizing the risk of recurrence. Further surgical interventions, with their potential risk even in the most experienced hands, are therefore avoided.

Figure 8.17 Right ear. Large epitympanic erosion with cholesteatoma and polypoid tissue that covers the head of the malleus. The pars tensa is intact.

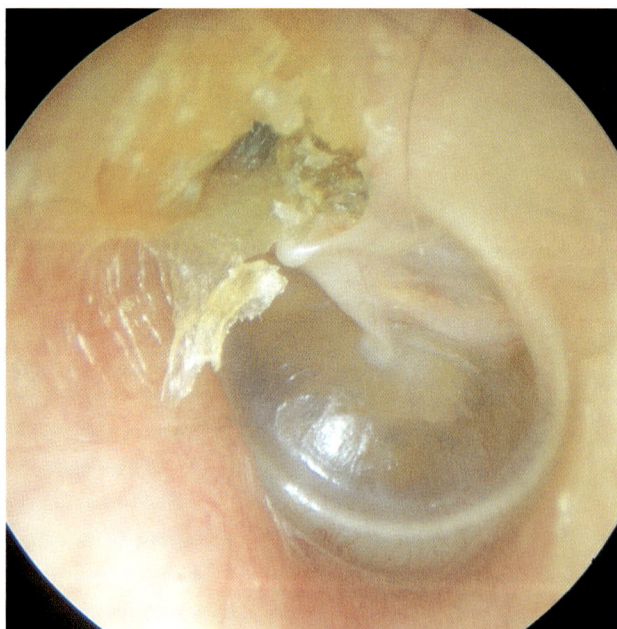

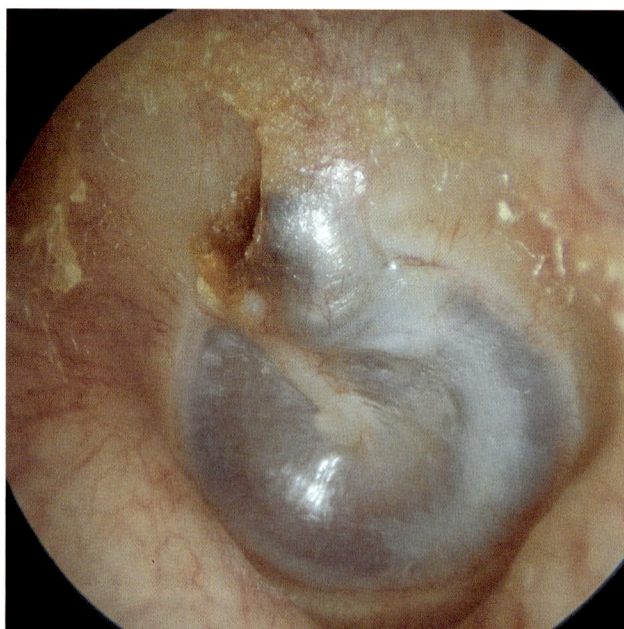

Figure 8.18 Left ear. Epitympanic cholesteatoma. Extensive erosion of the scutum with excessive cholesteatomatous debris. The pars tensa shows grade I atelectasis with catarrhal middle ear effusion.

Figure 8.19 Left ear. Cystic retrotympanic cholesteatoma situ-ated posterior to the malleus. The tympanic membrane shows bulging at the level of the pars flaccida and slight retraction with tympanosclerosis in the posterior quadrants.

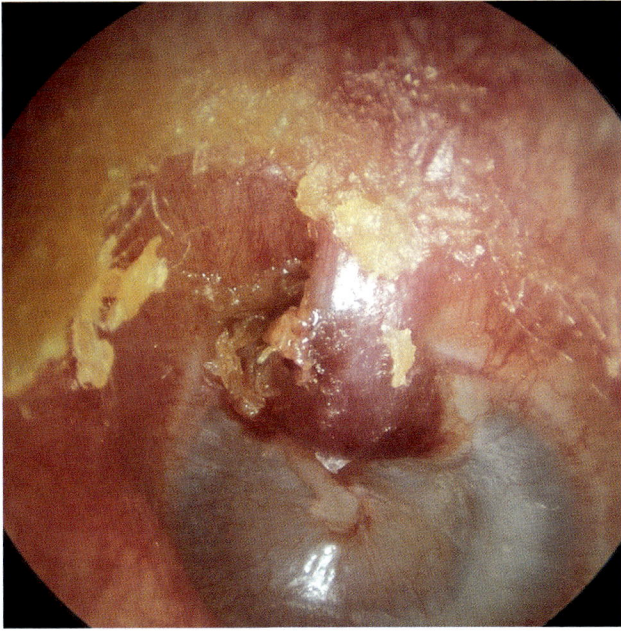

Figure 8.**20** Same case as in Figure 8.**19** during an acute inflammatory episode. Note the increase in size of the cholesteatomatous cyst.

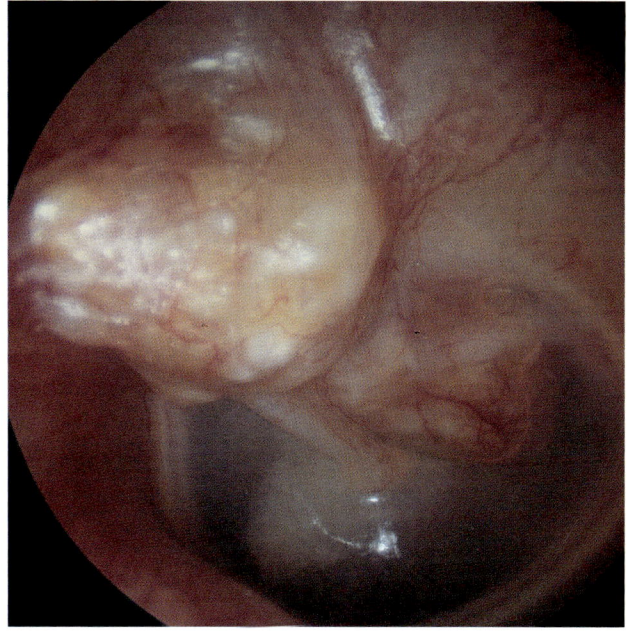

Figure 8.**21** Left ear. Epitympanic erosion occupied by a cholesteatomatous mass that protrudes into the external auditory canal. The mass is visible behind the posterior quadrant of the pars tensa. It engulfs the ossicular chain and extends towards the promontory and the hypotympanum.

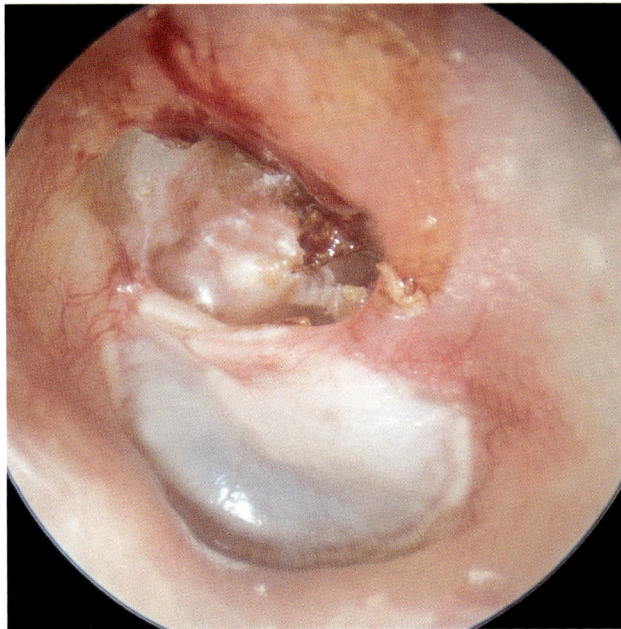

Figure 8.**22** Left ear. A large epitympanic erosion is seen with epidermization of the attic and posterior mesotympanum. The cholesteatoma, visible in transparency, causes bulging of the tympanic membrane in the posterior inferior quadrants. Resorption of the incus and head of the malleus is discernible.

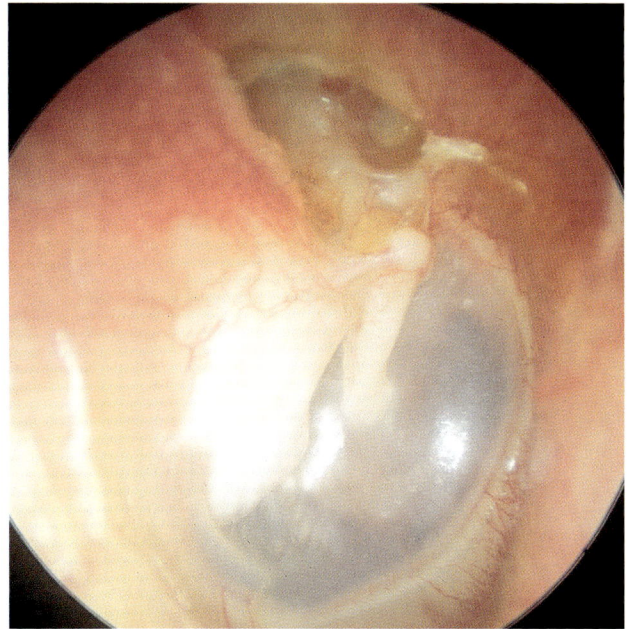

Figure 8.**23** Right ear. Epitympanic erosion with cholesteatoma. Extension of the cholesteatoma into the mesotympanum is seen through the bulging posterior quadrants of the tympanic membrane.

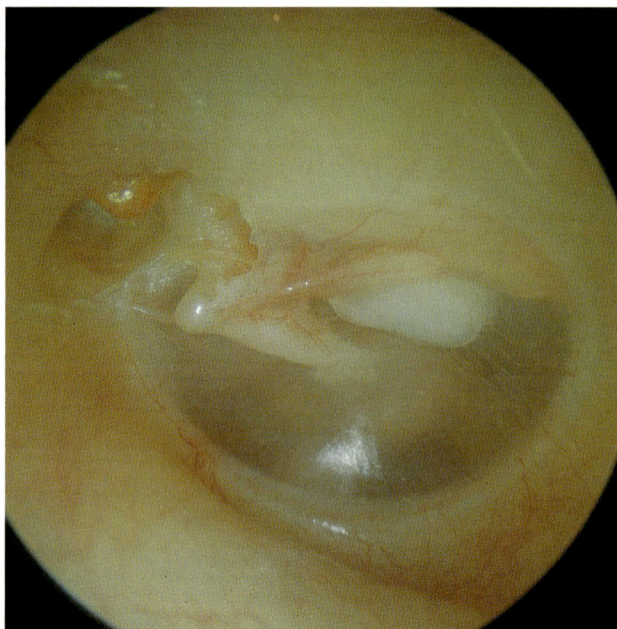

Figure 8.**24**   Left ear. Epitympanic erosion with cholesteatoma. Extension of the cholesteatoma into the mesotympanum (visible through the transparent pars tensa).

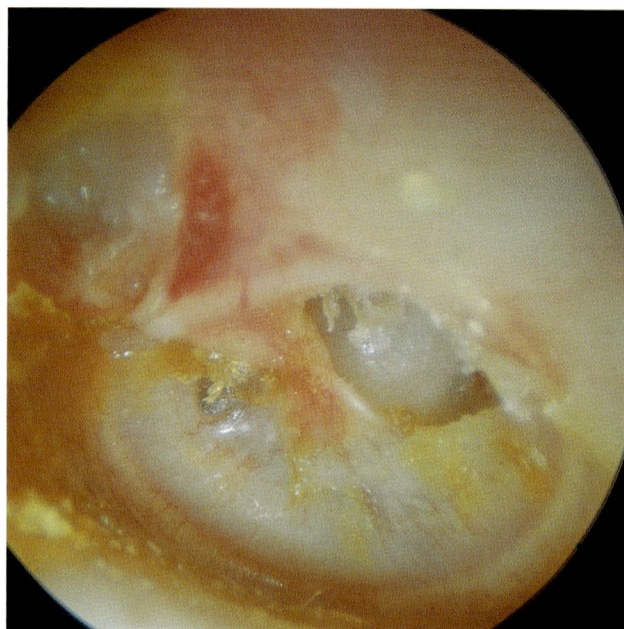

Figure 8.**25**   Left ear. Epitympanic erosion with cholesteatoma. Epidermization of the posterior mesotympanum is seen through a posterior perforation of the tympanic membrane. The tympanic membrane residue has a whitish color. This can be either due to tympanosclerosis or to epidermization of the medial surface of the tympanic membrane. Examination under the microscope can, in many cases, determine the exact cause.

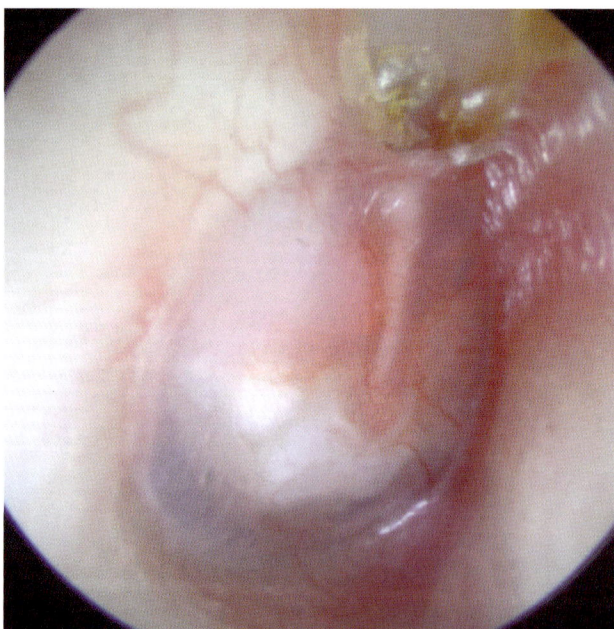

Figure 8.**26**   Right ear. Epitympanic erosion, with cholesteatoma extending into the middle ear (clearly visible through the tympanic membrane).

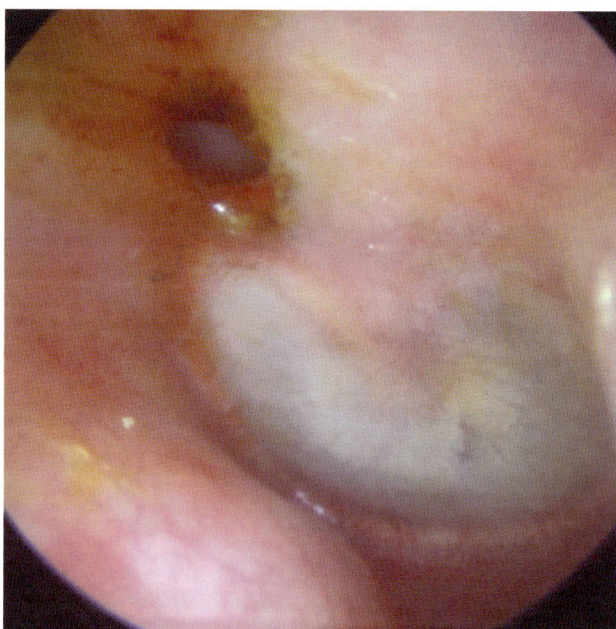

Figure 8.**27**   Left ear. Epitympanic erosion with fetid otorrhea. The head of the malleus is eroded.

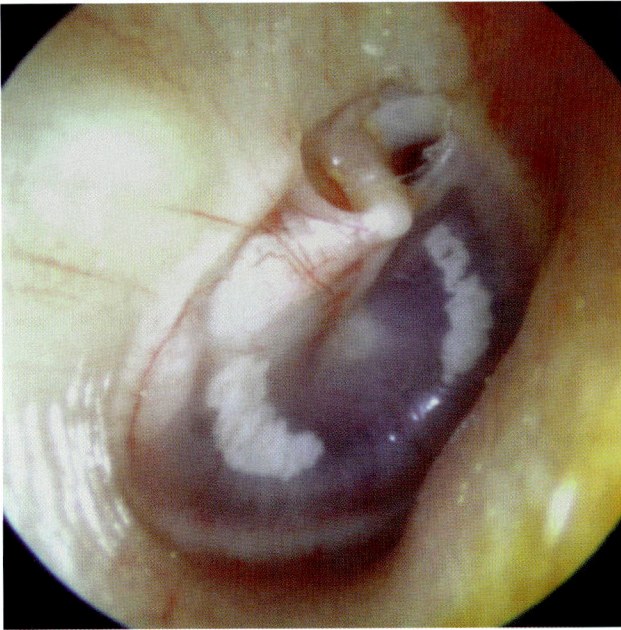

Figure 8.**28** Epitympanic retraction pocket, with extension of the cholesteatoma into the posterior mesotympanum. The posterior quadrant of the tympanic membrane is bulging. Some tympanosclerotic masses are present in the tympanic membrane.

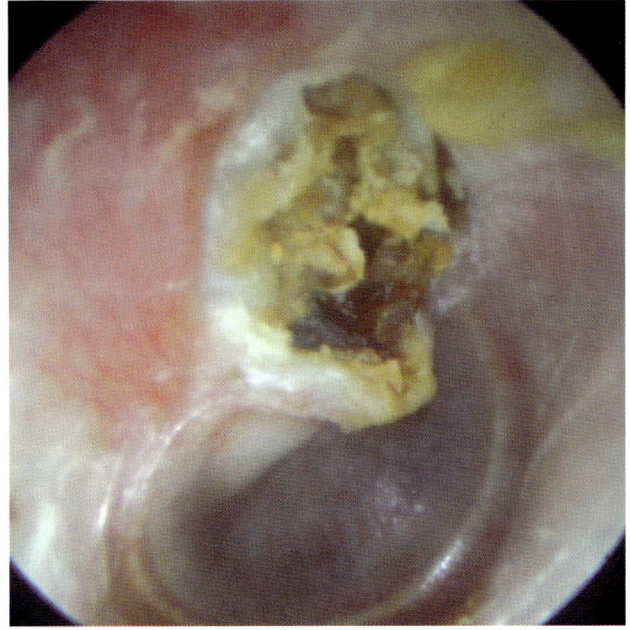

Figure 8.**29** Right ear. Large erosion of the scutum, with cholesteatomatous debris. The pars tensa is normal, with some middle ear effusion. Extension of the cholesteatoma into the mesotympanum is seen through the posterior quadrant of the tympanic membrane. Due to the large erosion, an open tympanoplasty is indicated.

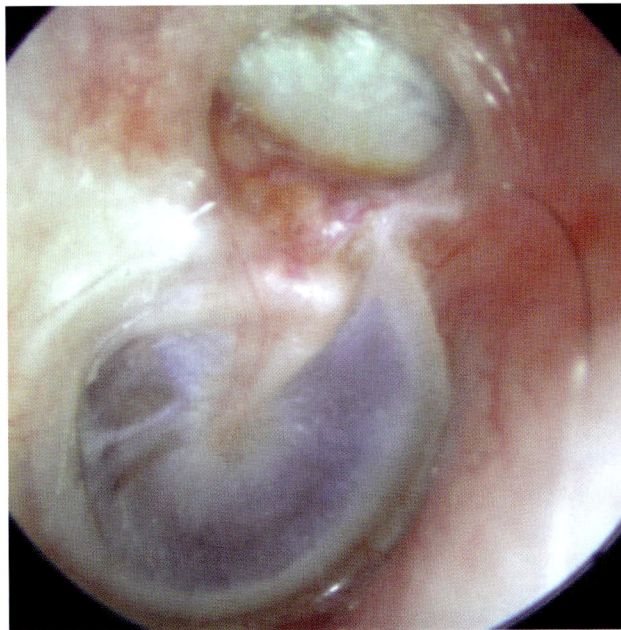

Figure 8.**30** Right ear. Extensive erosion of the scutum, with a cholesteatoma sac bulging out. The pars tensa is normal. The hearing is normal. In this case, a modified Bondy technique is indicated.

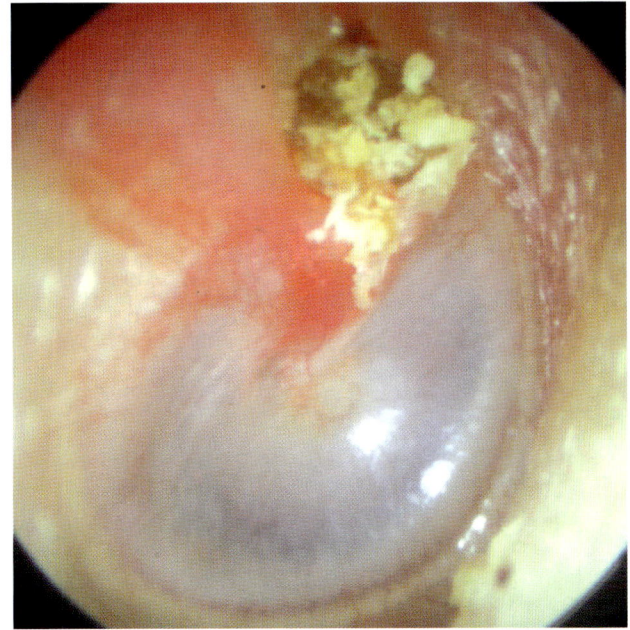

Figure 8.**31** Right ear. Erosion of the scutum, with cholesteatomatous debris. The pars tensa is normal, and the patient's hearing was normal. As in the previous case, a modified Bondy technique is indicated.

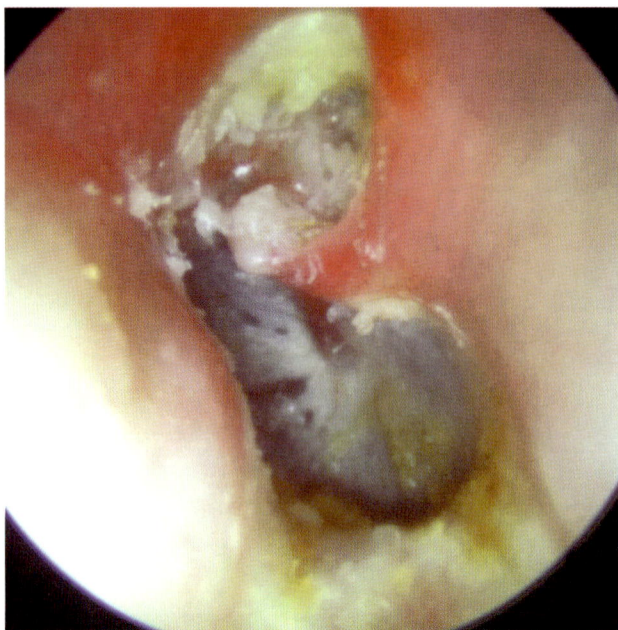

Figure 8.**32**   Left ear. Extensive erosion of the scutum, with cholesteatomatous debris. The skin surrounding the erosion is hyperemic. An open tympanoplasty is indicated.

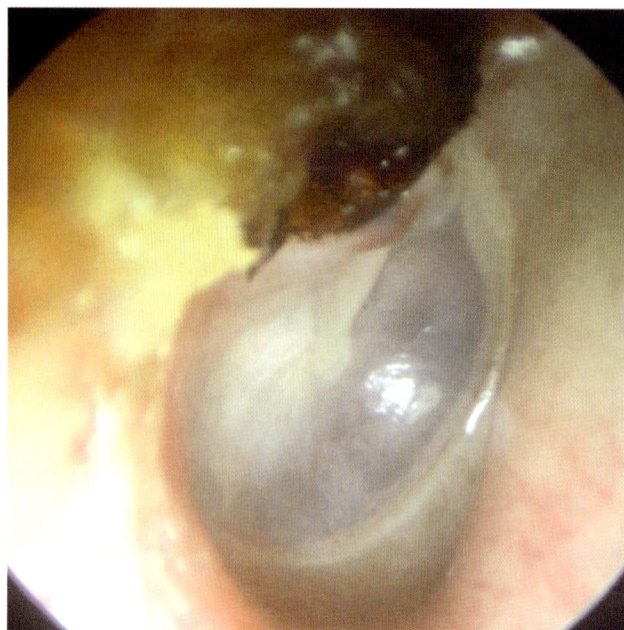

Figure 8.**33**   Right ear. Very large erosion of the scutum with cholesteatomatous debris. The head and part of the handle of the malleus have been resorbed. The pars tensa is normal.

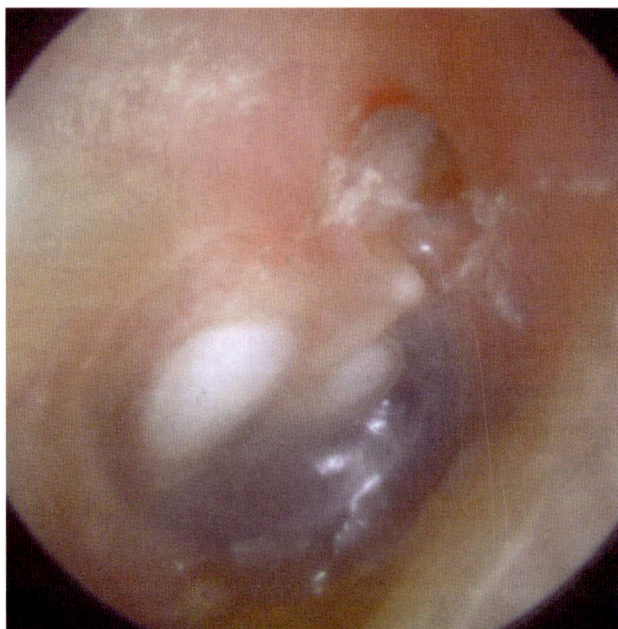

Figure 8.**34**   Epitympanic cholesteatoma, with a small erosion of the scutum. Extension of the cholesteatoma into the posterior mesotympanum and anteriorly to the malleus is seen through the pars tensa. A combined-approach tympanoplasty in two stages is indicated.

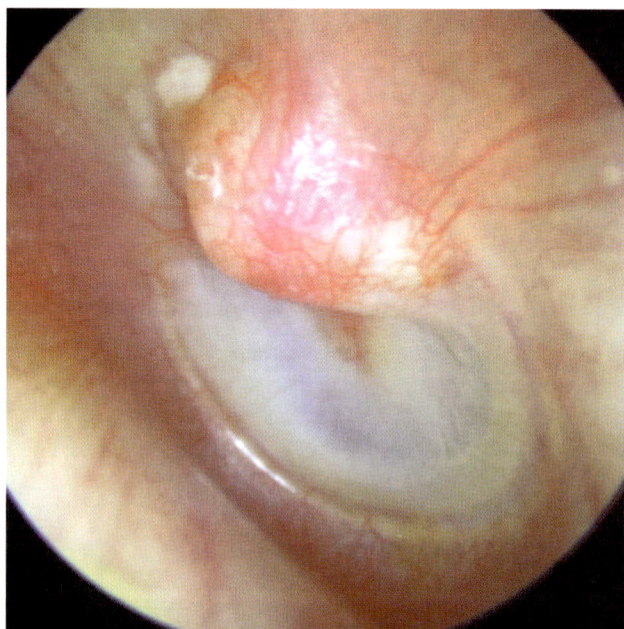

Figure 8.**35**   Left ear. The epitympanic area is occupied by a cholesteatoma mass protruding into the external auditor canal. The skin is hypervascularized.

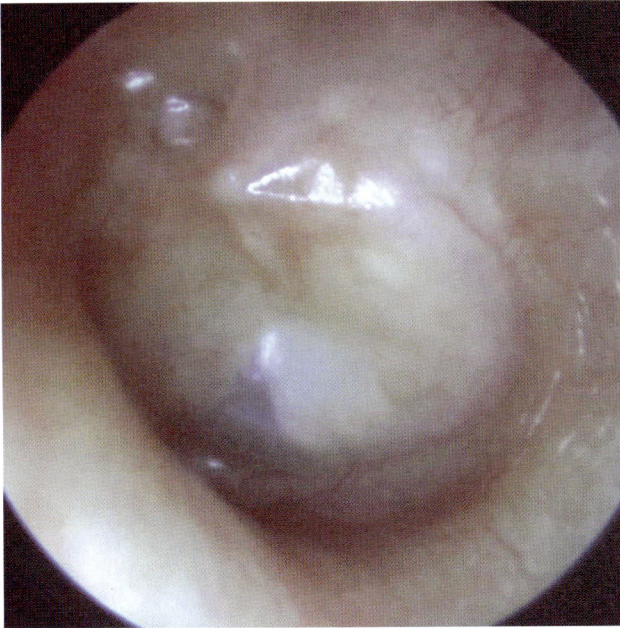

Figure 8.**36** Small epitympanic retraction pocket, with cholesteatoma, extending into the anterior and posterior mesotympanum (visible through the pars tensa). A closed combined-approach tympanoplasty is indicated.

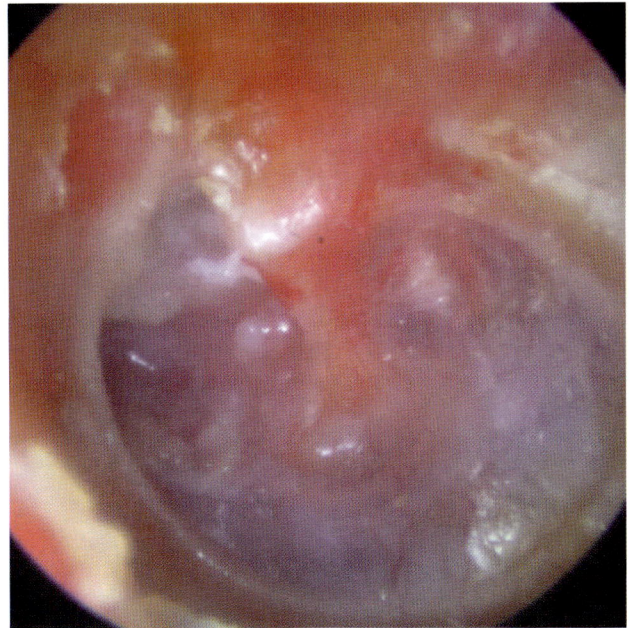

Figure 8.**37** Anterior epitympanic retraction pocket, with cholesteatomatous debris and peritubal atelectasia. An open tympanoplasty is indicated.

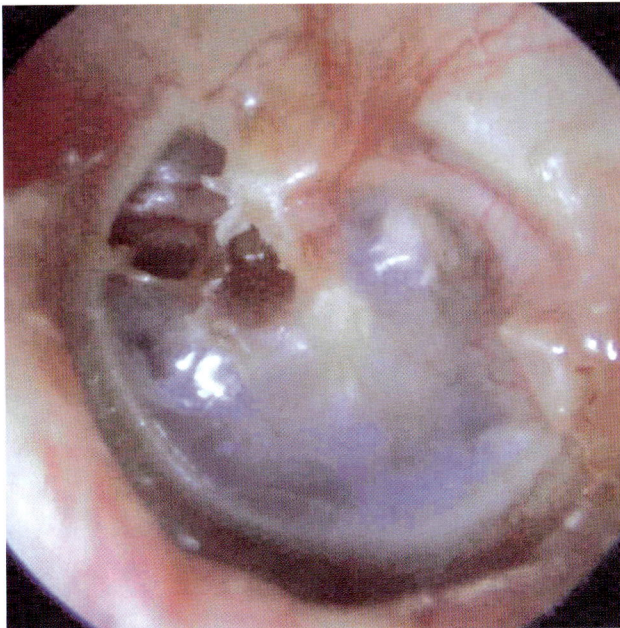

Figure 8.**38** Left ear. An anteromalleolar retraction pocket is present, combined with perforation and cholesteatomatous debris around the handle of the malleus. Due to the absence of any bony erosion and the normal pars tensa, a combined-approach tympanoplasty is indicated.

Summary

An epitympanic retraction pocket should be regularly checked with otomicroscopy. The 30° rigid endoscope allows visualization of the extent of the retraction pocket that can be difficult with the microscope. When progression of the epithelium into the epitympanum cannot be controlled, the presence of cholesteatoma is considered. In such cases, surgery should be performed. Whenever a minor epitympanic erosion is present, we adopt a closed technique with reconstruction of the attic using cartilage and bone paste. This technique is valid particularly in children, in whom the mastoid is usually very pneumatized. Frequently, surgery is staged in these cases.

When a marked attic erosion is present, especially in adults, we perform an open technique to avoid cholesteatoma recurrence that can occur due to absorption of the material used for reconstruction of the attic defect. When preoperative hearing is normal in the presence of attic cholesteatoma with large bony erosion, we perform an open tympanoplasty in the form of a modified Bondy technique. This technique allows single-stage eradication of the disease with conservation of the normal preoperative hearing.

Mesotympanic Cholesteatoma

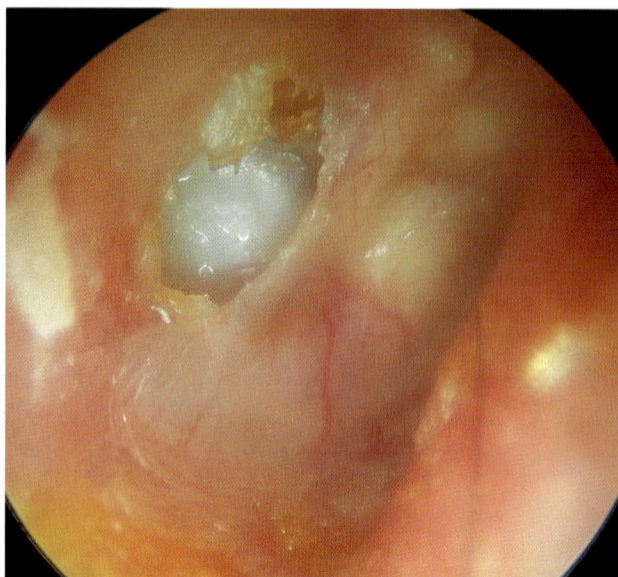

Figure 8.**39** Right ear. Mesotympanic cholesteatoma. The epithelial squamae can be seen through the retromalleolar perforation. Anterior to the malleus, the cholesteatomatous mass causes bulging and whitish coloration of the tympanic membrane without perforating it. The entire middle ear is filled with cholesteatoma in this case.

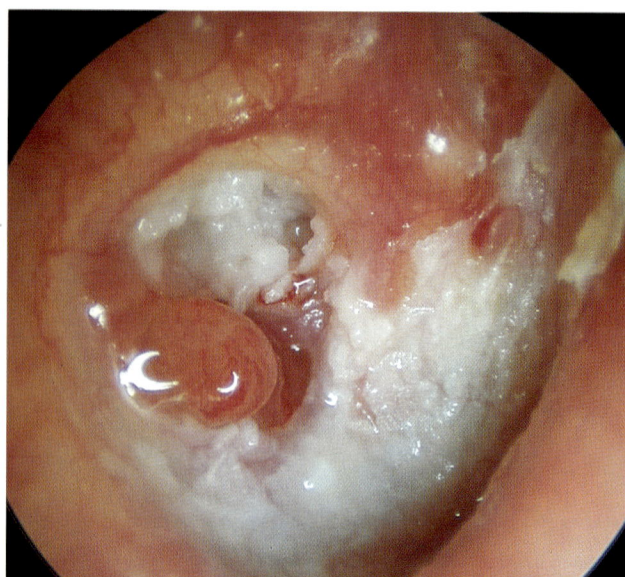

Figure 8.**40** Right ear. Posterior mesotympanic cholesteatoma associated with a polyp are seen at the level of the oval window. There is evidence of discharge.

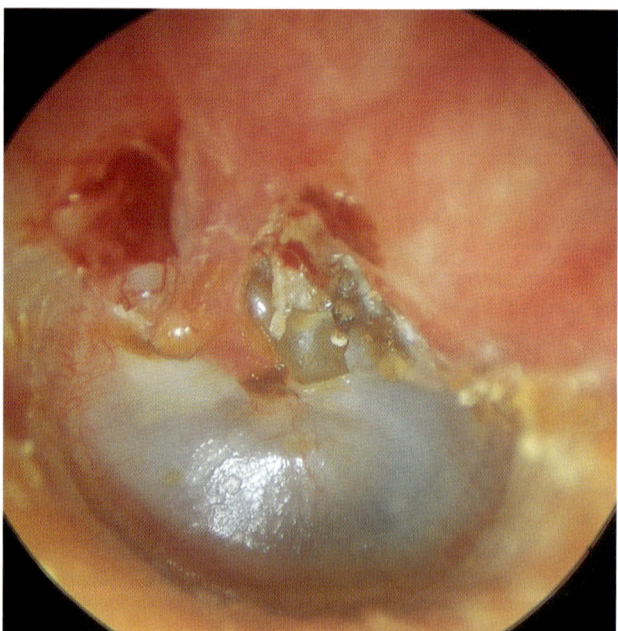

Figure 8.**41** Left ear. Small epitympanic erosion and a mesotympanic retraction pocket with wax and cholesteatomatous squamae. Extension of the cholesteatomatous mass into the anteromalleolar region is seen through the retracted tympanic membrane.

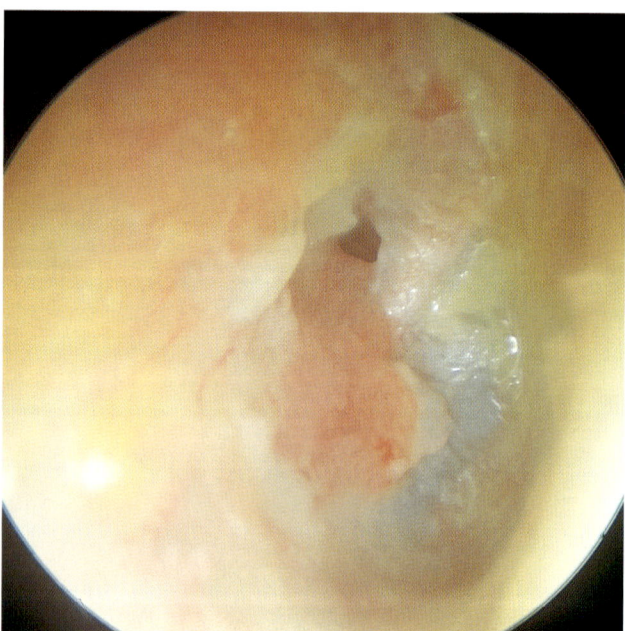

Figure 8.**42** Right ear. A child with mesotympanic retraction and posterosuperior perforation through which cholesteatomatous debris and inflammatory tissue are visible. Purulent discharge is observed. The patient was operated on using a staged closed tympanoplasty.

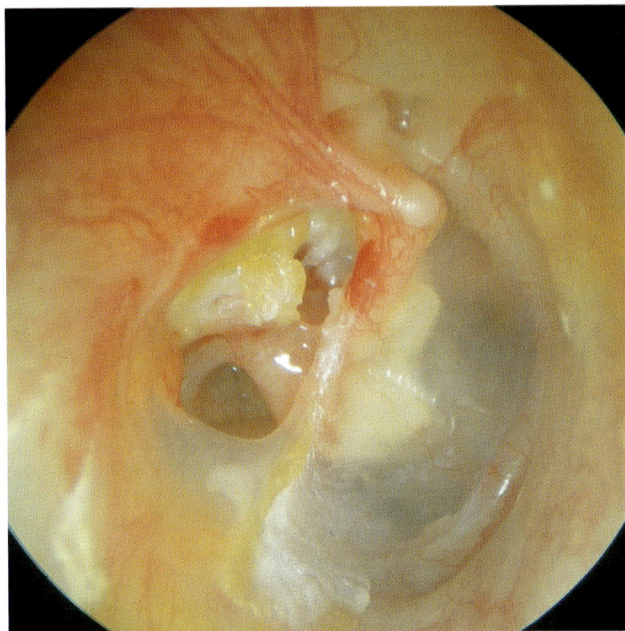

Figure 8.**43** Right ear. Posterior perforation with choleste-atoma in the posterior mesotympanum. The cholesteatomatous squamae cover the region of the oval window extending towards the attic and progress anterior to and under the handle of the malleus. The promontory and the round window are visible through the perforation.

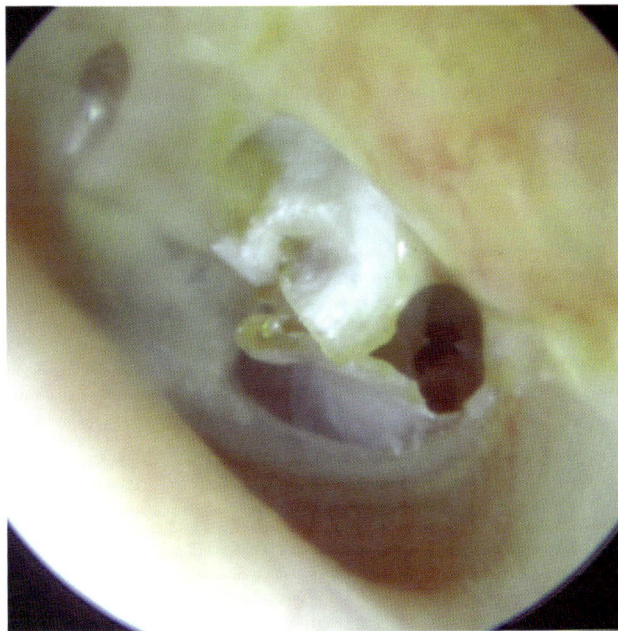

Figure 8.**44** Posterior mesotympanic perforation with cho-lesteatoma. A combined-approach tympanoplasty is indicated.

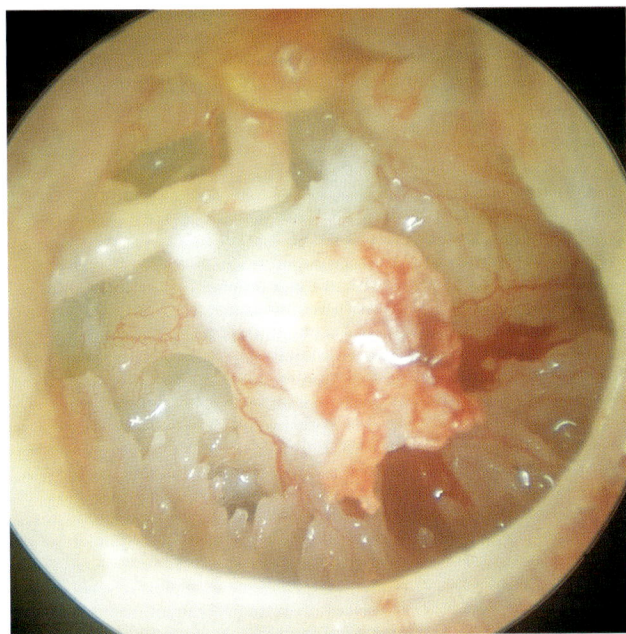

Figure 8.**45** Right ear. Total tympanic membrane perforation. The handle of the malleus is absent. The long process of the incus and part of the stapes are covered by cholesteatoma, which also involves the promontory. The round window, hypotympanic air cells, and tubal orifice are free of pathology. In these cases, a staged closed tympanoplasty can be performed.

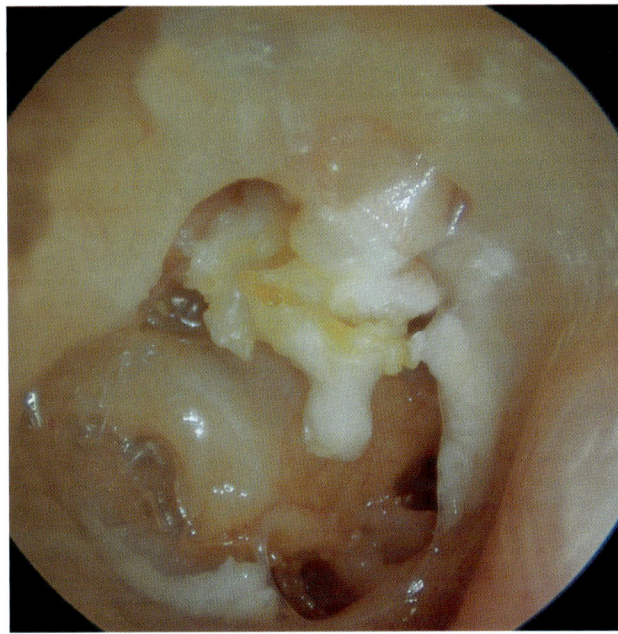

Figure 8.**46** Right ear. Total perforation of the tympanic mem-brane. A cholesteatoma completely covers the handle of the malleus and the incudostapedial joint.

Summary

The presence of a posterior mesotympanic retraction pocket is usually associated with erosion of the ossicular chain. Surgery is indicated in these cases. The retraction pocket is completely removed after performing canalplasty of the posterior canal wall. In the same stage, the tympanic membrane is grafted, the posterosuperior quadrant of the tympanic membrane is reinforced, and middle ear aeration is restored using Silastic sheeting. One year later, if the tympanic membrane position remains normal (i.e., not retracted), the ossicular chain is reconstructed.

When an extensive erosion of the posterior wall is present, a modified radical mastoidectomy is indicated in the elderly, whereas a staged open tympanoplasty is performed in younger patients. The same strategy is also followed in patients presenting with bilateral cholesteatoma.

Cholesteatoma Associated with Atelectasis

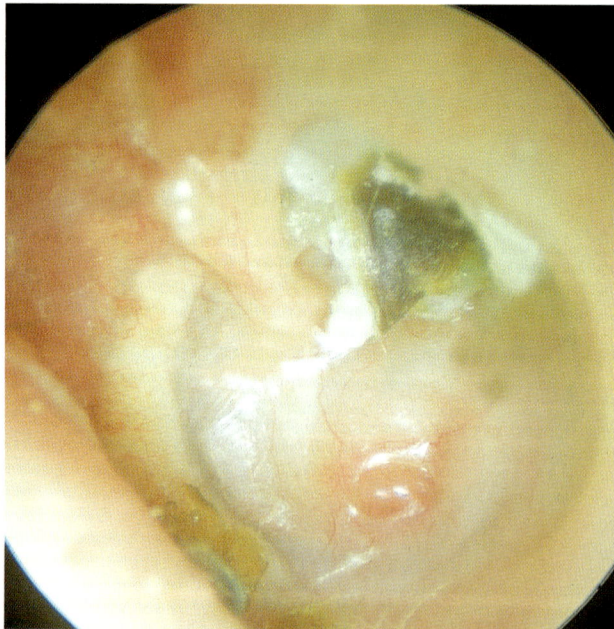

Figure 8.**47**   Left ear. Grade IV tympanic membrane atelectasis with posterosuperior mesotympanic retraction pocket. A mixture of wax and cholesteatomatous debris is seen. The middle ear mucosa is visible because of the absence of the epithelial layer.

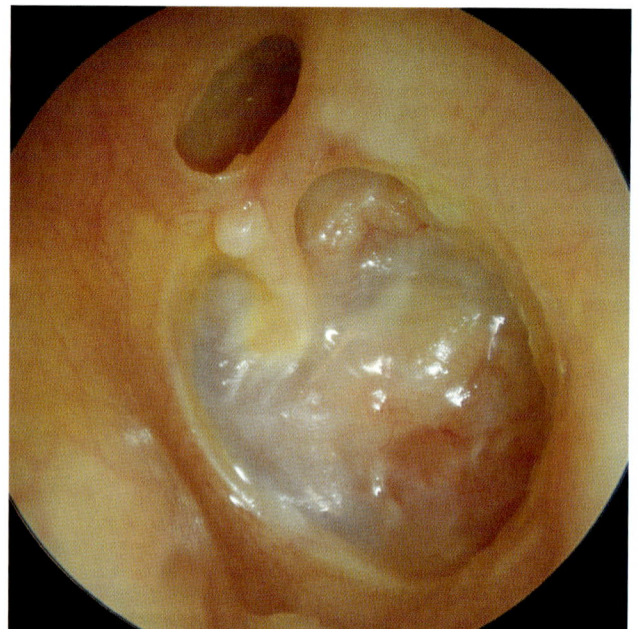

Figure 8.**48**   Left ear. Epitympanic erosion through which a cholesteatoma is shown filling the attic and causing erosion of the head of the malleus. A grade IV atelectasis of the tympanic membrane (adhesive otitis) is seen, with formation of polypoidal granulation tissue in the middle ear. In the region posterior to the malleus, the cholesteatoma engulfs the ossicular chain.

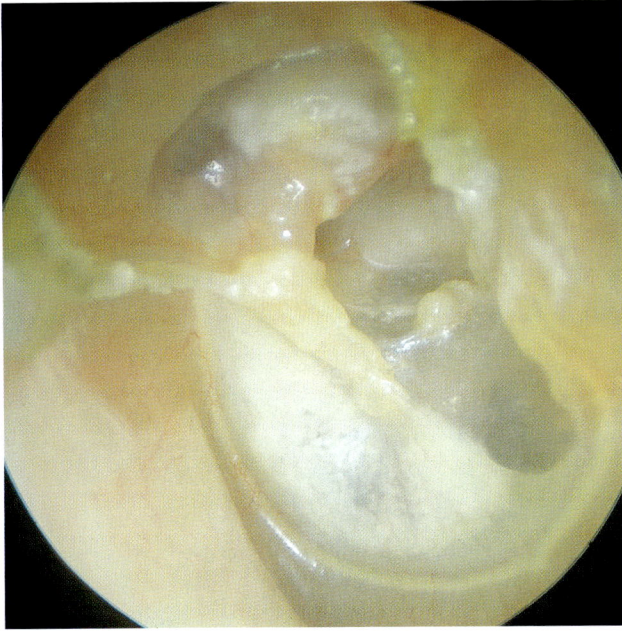

Figure 8.**49** Left ear. Epitympanic erosion with cholesteatoma associated with atelectasis of the tympanic membrane. The incus is absent. A natural myringostapedopexy has been created. The second portion of the facial nerve is seen superior to the stapes; inferiorly the round window is noted. The anterior part of the tympanic membrane is affected with tympanosclerosis. In these cases, as hearing loss is mild (< 30 dB), a modified radical mastoidectomy is indicated to maintain the normal preoperative hearing level obtained as a result of the spontaneous myringostapedopexy.

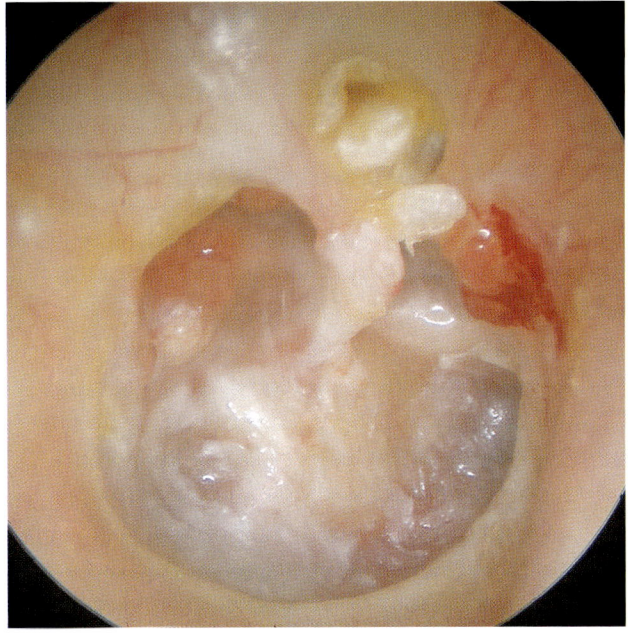

Figure 8.**50** Right ear. Epitympanic cholesteatoma associated with complete atelectasis of the tympanic membrane (see CT scan, Fig. 8.**51**).

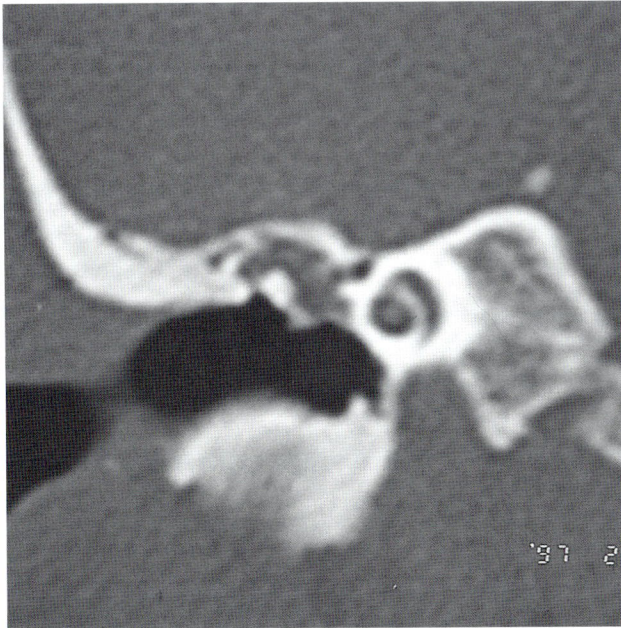

Figure 8.**51** CT scan of the previous case. An epitympanic cholesteatoma is found. Adhesions between the tympanic membrane and the promontory can be observed. This 45-year-old woman underwent a modified radical mastoidectomy with no interference in the middle ear.

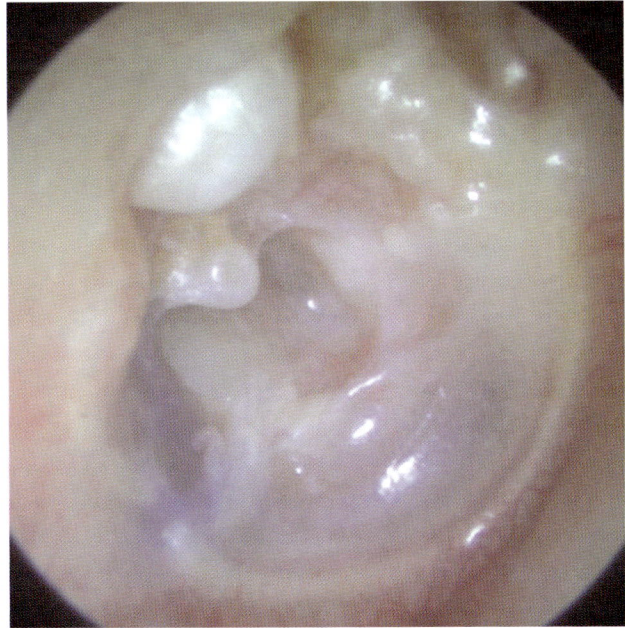

Figure 8.**52** Right ear. Epitympanic erosion and posterior retraction of the pars tensa. The malleus and incus are absent. The stapes is present and intact. There is a mesotympanic pearl located anterosuperiorly to the stapes.

Summary

In adult patients with extended epitympanic erosion or with bilateral cholesteatoma, we prefer to perform an open technique. In all cases of spontaneous tympanostapedopexy with normal preoperative hearing or elderly patients with normal contralateral hearing, we prefer to leave the atelectatic tympanic membrane untouched after having verified the absence of any middle ear cholesteatoma. In the presence of mesotympanic cholesteatoma, staging is indicated. In the first operation a closed tympanoplasty is performed with reconstruction of the tympanic membrane, and a Silastic sheet is positioned in the middle ear. Silastic favors regeneration of the middle ear mucosa and prevents the formation of adhesions. In the second stage, performed 6 to 8 months later, the middle ear is checked for the presence of any residual cholesteatoma. The ossicular chain is then reconstructed using, preferably, an autologous incus. In children we always try to perform a staged closed tympanoplasty. If a recurrent cholesteatoma (epitympanic retraction pocket) is encountered in the second stage, we do not hesitate to switch to an open technique.

Cholesteatoma Associated with Complications

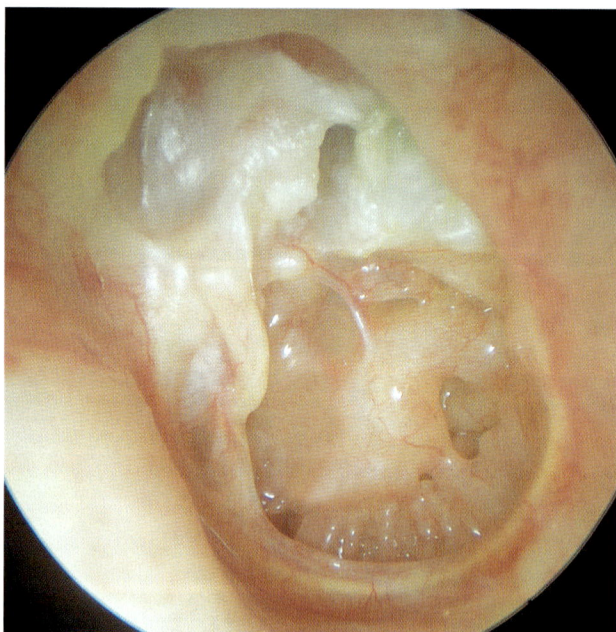

Figure 8.**53**   Left ear. Large epitympanic perforation with pars tensa perforation. Cholesteatomatous squamae are present in the attic, whereas the middle ear is completely free. The handle of the malleus is present. The promontory, round window, and hypotympanic air cells are covered with normal mucosa. The tympanic annulus is intact. During surgery, a fistula of the lateral semicircular canal was encountered (see Fig 8.**54**). In such cases, because of the presence of marked epitympanic erosion and of the fistula, an open tympanoplasty is preferred.

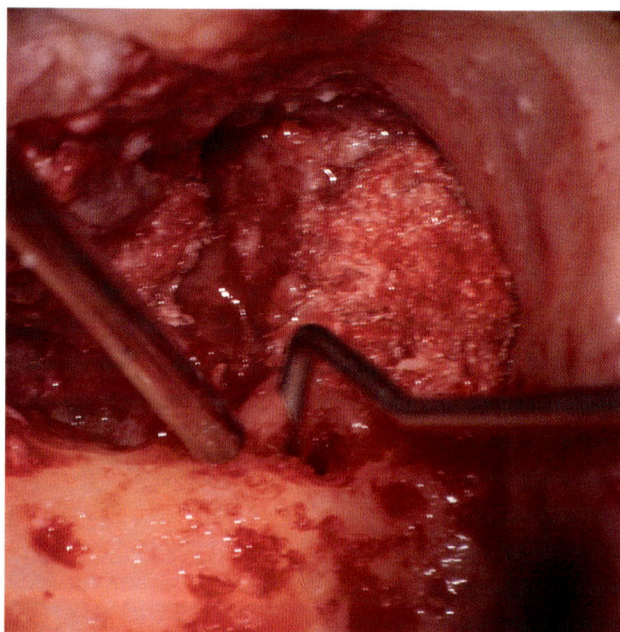

Figure 8.**54**   Intraoperative view of the previous case. A fistula of the lateral semicircular canal is clearly seen.

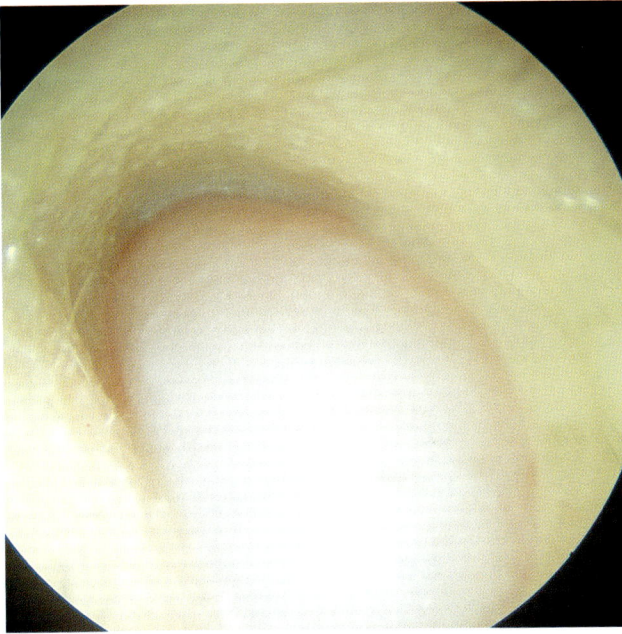

Figure 8.**55** Left ear. Large polyp obstructing the external auditory canal. The patient complained of fetid otorrhea, hearing loss, and vertigo. A high-resolution CT scan of the temporal bone was ordered (see Fig. 8.**56**). A CT scan of the temporal bone should always be ordered in patients with chronic suppurative otitis media suffering from vertigo and/or instability.

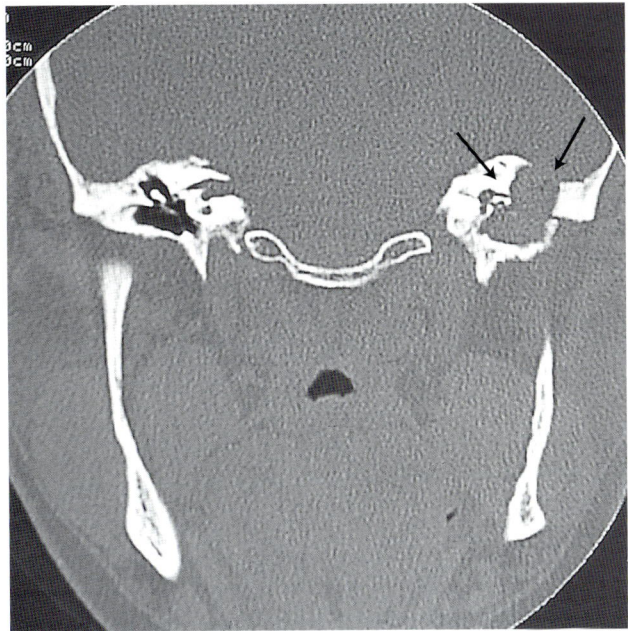

Figure 8.**56** CT scan of the previous case. A huge cholesteatoma causing a fistula of the lateral semicircular canal and erosion of the tegmen can be seen.

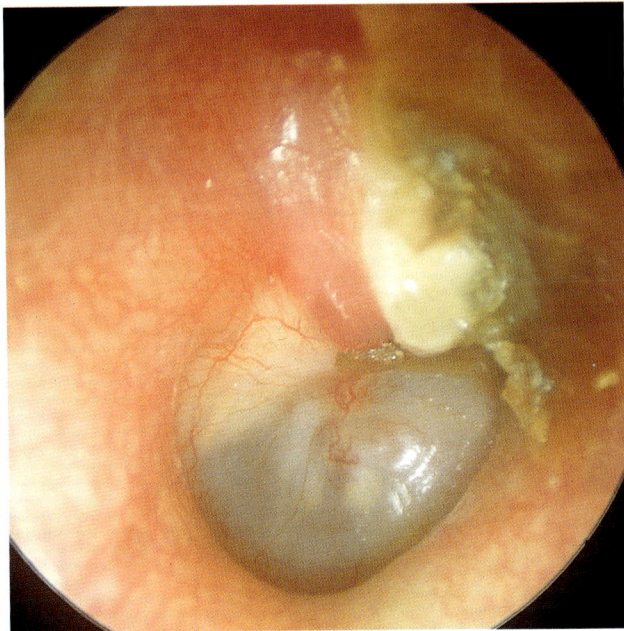

Figure 8.**57** Right ear. Epi- and mesotympanic cholesteatoma. The cholesteatomatous debris protruded through the epitympanic erosion. In the posterosuperior quadrant, the cholesteatomatous sac can be seen in transparency, causing bulging of the tympanic membrane. The skin surrounding the attic erosion is hyperemic. The pars tensa is intact. The patient complained of frequent episodes of vertigo. A CT scan (see Fig. 8.**58**) demonstrated the presence of a fistula of the lateral semicircular canal.

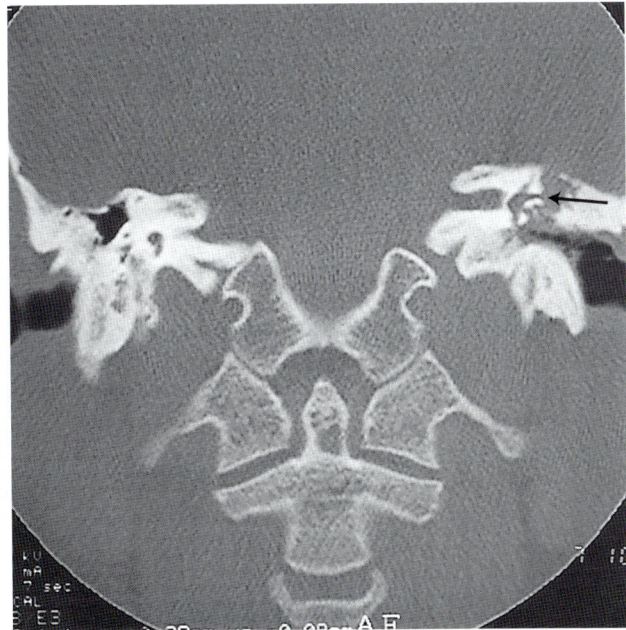

Figure 8.**58** CT scan of the previous case. The interruption of the lateral semicircular canal caused by the cholesteatoma is apparent.

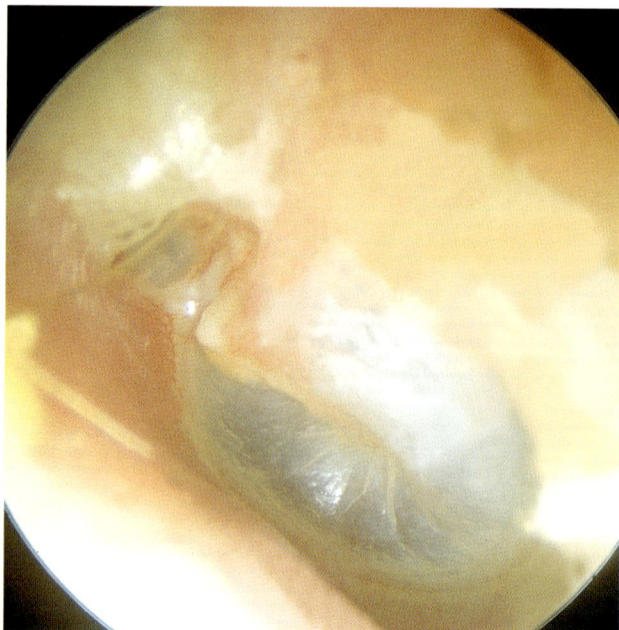

Figure 8.**59**   Left ear. Small epitympanic retraction pocket in a patient presenting with hearing loss, tinnitus, and recurrent episodes of otitis media with effusion. The contralateral ear had been operated on elsewhere using an open tympanoplasty that resulted in total hearing loss and facial nerve paralysis. A CT scan of the temporal bone revealed the presence of an epitympanic cholesteatoma that caused a fistula of the superior semicircular canal and erosion of the tegmen (see Fig. 8.**60**). The patient

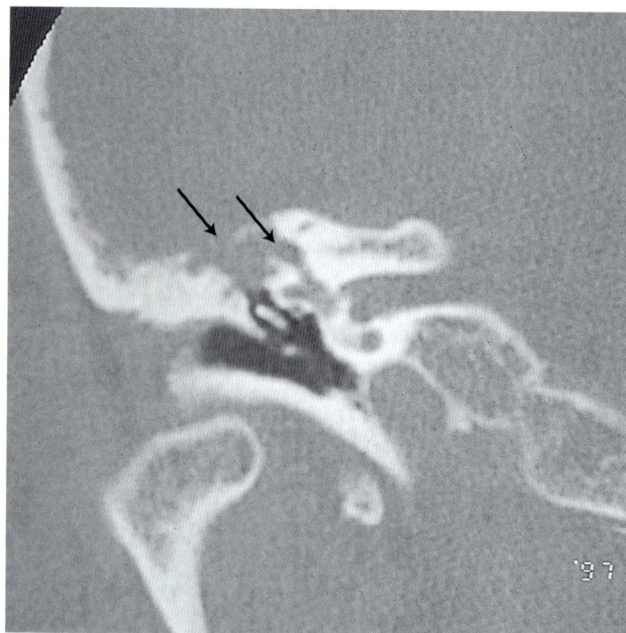

underwent open tympanoplasty. Being the only hearing ear, the cholesteatoma matrix was left over the fistula, whereas the tegmental erosion was repaired using cartilage to avoid a meningo-encephalic herniation (see Chapter 12).

Figure 8.**60**   CT scan of the previous case. Cholesteatoma caused a fistula of the superior semicircular canal and erosion of the tegmen.

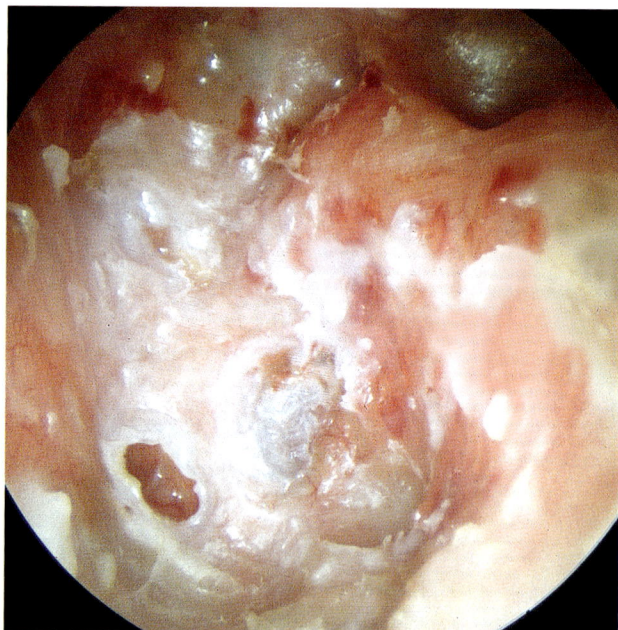

Figure 8.**61**   Left ear. This patient had already undergone bilateral radical mastoidectomy elsewhere. He presented with profound bilateral hearing loss and fetid otorrhea from his left ear. During revision surgery, a cholesteatoma causing a cochlear fistula was found. This patient suffered profound hearing loss in the other ear, thus the cholesteatoma matrix was left over the fistula to avoid deaf ear.

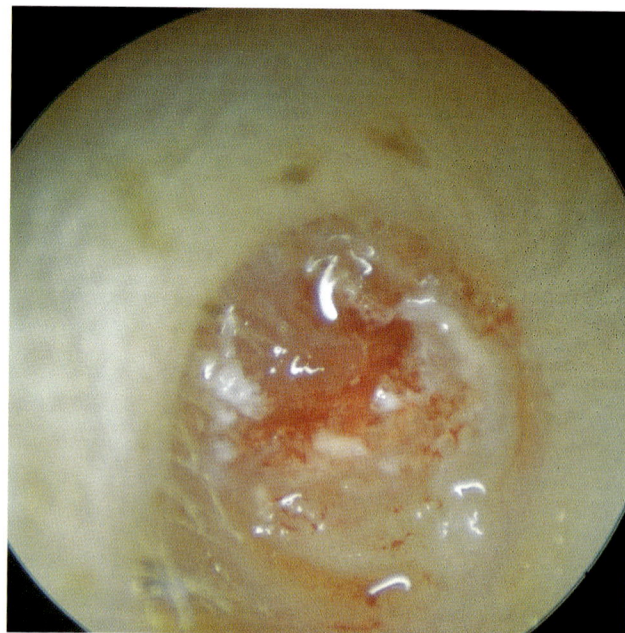

Figure 8.**62**   Polyp in the external auditory canal with purulent discharge. A cholesteatoma is frequently found behind such a polyp. In such cases, biopsy is not indicated as a CT scan is often used to differentiate cholesteatoma from other pathologies (glomus, carcinoid, or carcinoma). A tympanoplasty revealed the presence of a large cholesteatoma occupying the attic and mesotympanum.

Summary

At present, with the diagnostic methods at hand and increased medical care, it is very rare to find a cholesteatoma with intracranial complications (e.g., meningitis, brain abscess, lateral sinus thrombophlebitis, etc.). However, cases of cholesteatoma with massive bone destruction, labyrinthine fistulas, severe sensorineural hearing loss resulting in deaf ear, and facial nerve paralysis are not infrequently encountered. In general, it is not necessary to order a CT scan to diagnose a cholesteatoma. However, in the presence of headache, vertigo, facial nerve paralysis, severe sensorineural hearing loss, or sudden deafness, a high-resolution CT scan of the temporal bone becomes highly important. Axial and coronal cuts without contrast are required. When intracranial complications are suspected, contrast injection is also needed.

A labyrinthine fistula is found in less than 10% of cases. The lateral semicircular canal, being the most superficial, is the most commonly involved. Treatment of a labyrinthine fistula depends on the type (bony or membranous) and size of the fistula.

A tegmental erosion can be repaired using cartilage and bone paste.

Facial nerve paralysis is either due to infection of the exposed nerve or secondary to compression by the cholesteatoma. In the majority of cases, removing the cholesteatoma and clearing the infection are sufficient for the paralysis to resolve. It is very rare to find fibrosis or thinning of the nerve. In these cases, facial nerve reconstruction varies from rerouting and end-to-end anastomosis to nerve grafting, according to the degree of injury and length of the injured segment.

Surgical Treatment of Cholesteatoma: Individualized Technique

Various techniques for cholesteatoma surgery have been developed, practiced, criticized, and favored by different otologists. The current dilemma regarding the choice of technique reflects differences of opinion between various schools of thinking in otology. However, both the open and closed techniques have now been individualized, and the choice of procedure can be made in accordance with certain indications in order to optimize the results.

Until the mid-1980s, we were very strong proponents of closed cavity techniques. However, we now use open procedures in a large number of cholesteatoma cases and plan the operation in an individualized manner, on a case-by-case basis.

A modified Bondy mastoidectomy is indicated in epitympanic cholesteatoma when the patient has good hearing and an intact ossicular chain and pars tensa, thus allowing one-stage mastoid cavity exteriorization with removal of the cholesteatoma while preserving the preoperative hearing levels.

We use both the open and closed techniques in patients with a labyrinthine fistula. The cholesteatoma matrix is generally left over the fistula site in open cavity cases, while in closed cavity cases, the matrix is removed with small fistulas, and a second-look operation is carried out after 6 months. We prefer an open technique in patients who have a labyrinthine fistula in the only hearing ear, in those with small mastoids, and in any other situation in which an open procedure is indicated.

We generally prefer the closed techniques in patients with extensively pneumatized mastoids and in children, as we prefer not to create a cavity in order to prevent the possible later limitations of activity that may result. However, we do not hesitate to carry out a switch to open cavities in these patients, either during second-stage surgery or whenever there is recurrent disease. Difficulties have been encountered with regard to cavity care and water tolerance in some cases, but the incidence of this is very low in our hands. We attribute this to the effective reduction of the cavity size achieved using the surgical technique we have adopted.

Care is taken to remove all the overhanging margins, to amputate the mastoid tip when an extensively pneumatized mastoid is present, and to create a round cavity; all of these procedures help the prolapse of the adjacent tissues into the cavity, thereby genuinely reducing the size of the cavity.

Canal Wall Up (Closed) Tympanoplasty

Indications

- Chronic suppurative otitis media with cholesteatoma in children and in patients with highly pneumatized mastoids.
- Minor epitympanic erosion.
- Mesotympanic cholesteatoma.

In chronic suppurative otitis media without cholesteatoma, tympanoplasty without mastoidectomy produces the same results as mastoidectomy with regard to the rate of graft failure and postoperative hearing status. We only carry out mastoidectomy in cases in which inspection of the mastoid cavity is required.

In all patients with a spontaneous tympanostapedopexy with normal preoperative hearing, and in elderly patients with an air–bone gap with a diseased ear but normal contralateral hearing, we prefer to leave the atelectatic tympanic membrane untouched after having verified the absence of any middle ear cholesteatoma.

Whenever minor epitympanic erosion is present, we use a closed technique, with reconstruction of the attic using cartilage and bone paste.

There is no single procedure that can be used to treat all cases of cholesteatoma. The surgeon should be flexible and well prepared to choose a procedure that is suitable for the specific patient. In general, we use open tympanoplasty for most cases of cholesteatoma, since the closed technique results in a higher recurrence rate compared with the open one. Surgical intervention for cholesteatoma using closed tympanoplasty should be completed with a second-stage operation, since the purpose of the surgery is not only to reconstruct the sound transmission system, but also to eradicate any residual cholesteatoma. Currently, we apply the closed technique only in selected cases.

In patients with a very pneumatized mastoid, closed tympanoplasty is also indicated to prevent a very large cavity. In children, we try to perform a staged closed tympanoplasty because of children's highly cellular mastoids and in an attempt to preserve the anatomy of the ear as much as possible. However, even in such cases, if there is a large epitympanic erosion or surgery reveals intensive involvement of the middle ear by cholesteatoma, we apply the open technique. Open tympanoplasty is also chosen for the only hearing ear. When there is a mesotympanic cholesteatoma, especially in young patients, closed tympanoplasty may be indicated. In the first operation, a closed tympanoplasty is performed with reconstruction of the tympanic membrane, and a Silastic sheet is positioned in the middle ear. Silastic promotes regeneration of the middle ear mucosa and prevents the formation of adhesions. However, if the posterior wall interferes with the view of the cholesteatoma matrix—for example, in relation to its extension toward the eustachian tube—open tympanoplasty is used, especially in older patients.

If it turns out that open tympanoplasty is indicated, there is little difficulty in converting the technique by removing the posterior wall. The time spent on canalplasty and tympanotomies is worthwhile for the patient.

In the second stage, usually performed about 10–12 months later, the middle ear and mastoid cavity are checked for eradication of any residual cholesteatoma. The ossicular chain is then reconstructed, preferably using an autologous incus. If a recurrent cholesteatoma (epitympanic retraction pocket) or absorption of the posterior canal wall is encountered in the second stage, we do not hesitate to switch to an open cavity.

Regular otoscopic follow-up is essential to identify the formation of a retraction pocket or recurrent cholesteatoma. If those occur, there should be no hesitation in switching to an open tympanoplasty, since we believe these indicate persistence of the underlying pathogenesis even after the previous tympanoplasty.

Surgical Technique

The technique used for mastoidectomy in closed tympanoplasty should be the same as for open tympanoplasty. The only difference from the open technique is preservation of posterior canal wall, which may impede the view of the tympanic membrane. Adequate saucerization of the mastoid cavity, with complete drilling of the sinodural angle and bony overhang on the cavity edges, should be carried out before posterior epitympanotomy and posterior tympanotomy. The saucerized cavity maximizes the surgical view and surgical angle. Canalplasty may be required to obtain adequate visualization of the tympanic membrane. The canal wall should therefore not be thinned at the outset.

A meatal skin flap is elevated medially, and the meatal bone is calibrated if necessary. To obtain better control of any pathology and to facilitate reconstruction, it is important to be able to visualize the entire annulus without moving the microscope.

The attic is opened from behind, with the superior wall of the external auditory canal being left intact. The direction of the drilling should be from medial to lateral. The posterior atticotomy should have sufficient anterior extension to allow the whole attic to be visualized.

The utmost care should be taken not to touch the ossicular chain with the burr. If there is any risk, the incudostapedial joint should be disarticulated first. In this case, reconstruction of the ossicular chain may be performed either at the end of the procedure or during the second-stage operation, depending on the pathology. Care should be taken not to fenestrate the superior wall of the external auditory canal. If this occurs, reconstruction with cartilage and bone paste is carried out.

A retraction pocket with a small epitympanic erosion can be dissected and pushed back to the external auditory canal from the posterior cavity using a small cottonoid. If there is attic cholesteatoma, the head of the malleus is cut and the cog is removed with either a burr or a curette to open the anterior attic recess.

In cases of retraction pocket and attic cholesteatoma, it is important in the closed technique to drill the invisible edge of the lateral attic wall, or to scratch it with a curette, to avoid leaving skin in the middle ear. However, one should avoid creating a large atticotomy, in order to avoid recurrence.

The posterior wall of the external auditory canal is thinned out. The final step is preferably carried out using a large diamond burr. It is important not to make the posterior wall of the external auditory canal too thin. Inadvertent opening and postoperative atrophy of the bony canal wall can lead to recurrent cholesteatoma, even a considerable time after surgery in cases of tubal insufficiency.

To avoid injury to the facial nerve, the third portion of the nerve is identified using a large cutting burr, parallel to the course of the nerve, and with continuous suction and ample irrigation. The nerve is only skeletonized, never exposed. Care should be taken not to open the ampulla of the lateral semicircular canal, which is located just medial to the facial nerve. The chorda tympani is also identified.

Using a diamond burr or a curette, the facial recess between the facial nerve and the chorda tympani is opened. The chordal crest can be seen in this step. A small buttress of bone is left intact posterior to the short process of the incus, to protect the ossicular chain from the burr.

The posterior tympanotomy allows control of the incudostapedial joint and the oval and round windows. It can be extended inferiorly to allow control of the hypotympanum, by cutting the chorda tympani.

In order to ventilate the epitympanum via the supratubal recess, the overhanging cog is removed with a curette after the malleus head has been mobilized.

Medium to thick Silastic sheeting—shaped to cover the medial wall of the middle ear, including the tubal orifice, the epitympanum, the opened facial recess, and the mastoid—is inserted from the posterior cavity in cases of cholesteatoma, atelectatic ear and extensive defect of mucosa in the medial wall. The Silastic sheeting helps avoid adhesions between the graft and the denuded tympanic wall and promotes good mucosal regeneration.

The eustachian tube is blocked with small pieces of Gelfoam, and the tympanic cavity is filled with the same material. Any defect in the tympanic membrane is reconstructed with the temporalis fascia.

At the end of the procedure, the external auditory canal is packed with small pieces of Gelfoam.

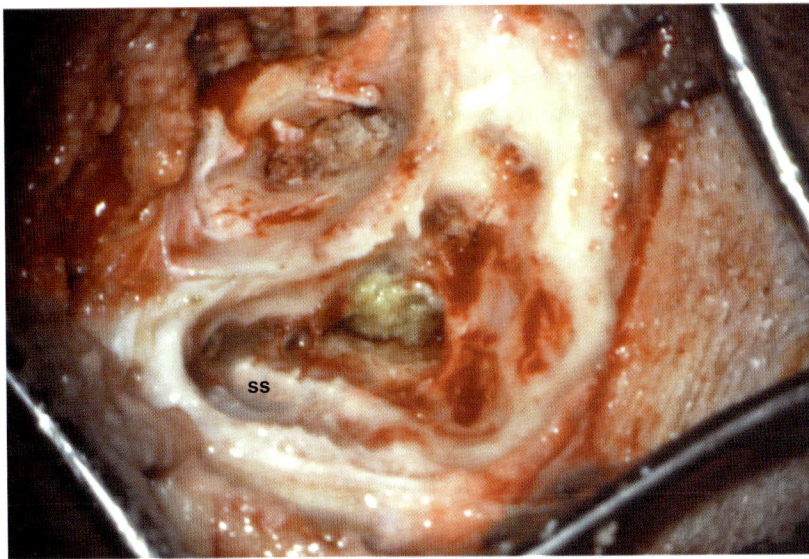

Figure 8.**63** Left ear. A retroauricular incision and the first steps of a cortical mastoidectomy have been performed. Cholesteatomatous debris is visible in the antrum.

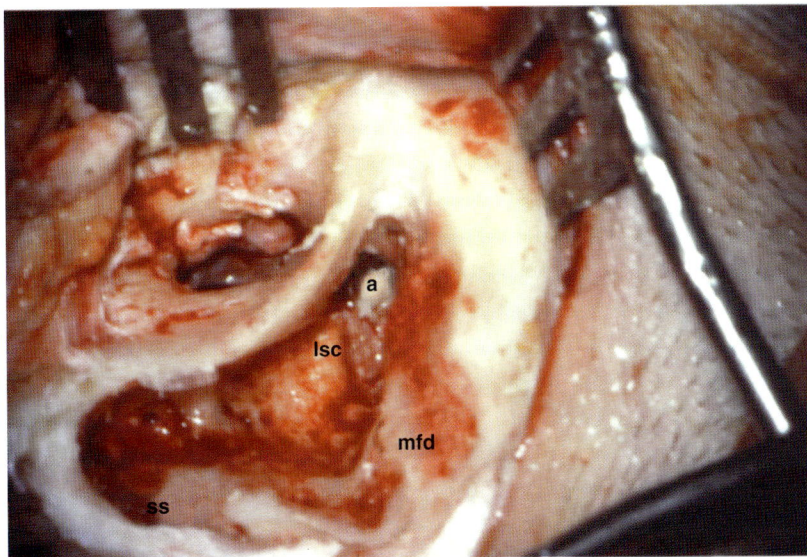

Figure 8.**64** The antrum has been opened, as well as the aditus.

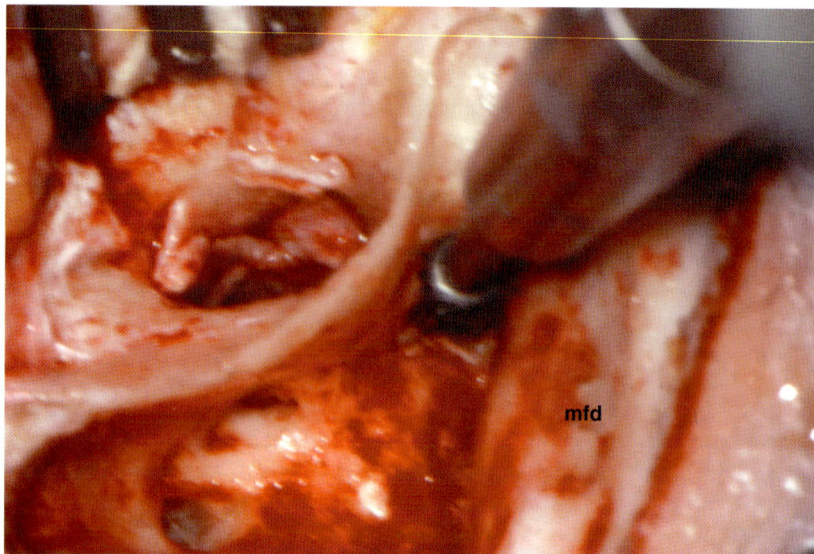

Figure 8.**65**   The bone covering the epitympanic recess is removed with the cutting burr.

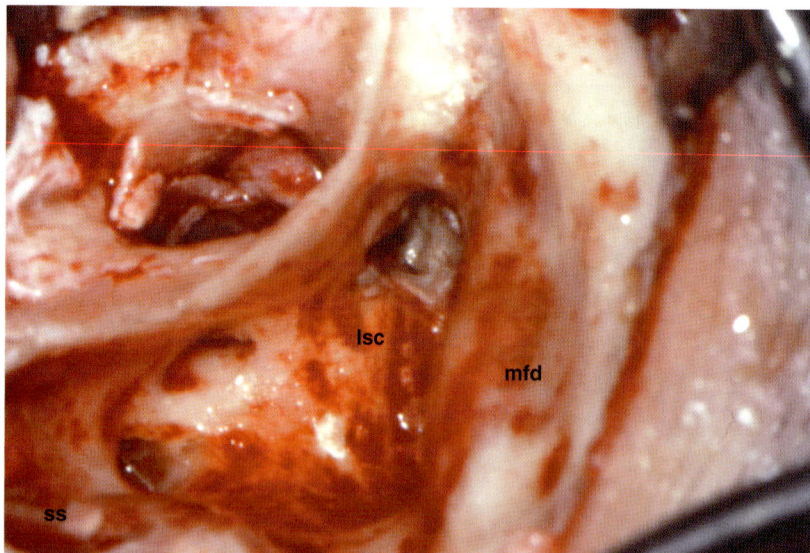

Figure 8.**66**   The cholesteatomatous matrix covers the lateral semicircular canal and epitympanum.

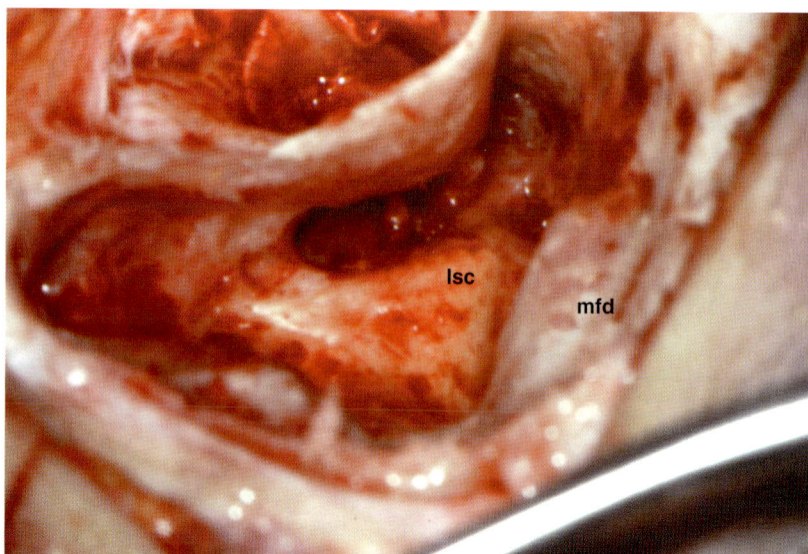

Figure 8.**67**   The cholesteatoma matrix has been removed. The posterior tympanotomy (PTT) is completed. There is a thick posterior canal wall. The head of the stapes and round window are seen through the PTT.

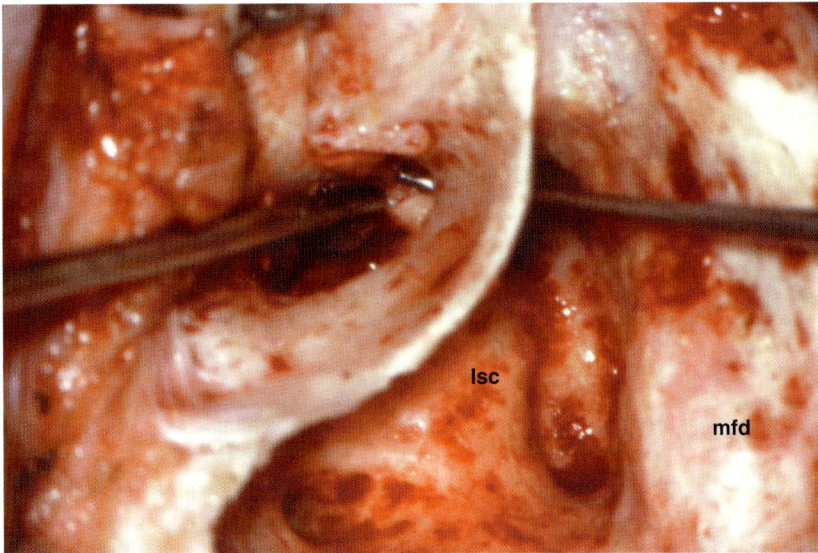

Figure 8.**68** Using a combined approach, a special instrument (the tympanic sinus raspatory) and a suction tip are used to remove the skin from the anterior part of the epitympanic area.

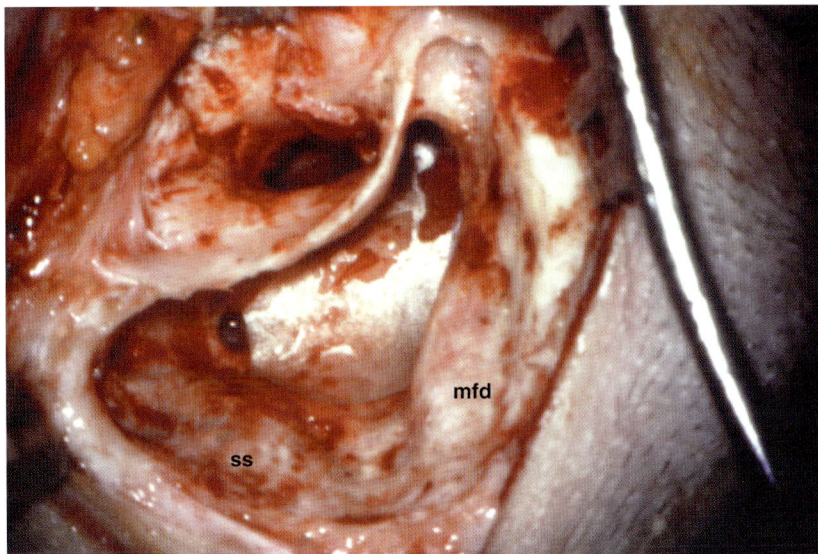

Figure 8.**69** A large Silastic sheet is introduced through the posterior tympanotomy.

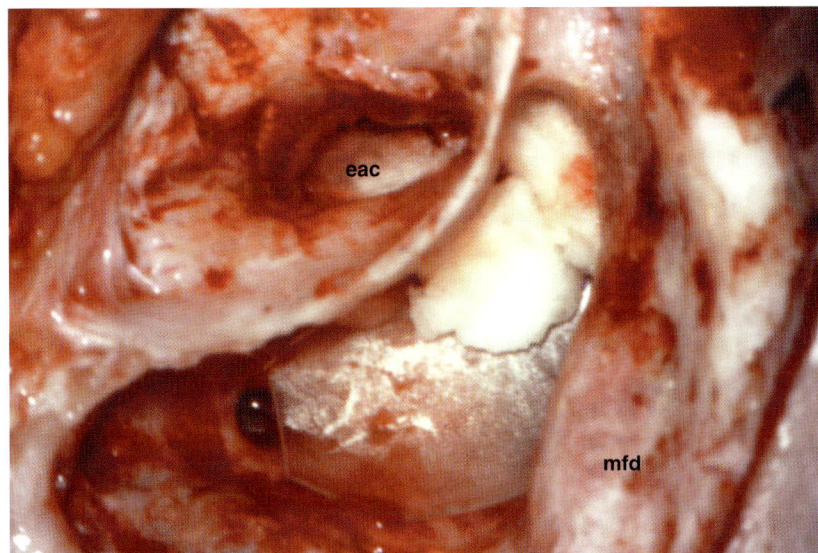

Figure 8.**70** The middle ear and epitympanic area are obliterated with Gelfoam.

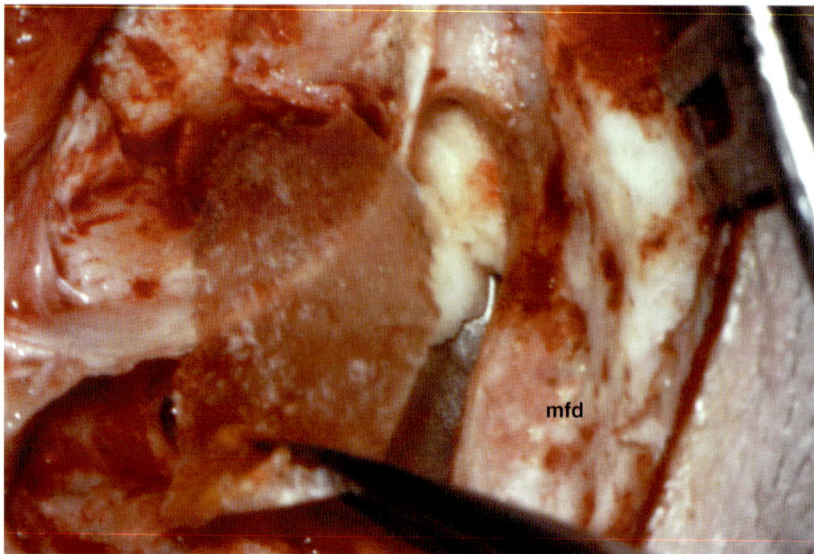

Figure 8.**71**   Dry temporalis fascia is used to reconstruct the tympanic membrane.

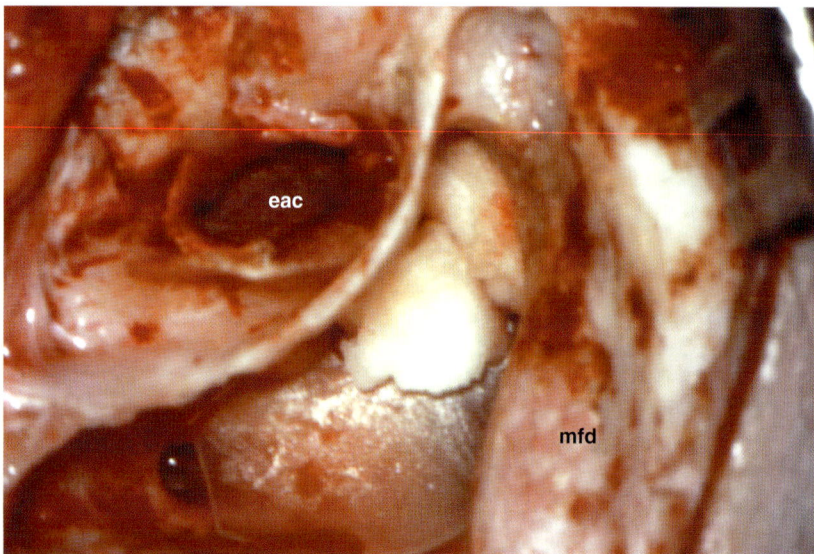

Figure 8.**72**   The tympanic membrane has been reconstructed using the underlay technique.

Canal Wall Down (Open) Tympanoplasty

Indications

• Cholesteatoma, in cases of:
  – Contracted mastoid
  – Large epitympanic erosions
  – Recurrence after closed tympanoplasty
  – Bilateral cholesteatoma
  – Cleft palate, or in Down's syndrome
  – The only hearing ear
  – Large labyrinthine fistula
  – Severe sensorineural hearing loss

• Some cases of benign tumor involving the middle ear and mastoid.

• Some cases of early malignancy of the external auditory canal.

Closed procedures, in comparison, do produce a dry ear, but are potentially unsafe due to the higher incidence of recurrent and residual disease. A well-performed primary open procedure usually avoids the need for any further surgical interventions, in contrast to the necessary preplanned second-look staged operation after closed cavity techniques. An adequate meatoplasty, which is a hallmark of a successful open procedure, is not cosmetically unacceptable to most of our patients. The hearing results are more or less same in open and closed procedures, and they depend on the availability of the stapes superstructure to reconstruct the sound transmission mechanism. Although we currently use the open procedure is more frequently, one should not be dogmatic about the technique to be adopted. By individualizing the surgery for cholesteatoma, we can now obtain the desired results in the majority of cases. However, since most of the theoretical advantages offered by closed techniques are overruled by those of open procedures, we have come to strongly believe that a proper open technique is a rational and logical approach in dealing with many cases of cholesteatoma, as we can achieve the primary goals of cholesteatoma surgery and extend the long-term benefit for the patient.

Surgical Technique

Local anesthesia (2% lidocaine and 1 : 100 000 epinephrine) is used in 95% of cases. General anesthesia is required in the remainder, when the patients are young or apprehensive. Using a postauricular skin incision, temporalis fascia is harvested for graft material.

The bone over the tegmen is thinned out in order to identify the middle fossa dura through the bone. Disease over the dura, if present, is gently removed. If there is any doubt about residual matrix on the dura, it is coagulated using bipolar cautery, as previously described by Sanna et al. (1993a). The air cells behind the sigmoid sinus are removed, and the sinodural angle is opened widely.

Usually, the antrum requires wide opening. The posterior canal wall is removed. The perilabyrinthine and the mastoid tip cells are also removed, and the mastoid tip is resected if it is pneumatized. The technique followed for excision of the mastoid tip is to create a fracture line lateral to the stylomastoid foramen, thereby avoiding any traction on the facial nerve in the process of removing the mastoid tip. With the help of a rongeur, the mastoid tip is mobilized and rotated outward in a clockwise fashion. The digastric muscle on the medial surface of the mastoid tip is dissected, and the sternomastoid muscle attachments are cut with the help of scissors. This amputation of the mastoid tip helps reduce the size of the cavity by 50%, and also avoids the sink-trap effect. The facial nerve should be distinguished from the disease. The two consistent structures for identifying the facial nerve are the cochleariform process and the digastric ridge. The digastric ridge is identified and then followed to the stylomastoid foramen. The ossicles are usually absent. The anterior buttress and the bony spur superior to the cochleariform process are removed along with the anterior attic cells. The zygomatic air cells are exteriorized, thereby removing all the air cells in the epitympanic space and the supratubal recess. The skin of the anterior and inferior bony ear canal is reflected towards the annulus and protected with aluminum foil. The ear canal is enlarged, with care being taken not to uncover the capsule of the temporomandibular joint. The tympanic membrane is then inspected, as usually there is some residual anterior and inferior tympanic membrane present.

The posterior buttress and the facial ridge are lowered to the floor of the external ear canal or the facial nerve itself. The disease is then cleared from the facial recess, sinus tympani and hypotympanum. At the end of the procedure, the cavity edges are smooth, rounded, and well saucerized. The appearance of white cortical bone signifies total exteriorization of all accessible air cells. The cavity, if even large, is not obliterated. We are not in favor of using any subcutaneous or muscle flaps, because of postoperative atrophy.

One of the most important steps in creating a trouble-free cavity is obtaining a wide meatus, to provide an adequate surface–volume ratio for aeration, epithelial stability, and good postoperative visualization of the cavity. The size of the meatus varies with the size of mastoid cavity. The conchal incision is made in an anterior to posterior direction, with the help of a nasal speculum. The conchal cartilage is further exposed by dissecting the skin from it. The cartilage on each side of the incision is excised in a triangular fashion. The skin flaps are sutured together with the subcutaneous tissue, so as to lie on the posterosuperior and posteroinferior aspects of the mastoid cavity. These skin flaps cover the remaining edge of the conchal cartilage, thereby preventing the possibility of perichondritis.

In cases in which staged procedures are necessary, medium-thickness Silastic is placed on the promontory, with a long extension into the eustachian tube orifice.

Temporalis fascia is placed on the Gelfoam bed medial to the annulus, spreading over to cover the facial ridge, epitympanum, and mastoid cavity. The residual tympanic membrane and canal skin are placed over it. The cavity and the ear canal are then filled with Gelfoam. The postauricular incision is sutured in layers, and a mastoid bandage is applied.

Modified Bondy Technique

Indications

- Epitympanic cholesteatoma with an intact tympanic membrane, ossicular chain, and middle ear.
- Epitympanic cholesteatoma in the better-hearing or only hearing ear with a slightly damaged ossicular chain.

  A modified Bondy technique is indicated in patients who have cholesteatoma arising from the epitympanic retraction pocket and an intact tympano-ossicular system, good hearing, and a mesotympanum free of disease.

Surgical Technique

The surgery is carried out in a such a way as to optimize the results and avoid a preoperative draining cavity. The authors prefer to carry out the procedure with the patient under local anesthesia. The mastoid is exposed through a postauricular incision. The posterior canal skin is saved as a vascular strip. A simple mastoidectomy is performed after the middle fossa and sinus plates have been identified. All of the air cells are removed, with particular attention being given to the perilabyrinthine and retrosigmoid air cells to avoid the formation of a mucous cyst postoperatively. The sinodural angle is opened as widely as possible, to allow proper aeration of this narrow angle. The facial bridge is removed after elevation of the meatal skin from the bone in order to create a smooth superior wall along the tegmen antri and middle fossa. Special care is taken to avoid contact with the intact ossicular chain while the facial bridge and anterior and posterior buttresses are being removed. The facial ridge is lowered, to create a round cavity instead of a kidney-shaped cavity (Figure 8.**75**). The anterior wall of the external canal is widened after the meatal flap has been elevated. An aluminum plate is used to protect the meatal flap and tympanic membrane during drilling. The cavity is saucerized to form a smooth wall and rounded margins (Figure 8.**74**).

To avoid retraction around the ossicles postoperatively, part of the lateral attic wall is reconstructed with cartilage and bone paste. In some cases, a piece of cartilage is put over the long process of the incus to prevent retraction around it.

For meatoplasty, an incision is made in the skin in the middle of the concha to create two triangular flaps. A piece of the cartilage of the posterior canal and concha is excised for meatoplasty, depending on the size of the cavity. The skin flaps are turned in and sutured in place to line part of the cavity. The postauricular incision is closed in two layers.

In the Bondy operation, the mastoid cavity is exteriorized without disturbing the normal middle ear contents. Incomplete mastoid air cell removal and insufficient lowering of the facial ridge were the drawbacks of the procedure when it was introduced. These can be easily avoided in a properly performed mastoidectomy, with the better facilities for magnification and illumination that are now available.

The risk of the procedure is sensorineural hearing loss due to acoustic trauma, as the ossicular chain remains intact during drilling. In experienced hands, this risk is easily avoided with careful drilling close to the ossicles. There are no risks other than those with other open mastoidectomy procedures, such as problems relating to the cavity. Preservation of good preoperative hearing is not possible with all techniques. A modified Bondy technique is the only procedure that allows preservation of good preoperative hearing in one stage in patients with epitympanic cholesteatoma and an intact ossicular chain and pars tensa.

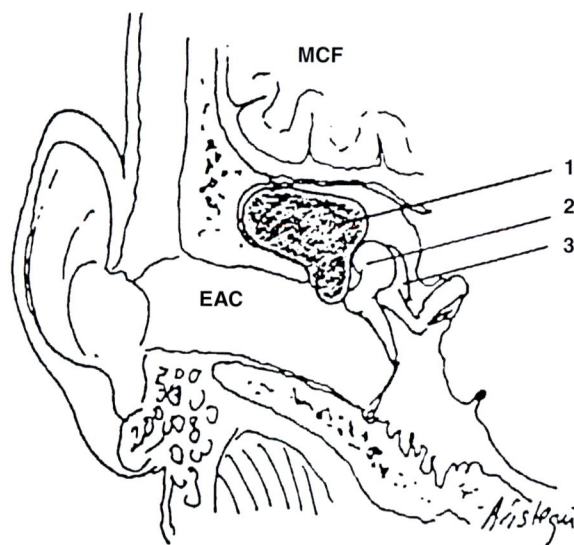

Figure 8.**73**   A typical indication for the Bondy technique for cholesteatoma. The epitympanic cholesteatoma lies laterally to the malleus and the incus.

EAC: External auditory canal
MCF: Middle cranial fossa
1:   Epitympanic cholesteatoma
2:   Malleus
3:   Incus

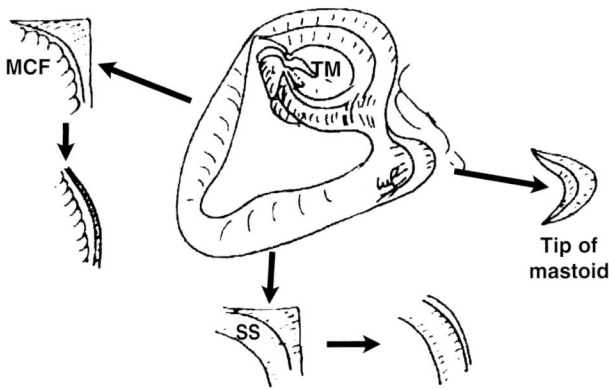

Figure 8.**74**   The cavity is saucerized to form a smooth wall and rounded margins.

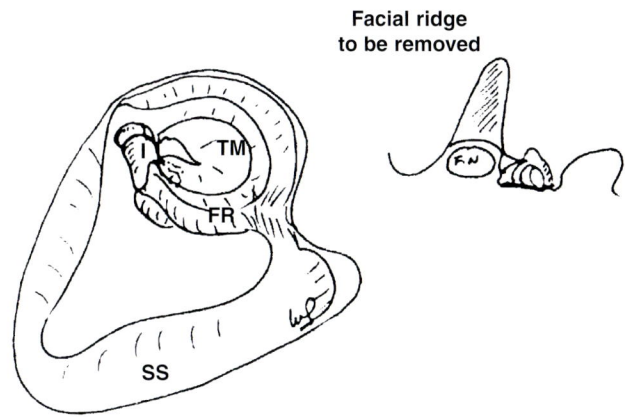

Figure 8.**75**   The facial ridge is lowered to create a round cavity.

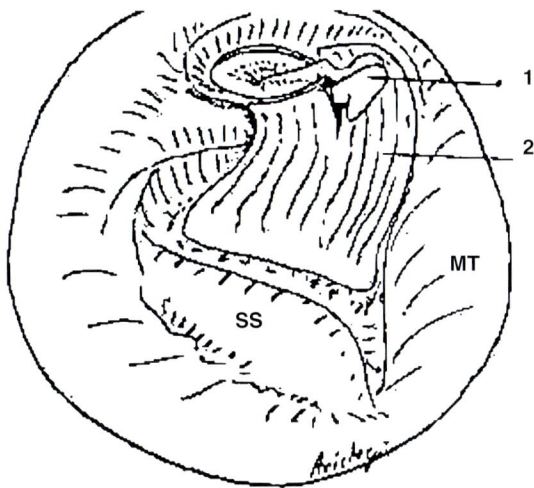

Figure 8.**76**   Fascia is inserted with two anterior tongues, one under the incus body and the other between the handle of the malleus and the long process of the incus.

1:   Incus
2:   Fascia

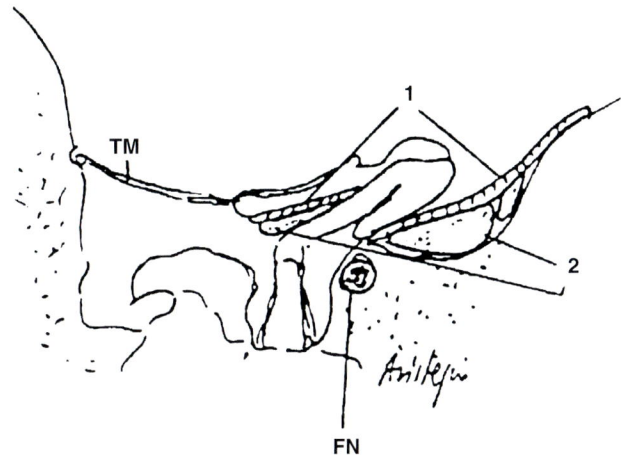

Figure 8.**77**   A sagittal view, showing the position of the fascia as described in Fig. 8.**76**.

1 : Fascia
2 : Cartilage
FN: Facial nerve

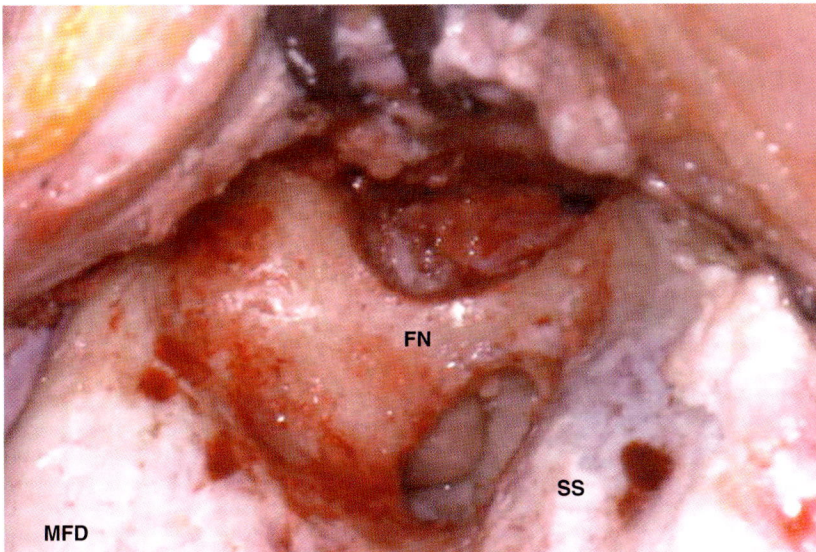

Figure 8.**78**   The initial surgical step. The bony overhangs are drilled on the middle fossa dura and sigmoid sinus.

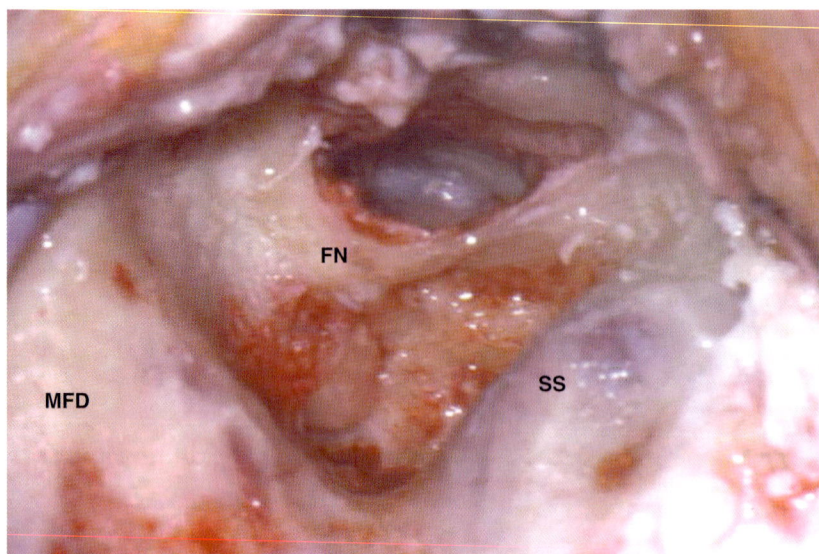

Figure 8.**79** The facial ridge must be lowered as far as the annulus.

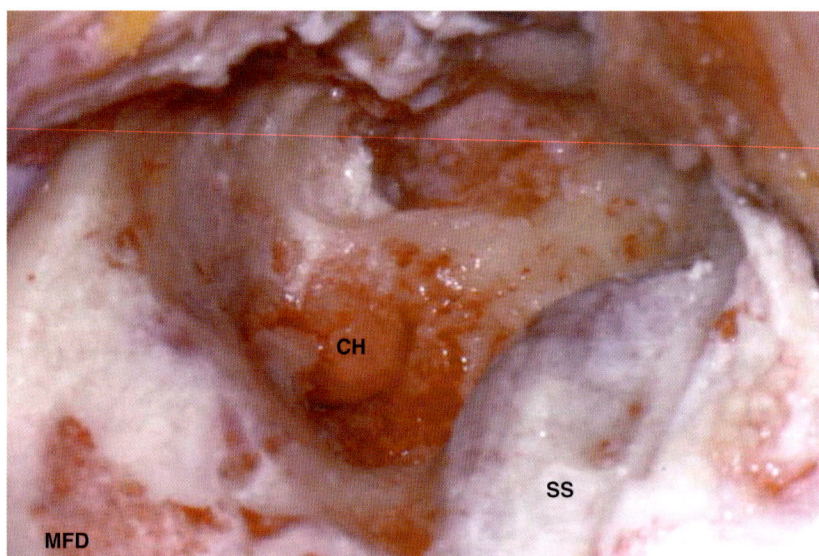

Figure 8.**80** The sinus dural angle is opened. Cholesteatoma is present in the attic.

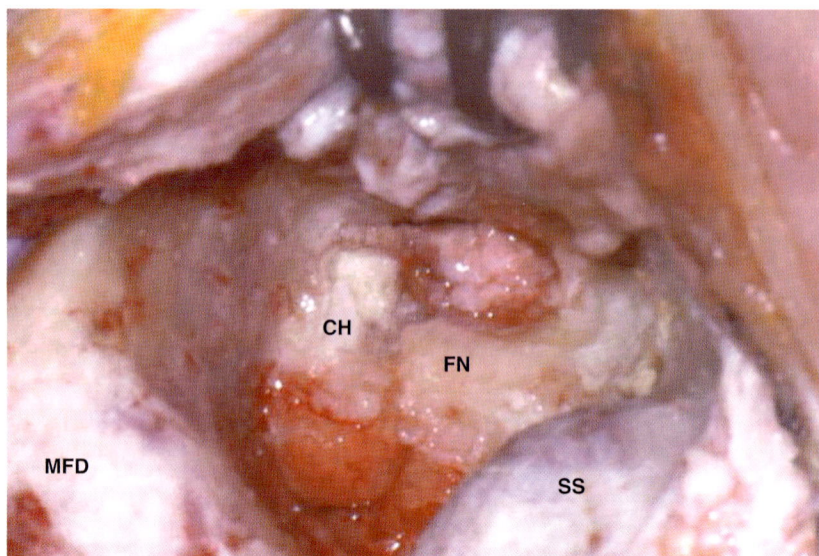

Figure 8.**81** Further drilling over the middle fossa dura and on the facial ridge exposes the cholesteatoma better.

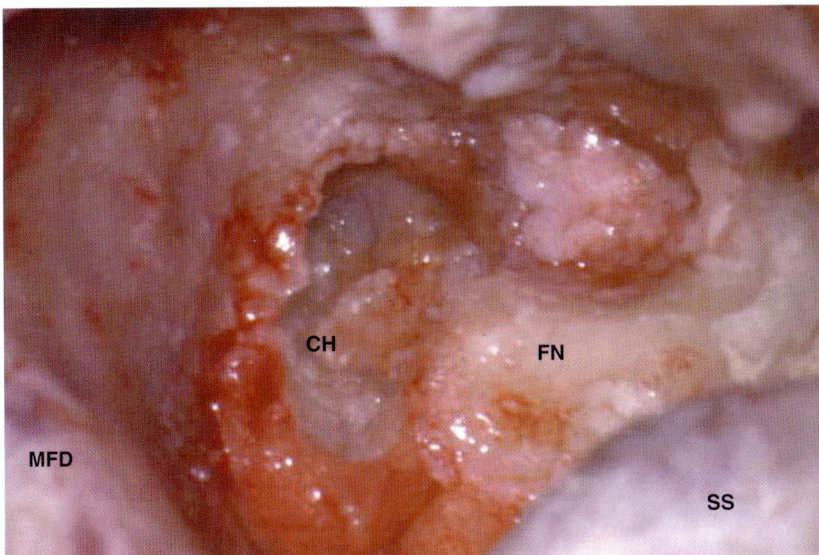

Figure 8.**82** The cholesteatoma is removed from the attic.

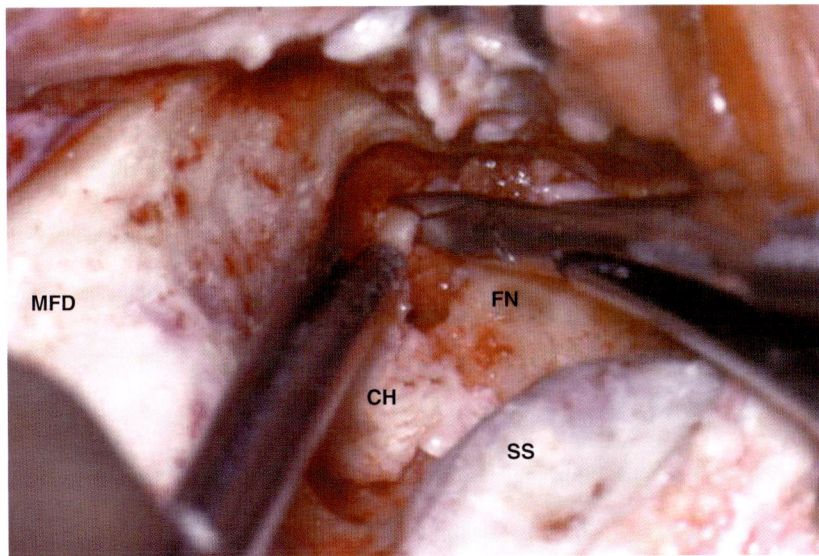

Figure 8.**83** Drilling is carried out until the whole of the attic has been checked.

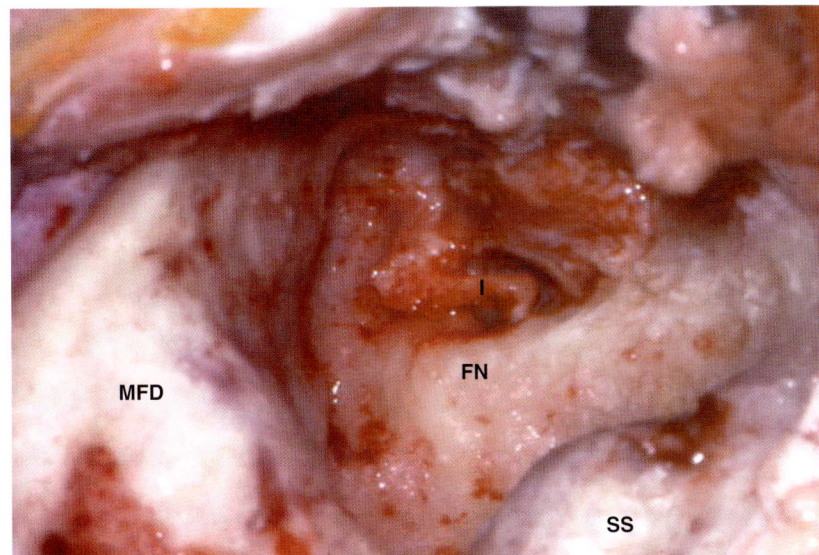

Figure 8.**84** After removal of the cholesteatoma, the ossicular chain is left intact.

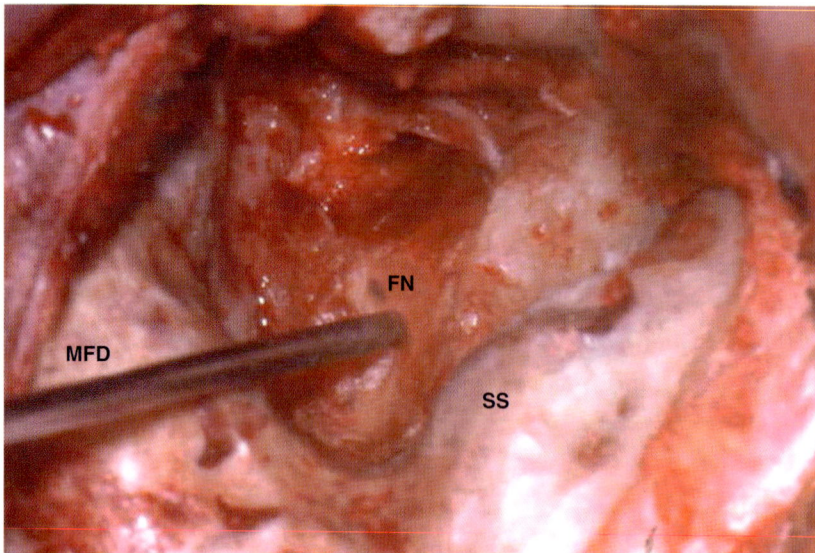

Figure 8.**85**   The fascia is inserted with the two anterior tongues, one under the incus body and the other between the handle of the malleus and the long process of the incus.

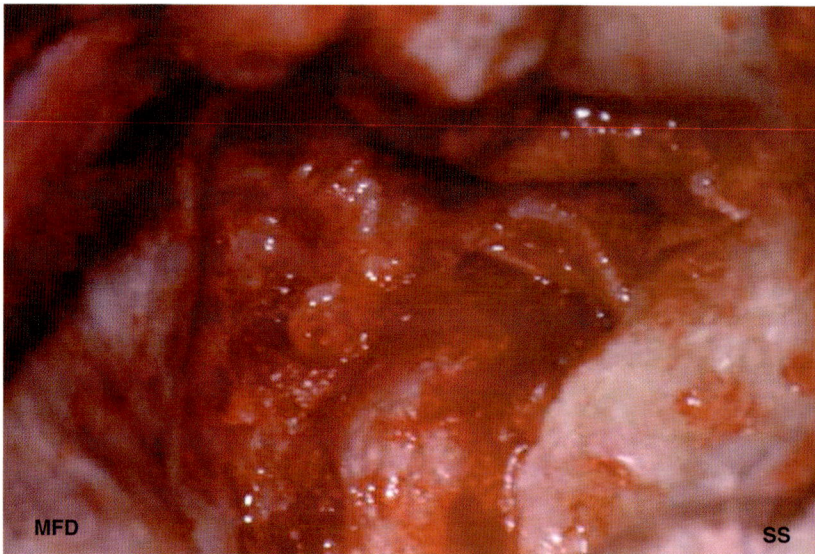

Figure 8.**86**   With greater magnification, the correct positioning of the fascia in surgical activity is clearly seen.

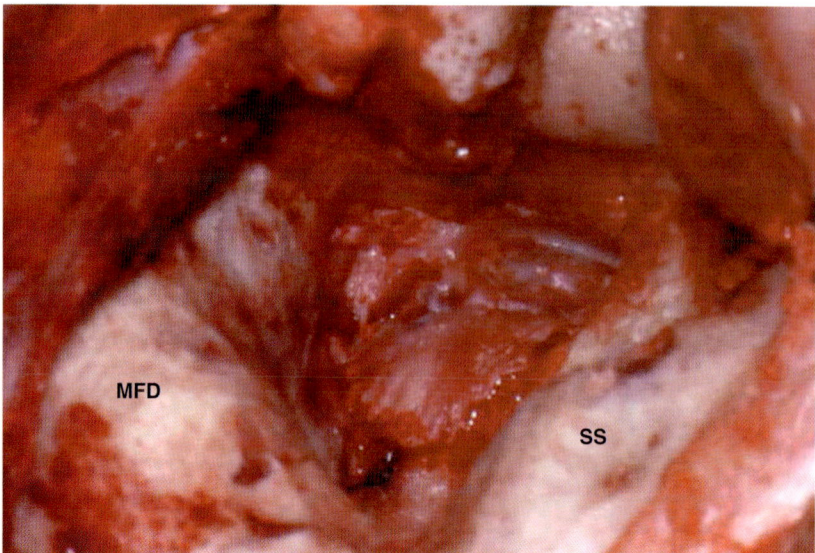

Figure 8.**87**   View of the surgical cavity as it appears at the end of the procedures.

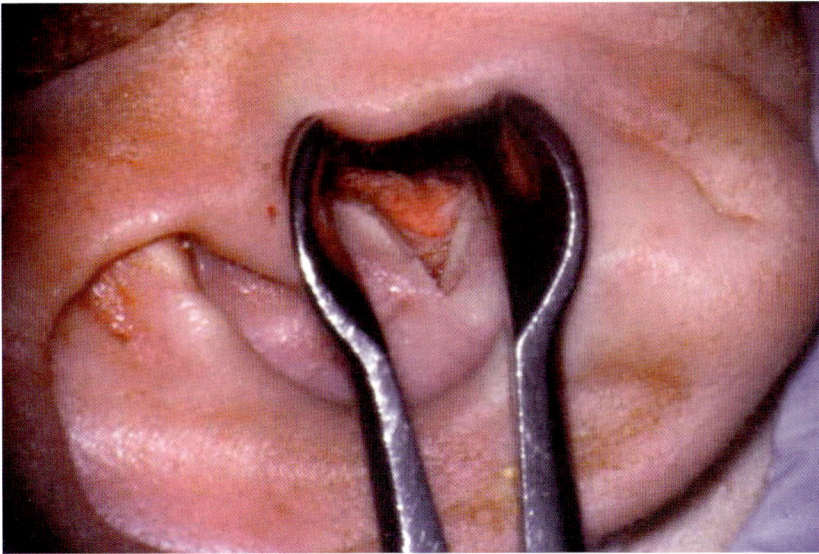

Figure 8.**88**   A meatoplasty is carried out in accordance with the size of the cavity.

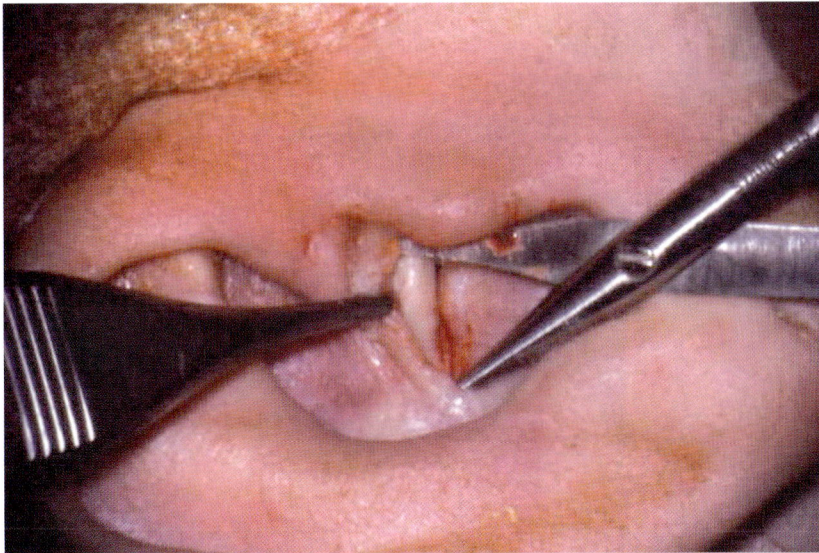

Figure 8.**89**   A superior triangle of cartilage is removed.

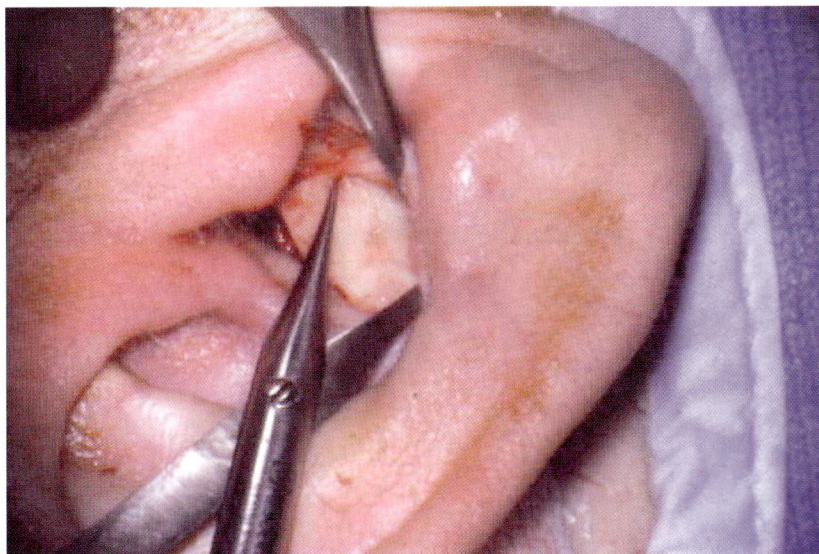

Figure 8.**90**   An inferior triangle of cartilage is also removed.

9 Congenital Cholesteatoma of the Middle Ear

Congenital cholesteatoma is defined as an epidermoid cyst that develops behind an intact tympanic membrane in a patient with no history of otorrhea, trauma, or previous ear surgery. Michaels studied fetal temporal bones and demonstrated the presence of an epidermoid structure between 10 and 33 weeks of gestation. This structure tends to involute spontaneously until it completely disappears. Michaels hypothesized that the persistence of this structure could act as an anlage and lead to congenital cholesteatoma. The fact that the most classic location of congenital cholesteatoma, namely in the anterosuperior part of the tympanum, corresponds to the site of the fetal Michaels structure supports this theory. In our cases, however, and contrary to the few studies reported in the literature (Derlacki and Clemis 1965, Friedberg 1994, Levenson et al. 1989, Cohen 1987), the most common site of congenital cholesteatoma was the posterior mesotympanum (see Table 9.1).

As no existing theory can truly explain the origin of congenital cholesteatoma in the posterior location, a strong conjecture can be made that these lesions might represent a different entity from those of the anterior location and may originate from epithelial cell rests that are trapped in the posterior mesotympanum during the development of the temporal bone. Diagnosis is either occasional in the asymptomatic patient, or the patient may complain of hearing loss due to erosion of the ossicular chain or of recurrent attacks of secretory otitis media due to occlusion of the tubal orifice by the cholesteatomatous mass. A high degree of suspicion and thorough examination are essential in detecting the presence of these lesions.

Table 9.1 Classification of congenital cholesteatoma of the middle ear

Type	Location	Percent
Type A	Mesotympanic	52.27
Type A1	Premalleolar	4.54
Type A2	Retromalleolar	46.72
Type B	Epitympanic	6.81
Type A/B	Mixed	40.90

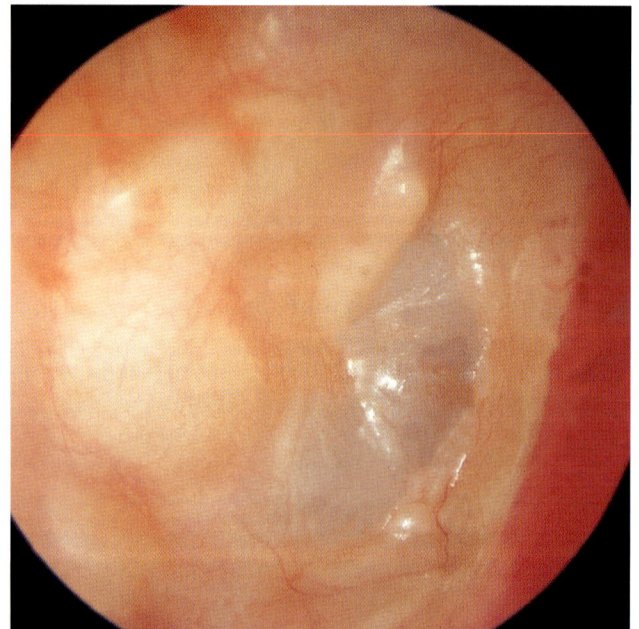

Figure 9.1 Right ear. Congenital cholesteatoma seen as a white retrotympanic mass causing bulging of the posterior quadrants of the tympanic membrane. Neither drum perforation nor bony erosion are detected.

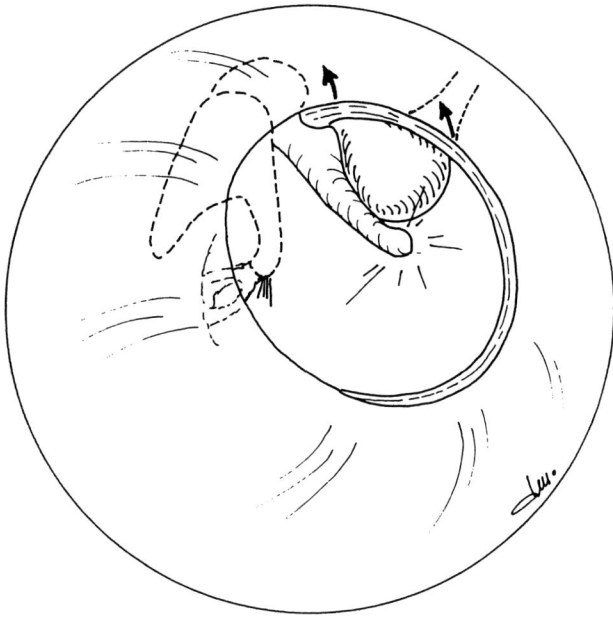

Figure 9.**2**   Type A1 congenital cholesteatoma.

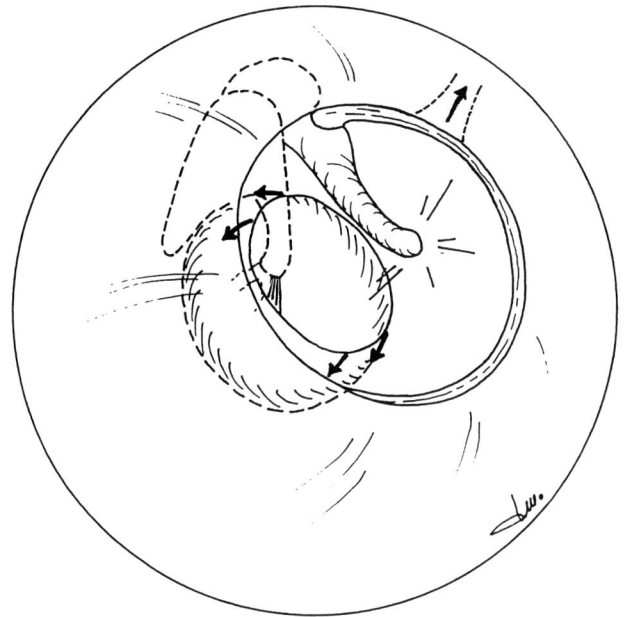

Figure 9.**3**   Type A2 congenital cholesteatoma.

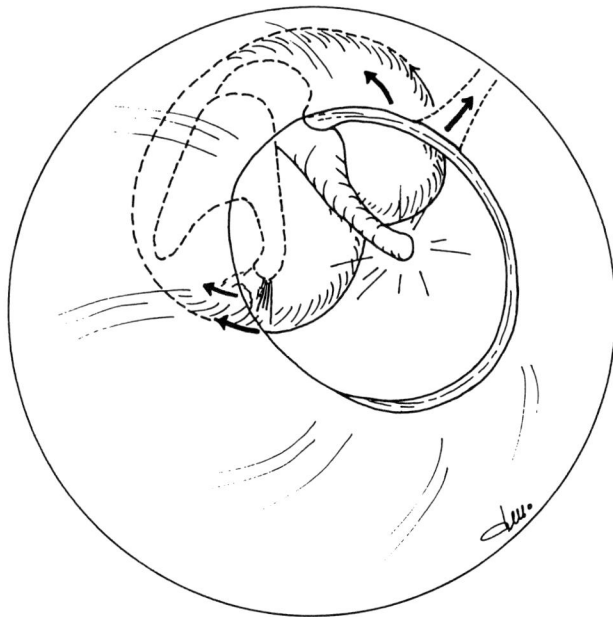

Figure 9.**4**   Type B congenital cholesteatoma.

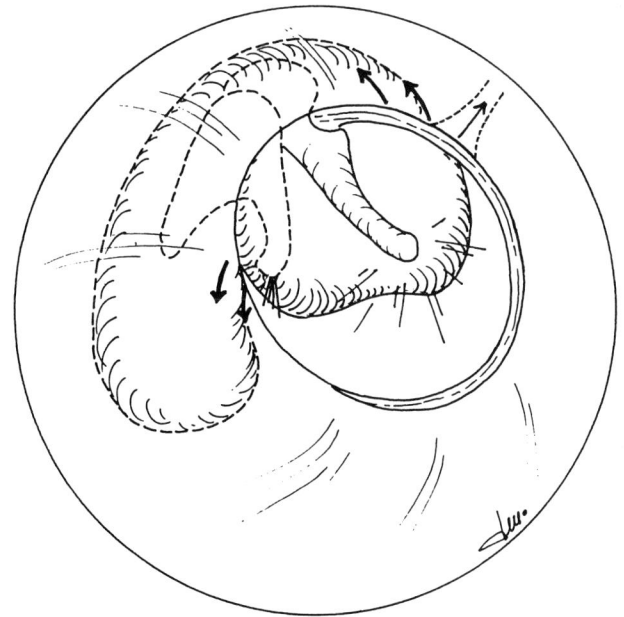

Figure 9.**5**   Type A/B congenital cholesteatoma.

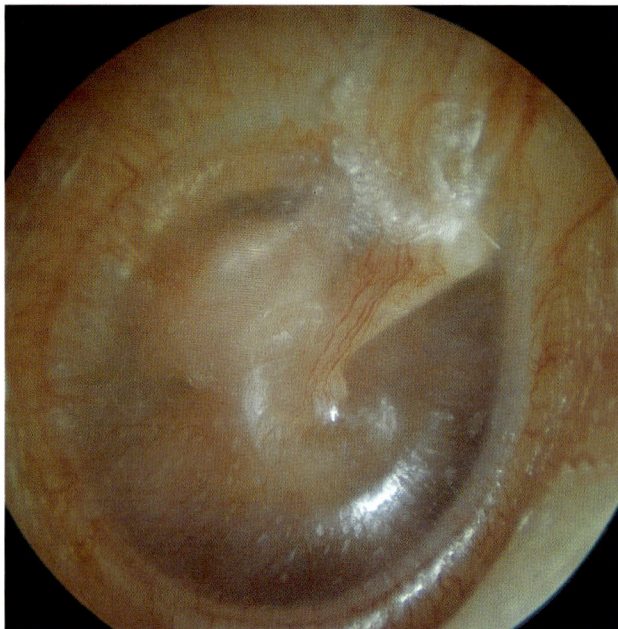

Figure 9.**6** Right ear. A small whitish retrotympanic mass is clearly seen. The mass lies posterior to the malleus (type A2). By definition, a cholesteatoma is considered congenital when the tympanic membrane is intact and there is no history of otorrhea or previous ear operations (including myringotomy or ventilation tube insertion).

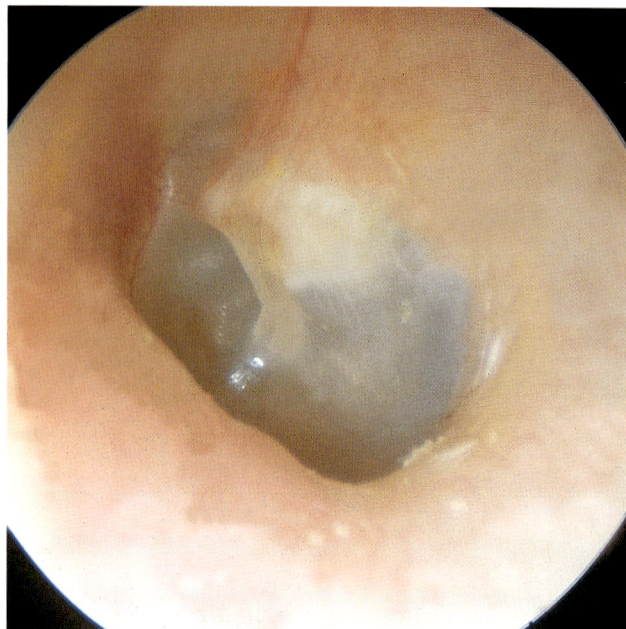

Figure 9.**7** Left ear. A case similar to that in Figure 9.**6**. The cholesteatoma caused erosion of the long process of the incus with resultant conductive hearing loss.

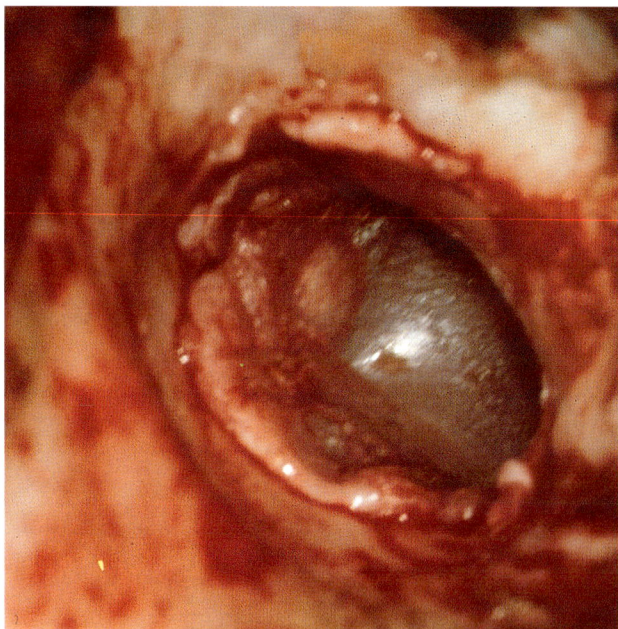

Figure 9.**8** Right ear, intraoperative view. A small premalleolar congenital cholesteatoma (type A1) can be seen behind the intact tympanic membrane.

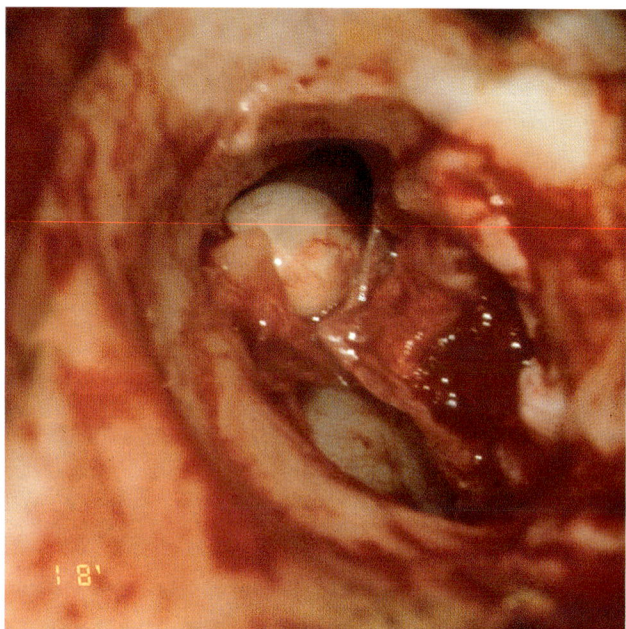

Figure 9.**9** Same case, intraoperatively, after elevation of the tympanomeatal flap.

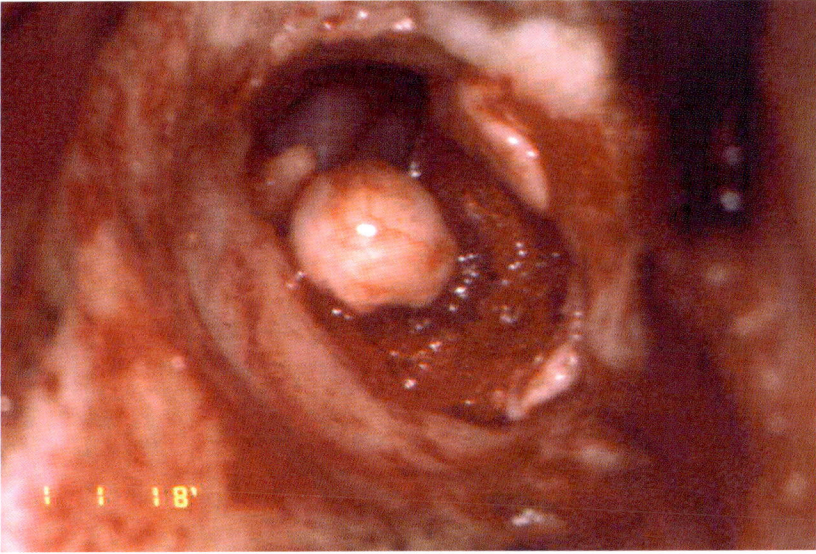

Figure 9.**10**   The cholesteatoma pearl has been almost completely removed.

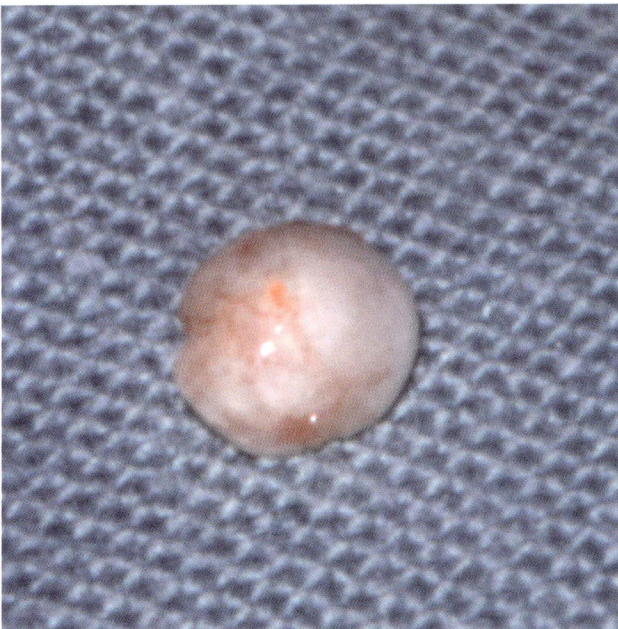

Figure 9.**11**   The cholesteatoma pearl has been removed.

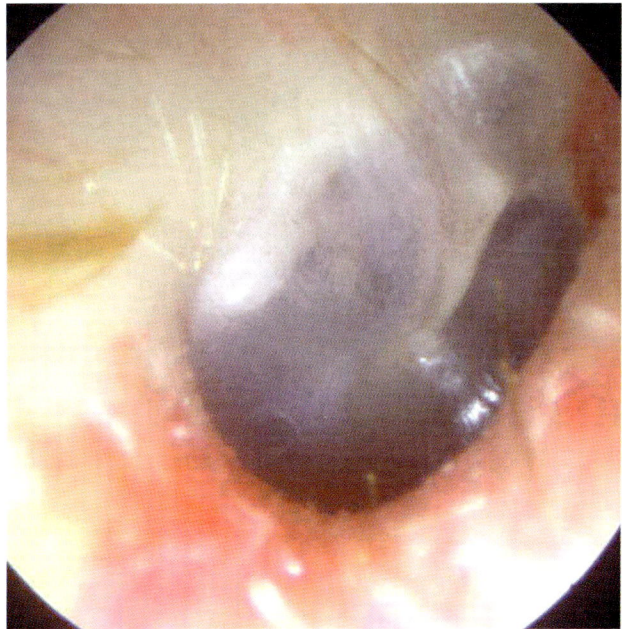

Figure 9.**12**   Right ear. Type A2 congenital cholesteatoma. The cholesteatoma caused erosion of the long process of the incus and the stapes superstructure, with resultant conductive hearing loss.

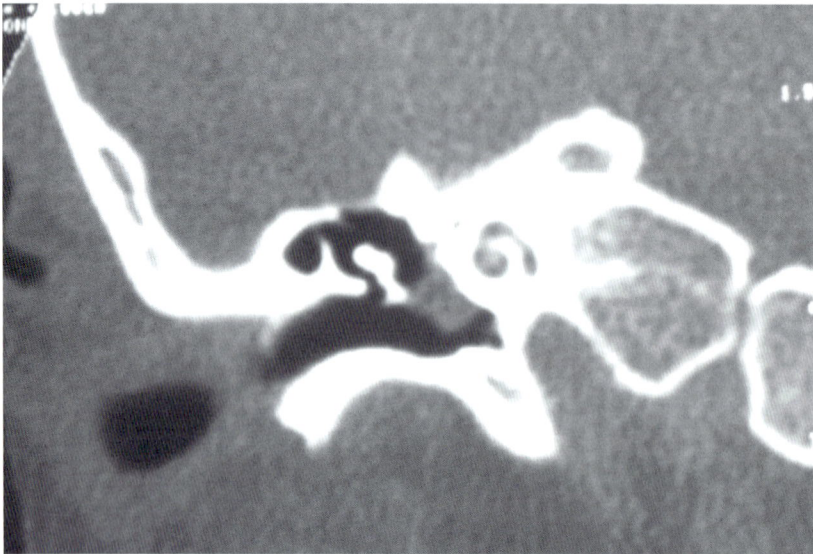

Figure 9.**13**   CT scan of the same patient. The cholesteatoma pearl is clearly visible at the level of oval window. The mastoid and middle ear are completely free. A retroauricular transmeatal approach with ossicular reconstruction in one stage was performed.

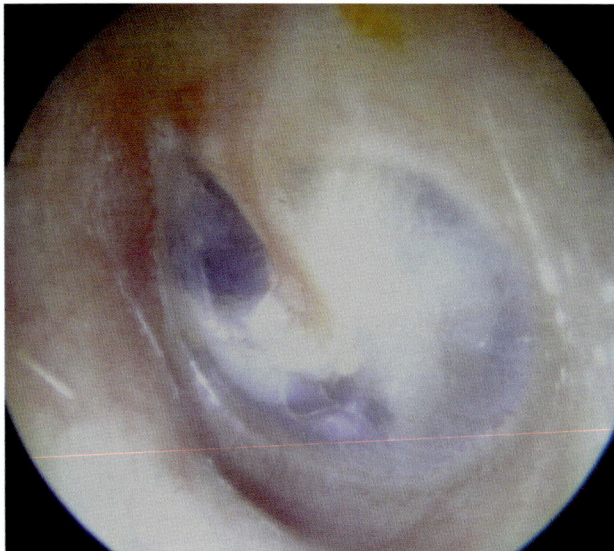

Figure 9.**14**   Left ear. Type A2 retromalleolar congenital cholesteatoma. The pearls extend anteriorly to the umbo.

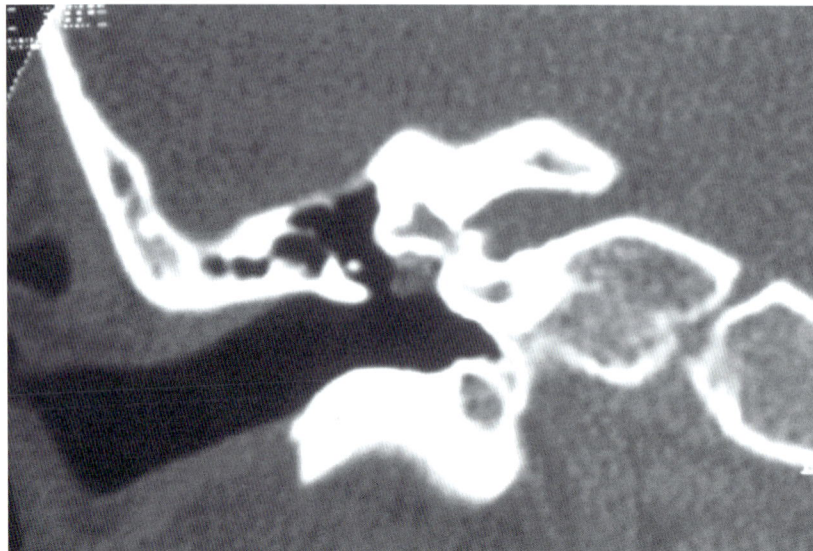

Figure 9.**15**   CT scan of the same patient as in Fig. 9.**14**, with a small congenital cholesteatoma localized in the mesotympanum.

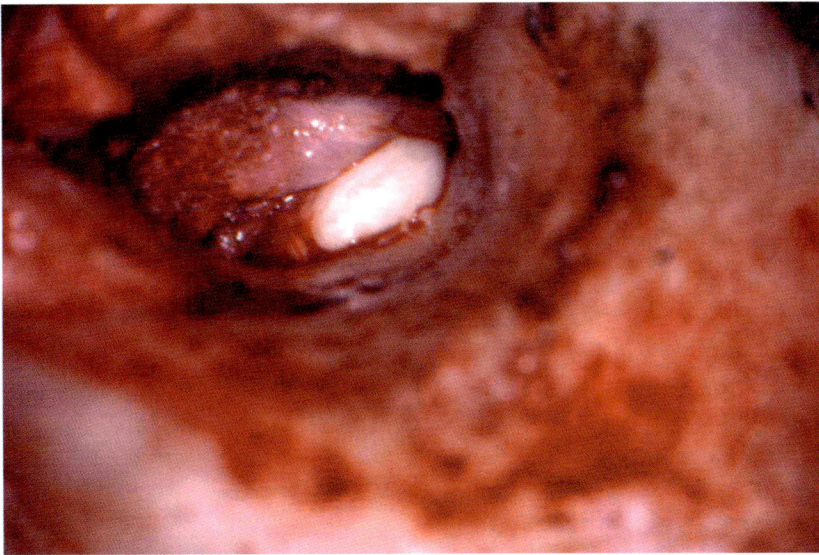

Figure 9.**16**   Left ear. First stage canal wall up tympanoplasty of the patient in Fig. 9.**14**. A postero-auricular incision has been made and a tympanomeatal flap has been created. The cholesteatoma cyst is clearly visible.

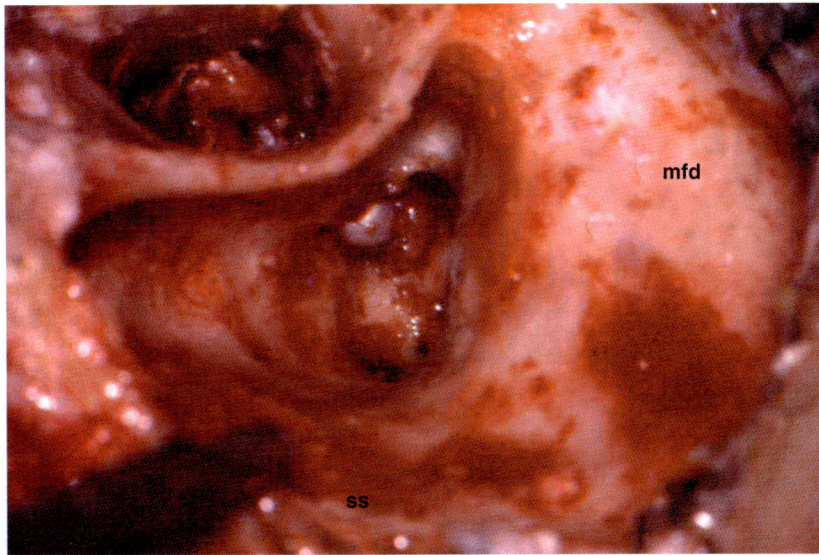

Figure 9.**17**   Left ear. A subtotal mastoidectomy has been carried out, and the posterior wall of the external auditory canal is preserved. The cholesteatoma appears at the level of the short process of the incus.

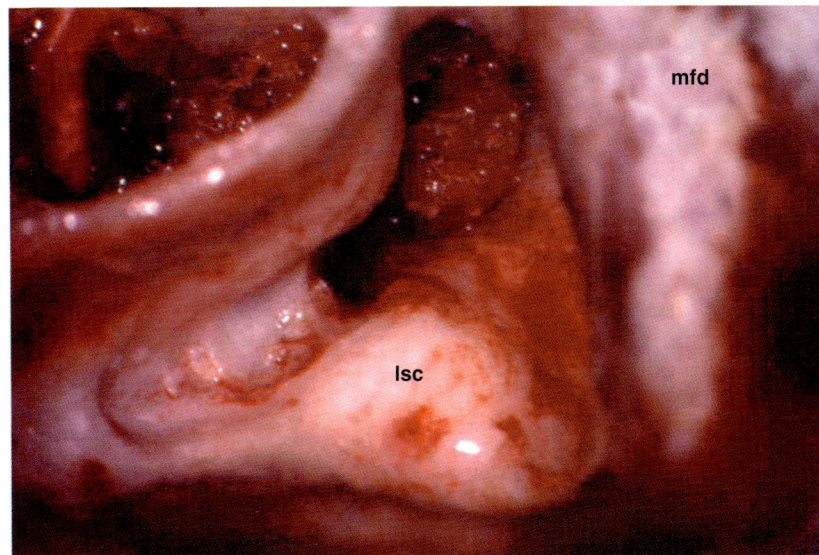

Figure 9.**18**   The posterior tympanotomy has been started.

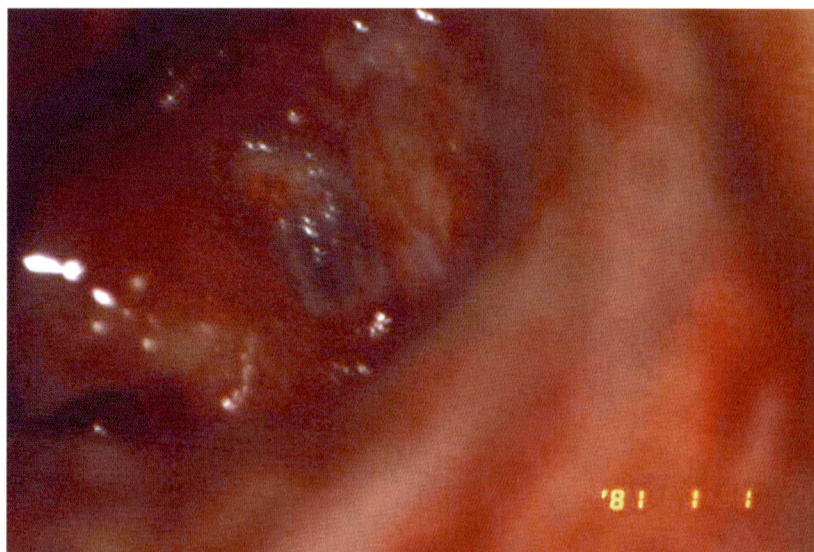

Figure 9.**19** The stapes superstructure is missing, as often happens in type A2 and A/B congenital cholesteatoma.

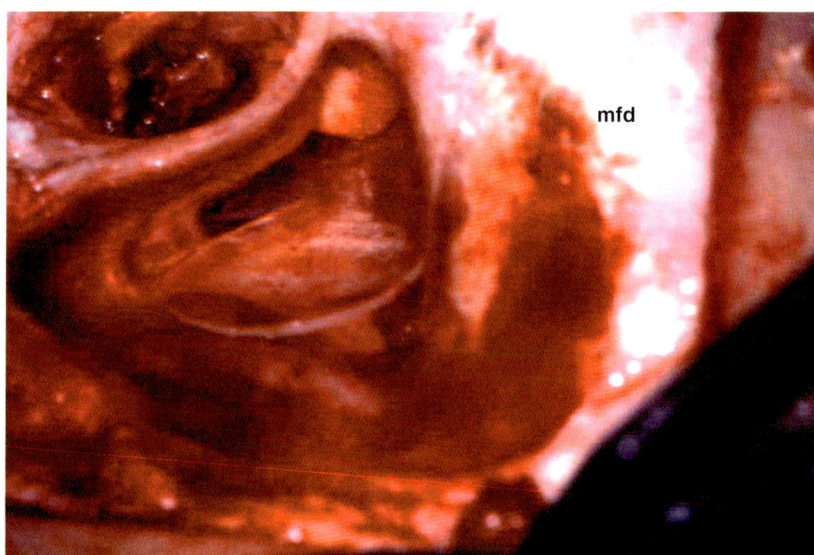

Figure 9.**20** Removal of the cholesteatoma has been completed. A Silastic sheet is inserted through the posterior tympanotomy. The functional second-stage procedure to control the cavity and carry out ossicular reconstruction is planned after an interval of 12 months.

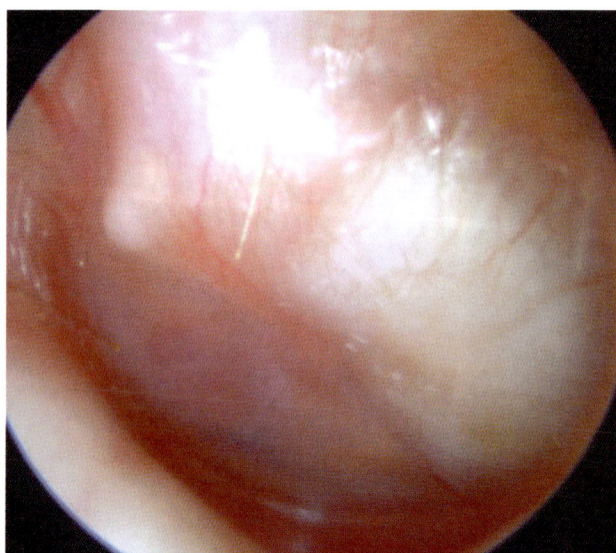

Figure 9.**21** Left ear. Type A/B congenital cholesteatoma. The cholesteatoma is seen as a white retrotympanic mass, causing bulging of the posterior quadrant of the tympanic membrane. A combined-approach tympanoplasty in two stages is indicated.

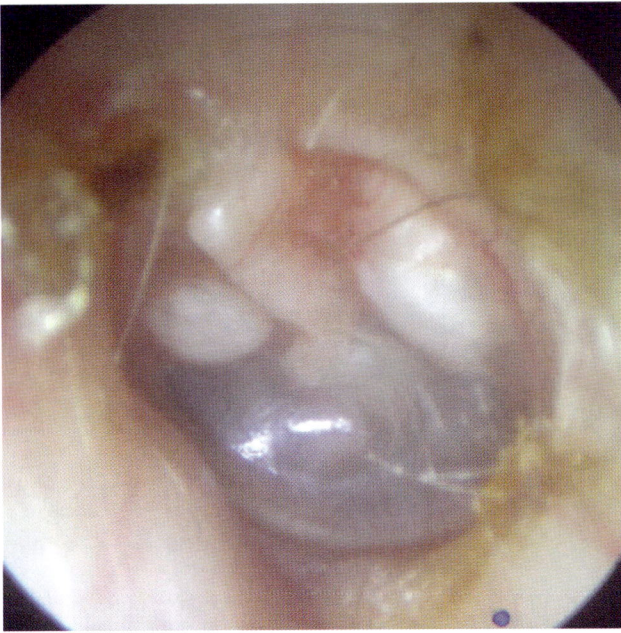

Figure 9.**22**   Left ear. Congenital cholesteatoma type A/B with two white masses anterior and posterior to the handle of the malleus. Neither perforation nor bony erosion is evident. The tympanic membrane is perfectly normal. A combined-approach tympanoplasty is indicated.

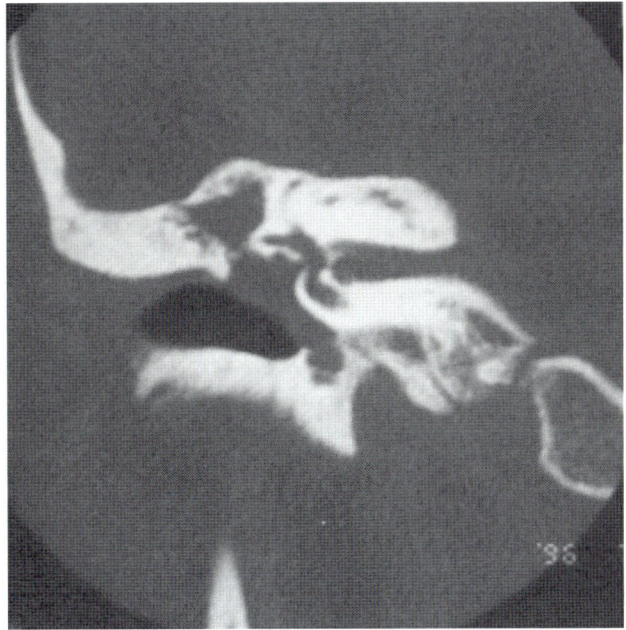

Figure 9.**23**   CT scan of type A/B congenital cholesteatoma. The hypotympanum and mastoid are completely filled with cholesteatoma. The incus and stapes are absent.

Summary

Congenital cholesteatoma of the middle ear is an infrequent pathology during infancy and childhood. It presents behind an intact tympanic membrane, either anterior or posterior to the handle of the malleus.

Anterosuperior cholesteatoma can be removed through an extended tympanotomy that permits the preservation of the tympanic membrane and ossicular chain integrity. Posterior cholesteatoma, however, requires a staged closed tympanoplasty. The second stage serves to check for any residual cholesteatoma. The ossicular chain, which is generally eroded in the posterior type, can be reconstructed at this stage.

10 Petrous Bone Cholesteatoma

Unlike middle ear cholesteatoma, petrous bone cholesteatoma represents an epidermoid cyst that involves the petrous part of the temporal bone. This type of cholesteatoma involves and/or is related to very important structures (namely, the facial nerve, posterior labyrinth, cochlea, internal carotid artery, internal auditory canal, and posterior and middle fossa dura); therefore, the management of such lesions should be performed in centers specialized in otoneurology and skull base surgery. The main presenting symptom is fetid otorrhea, which frequently recurs in an open mastoid cavity. The second most common symptom is progressive facial nerve palsy, which occurs in more than 50% of cases. Hearing loss can be conductive, sensorineural, or mixed. About 50% of cases complain of vertigo, but it is rarely the motive for the patient's visit to the doctor. Otoscopy may be irrelevant or only demonstrates pars flaccida perforation or an open mastoid cavity with evidence of suppurative discharge. A computed tomography (CT) scan and magnetic resonance imaging (MRI) are fundamental to evaluate the extension of the lesion and to determine the surgical approach.

Petrous bone cholesteatoma is defined as congenital when it develops from epithelial cell rests entrapped in the petrous bone during embryological development. In such cases, the first symptoms are facial nerve paralysis, vertigo, and deaf ear due to invasion of the facial nerve and labyrinth. This type represents about 3% of all cases of cholesteatoma and is localized at the level of the petrous apex.

Petrous bone cholesteatoma is defined as acquired when a middle ear cholesteatoma follows the cell tracts of the temporal bone in a lateral to medial direction and invades the underlying structures. The most frequent symptoms in such cases are fetid otorrhea, followed by hearing loss (conductive, perceptive, or mixed), facial nerve paralysis, and vertigo.

The iatrogenic form also develops in an old radical cavity or as a late occurrence following tympanoplasty. The most common symptoms in such cases are also fetid otorrhea, facial nerve paralysis, hearing loss, and vertigo.

We classify petrous bone cholesteatoma into five types according to its localization and extension: supralabyrinthine, infralabyrinthine, massive labyrinthine, infralabyrinthine apical, and apical.

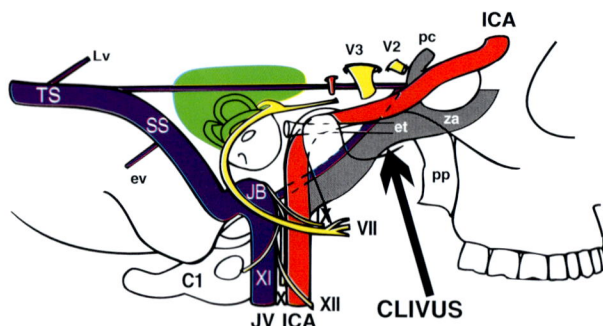

Figure 10.1 The supralabyrinthine type of petrous bone cholesteatoma is centered on the region of the geniculate ganglion. Most frequently, it extends anteriorly towards the basal turn of the cochlea and the internal carotid artery. Less commonly, it grows towards the retrolabyrinthine air cells. This localization is typical of congenital cholesteatoma of the petrous bone. It may also arise due to a deep growth of an epitympanic cholesteatoma.

TS:	Transverse sinus	pc:	Posterior clinoid
Lv:	Labbé's vein	V2:	Trigeminal 2
SS:	Sigmoid sinus	V3:	Trigeminal 3
ev:	Emissary vein	C1:	First cervical vertebra
JB:	Jugular bulb	VII:	Facial nerve
JV:	Jugular vein	IX:	Glossopharyngeal nerve
ICA:	Internal carotid artery	X:	Vagus nerve
pp:	Pterygoid processes	XI:	Spinal accessory nerve
za:	Zygomatic arc	XII:	Hypoglossal nerve
et:	Eustachian tube		

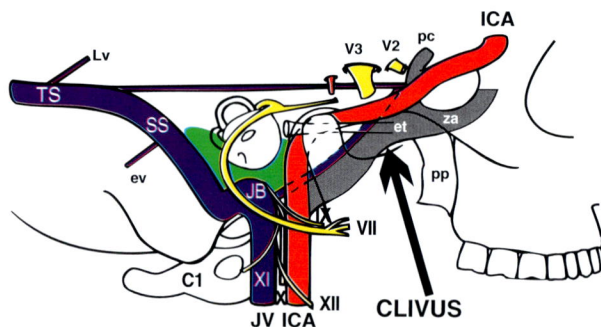

Figure 10.2 The infralabyrinthine type of petrous bone cholesteatoma is usually encountered in an old radical mastoid cavity. It is localized in the region of the hypotympanum and the infralabyrinthine air cells. It may extend posteriorly towards the posterior cranial fossa or anteriorly towards the internal carotid artery, petrous apex, and clivus.

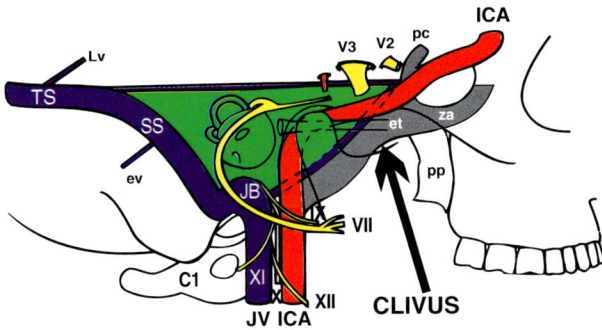

Figure 10.**3** The massive labyrinthine type of petrous bone cholesteatoma largely involves the posterior labyrinth and the cochlea. It may extend anteriorly towards the internal carotid artery, medially towards the internal auditory canal, posteriorly towards the posterior fossa, or inferiorly towards the infralabyrinthine compartment. Abbreviations are given in Figure 10.**1**.

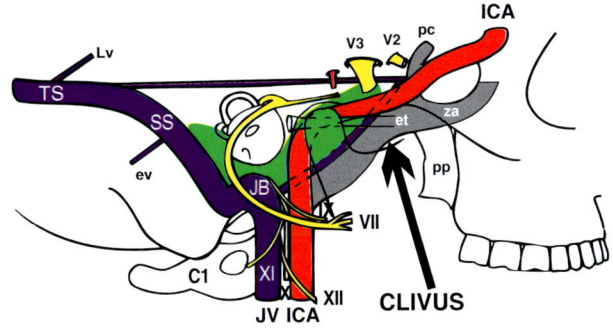

Figure 10.**4** The infralabyrinthine apical type of petrous bone cholesteatoma originates from the infralabyrinthine or apical compartments. When it originates from the former, it extends into the petrous apex. In some cases it may grow towards the sphenoid sinus or the horizontal portion of the internal carotid artery.

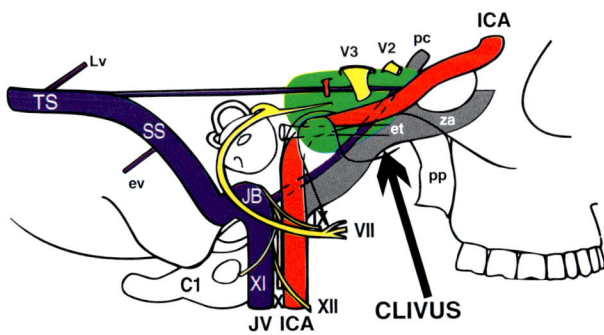

Figure 10.**5** The apical type of petrous bone cholesteatoma is a rare congenital lesion. It may solely involve the apical compartment, causing erosion of it. It may involve the trigeminal nerve or more posteriorly the posterior cranial fossa. It may also engulf the horizontal portion of the internal carotid artery.

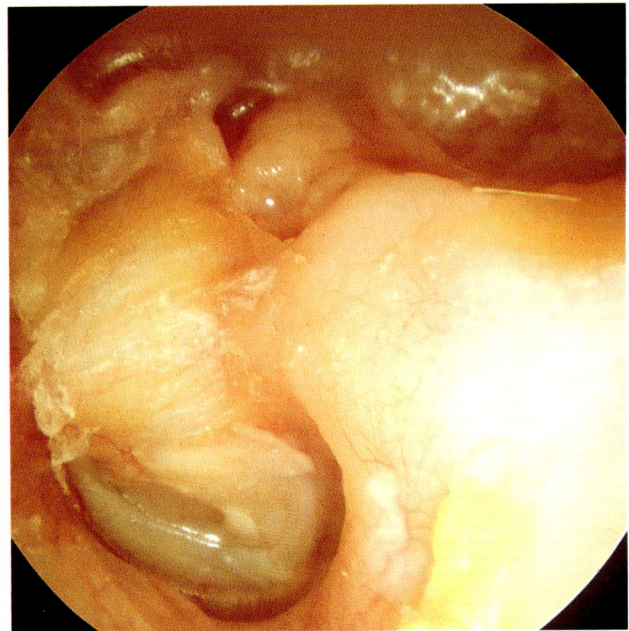

Figure 10.**6** Left acquired or iatrogenic supralabyrinthine petrous bone cholesteatoma in a radical cavity. A whitish retrotympanic mass is seen at the level of the second portion of the facial nerve. The patient presented with progressive facial nerve paralysis and total hearing loss. A correct diagnosis depends not only on otoscopy but also on the symptomatology (facial paralysis, anacusis) and a high-resolution CT scan.

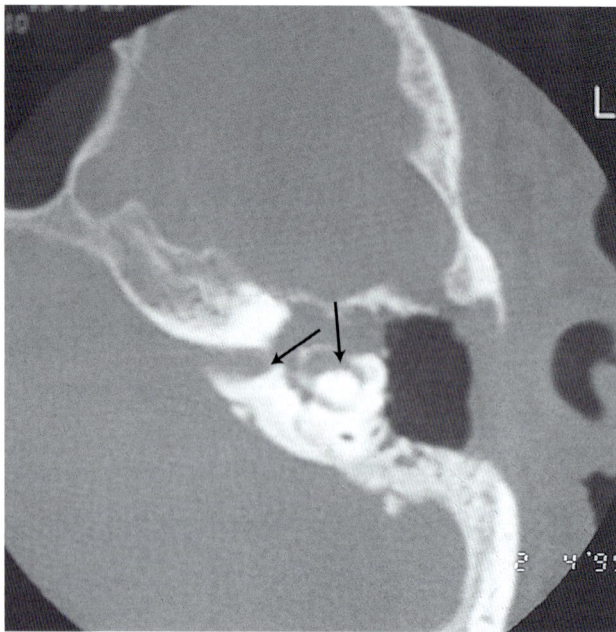

Figure 10.**7**   CT scan of the case presented in Figure 10.**6**, axial section. Involvement of the lateral semicircular canal and the vestibule is well visualized. The cholesteatoma invades the cochlea anteriorly, while medially it reaches the fundus of the internal auditory canal. The posterior semicircular canal is not invaded.

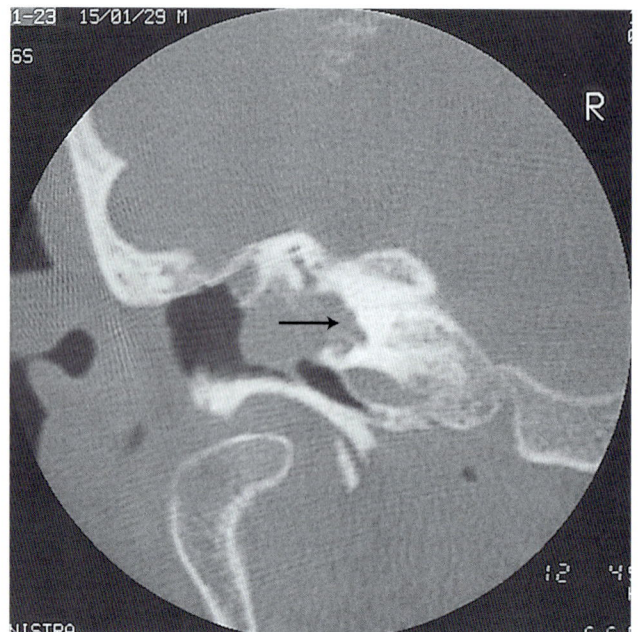

Figure 10.**8**   CT scan of the case presented in Figure 10.**6**, coronal section. The medial extension of the cholesteatoma can be appreciated.

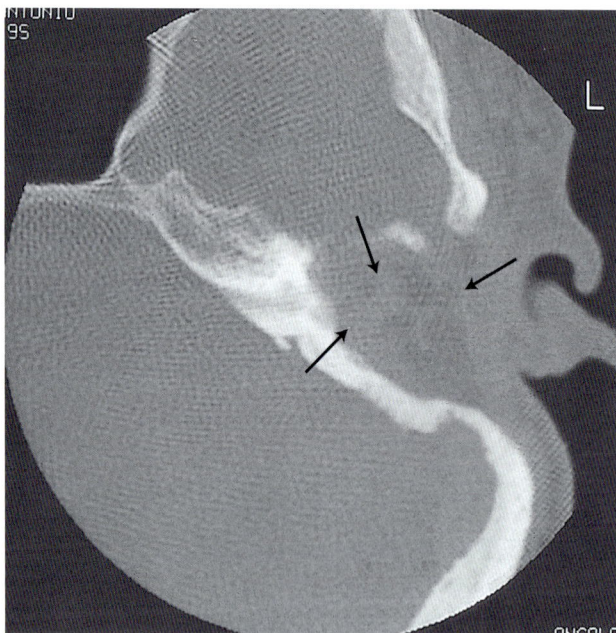

Figure 10.**9**   Postoperative CT scan. A transcochlear approach was performed and the operative cavity was obliterated with abdominal fat.

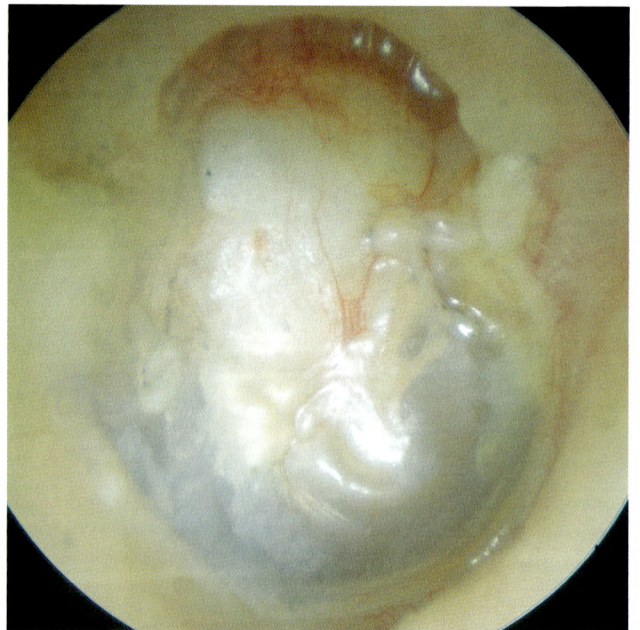

Figure 10.**10**   Right acquired supralabyrinthine petrous bone cholesteatoma. A whitish mass is present in the mastoid cavity of an open tympanoplasty. The mass occupies the whole epitympanum and extends inferiorly behind the tympanic membrane. The patient presented with ipsilateral facial paralysis and conductive hearing loss.

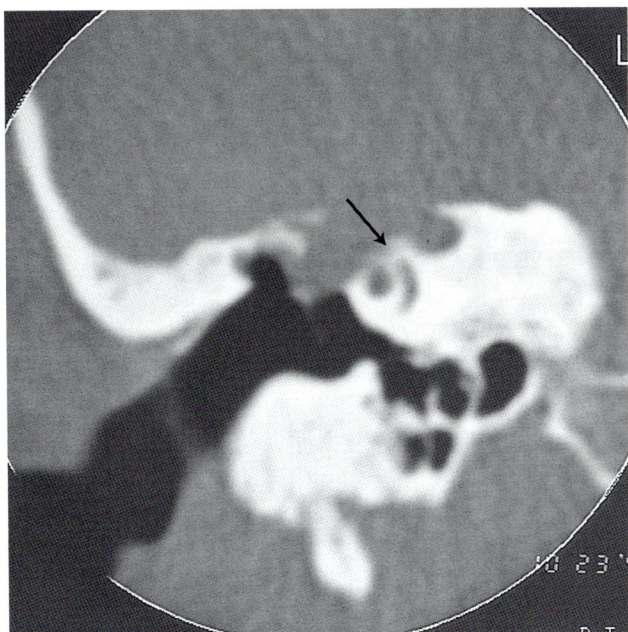

Figure 10.**11**   CT scan of the case presented in Figure 10.**10**. The cholesteatoma invades the cochlea. Total removal of the pathology was accomplished using a transcochlear approach with obliteration of the operative defect using abdominal fat. The external auditory canal was closed as a cul-de-sac. The facial nerve was infiltrated at the level of the geniculate ganglion and was repaired using a sural nerve graft.

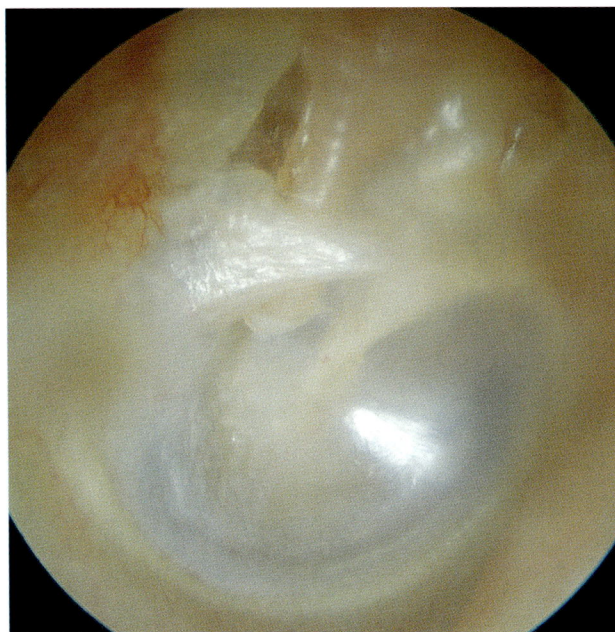

Figure 10.**12**   Another example of right acquired supralabyrinthine petrous bone cholesteatoma. The patient presented with right facial nerve paralysis. Otoscopy reveals a right epitympanic erosion.

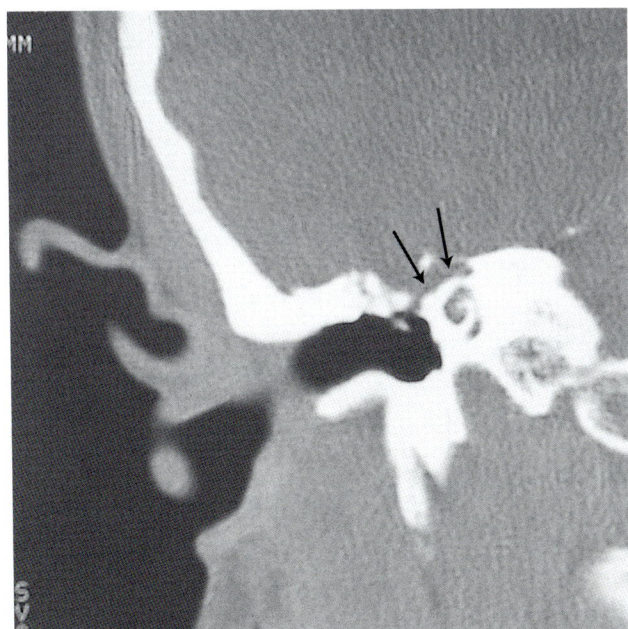

Figure 10.**13**   CT scan of the case presented in Figure 10.**12**, coronal view. Typical location and erosion of acquired small supralabyrinthine petrous bone cholesteatoma.

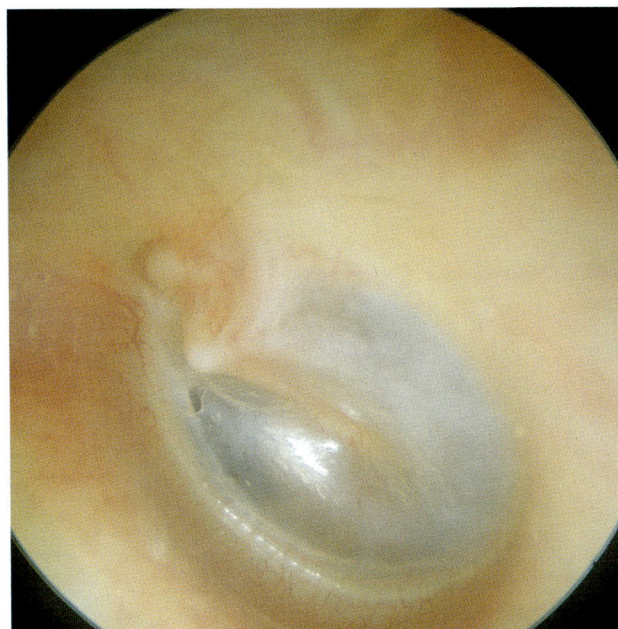

Figure 10.**14**   Left congenital supralabyrinthine petrous bone cholesteatoma with extension towards the apex. Otoscopy is negative. The patient complained of progressive facial nerve paralysis of 5 years' duration as well as conductive hearing loss.

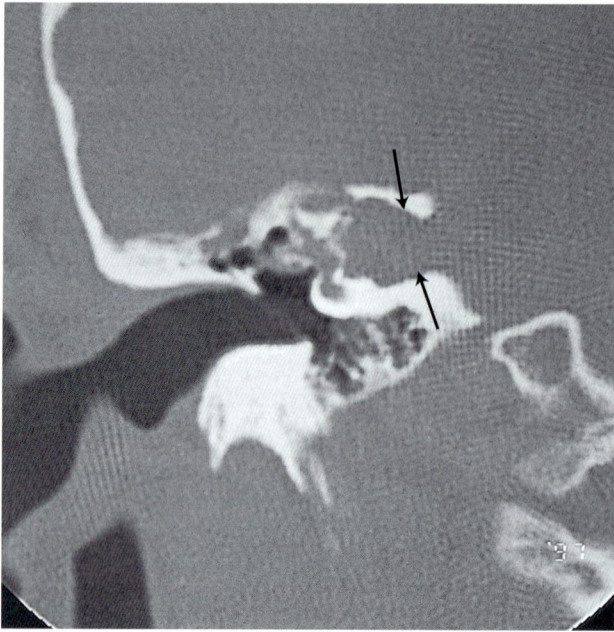

Figure 10.**15**   CT scan of the case presented in Figure 10.**14**. Coronal view showing extension of the cholesteatoma into the internal auditory canal.

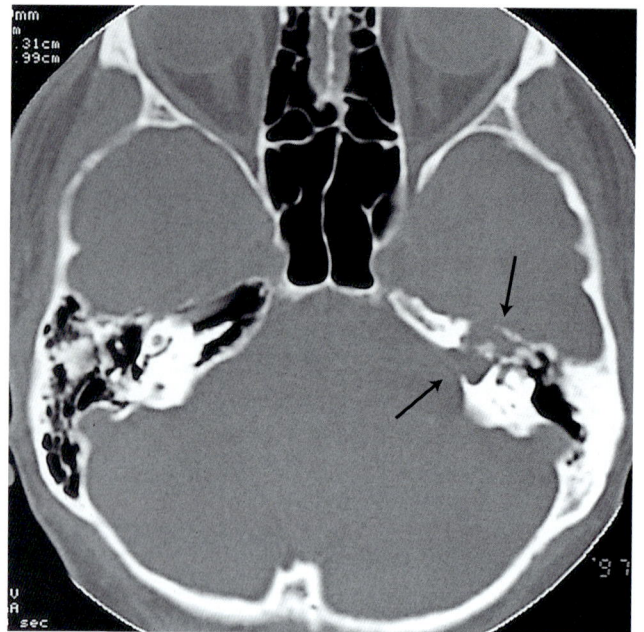

Figure 10.**16**   CT scan of the case presented in Figure 10.**14**. Axial view showing cholesteatoma extending into the petrous apex.

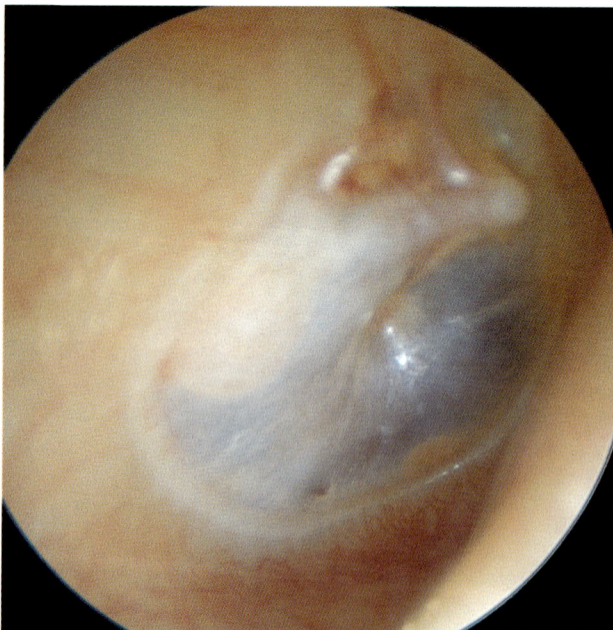

Figure 10.**17**   Right congenital infralabyrinthine apical petrous bone cholesteatoma in a 30-year-old female patient. In the posterosuperior quadrant a white retrotympanic view is observed. The patient had been suffering from right anacusis since childhood and instability of 1 year duration. The facial nerve was normal.

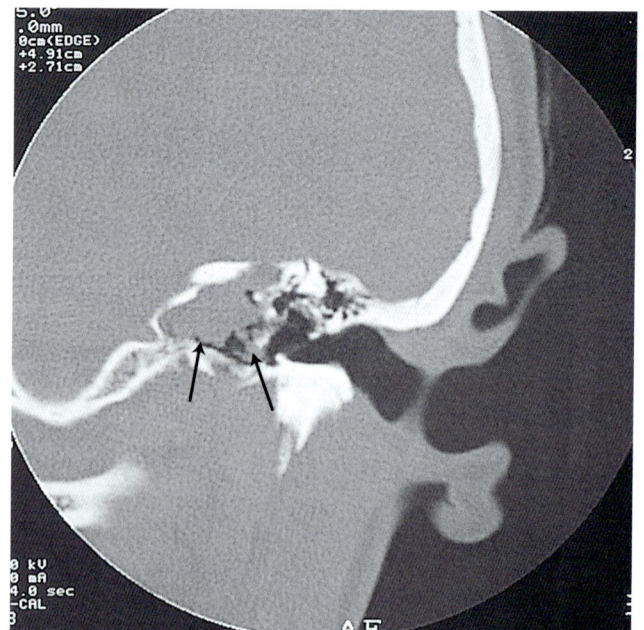

Figure 10.**18**   CT scan of the case presented in Figure 10.**17**. Coronal view demonstrating the involvement of the infralabyrinthine apical compartment by the cholesteatoma.

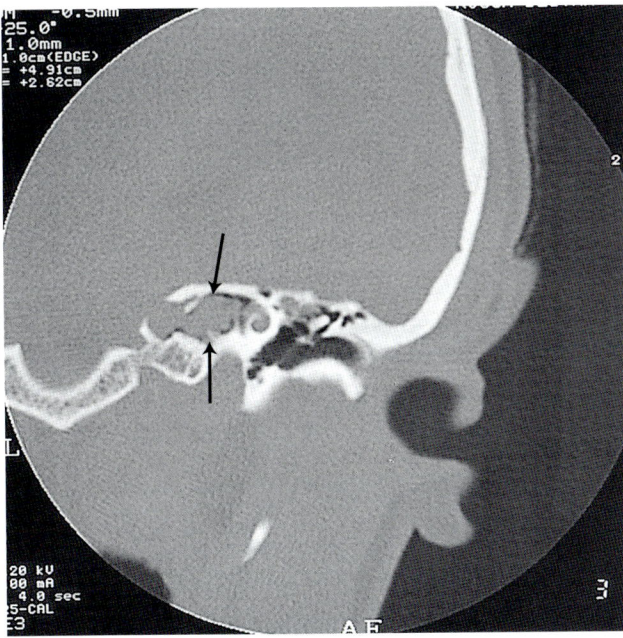

Figure 10.**19**   CT scan of the case presented in Figure 10.**17**. A more anterior coronal view at the level of the cochlea.

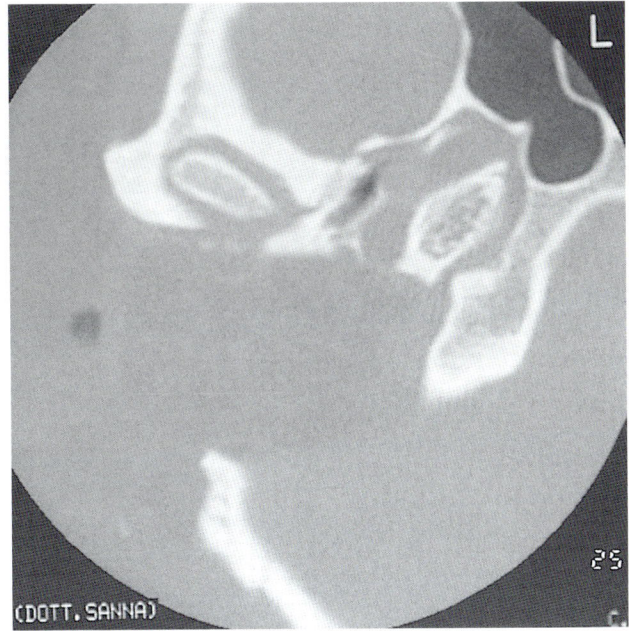

Figure 10.**20**   Postoperative CT scan showing total removal of the cholesteatoma through the transcochlear approach and obliteration of the operative cavity using abdominal fat.

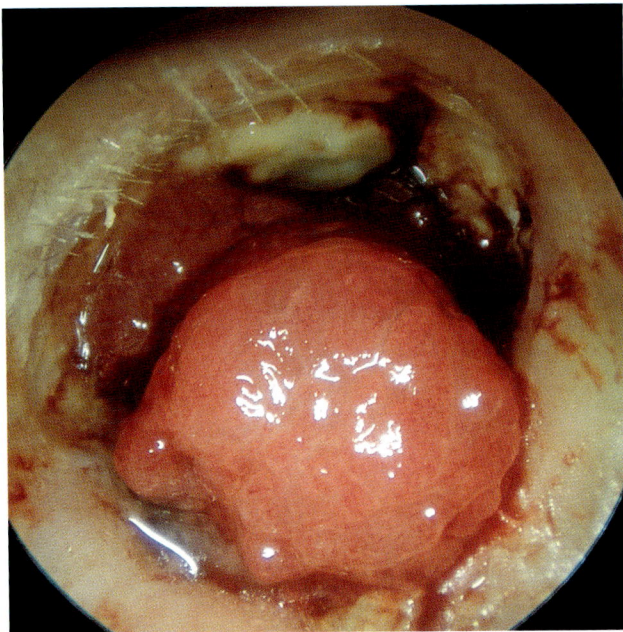

Figure 10.**21**   Polyp in the external auditory canal in a patient who had undergone a tympanoplasty (see CT scan, Fig. 10.**22**). The patient presented with otorrhea and hearing loss.

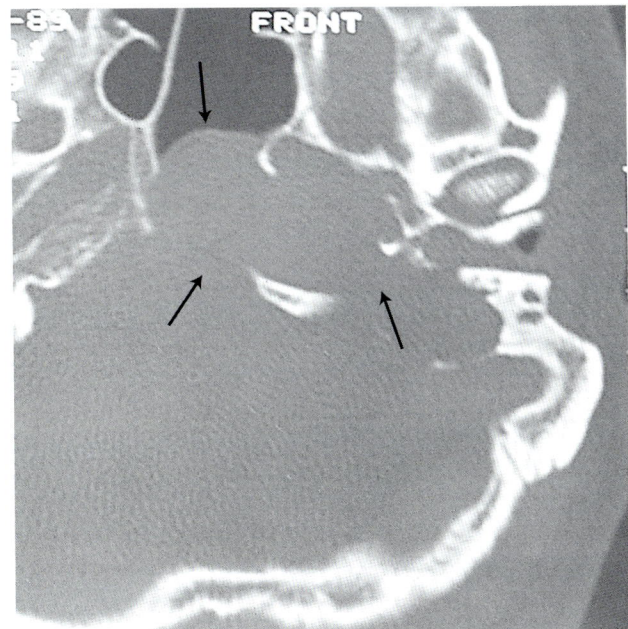

Figure 10.**22**   CT scan of the case presented in Figure 10.**21**. A large infralabyrinthine apical petrous bone cholesteatoma extending to the cavernous sinus and to the sphenoid sinus can be seen. Total removal was achieved using an infratemporal fossa approach type B.

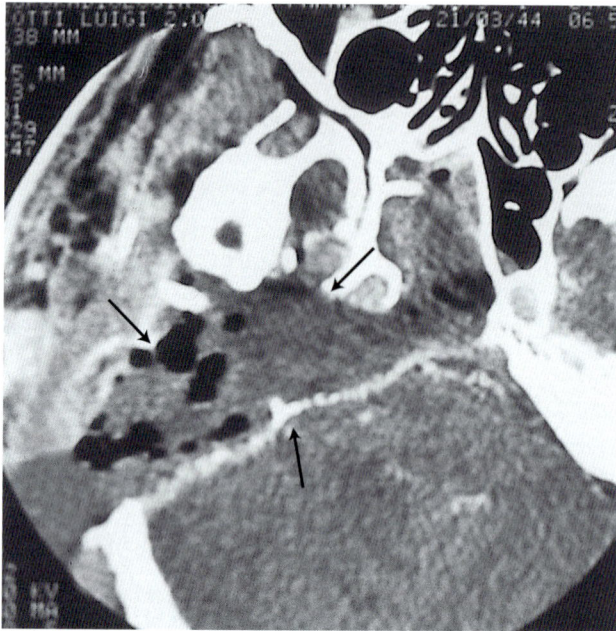

Figure 10.**23** Postoperative CT scan showing total removal.

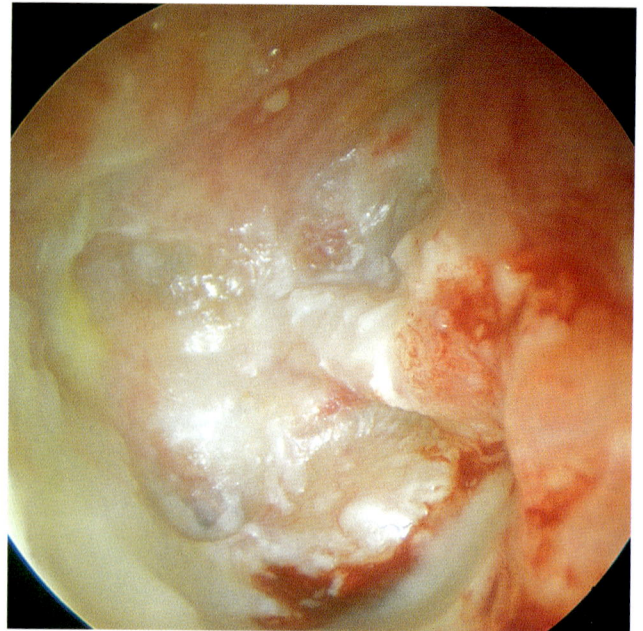

Figure 10.**24** Left acquired petrous bone cholesteatoma of the massive type. The patient had complained of fetid otorrhea and hearing loss since early childhood. Six months before presentation, he had started to experience facial nerve paralysis. A radical mastoidectomy was performed in another center with partial removal of the pathology. The second and third portions of the facial nerve can be observed in the mastoid cavity. The patient underwent surgery using a transcochlear approach to obliterate of the cavity with abdo-minal fat.

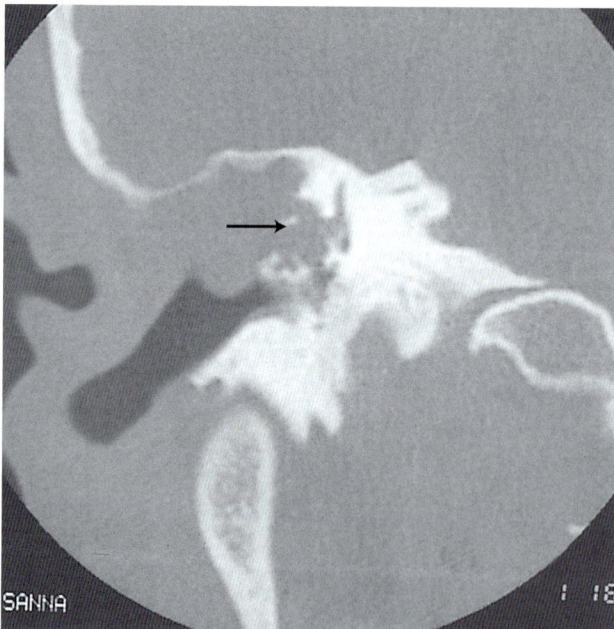

Figure 10.**25** CT scan of the case presented in Figure 10.**24**, demonstrating cholesteatoma invading the labyrinth.

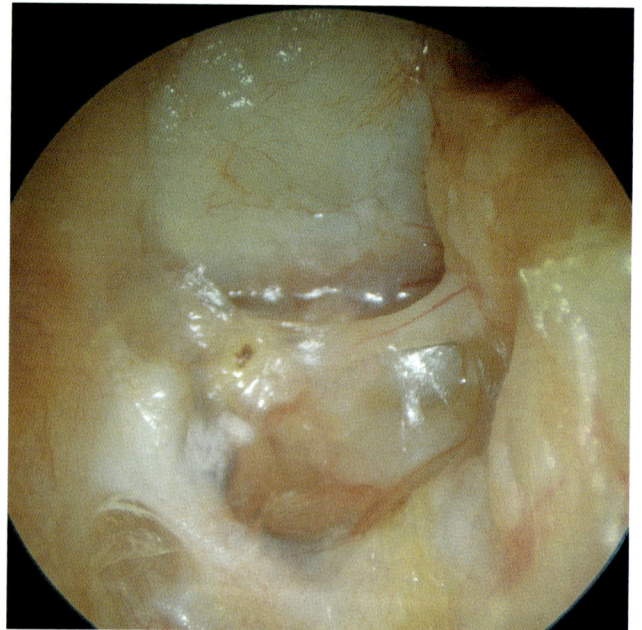

Figure 10.**26** Left radical mastoid cavity. This patient was operated on using a combined middle cranial fossa and transmastoid approach for the removal of a petrous bone cholesteatoma. The facial nerve was left as a bridge in the middle of the cavity. On follow-up, the patient complained of recurrent episodes of facial nerve paralysis due to accumulation of cerumen and debris in the cavity. Therefore, the patient underwent a second operation for obliteration of the cavity with abdominal fat and closure of the external auditory canal as a cul-de-sac.

Surgical Management

The ideal treatment for petrous bone cholesteatomas is radical surgical removal, although destruction of the labyrinth and rerouting of the facial nerve may be required. This approach may have to be modified, depending on the status of the contralateral ear. The choice of the actual surgical approach is based on the location and extent of the lesion, but it must provide adequate and safe exposure of the middle and posterior fossa dura, carotid artery, lateral sinus and jugular bulb, and facial nerve.

Our approach to the management of petrous bone cholesteatoma has been developing since 1984, and the present guidelines can be summarized as follows.

- Radical petromastoid exenteration with marsupialization of the cavity is carried out only in cases of infralabyrinthine cholesteatoma with limited extension.
- Radical petromastoid exenteration with closure of the eustachian tube, obliteration of the cavity with abdominal fat, and blind sac closure of the external ear canal, is used in large and deep cavities resulting from infralabyrinthine cholesteatomas.
- We use the middle cranial fossa approach only for small supralabyrinthine cholesteatomas without posterior or anterior extensions, when the hearing in the affected ear is normal.
- The modified transcochlear approach is used for massive labyrinthine, infralabyrinthine–apical, and apical cholesteatomas extending to the clivus, and in all cases of internal auditory canal involvement and cerebrospinal fluid (CSF) leak. The modified transcochlear approach is based on a wide petrosectomy with exposure and rerouting of the facial nerve, exposure of the middle and posterior cranial fossa dura, sigmoid sinus and jugular bulb, and petrous carotid artery. The external and middle ear are removed with blind sac closure of the external ear canal; the eustachian tube is closed, and the cavity is obliterated with abdominal fat.
- The type B infratemporal approach is used when petrous bone cholesteatoma has affected the horizontal portion of the internal carotid artery or the sphenoid sinus. This approach can be extended to the neck when the sigmoid sinus and jugular bulb are involved by cholesteatoma and are to be removed with ligature of the jugular vein in the neck.

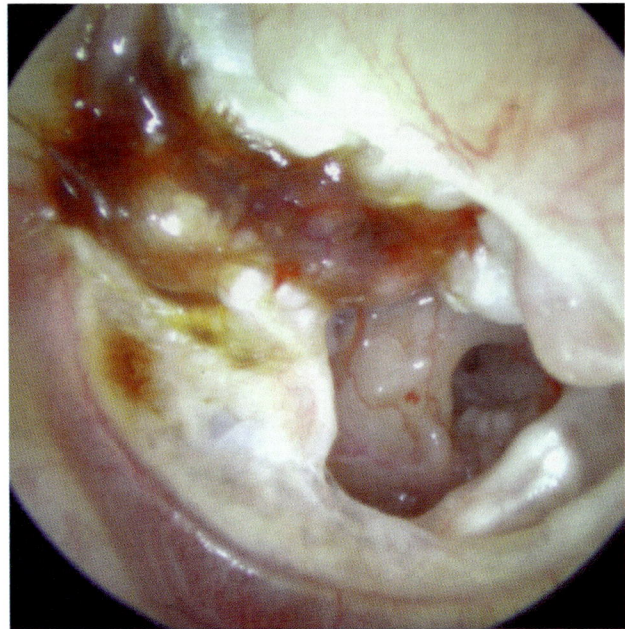

Figure 10.**27a** Left acquired petrous bone cholesteatoma. A subtotal tympanic perforation is present, with erosion of the scutum. Cholesteatoma debris is present in the mesotympanic area. The patient had suffered a sudden facial palsy 2 months before presentation. A left grade VI facial nerve palsy was found at the consultation.

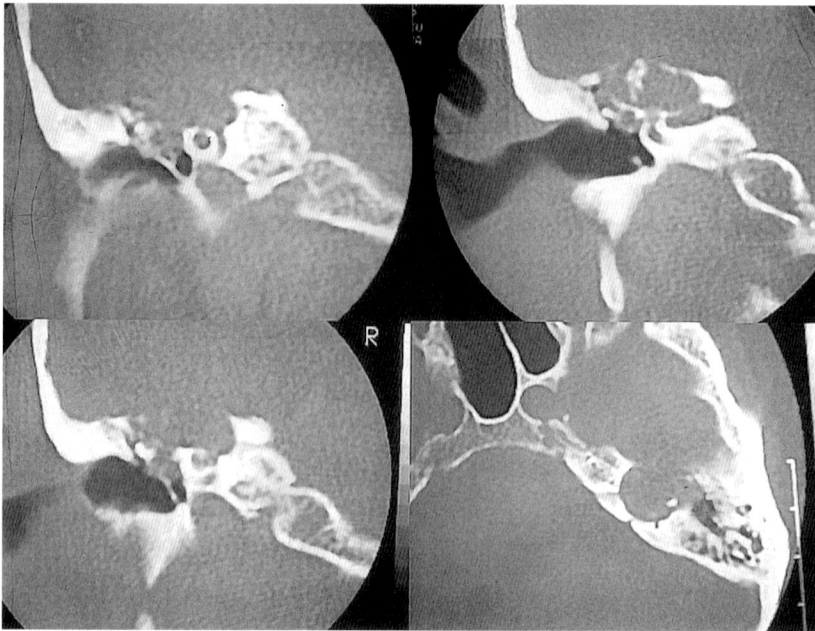

Figure 10.**27b**   Coronal and axial CT views in the same patient. A supralabyrinthine–apical cholesteatoma has produced erosion of the cochlea and roof of the internal auditory canal. However, bone conduction is normal.

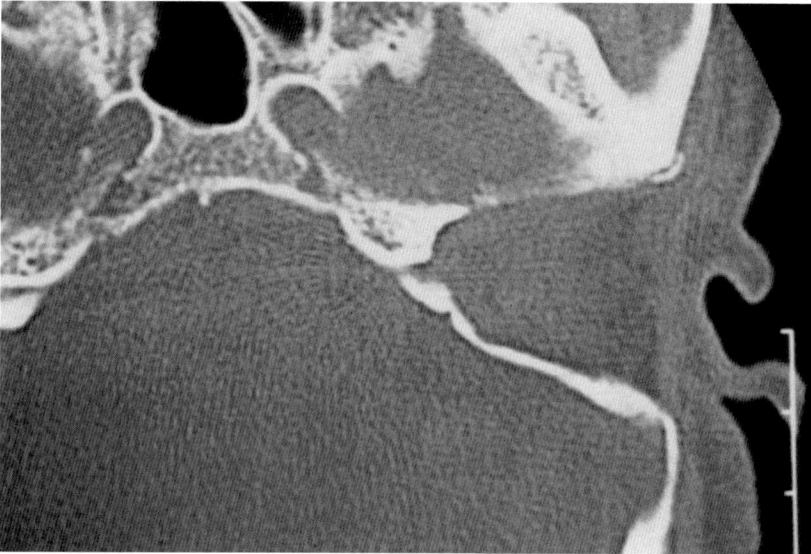

Figure 10.**27c**   Postoperative axial CT in the same patient. A modified type A transcochlear approach was used, with sural grafting of the facial nerve.

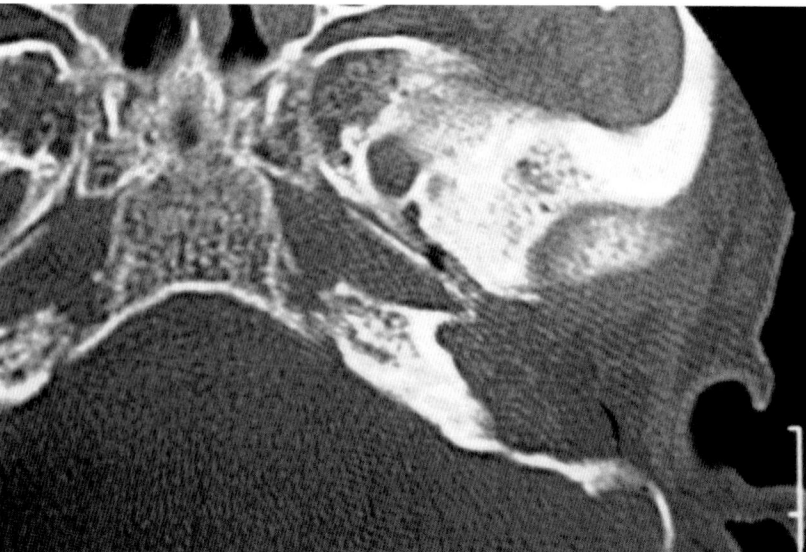

Figure 10.**27d**   The cavity has been completely filled with abdominal fat. No residual cholesteatoma is seen.

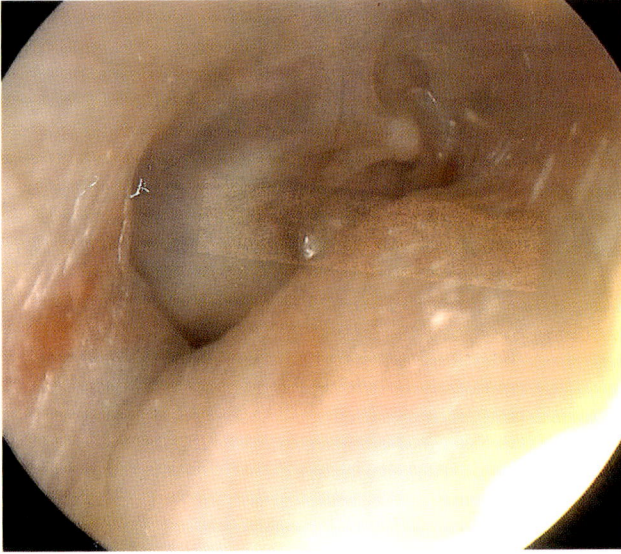

Figure 10.**28a** Right ear. Congenital petrous bone cholesteatoma. The tympanic membrane is normal. A white retrotympanic mass is clearly visible in the posteroinferior quadrant. The patient complained of progressive hearing loss since 15 years, and had had progressive facial nerve palsy since 1 year. A grade VI facial nerve palsy was found at the consultation.

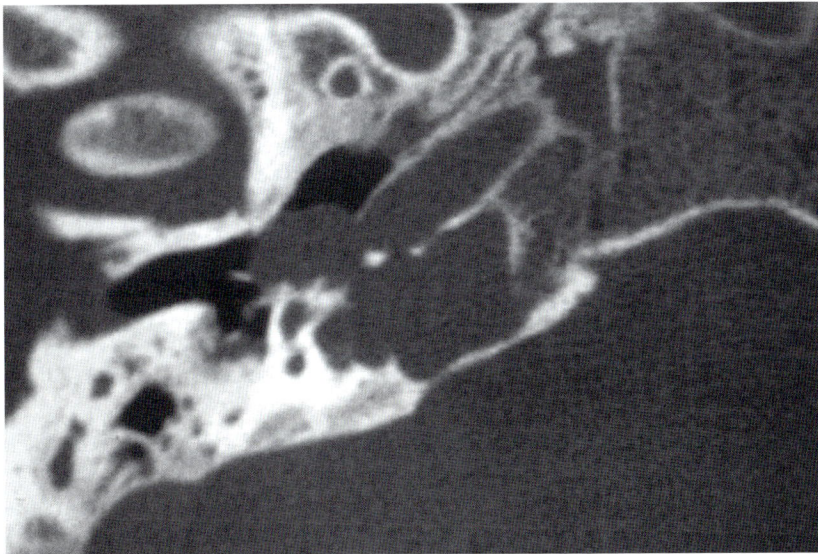

Figure 10.**28b** Axial CT in the same patient. A cholesteatomatous mass is seen in the infralabyrinthine apical compartment, eroding the horizontal bony canal of the internal carotid artery.

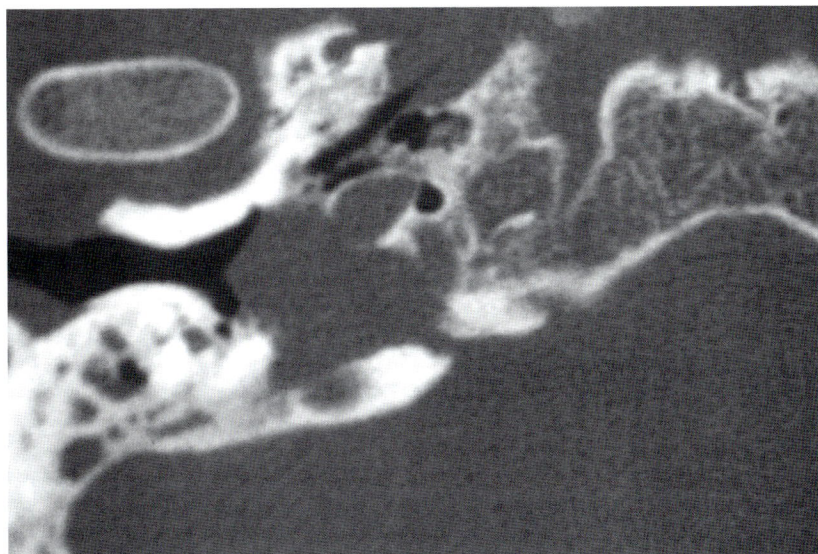

Figure 10.**28c** Axial CT. The cholesteatoma mass is eroding the bony canal of the vertical portion of the internal carotid artery.

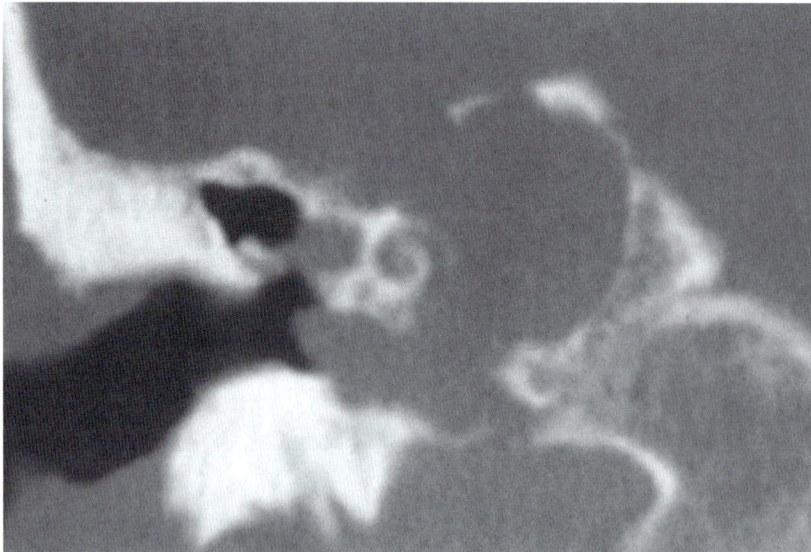

Figure 10.**28d**   Coronal CT. The cholesteatoma mass has completely engulfed the cochlea and is eroding it. A massive labyrinthine petrous bone cholesteatoma was diagnosed.

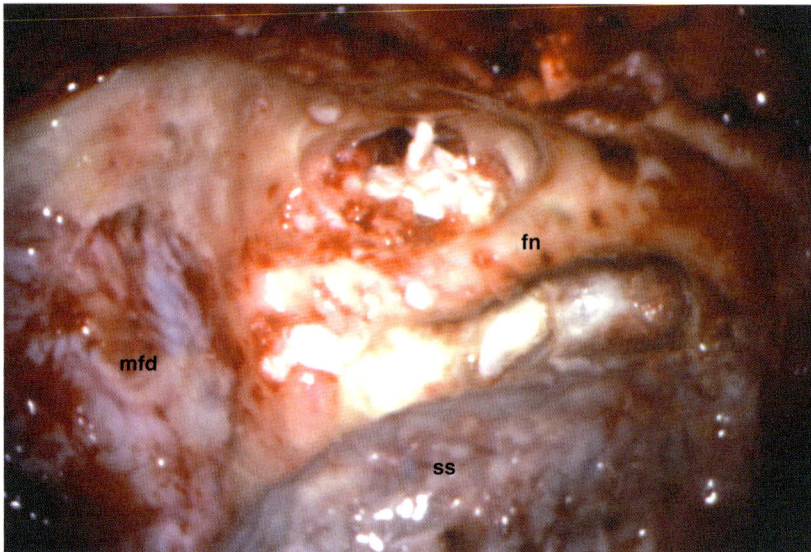

Figure 10.**29a**   A modified type A transcochlear approach has been performed in this case (same patient as in Fig. 10.**28a**). The external auditory canal has been closed in a cul-de-sac fashion. The tympanic membrane has been removed, as well as the posterior canal wall. The middle fossa plate and sigmoid sinus have been skeletonized, as well as the fallopian canal. The cholesteatoma mass occupied the promontory and posterior labyrinth, and has completely engulfed the second portion of the facial nerve.

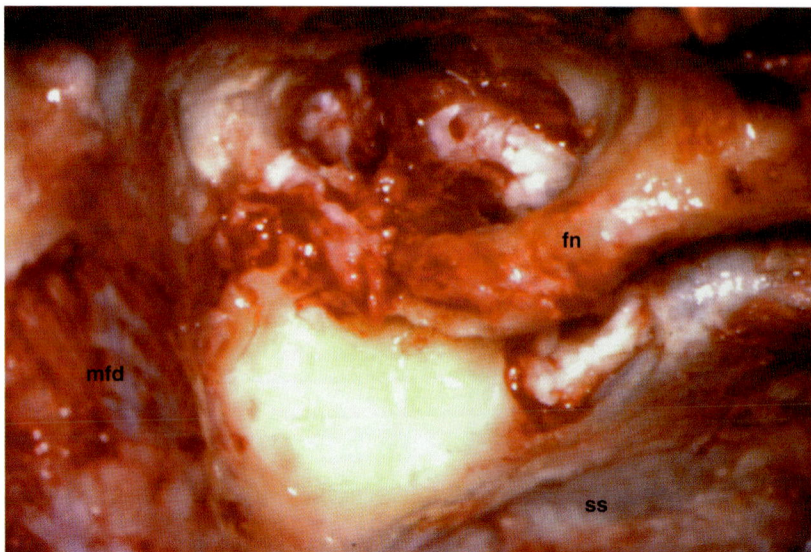

Figure 10.**29b**   The cholesteatomatous mass has been partially debulked. Interruption of the facial nerve is seen at the level of the second genu.

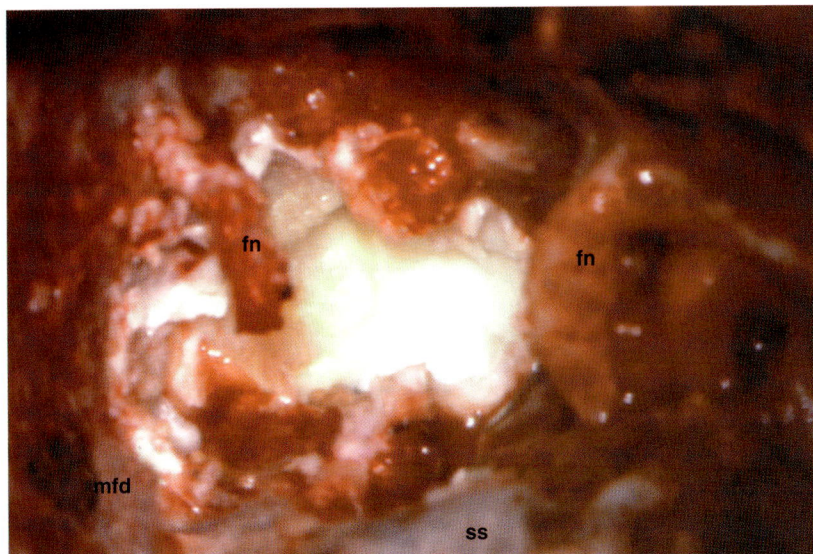

Figure 10.**29c** The third portion of the facial nerve has been rerouted posteriorly. The second portion is still present, but the first portion is absent. The cholesteatoma mass occupies the apical compartment and spreading toward the vertical portion of the carotid artery.

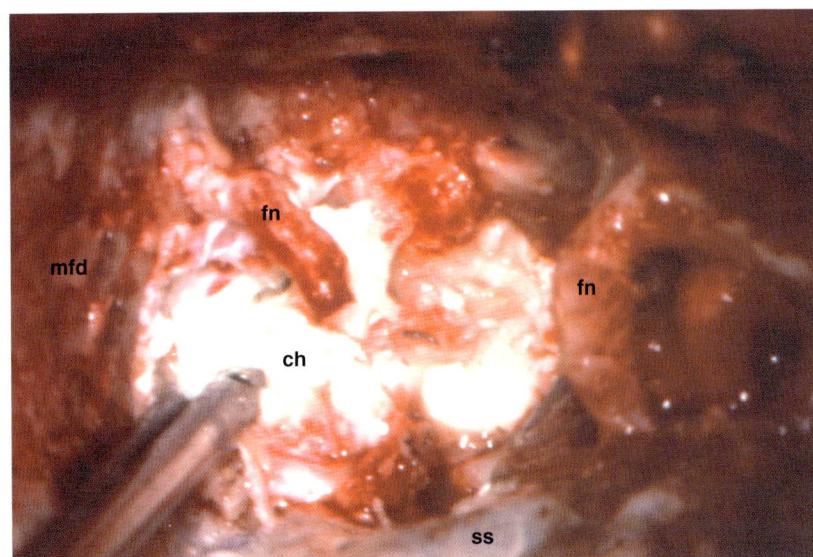

Figure 10.**29d** Next surgical step in the same case. A suction–irrigation tube is used to debulk the cholesteatomatous debris.

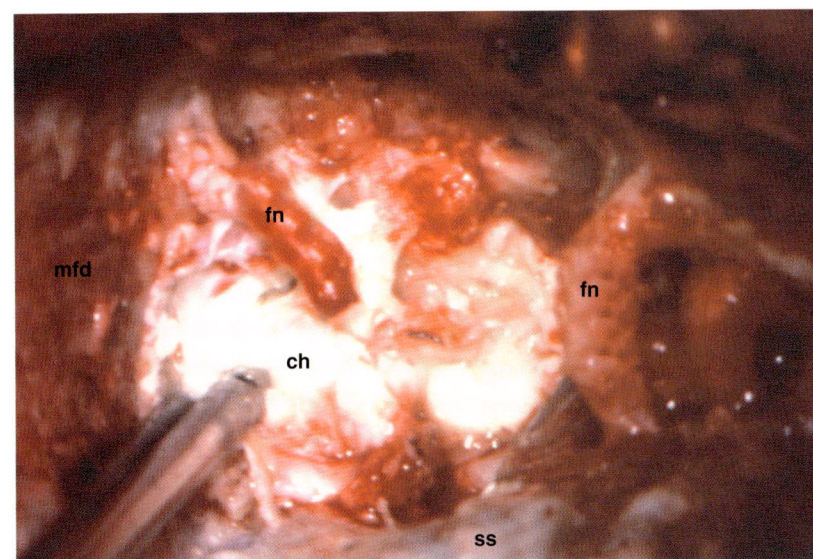

Figure 10.**29e** The geniculate ganglion and second portion of the facial nerve have been removed, and it is clearly seen that the first portion is absent. The cholesteatoma mass is still in place.

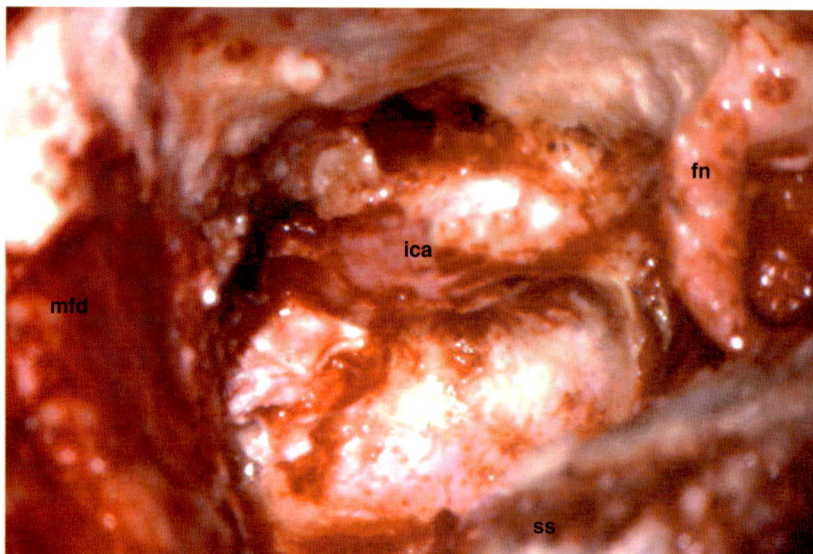

Figure 10.**29f**   The cholesteatoma mass has been almost completely removed. There is still a small piece adhering to the genu of the internal carotid artery.

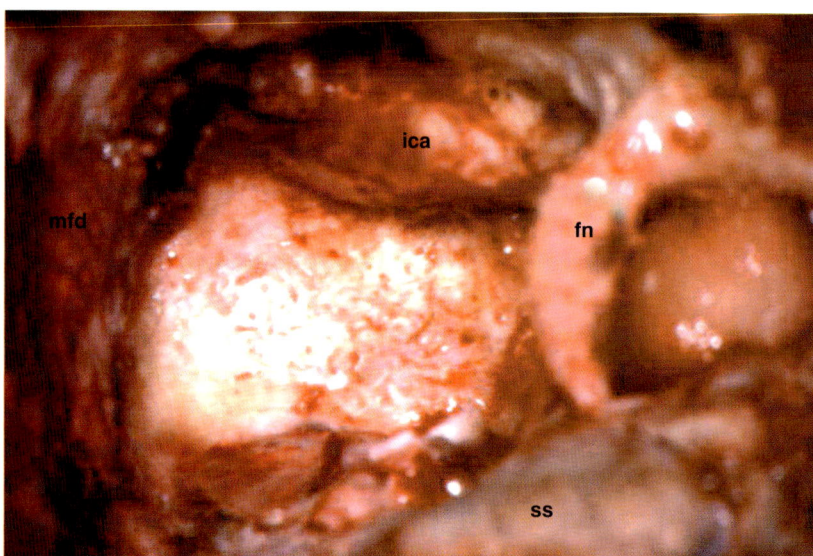

Figure 10.**29g**   Total removal of the cholesteatoma mass has been accomplished.

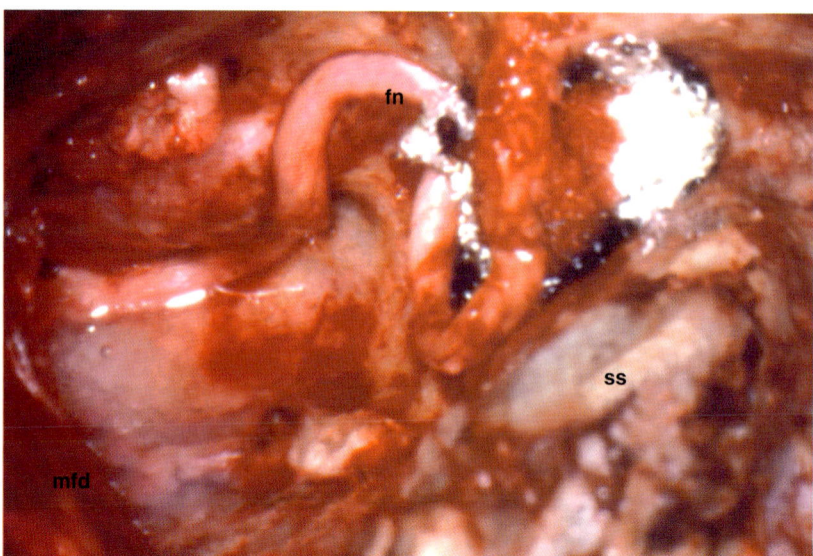

Figure 10.**29h**   A long sural nerve graft has been used to reconstruct the continuity of the facial nerve from the internal auditory canal to the third portion of the facial nerve. The graft has been secured with tissue adhesive in the internal auditory canal.

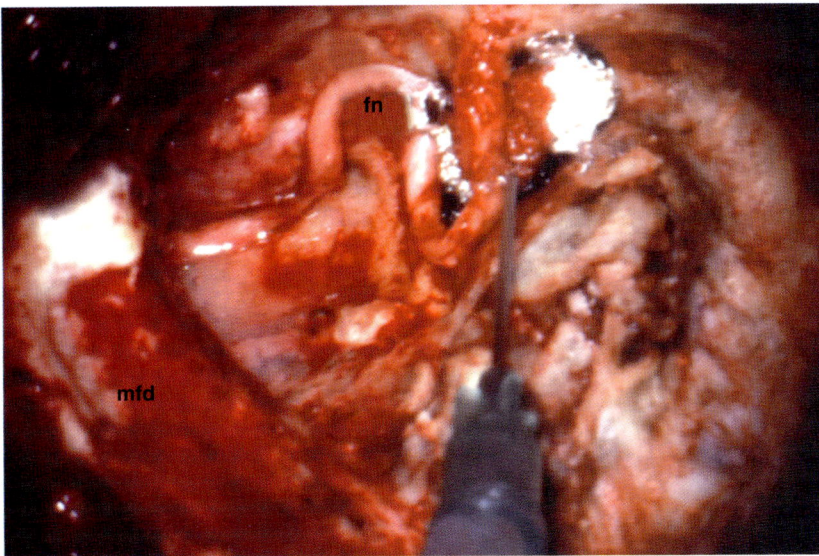

Figure 10.**29i** Tissue adhesive in the area of the anastomosis with the third portion of the facial nerve. Obliteration of the cavity has been carried out using abdominal fat.

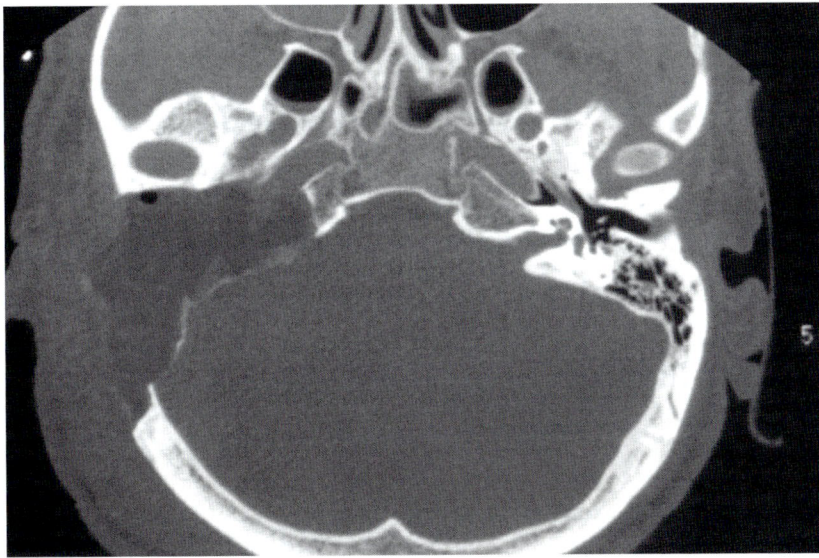

Figure 10.**29j** Postoperative CT in the same patient. The cavity has been obliterated with abdominal fat. The first portion of the horizontal internal carotid artery is surrounded by the fat.

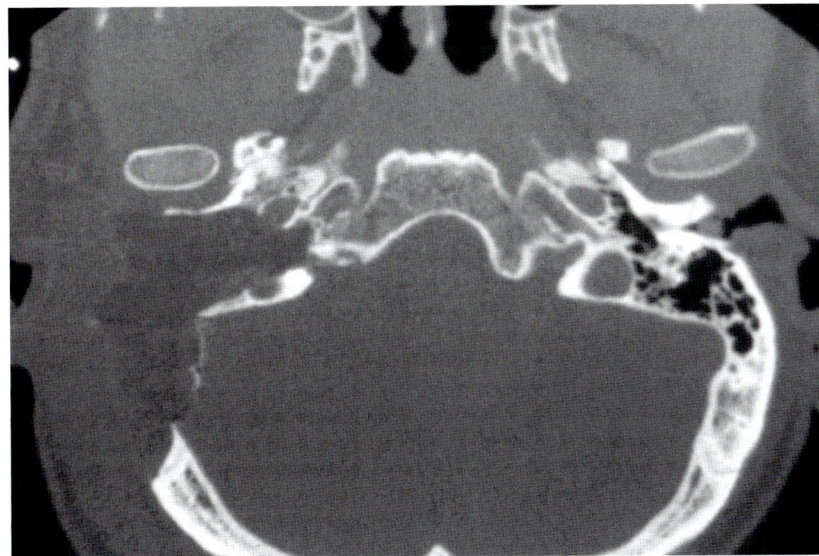

Figure 10.**29k** Postoperative CT. The external auditory canal is closed using a blind sac technique. The cavity has been obliterated with abdominal fat. The vertical portion of the internal carotid artery is seen.

Problems in Surgery

Surgical removal versus inner ear function preservation. At the beginning of our surgical experience, we attempted to preserve inner ear function despite labyrinthine involvement by petrous bone cholesteatoma. However, the results showed that we were rarely able to preserve hearing. We therefore do not hesitate now to remove the otic capsule when necessary. Of course, the status of the contralateral ear affects the therapeutic approach; when the ear with petrous bone cholesteatoma is the only hearing ear, it is managed with regular radiographic follow-up examinations and watchful waiting.

Facial nerve involvement. Involvement of the facial nerve poses particular problems. In some instances, the cholesteatoma can be easily dissected, and simple decompression is the treatment of choice. When preoperative facial palsy is present, the involved segment may be compressed but anatomically intact, interrupted, or replaced by fibrous degeneration. If it is intact, the nerve can be freed and decompressed. If it is interrupted, continuity is reestablished by rerouting and direct anastomosis, or using a cable graft. If it has been replaced by fibrous degeneration, the degenerated part is removed and continuity is reestablished using the methods mentioned above. If facial nerve palsy has been present for more than 2 years, a hypoglossal–facial anastomosis is carried out.

Carotid artery involvement. The surgeon should plan an approach that allows complete control of the artery. When the horizontal portion is involved, only the type B infratemporal fossa approach with downward dislocation of the mandible provides direct control of the vessel.

Dissection of the matrix from the artery poses no particular problems, but requires extreme caution and skill.

Sigmoid sinus and jugular bulb involvement. Complete removal of pathologic tissue from the sigmoid sinus is difficult, and the problems increase if the jugular bulb is involved, because of its fragility. In such cases, it is necessary to ligate the sigmoid sinus and the jugular vein. This allows removal of the dome of the jugular bulb and the external wall of the sigmoid sinus covered by matrix. Cranial nerves IX, X, XI, and XII are identified and preserved. Bleeding from the inferior petrosal sinus is controlled by packing it with Surgicel.

Dural involvement. Dural involvement occurs very often and makes radical removal of pathologic lesions a challenging procedure for the otologist. The matrix can be so adherent to the dura that removal is nearly impossible, and even a skilled surgeon is unable to distinguish between them. In this case, the surgeon has three options: firstly, if the cavity is not infected, the involved dura can be removed and the defect can be closed with fascia; secondly, one can use 90% ethyl alcohol, as proposed by Fisch; thirdly, bipolar coagulation of all the suspected portions of dura mater can be used to destroy all the possible remnants of cholesteatoma matrix (this is our method of choice). This method can be used in all instances, without exceptions.

Cerebrospinal fluid leaks may result from dural tears occurring during matrix removal. The leaks are stopped by inserting a free muscular flap into the subarachnoid space through the dural opening. Large dural tears are repaired with muscle plugs and suturing of the dural margins over the muscle.

Summary

When a patient presents with hearing loss (sensorineural or mixed) and/or facial nerve paralysis with or without a retrotympanic mass, the probability of petrous bone cholesteatoma should be considered. In such cases, it is necessary to perform a high-resolution CT scan of the temporal bone.

The ideal treatment for petrous bone cholesteatoma is radical surgical removal, although destruction of the labyrinth and rerouting of the facial nerve may be required. The status of the contralateral ear must also be considered.

The modified transcochlear approach is the most appropriate for the removal of petrous bone cholesteatoma. This approach offers direct lateral access to the petrous bone and allows the removal of all types of petrous bone cholesteatoma with their possible extension into the clivus or sphenoid sinus. In addition, it has the advantage of minimizing the occurrence of cerebral spinal fluid (CSF) leak and allows control of the different vital structures, including the internal carotid artery. Closure of the external auditory canal as a cul-de-sac and obliteration of the operative cavity with abdominal fat avoids the risk of infection and the need for frequent toilet of a very deep cavity.

The middle cranial fossa approach and the radical mastoidectomy can be used in cases with non-compromised inner ear function. The former is utilized in small supralabyrinthine cholesteatoma, while the latter is utilized in small infralabyrinthine cholesteatoma with no involvement of the internal carotid artery.

11 Glomus Tumors (Chemodectomas)

The glomus body was first described by Guild in 1941 as a small highly vascular mass of epithelioid cells located in the region of the adventitia of the jugular bulb. In 1953, Guild described glomus formations along the tympanic branches of the glossopharyngeal and vagus nerves (Jacobson's and Arnold's nerves, respectively).

Glomus bodies are mainly found in the tympanic region, jugular bulb, at the carotid bifurcation, and related to the vagus nerve. They are classified as paraganglia that are derived from the neural crest. While the carotid and vagal bodies function as chemoreceptors stimulated by the changes in the oxygen tension, tympanic and jugular bulb paraganglia do not exhibit this function.

The term *glomus tympanicum* is reserved for tumors that originate from the mesotympanum, while the term *glomus jugulare* is attributed to those cases that arise from the jugular bulb or the hypotympanum with secondary invasion of the bulb. These tumors are highly vascular and they derive the blood supply mainly from the ascending pharyngeal artery. It is claimed that they have a hereditary transmission as autosomal dominant traits with penetrance that increases with age.

In the majority of cases, the initial symptoms are hearing loss (conductive, sensorineural, or mixed) and pulsatile tinnitus synchronous with pulse. The tumor can extend into the labyrinth, causing vertigo of peripheral origin; towards the jugular foramen, leading to deficits of one or more of the lower cranial nerves (IX–XI); or towards the occipital condyle, leading to hypoglossal nerve paralysis. Patients suffering from preoperative affection of the lower cranial nerves have a better postoperative course as compensation of the contralateral side has already started. The contralateral vocal cord compensates by crossing the midline to meet the paralyzed cord, thereby markedly reducing the risk of aspiration pneumonia. On the other hand, patients with preoperative intact lower cranial nerves in whom the nerves are sacrificed during the operation suffer from deglutition problems in the postoperative course. Nasogastric feeding is used in such cases and oral feeding is resumed only when compensation from the contralateral side occurs. A useful alternative is vocal cord medialization either by Teflon injection or by medialization thyroplasty using cartilage or silicon.

The tumor can also extend into the petrous apex, leading to paralysis of the abducent nerve and trigeminal neuralgia, or invade the mastoid, resulting in facial nerve paralysis. Further extension can also occur in the external auditory canal. Tumors occupying the external auditory canal can lead to serous or purulent otorrhea due to irritation of the skin and retention of squamae and epithelial debris. Hemorrhagic discharge rarely occurs.

Fisch classified glomus tumors into four classes based on location and extension seen on high-resolution CT scans (see Table 11.1 and Figs. 11.1–11.6).

On otoscopy, a retrotympanic pulsatile mass is usually seen in the inferior quadrants. The mass is red or bordeaux red. In some cases the mass may have a reddish-blue color due to the presence of middle ear effusion secondary to eustachian tube blockage. The tumor may be seen as a polyp in the external auditory canal either due to erosion of the floor of the canal or to the tumor breaking through the tympanic membrane.

The diagnosis can be made clinically (history and otoscopic findings). Computed tomography (CT) with contrast, and magnetic resonance imaging (MRI) with gadolinium, allow exact definition of the tumor extension. Radiology also helps to differentiate between glomus tumors and other lesions such as aberrant carotid artery, high jugular bulb, cholesterol granuloma, or meningioma extending into the middle ear. Carotid and vertebral angiography allows identification of the arteries supplying the tumor; and they should be embolized before surgery to avoid excessive intraoperative bleeding.

In cases in which the horizontal carotid artery is engulfed by the tumor, the balloon occlusion test is indispensable for studying the perfusion by the contralateral carotid artery as well as for the safety of the closure of the involved carotid.

Table 11.1 Classification of glomus tumors according to Fisch (1978)

Class A:	Glomus tympanicum
Class B:	Tympanomastoid
Class C:	Glomus jugulare
C1:	Carotid foramen
C2:	Vertical ICA until genu
C3:	Horizontal ICA
C4:	ICA + FL
Class D:	Intracranial extension
De (1-2):	Intracranial extradural
Di (1-2):	Intracranial intradural

ICA = internal carotid artery; FL = anterior foramen lacerum

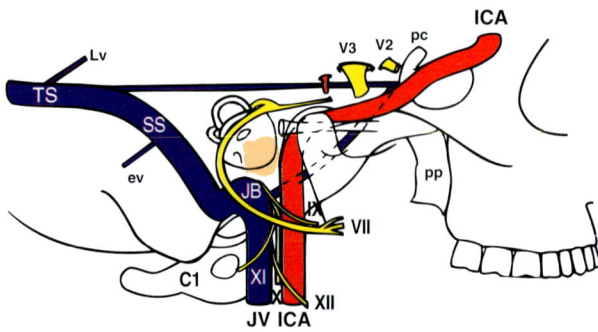

Figure 11.**1** The class A tumor originates from glomus formations along the course of Jacobson's nerve. They are localized to the middle ear. Abbreviations are given in Figure 10.**1**.

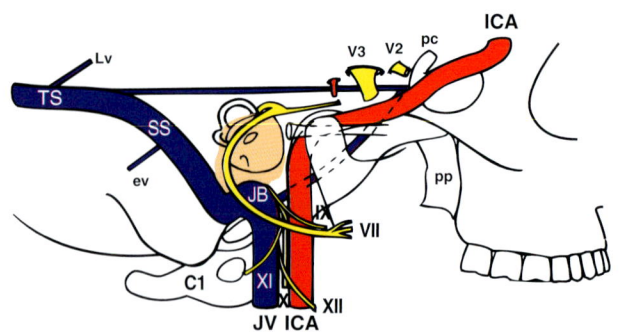

Figure 11.**2** The class B tumor originates at the level of the promontory and invades the hypotympanum without affecting the jugular bulb. The tumor also can extend into the mastoid and the retrofacial air cells.

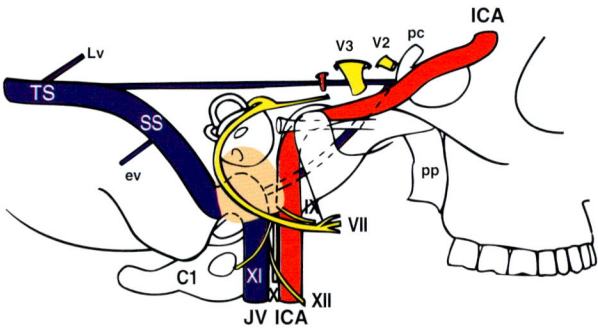

Figure 11.**3** The class C tumor originates in the dome of the jugular bulb and destroys the infralabyrinthine compartment. The tumor may spread in the following directions: inferiorly, along the internal jugular vein and cranial nerves IX–XII; superiorly, towards the otic capsule and the internal auditory canal; posteriorly, into the sigmoid sinus; anteriorly, to the internal carotid artery; more medially, to the petrous apex and the cavernous sinus; or lateral-

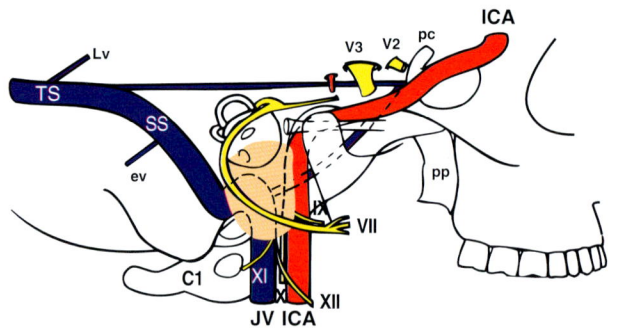

ly, to the hypotympanum and middle ear. Class C tumors are further subdivided according to the degree of erosion of the carotid canal. The C1 tumor erodes the carotid foramen without involvement of the carotid artery.

Figure 11.**4** The class C2 tumor erodes the vertical carotid canal up to the carotid genu.

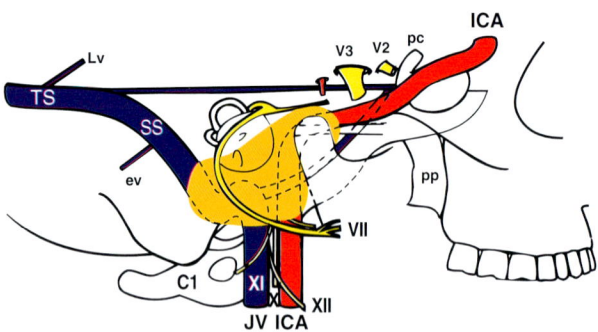

Figure 11.**5** The class C3 tumor involves the horizontal segment of the carotid.

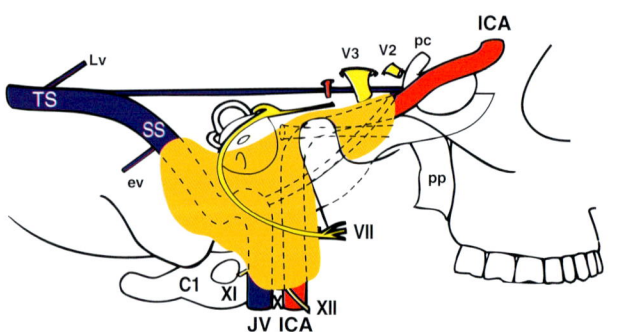

Figure 11.**6** The class C4 tumor grows to the anterior foramen lacerum and extends to the cavernous sinus. Class D indicates intracranial extension of the tumor. This might be extradural (De) or intradural (Di).

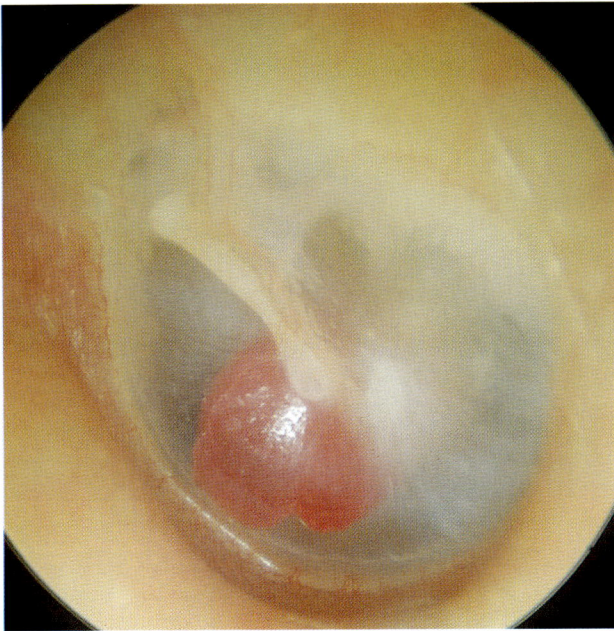

Figure 11.**7** Left ear. Glomus tympanicum or class A tumor. The small red mass behind the anteroinferior quadrant is localized on the promontory and does not extend towards the hypotympanum (see Fig. 11.**8**).

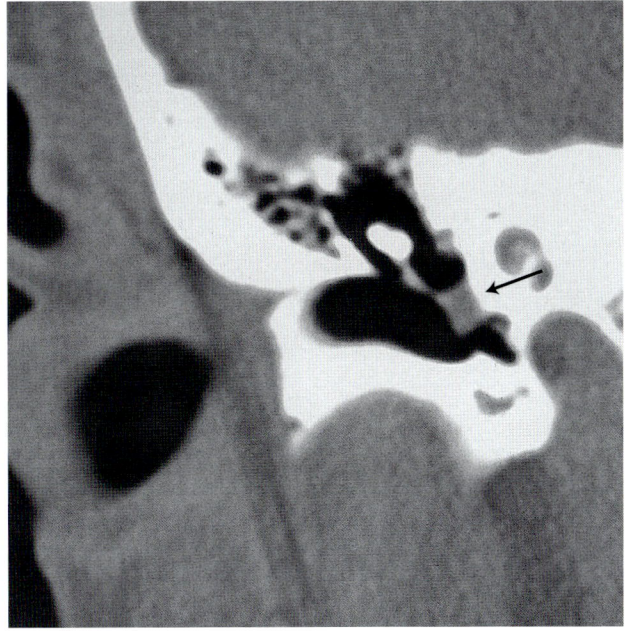

Figure 11.**8** CT scan of the case presented in Figure 11.**7**. The lesion is limited to the region of the promontory. There are no visible signs of bone erosion.

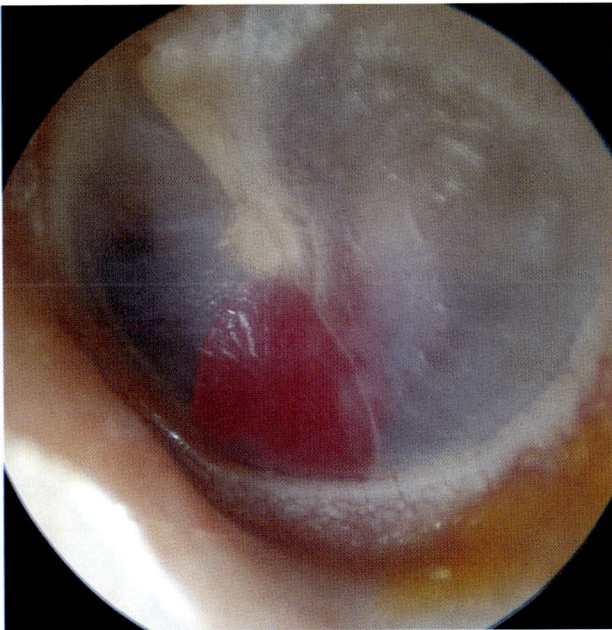

Figure 11.**9** Left ear. Class A glomus tumor. The tumor is again limited to the promontory (see Figs. 11.**10** and 11.**11**).

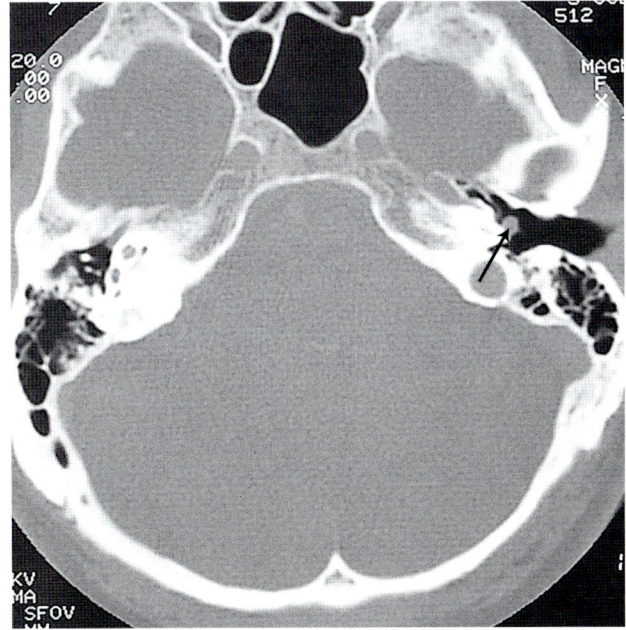

Figure 11.**10** CT scan of the case described in Figure 11.**9**.

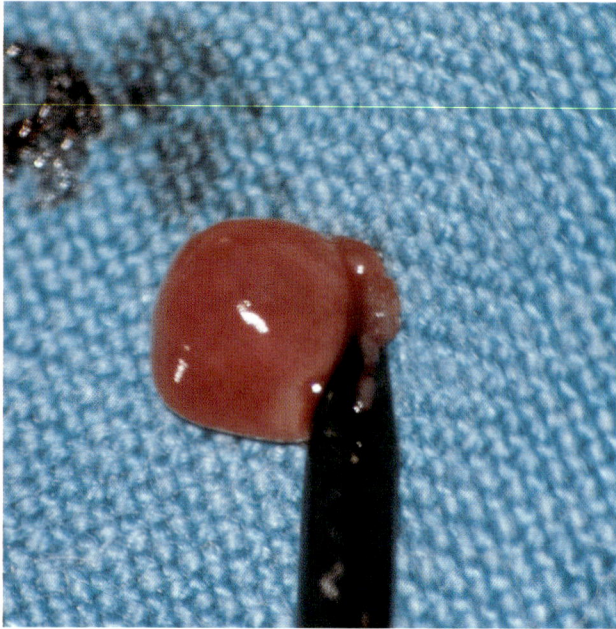

Figure 11.**11**   The tumor was removed using a transcanal approach after having bipolarly coagulated the tympanic arteries that supply the tumor.

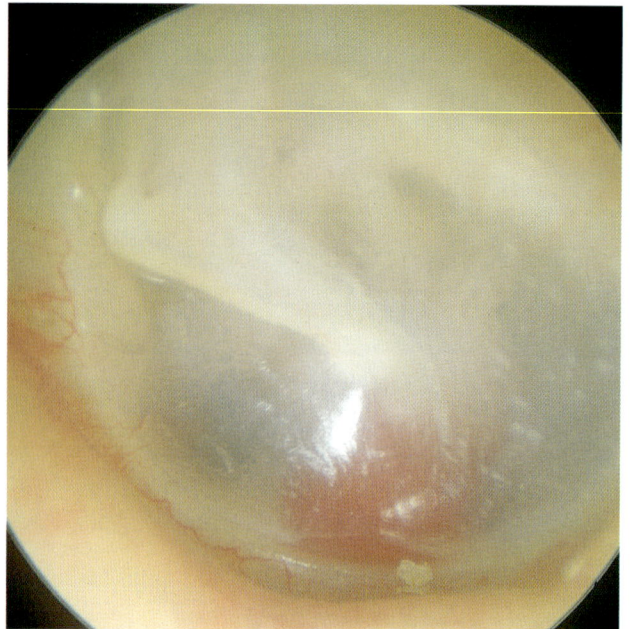

Figure 11.**12**   Left ear. Another example of a small class A glomus tumor.

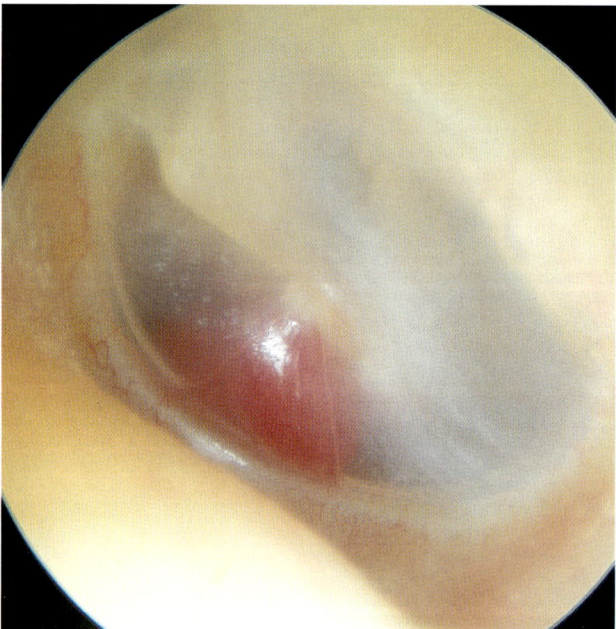

Figure 11.**13**   Left ear. This small glomus tympanicum tumor is situated in the anteroinferior quadrant of the middle ear near the tubal orifice. Further growth of the tumor can block the tubal orifice, leading to middle ear effusion.

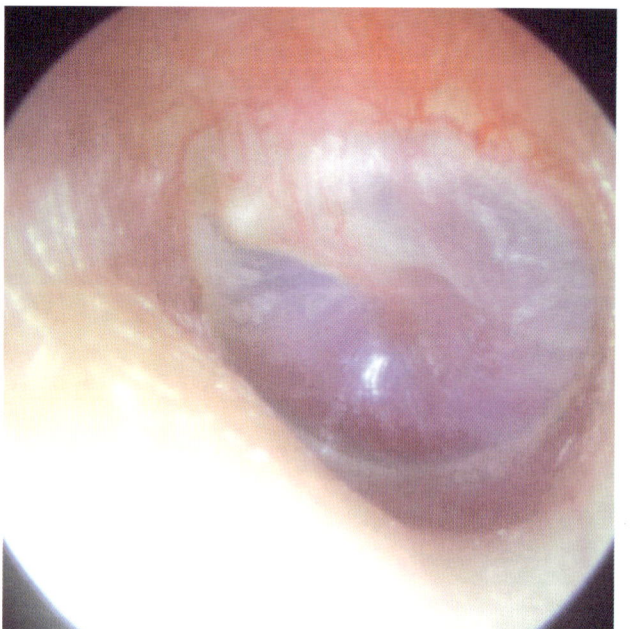

Figure 11.**14a**   Left ear. Class A glomus tumor. The mass is visible at the level of the inferior and anterior quadrant of the tympanic membrane.

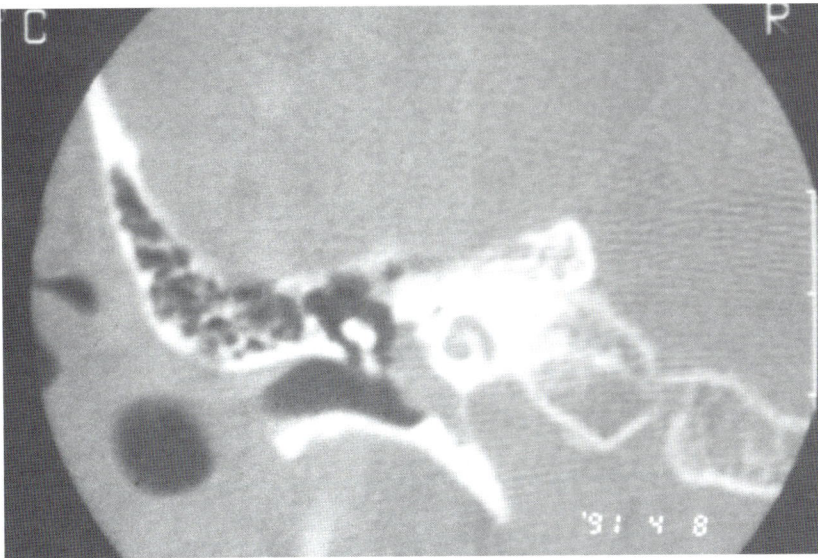

Figure 11.**14b** Coronal CT in the same patient. There is tumor extension toward the hypotympanum and the vertical portion of the internal carotid artery. There is no erosion of the bony plate covering the carotid artery.

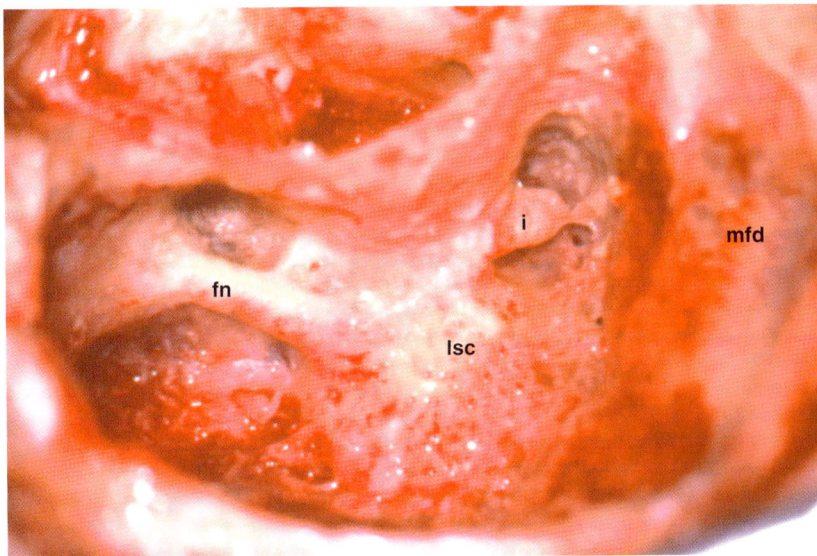

Figure 11.**14c** Total mastoidectomy has been carried out using a combined-approach tympanoplasty. The third portion of the facial nerve has been skeletonized, and the posterior tympanotomy starts at this point.

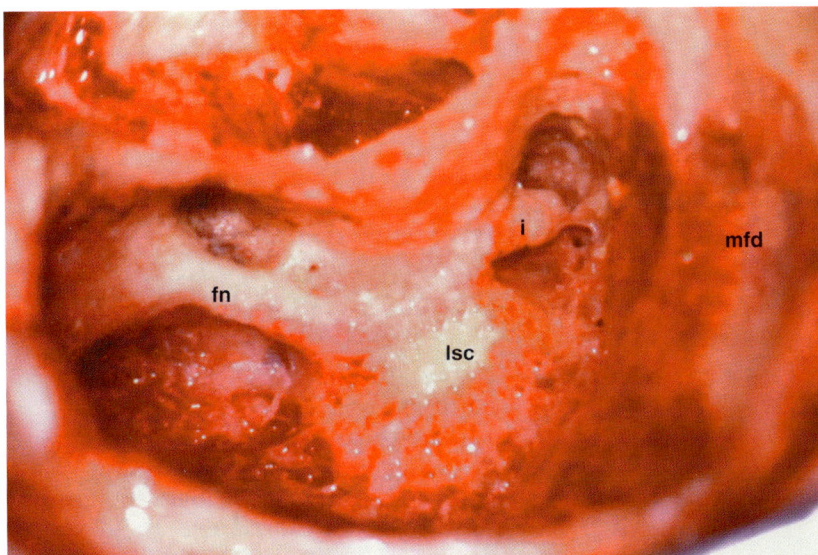

Figure 11.**14d** The posterior tympanotomy has almost been completed. The "buttress" is left to protect the incus.

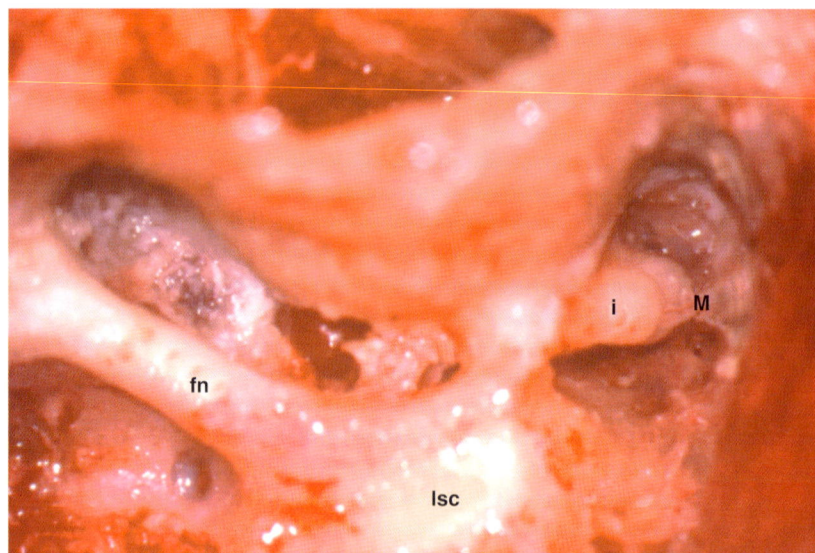

Figure 11.**14e** The posterior tympanotomy is now complete, and the tumor can be seen through the opening.

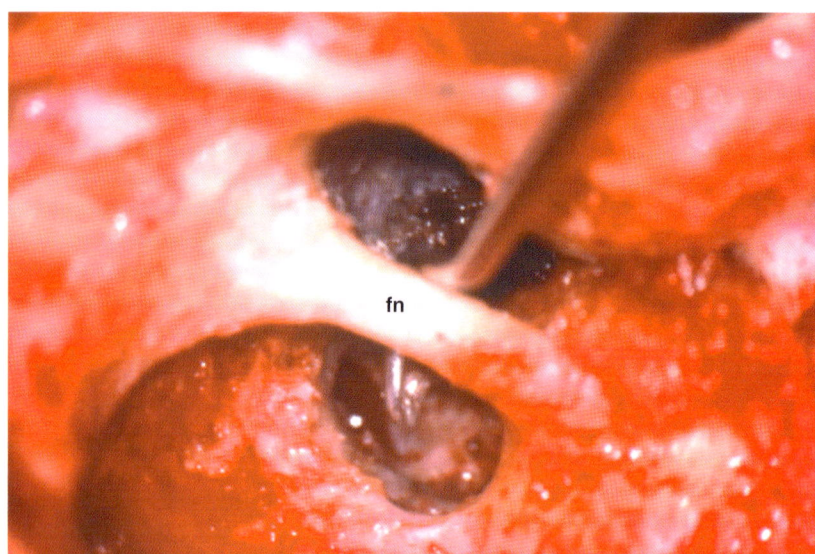

Figure 11.**14f** A subfacial recess tympanotomy is combined with the posterior tympanotomy to facilitate tumor removal.

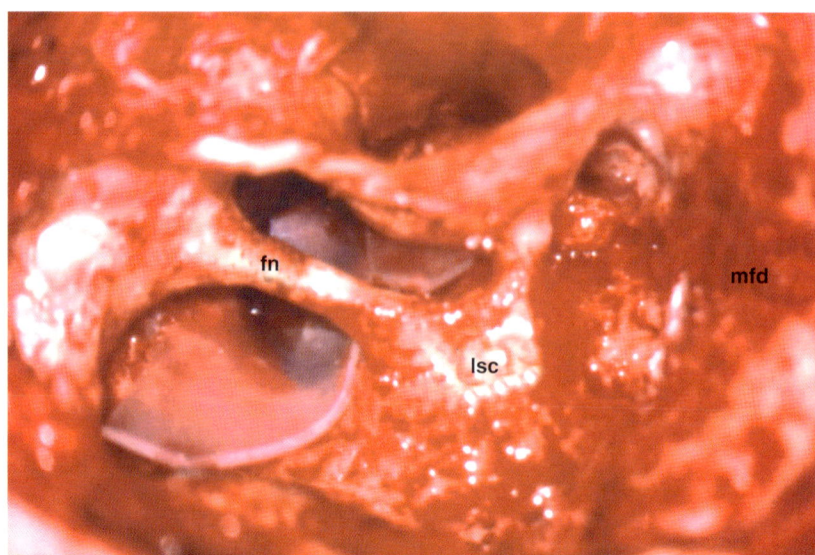

Figure 11.**14g** At the end of the procedure, a Silastic sheet is inserted under the third portion of the facial nerve, extending towards the hypotympanum and middle ear.

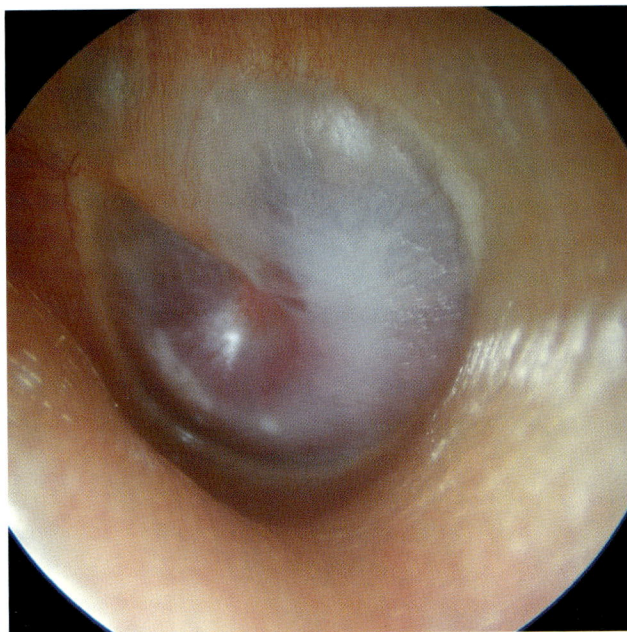

Figure 11.15 Left ear. Class B glomus tumor or hypotympanic tumor. The reddish mass is visible through the inferior quadrants of the tympanic membrane.

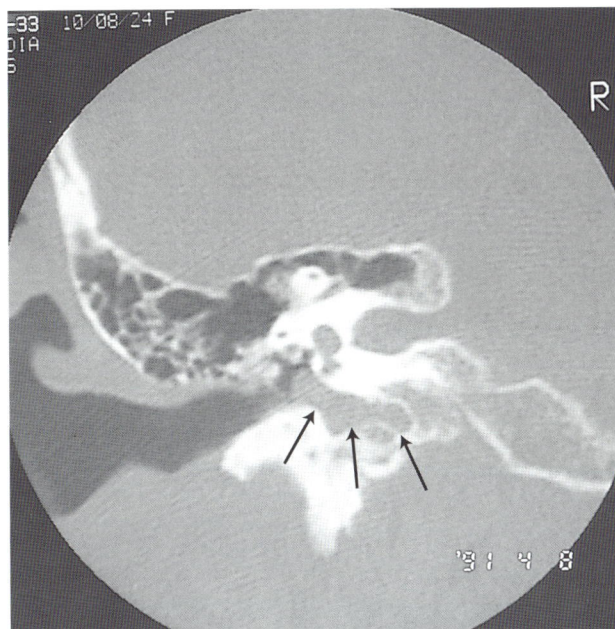

Figure 11.16 CT of the case presented in Figure 11.15. Tumor extension towards the hypotympanum is observed. There is no erosion of the bony plate covering the jugular bulb.

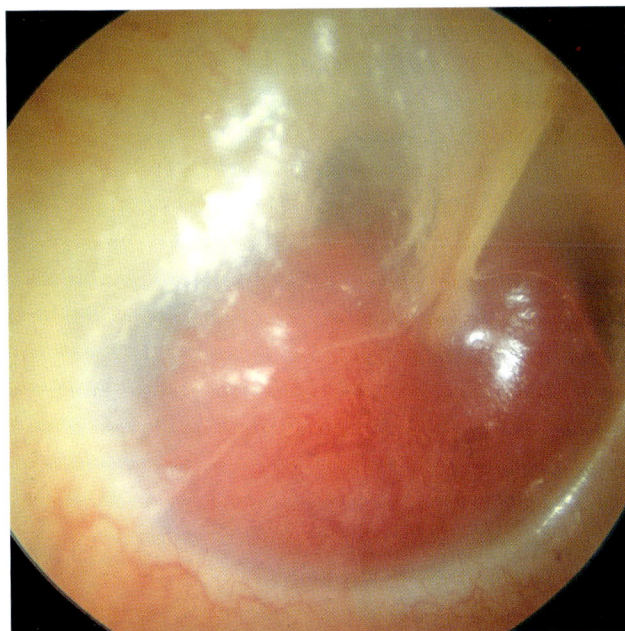

Figure 11.17 Right ear. Class B glomus tumor. The highly vascular red tumor mass pushes the tympanic membrane laterally. A middle ear effusion is present.

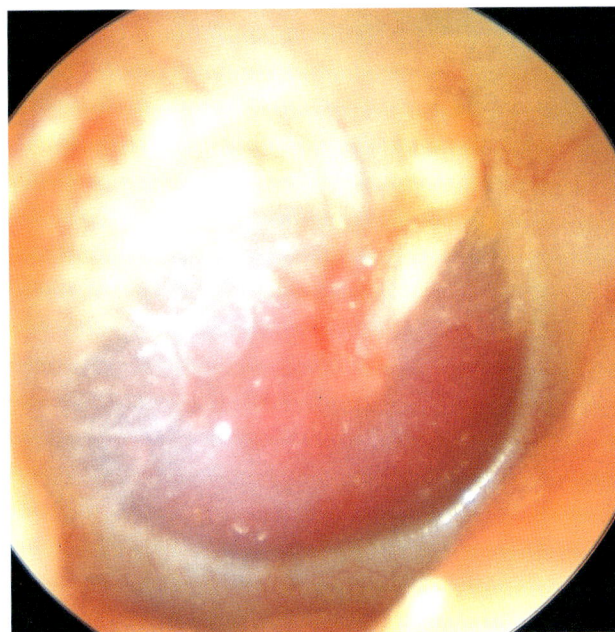

Figure 11.18 Right ear. Class B glomus tumor. An air–fluid level due to middle ear effusion is seen together with the tumor. A tympanoplasty removed all of the tumor while conserving the excellent preoperative hearing.

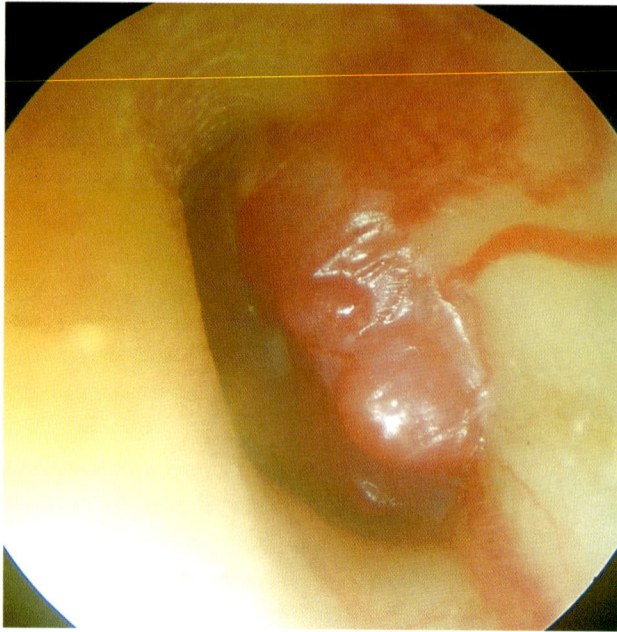

Figure 11.**19**   Left ear. Type B glomus tumor. The tumor causes bulging of the posterior quadrants of the tympanic membrane (see CT scan, Fig. 11.**20**).

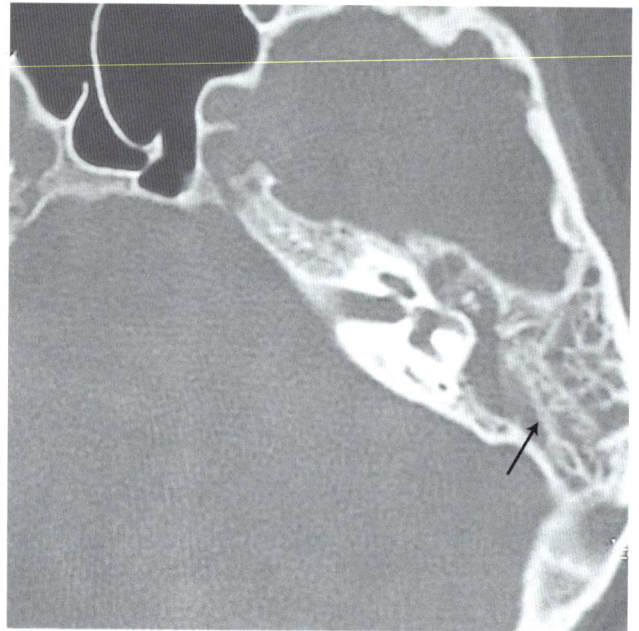

Figure 11.**20**   CT scan of the case in Figure 11.**19**. An axial section demonstrates the presence of effusion in the mastoid due to retention.

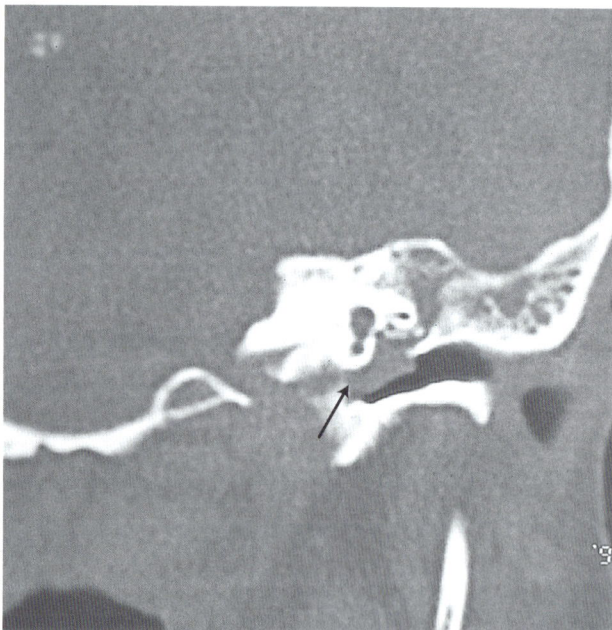

Figure 11.**21**   CT scan of the case in Figure 11.**19**. The tumor extends to the hypotympanum but does not erode the bone overlying the dome of the jugular bulb.

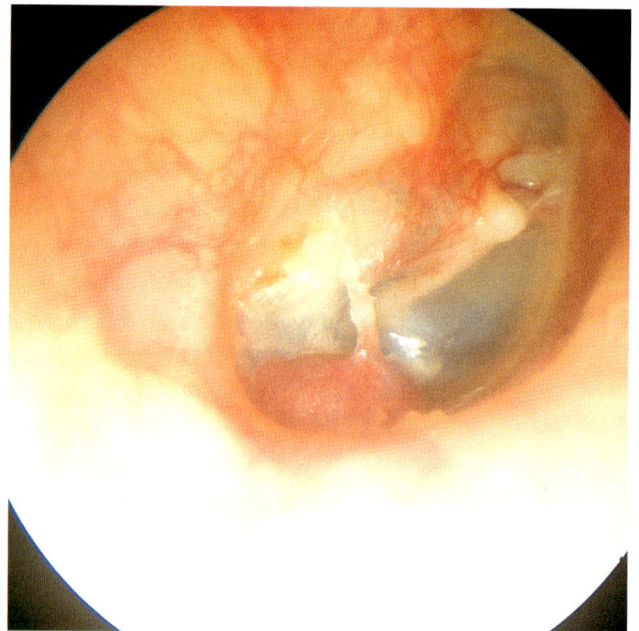

Figure 11.**22**   Right ear. Reddish mass protruding from the inferior wall of the external auditory canal.

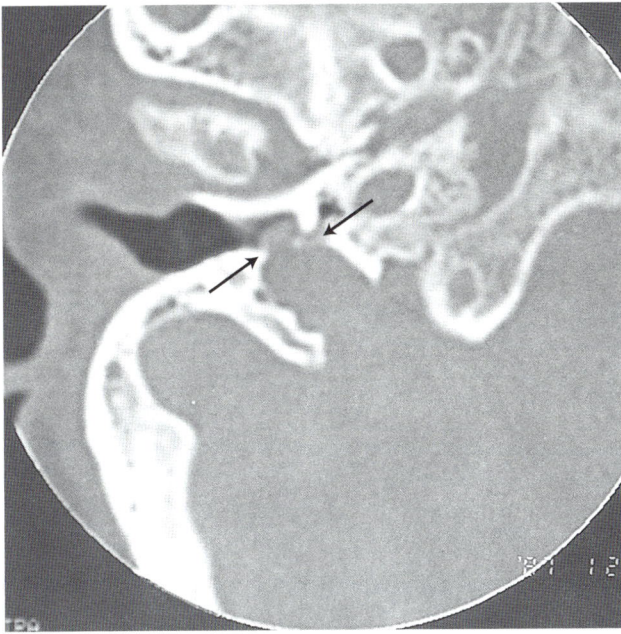

Figure 11.23 CT scan of the previous case. Axial view demonstrating the erosion caused by the tumor of the bone overlying the jugular bulb. This tumor can be considered an intermediate class between B and C. The tumor is localized in the hypotympanum and extends to the jugular bulb but does not invade it.

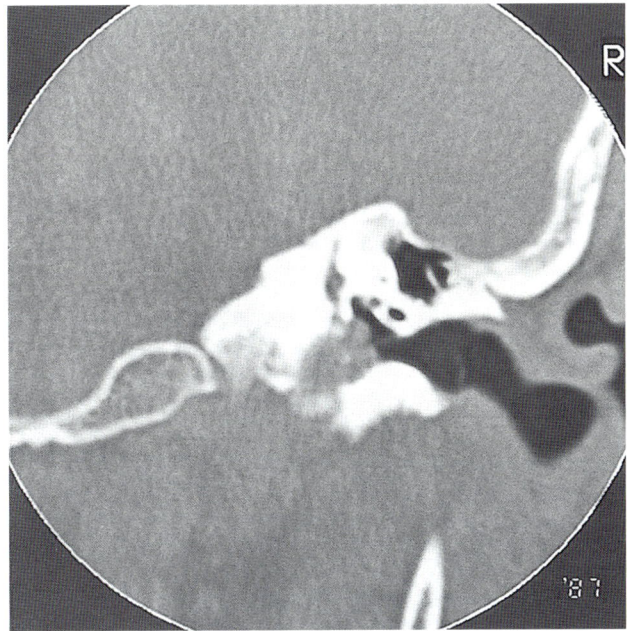

Figure 11.24 Coronal section giving a better view of the tumor extension towards the jugular bulb. Intraoperatively, no invasion of the bulb was noted and the integrity of the bulb was thus conserved.

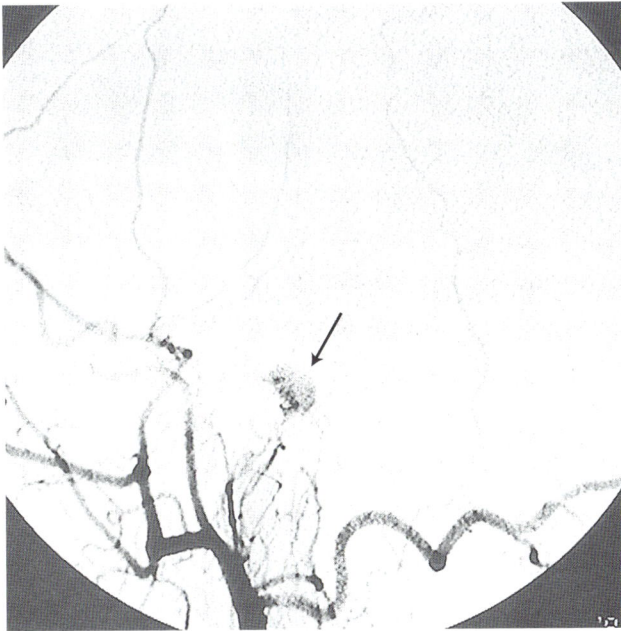

Figure 11.25 Angiography of the same case. The blood supply of the tumor (arrow) is derived from the ascending pharyngeal artery that is a branch of the external carotid artery.

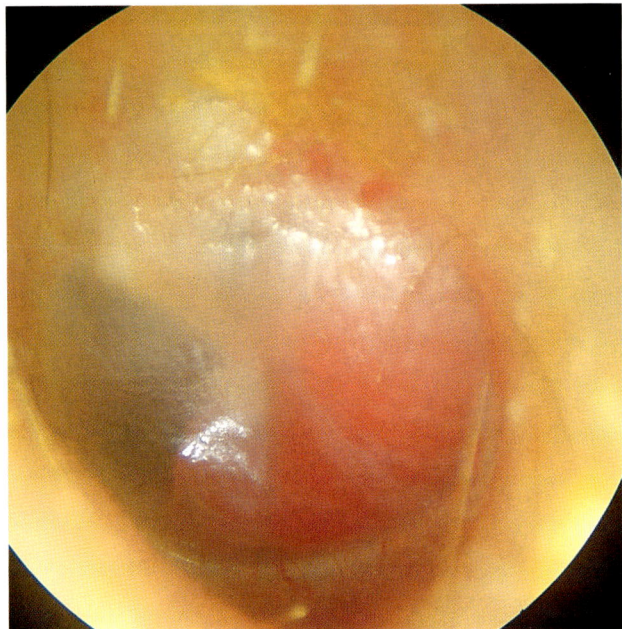

Figure 11.26 Left ear. Class C1 glomus tumor. The only complaint of the patient was ipsilateral pulsatile tinnitus of 4 years' duration (see following figures).

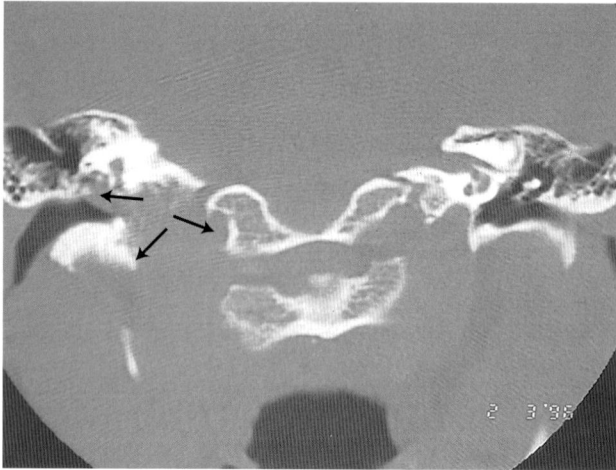

Figure 11.**27** CT scan, coronal view showing enlargement of the jugular foramen with extension of the tumor into the middle ear.

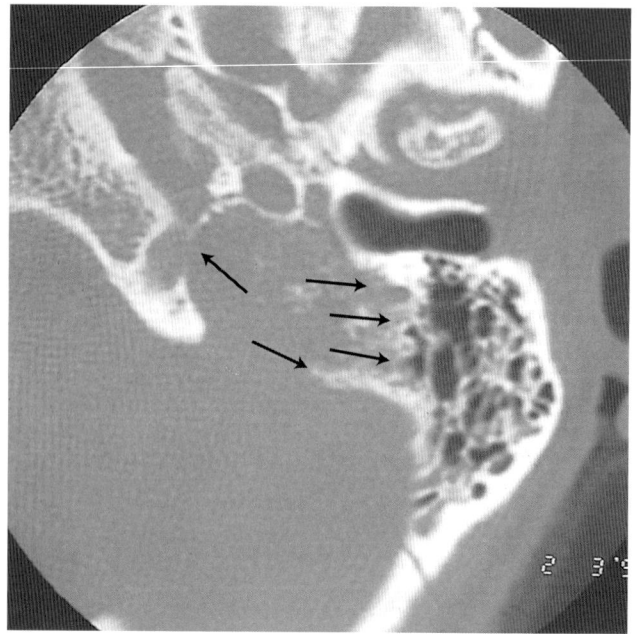

Figure 11.**28** CT scan, axial view. The jugular foramen is enlarged. Irregular erosion of the borders of the jugular foramen can be observed (differential diagnosis with lower cranial nerves' schwannoma).

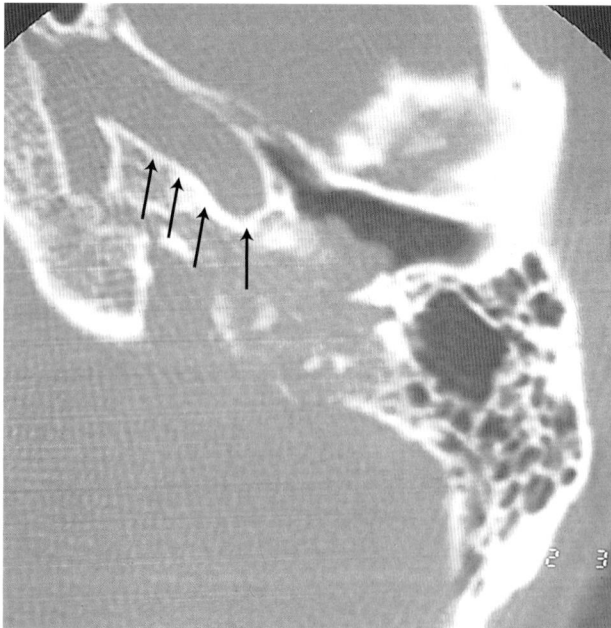

Figure 11.**29** Axial view demonstrates that the horizontal segment of the internal carotid artery is free of tumor.

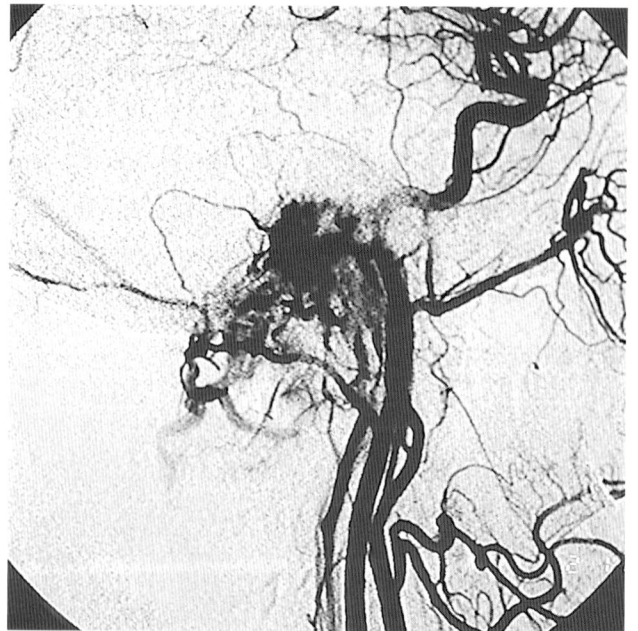

Figure 11.**30** Angiography demonstrating that the blood supply of the tumor comes from the ascending pharyngeal, the occipital, and the posterior auricular arteries.

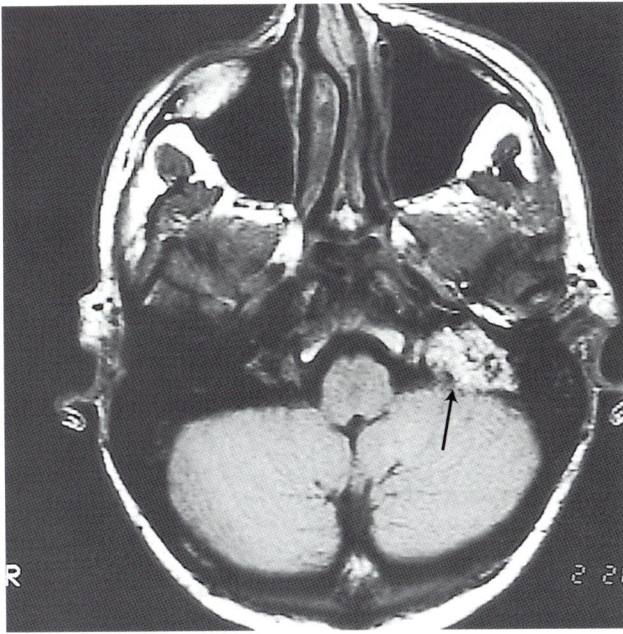

Figure 11.**31** MRI with gadolinium. The tumor is enhancing except for some flow-void zones corresponding to large vascular spaces. This picture is pathognomonic of glomus tumors.

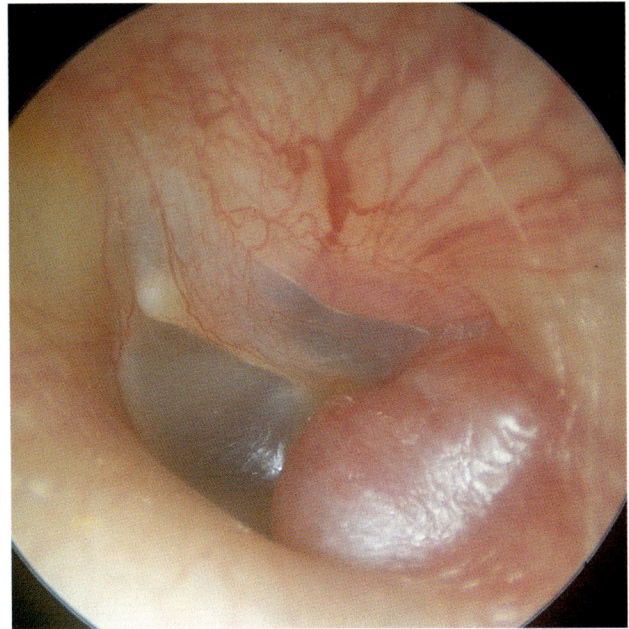

Figure 11.**32** Class C2 De2 glomus jugulare tumor of the left ear. The patient complained of pulsatile tinnitus, hearing loss, and 2 months before presentation started to suffer from dysphonia, dysphagia, and hypoglossal paresis. The involvement of the lower cranial nerves was progressive in nature. It resulted from compression by the slowly growing tumor.

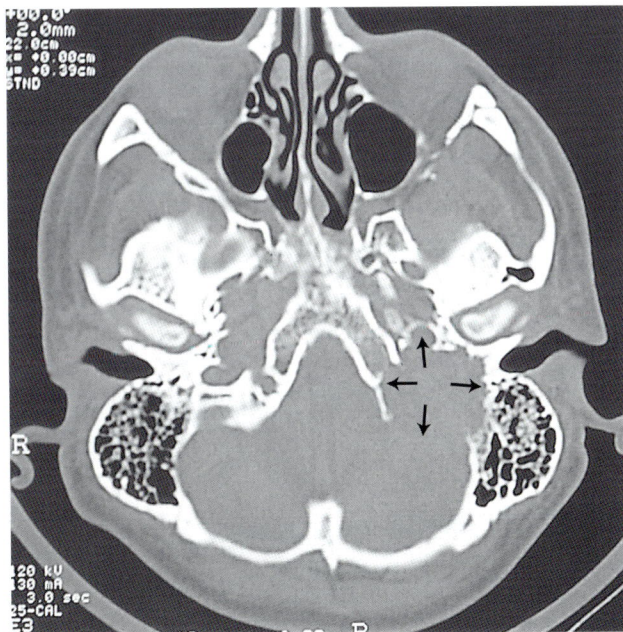

Figure 11.**33** CT scan of the case presented in Figure 11.**32**. The marked erosion of the jugular foramen and the vertical portion of the carotid canal can be appreciated.

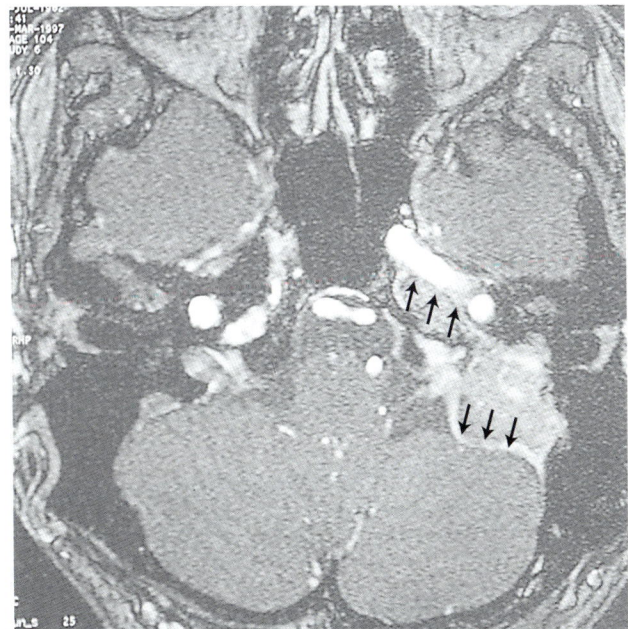

Figure 11.**34** MRI demonstrating tumor in contact with the medial aspect of the horizontal carotid artery and the posterior fossa dura without infiltrating it.

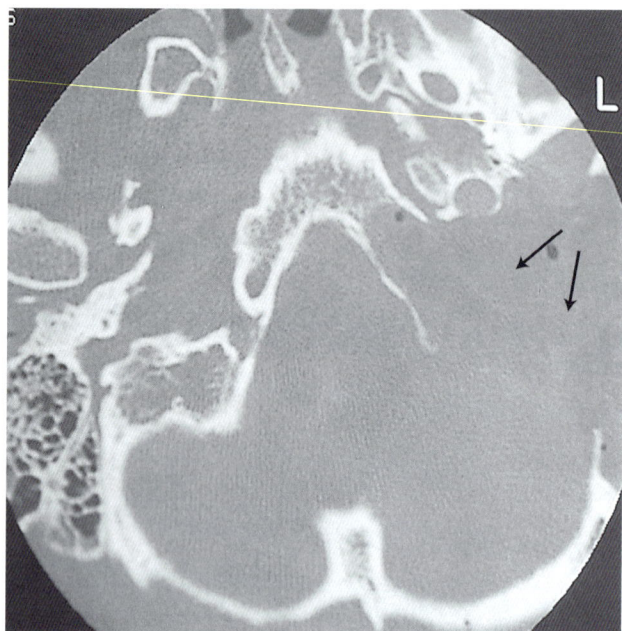

Figure 11.**35** Postoperative CT scan demonstrating tumor removal using an infratemporal fossa approach type A.

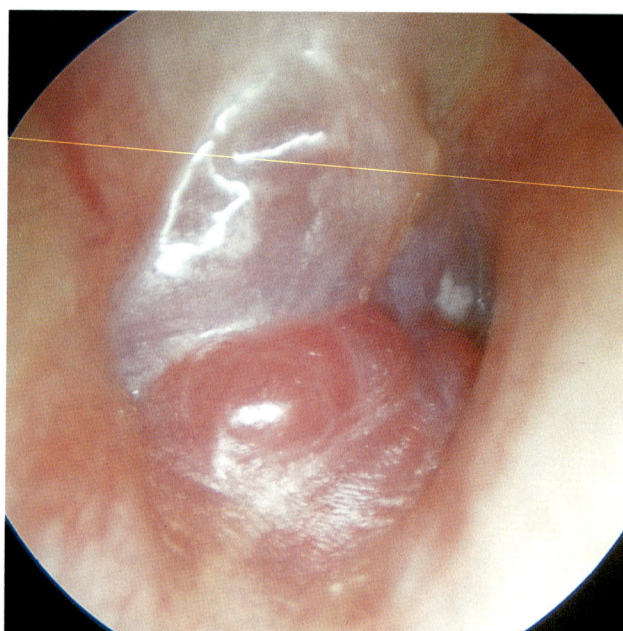

Figure 11.**36** Right ear. Class C3 Di2 glomus jugulare tumor. The patient complained of pulsatile tinnitus and mixed hearing loss of 12 months' duration.

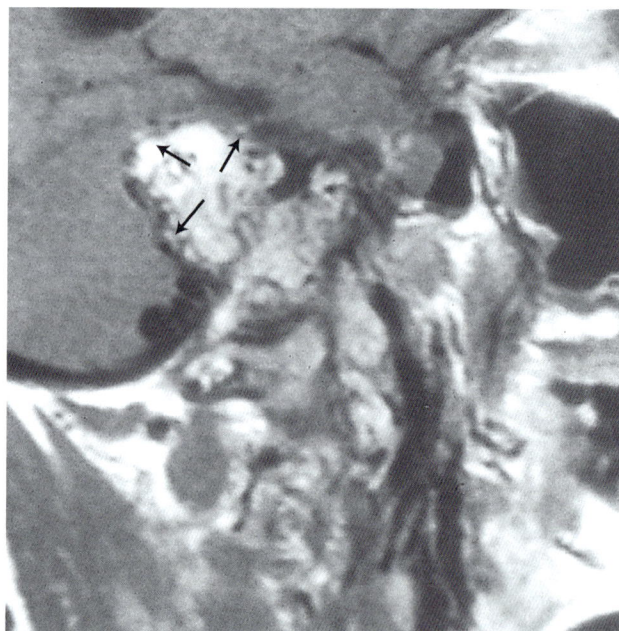

Figure 11.**37** MRI, sagittal view demonstrating intradural extension of the tumor.

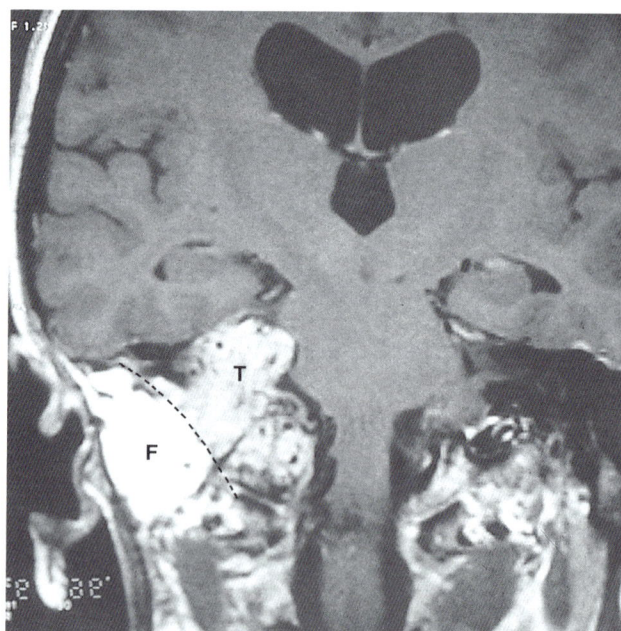

Figure 11.**38** MRI, coronal view after first-stage removal of the extradural component of the tumor using an infratemporal fossa approach type A. The fat (F) obliterating the operative cavity can be seen. The intradural tumor residue (T) is also observed. Staging is necessary in such cases to avoid communication between the subarachnoid space and the wide open neck spaces.

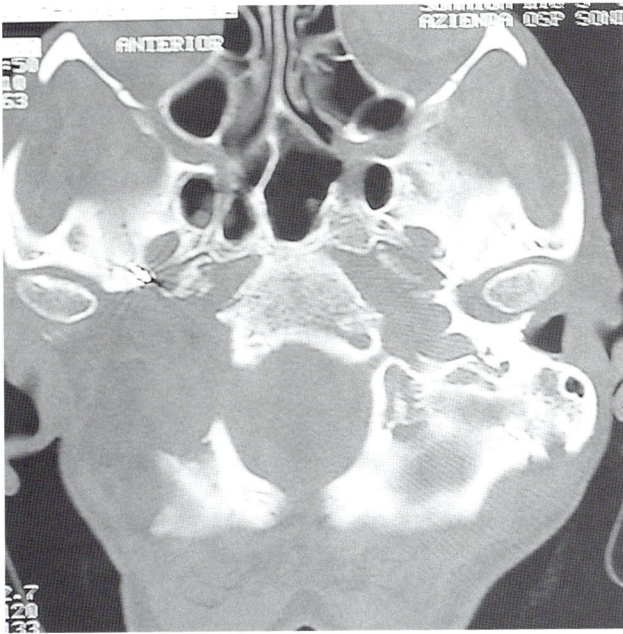

Figure 11.**39**   Postoperative CT scan after the second-stage removal of the tumor through a petro-occipital approach.

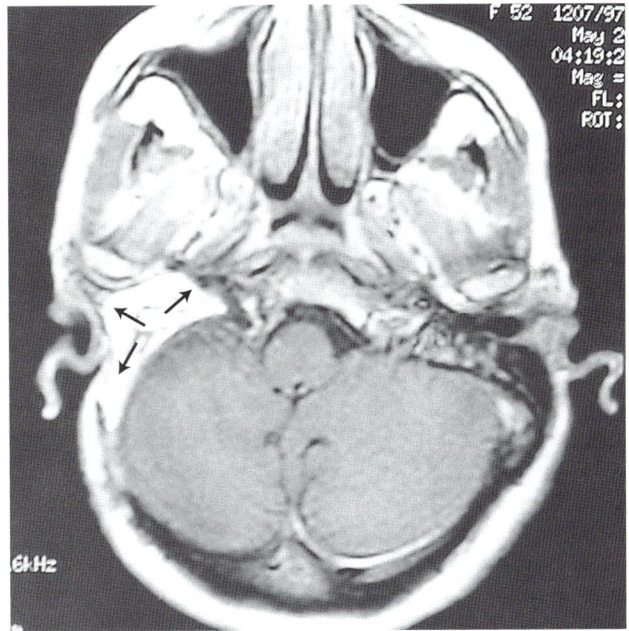

Figure 11.**40**   MRI demonstrating obliteration of the operative cavity with abdominal fat.

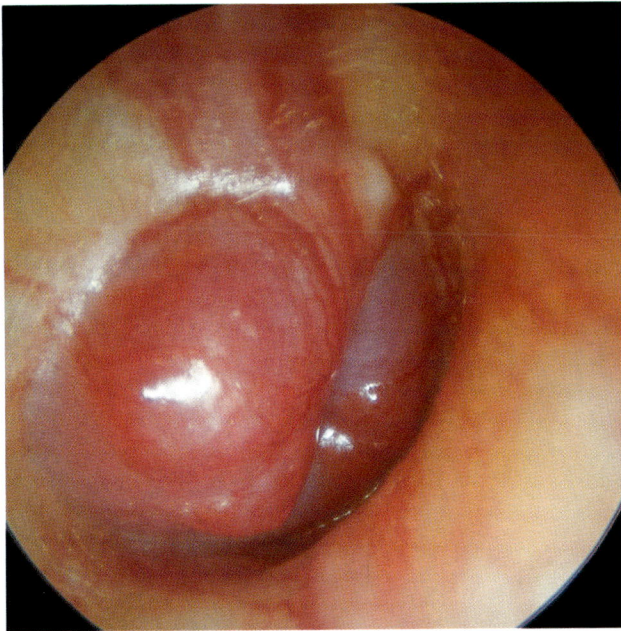

Figure 11.**41**   Right ear. Class C3 Di2 glomus jugulare tumor. The patient complained of ipsilateral total hearing loss, diplopia, grade IV facial paralysis, and dysphonia (see following figures).

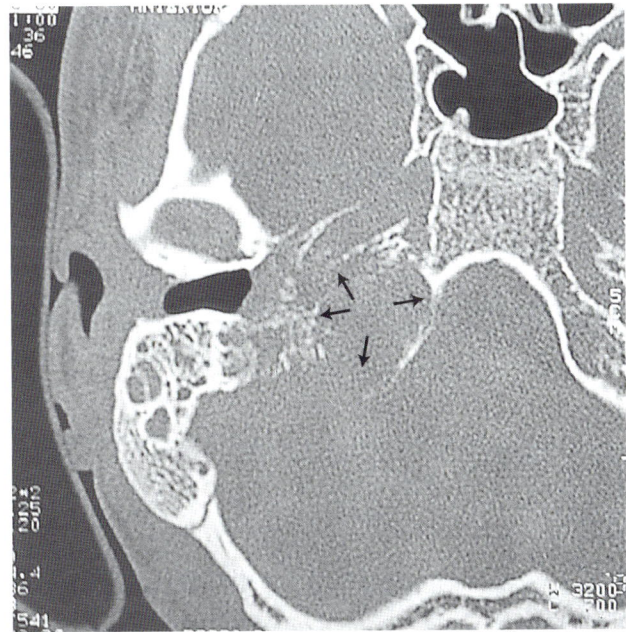

Figure 11.**42**   CT scan axial section demonstrating the involvement of the jugular foramen and the horizontal segment of the internal carotid artery. The artery was closed preoperatively with a balloon.

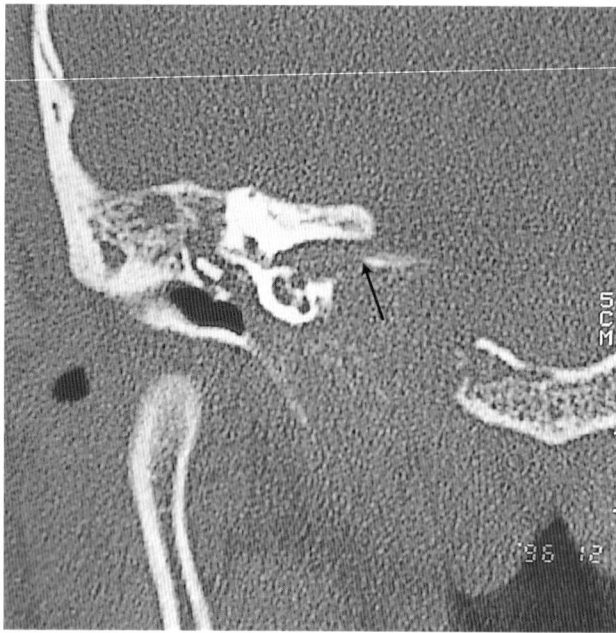

Figure 11.**43** CT scan, coronal section. The tumor involves the internal auditory canal.

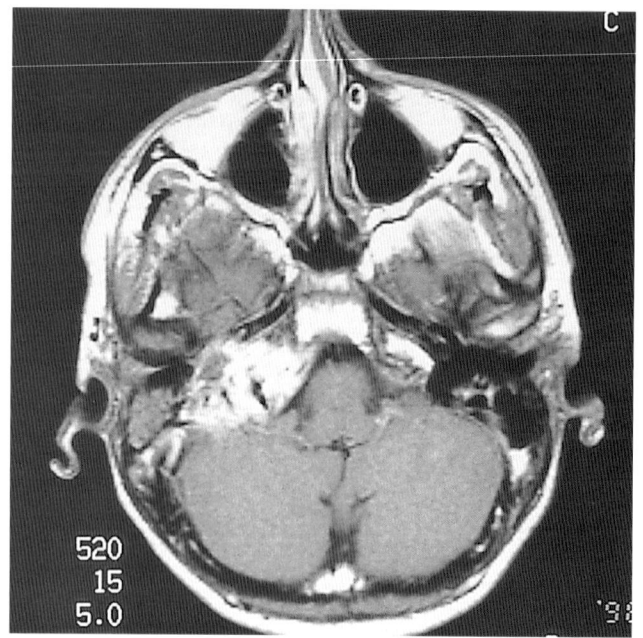

Figure 11.**44** MRI, axial view giving a global idea of the extra- and intradural extension of the tumor.

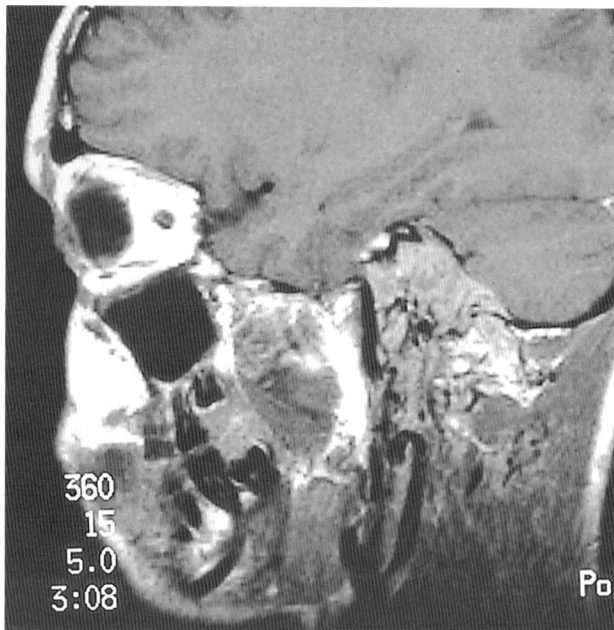

Figure 11.**45** MRI, sagittal view.

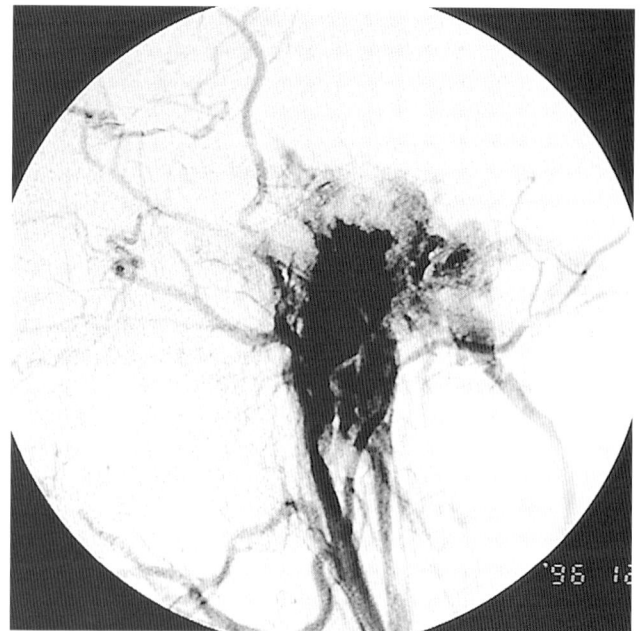

Figure 11.**46** Angiography before embolization.

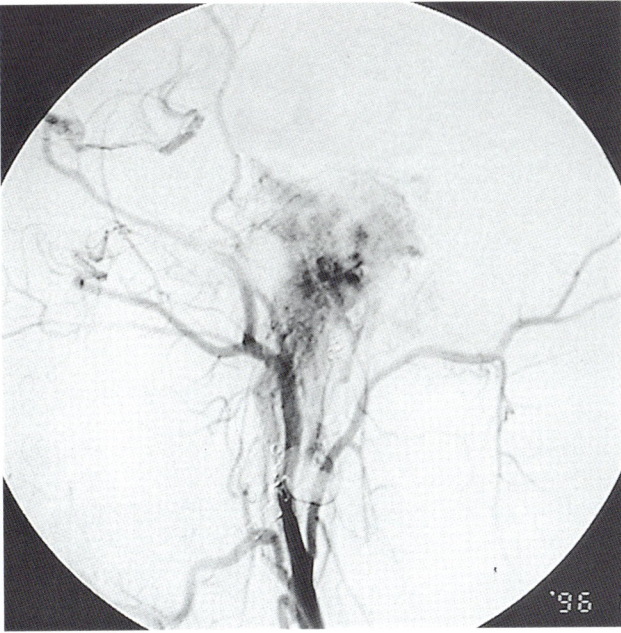

Figure 11.**47** Angiography showing marked reduction of the tumor vascularity following embolization.

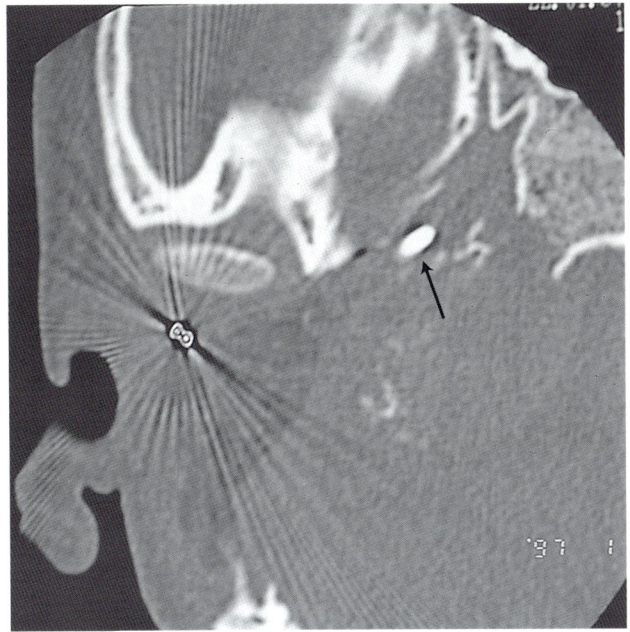

Figure 11.**48** CT scan performed after first-stage removal of the extradural part of the tumor using an infratemporal fossa approach type A. Staging is necessary to avoid communication between the subarachnoid spaces and the neck spaces. The balloon used for the closure of the internal carotid artery can be seen (arrow).

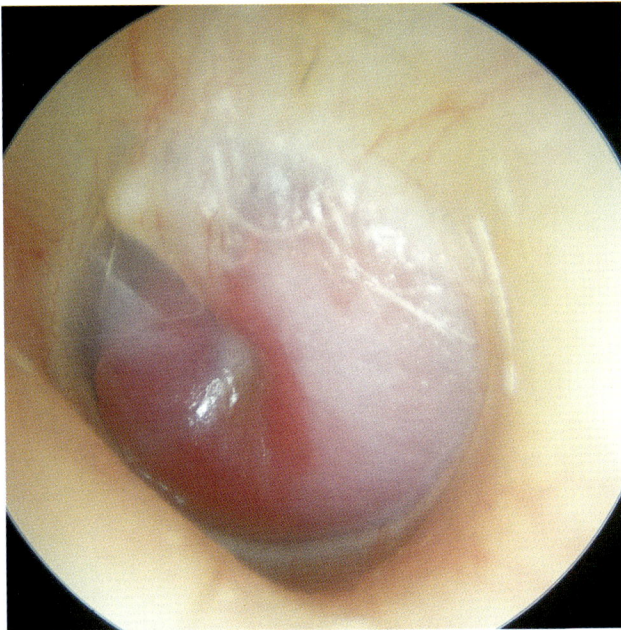

Figure 11.**49** Left ear. Class C2 Di2 glomus jugulare tumor. The patient complained of hearing loss and pulsatile tinnitus of 2 years' duration. He also had dysphonia, dysphagia, paralysis of the left half of the tongue, and paresis of the lower face.

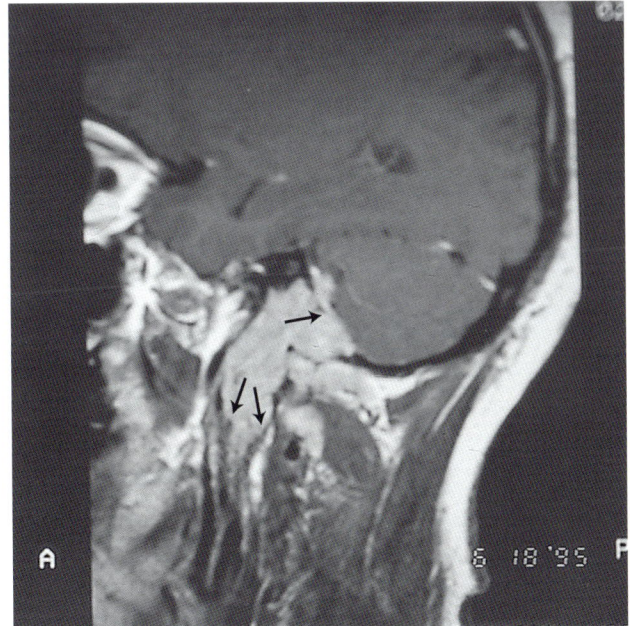

Figure 11.**50** MRI, sagittal view demonstrating the intradural extension of the tumor as well as the inferior extension towards C1 and C2.

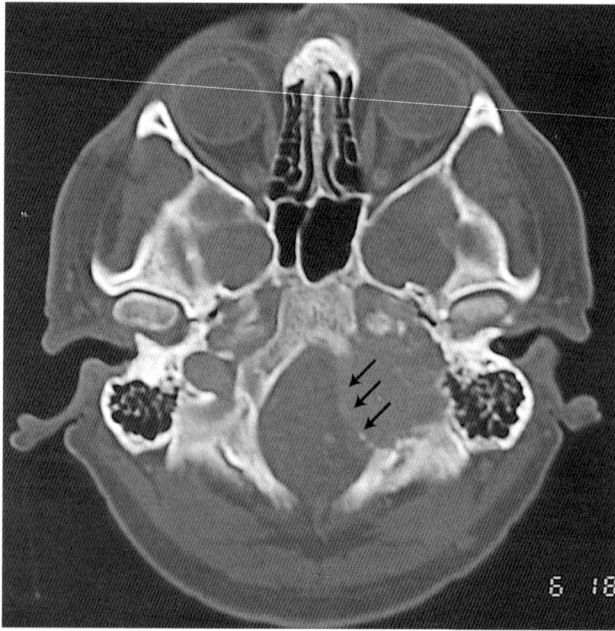

Figure 11.**51**   Preoperative CT scan. The jugular foramen is enlarged, with involvement of the foramen magnum.

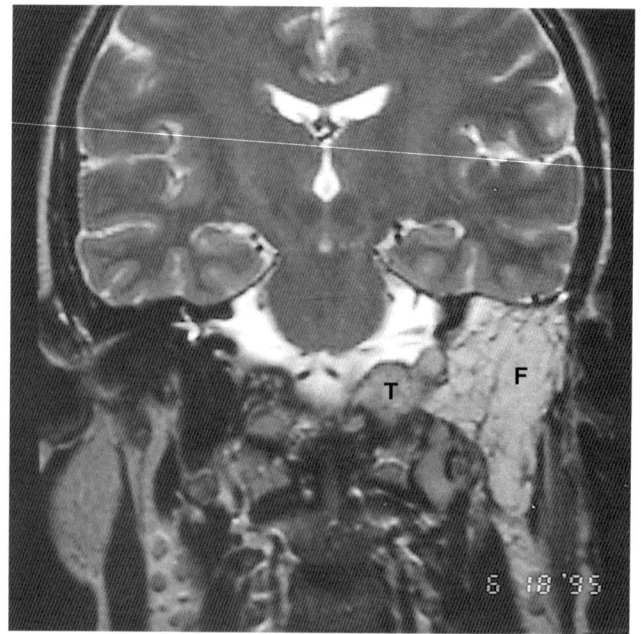

Figure 11.**52**   MRI with gadolinium after removal of the extradural part using an infratemporal fossa approach type A. Fat is seen obliterating the operative cavity (F). The intradural tumor residue at the level of the foramen magnum is noted (T).

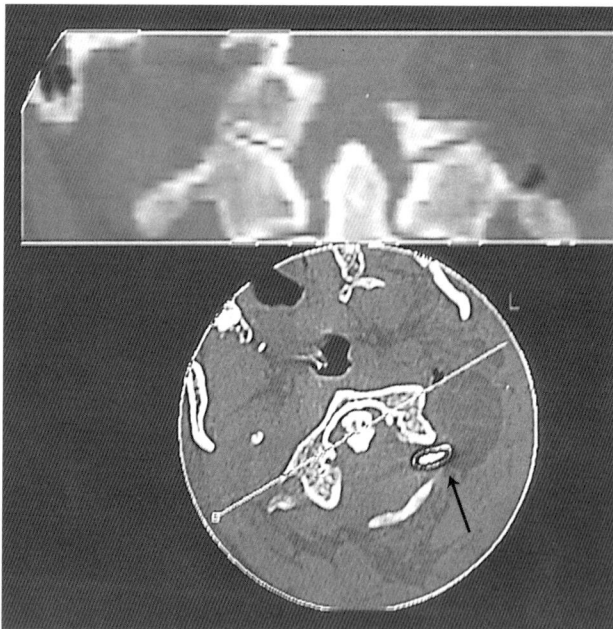

Figure 11.**53**   CT scan following the second-stage removal of the intradural portion of the tumor using an extreme lateral approach. The balloon used to close the vertebral artery is visible.

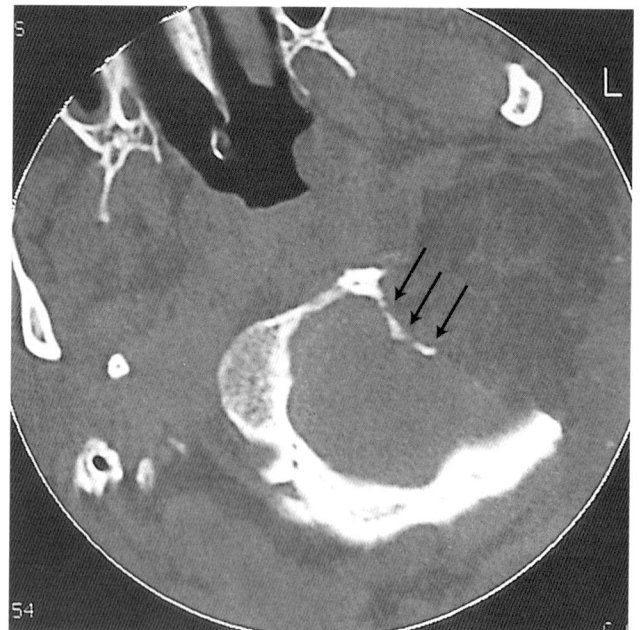

Figure 11.**54**   CT scan following the second-stage removal of the intradural portion of the tumor. The removal of a large part of the left occipital condyle is also shown.

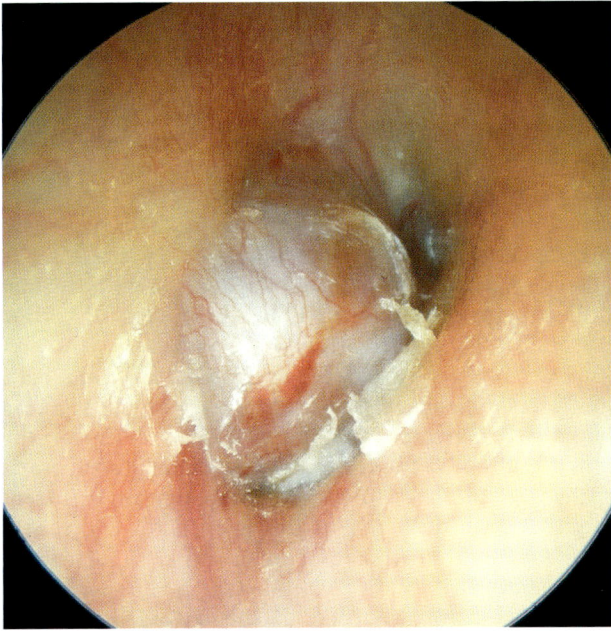

Figure 11.**55**   Another example of a large class C3 Di2 glomus tumor.

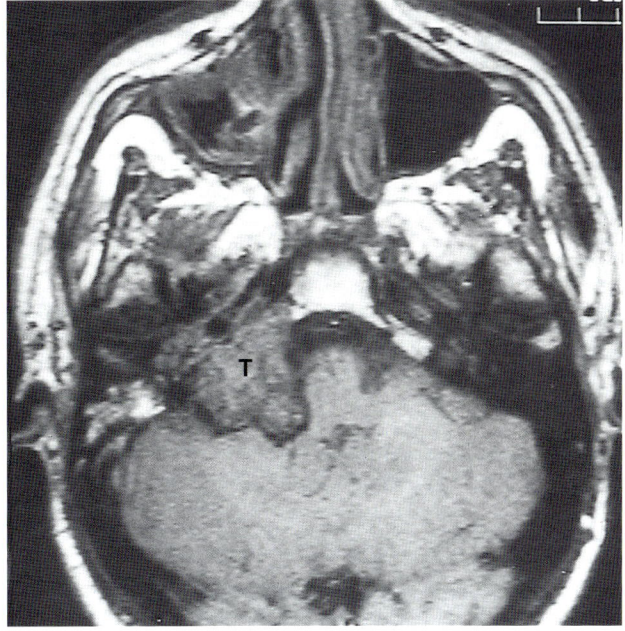

Figure 11.**56**   MRI of the case in Figure 11.**55** (T= tumor).

Type A Infratemporal Fossa Approach

The key point in this approach is the anterior transposition of the facial nerve, which provides optimal control of the infralabyrinthine and jugular foramen regions, as well as the vertical portion of the internal carotid artery.

Indications

The main indication for this approach is lesions of the jugular foramen–type C and D glomus jugulare tumors. We do not use this approach for neuromas or meningiomas of the jugular foramen, which we manage using the petro-occipital trans-sigmoid (POTS) approach, with preservation of middle ear function and without anterior transposition of the facial nerve.

Surgical Technique

A postauricular skin incision is performed. A small, anteriorly-based musculoperiosteal flap is elevated to help in closure afterwards. The skin of the external auditory canal is transected, elevated and closed using a blind sac.

The facial nerve is identified at its exit from the temporal bone. The main trunk is the perpendicular bisection of a line joining the cartilaginous pointer to the mastoid tip. The main trunk is traced in the parotid until the proximal parts of the temporal and zygomatic branches are identified.

The posterior belly of digastric muscle and the sternocleidomastoid muscle are divided close to their origin. The internal jugular vein and the external and internal carotid arteries are identified in the neck. The vessels are marked with umbilical tape.

The skin of the external auditory canal, the tympanic membrane, the malleus and the incus are removed. A canal wall down mastoidectomy is performed, with the removal of the bone anterior and posterior to the sigmoid sinus.

The facial nerve is skeletonized from the stylomastoid foramen to the geniculate ganglion. The last shell of bone is removed using a double-curved raspatory.

The stapes superstructure is preferably removed after cutting its crura with microscissors. The inferior tympanic bone is widely removed and the mastoid tip is amputated using a rongeur. A new fallopian canal is drilled in the root of the zygoma superior to the eustachian tube.

Using strong scissors, the facial nerve is freed at the level of the stylomastoid foramen. The soft tissue at this level are not separated from the nerve. The mastoid segment is next elevated using a Beaver knife to cut the fibrous attachments between the nerve and the fallopian canal.

The tympanic segment of the nerve is elevated carefully, using a curved raspatory, until the level of the geniculate ganglion is reached. A nontoothed forceps is used to hold the soft tissue surrounding the nerve at the stylomastoid foramen and the anterior rerouting is carried out. A tunnel is created in the parotid gland to lodge the transposed nerve. The tunnel is closed around

the nerve using two sutures. The nerve is fixed to the new bony canal, just above the eustachian tube, using fibrin glue.

Drilling of the infralabyrinthine cells is completed, and the vertical portion of the internal carotid artery is identified. The mandibular condyle is separated from the anterior wall of the external auditory canal using a large septal raspatory. To avoid injury to the facial nerve, we no longer use the Fisch infratemporal fossa retractor. The anterior wall of the external auditory canal is further drilled, completing the exposure of the vertical portion of the internal carotid artery.

The sinus is closed using Surgicel extraluminally and intraluminally. The proximal part of the sigmoid sinus is compressed extraluminally with Surgicel; the sinus is then opened and packed distally and proximally with two large pieces of Surgicel. With this technique, we avoid the use of a dural incision, which may lead to a higher risk of cerebrospinal fluid leakage postoperatively.

The structures attached to the styloid process are severed. This process is fractured using a rongeur and is then cut with strong scissors. The remaining fibrous tissue surrounding the internal carotid artery at its point of entry into the skull base is carefully removed using scissors.

The internal jugular vein in the neck is double-ligated and cut. The vein is elevated superiorly, with care being taken not to injure the related lower cranial nerves. If the eleventh nerve passes laterally, the vein has to be pulled under the nerve carefully to prevent it from being damaged. If necessary (as in the case of glomus jugulare tumors), the lateral wall of the sigmoid sinus can be removed. Removal continues down to the level of the jugular bulb. The lateral wall of the jugular bulb is opened. Bleeding usually occurs from the apertures of the inferior petrosal sinus and the condylar emissary vein. This is controlled by Surgicel packing. If there is limited intradural extension, the dura is opened without injury to the endolymphatic sac.

At the end of the procedure, the eustachian tube is closed with a piece of muscle. The dural opening is closed with a muscle plug. A transfixing suture is passed into one dural edge, through the muscle plug, and out from the other dural edge, and then tied. The cavity is obliterated using abdominal fat without rotating the temporalis muscle, which is to be sutured over the fat.

Rarely, there may be marked stenosis in the artery, or its wall may be too fragile due to previous radiotherapy or surgery. A balloon occlusion test is mandatory before removal of the carotid is attempted. At the beginning of our experience, carotid resection was carried out more frequently. We have adopted a less aggressive attitude nowadays, for fear of long-term consequences such as strokes, hemiplegia, and aneurysm of the contralateral internal carotid artery.

With large glomus tumors (C3, involving the horizontal internal carotid artery, or C4, reaching the anterior foramen lacerum and extending to the cavernous sinus), the approach is combined with a type B or C infratemporal fossa approach for removal of the tumor.

Summary

Because of the complex anatomy of the temporal bone and the structures at the base of the skull, as well as the invasiveness, rich vascularity, and aggressive behavior of glomus tumors, surgery for these difficult lesions is problematic.

Glomus tumors generally present with hearing loss and pulsatile tinnitus. When the lower cranial nerves are invaded, a jugular foramen syndrome becomes manifest.

Otoscopy usually reveals a reddish retrotympanic mass. A definitive diagnosis is obtained after neuroradiological studies are performed. These include a high-resolution CT scan with bony window, MRI with and without gadolinium, and digital subtraction angiography. Radiological studies are essential not only to confirm the diagnosis and define the exact tumor class, but also to properly evaluate these tumors. The neuroradiologist should be able to inform the surgeon about the following:

- Details of the osseous lesion
- Involvement of the jugular bulb and foramen
- Exact involvement of the temporal bone
- The presence of inner ear invasion
- The relationship between the fallopian canal and the tumor
- Carotid canal erosion and exact involvement of the internal carotid artery
- Invasion of the petrous apex and clivus
- Details regarding the relationship between the tumor and surrounding soft tissues, e.g.:
  - Degree of neck extension
  - Infratemporal fossa involvement
  - Intracranial and intradural extension

Radiology also helps to determine the superior and inferior extension of the tumor, the possibility of other associated lesions (e.g., contralateral glomus or carotid body tumor), as well as the patency of the contralateral sigmoid sinus and internal jugular vein.

In class C and D tumors, selective digital subtraction angiography is essential. Arteriography is performed for both ipsilateral and contralateral internal and external carotids and for the vertebrobasilar system. A study of the venous phase is also of great importance.

Arteriography of the external carotid artery defines the exact feeding vessels for further embolization. In all tumors of class C and D, embolization is fundamental.

Arteriography of the internal carotid artery shows vascularization from the caroticotympanic artery and from the cavernous branches of the artery as well as the exact status of arterial invasion by the tumor.

Study of the vertebrobasilar system demonstrates the vascularization of intracranial extension of the tumor from muscular, meningeal, and parenchymal (PICA, AICA) branches. Arterial supply from these latter branches indicates a definite intradural extension of the tumor. This study also provides indications for the possibility of embolizing muscular or meningeal branches.

When arteriography shows clear involvement of the internal carotid artery in its horizontal segment (C3 and C4 tumors), a balloon occlusion test to evaluate the collateral circulation and the possibility of sacrificing the artery is necessary. In some selected cases, when the temporary balloon occlusion test is negative, it might be necessary to perform a permanent closure of the artery 30 to 40 days before operation.

In 1978, Fisch classified these lesions into four types: A, B, C, and D. He introduced the type A infratemporal fossa approach for the management of tumors localized in the jugular foramen that were considered inoperable at that time due to the presence of the facial nerve in the middle of the operative field and the inaccessibility of the internal carotid artery and petrous apex. To overcome these obstacles, Fisch proposed anterior rerouting of the facial nerve, giving direct access to the whole intratemporal course of the internal carotid artery as well as an excellent control of the large venous sinuses. Hearing loss is the only permanent postoperative deficit in this approach and is the result of obliteration of the middle ear.

The type A infratemporal fossa approach is generally used for the removal of class C and D glomus tumors of the temporal bone according to the Fisch classification. In cases with intradural extension exceeding 2 cm in diameter, staging is indicated where the intradural part is removed in a second stage 6 to 8 months after the first operation. This surgical strategy avoids the high risk of having postoperative CSF leak should a single-stage removal be attempted. The reason for such a risk is the need to resect a wide area of the dura infiltrated by the tumor, and hence the subarachnoid space becomes widely connected to the open neck spaces. Using the staging strategy, we never experienced any CSF leak in our cases.

To sum up, the infratemporal fossa approach offers a wide access to the lateral skull base. The adequate exposure and systematic management of the important arteries and venous sinuses greatly reduces the intraoperative hemorrhage. An accurate preoperative study of the tumor extension, the preoperative tumor embolization, and the eventual closure of an invaded internal carotid artery (when feasible) by the neuroradiologist are prerequisites for successful surgery. Therefore, the collaboration between the neuroradiologist and the skull-base surgeon is of paramount importance. Lesions of the skull base are rare and very difficult to treat. Management of such cases should be restricted to specialized centers to avoid any serious problems.

12 Rare Retrotympanic Masses

Differential Diagnosis of Retrotympanic Masses

A variety of diseases can present as a mass behind an intact tympanic membrane. A detailed history of the patient, audiological assessment, and proper radiological evaluation are essential to reach a proper diagnosis. Table 12.1 summarizes the most common conditions causing a retrotympanic mass. For details of each condition, the reader is referred to the relevant chapters.

Table 12.1   Conditions that may present as a retrotympanic mass.

Anomalous anatomy
High jugular bulb
Aberrant carotid artery
Tumors and tumor-like conditions
Congenital cholesteatoma
Iatrogenic cholesteatoma
Glomus tumor
Facial nerve tumor (neuroma, hemangioma)
Carcinoid tumor
Adenoma, adenocarcinoma
Meningioma (primary or secondary to temporal bone invasion)
Rhabdomyosarcoma of the tensor tympani
Miscellaneous
Meningoencephalic herniation

Meningioma

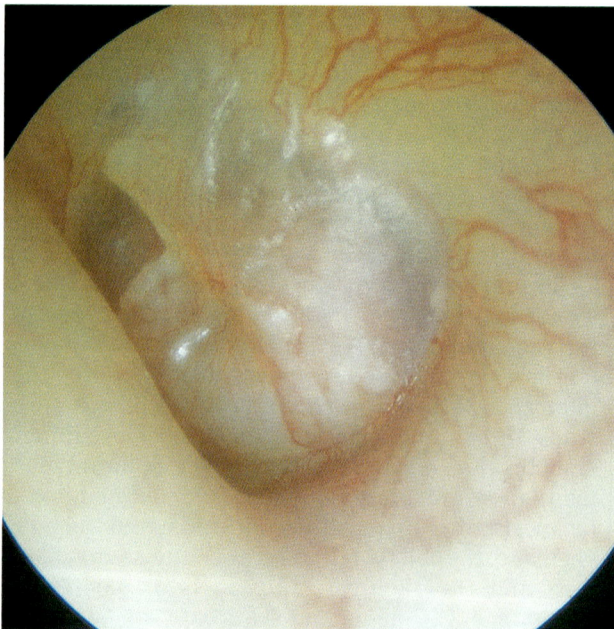

Figure 12.1   Left ear. This patient presented with dysphagia as her only symptom. A nonpulsating retrotympanic mass was noticed. The mass was whitish rather than the reddish color characteristic of glomus tumor. CT scan and MRI demonstrated an enplaque meningioma invading the posterior surface of the temporal bone.

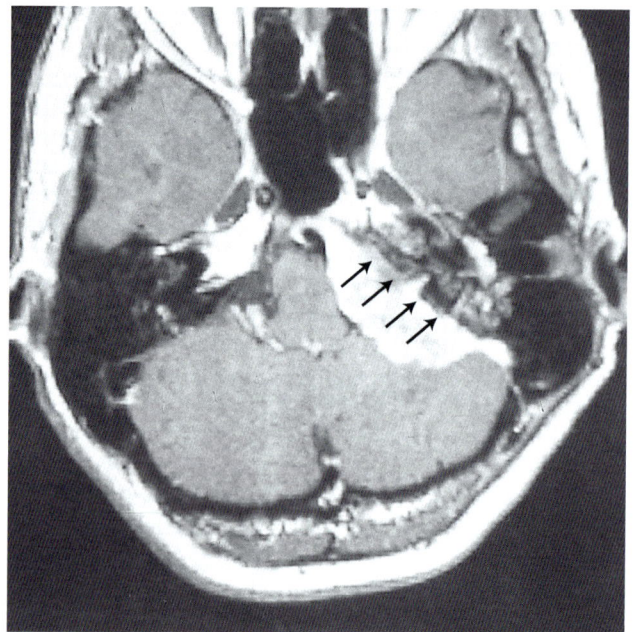

Figure 12.2   MRI of the case presented in Figure 12.1. Large posterior fossa meningioma located along the posterior surface of the petrous bone.

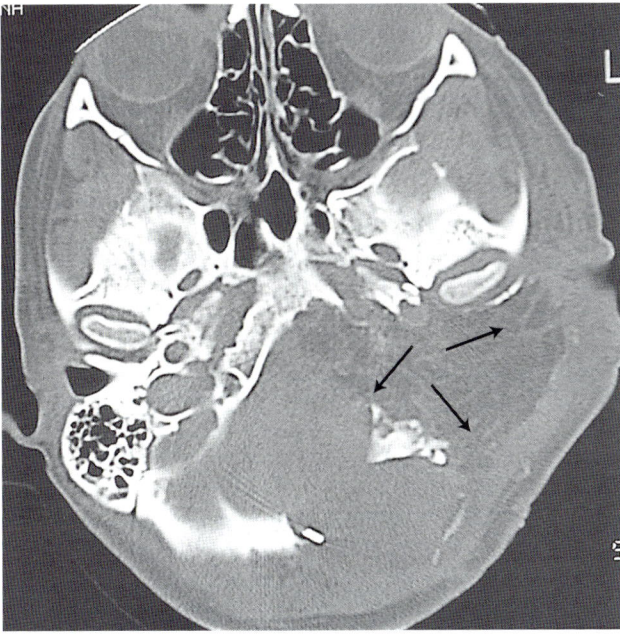

Figure 12.**3** Postoperative CT scan of the case described in Figure 12.**1**The tumor was removed using a modified transcochlear approach. The surgical cavity was obliterated using abdominal fat.

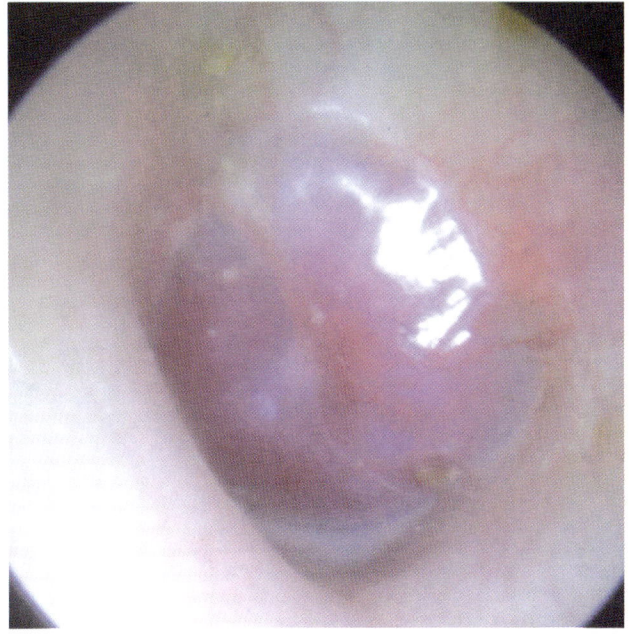

Figure 12.**4a** Left ear. A reddish mass is visible, behind the tympanic membrane. The patient was suffering from right conductive hearing loss, fullness, and tinnitus.

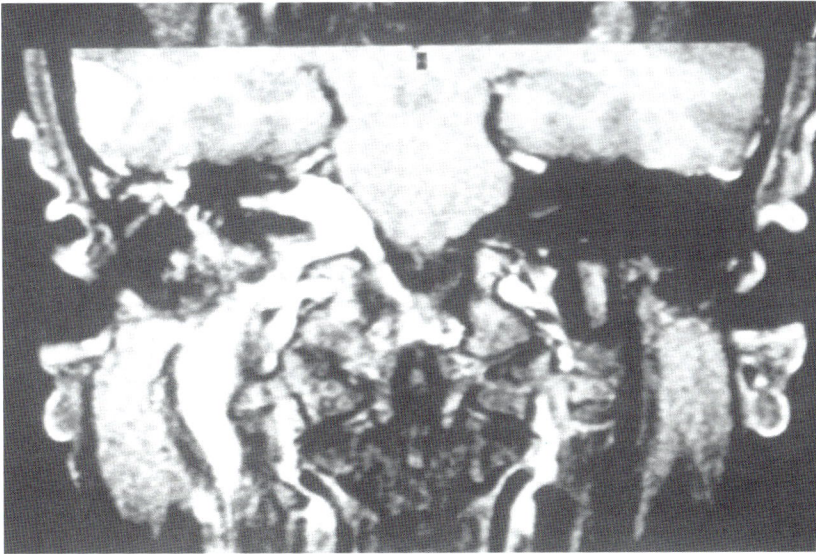

Figure 12.**4b** Coronal MRI. An en plaque meningioma is clearly visible, extending from the posterior fossa to the neck.

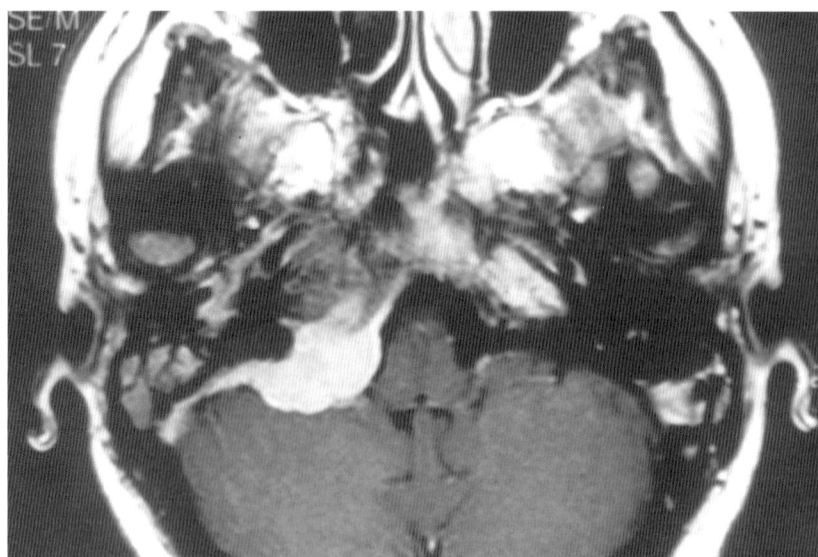

Figure 12.**4c** Axial MRI. The tumor is enhanced, showing the classic dural signs of a meningioma ("dura tails").

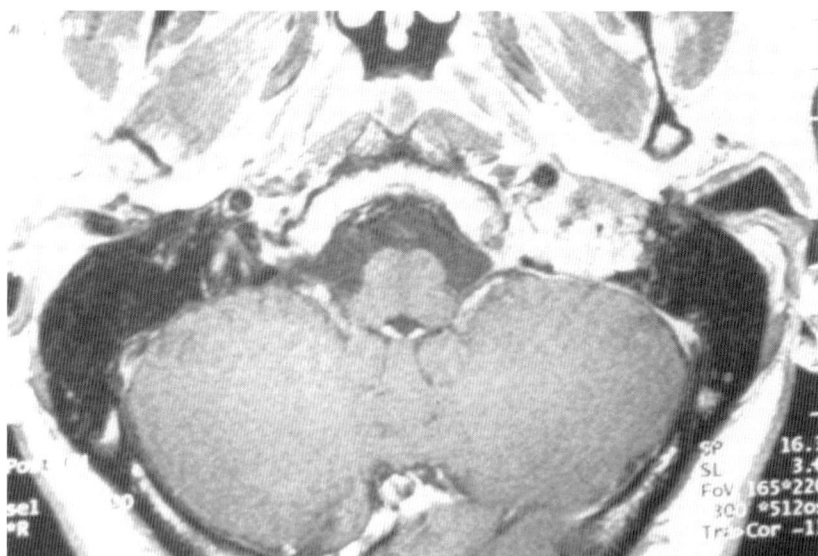

Figure 12.**4d** Axial MRI. The tumor involves the vertical portion of the ICA.

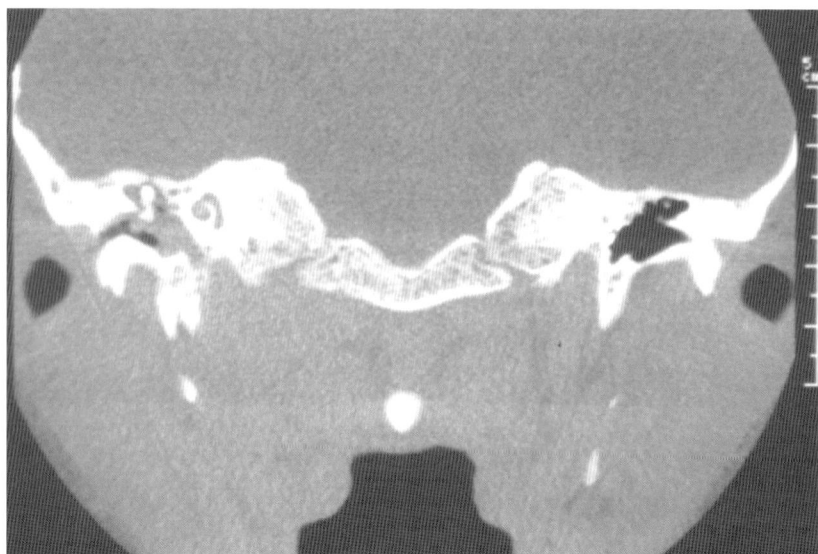

Figure 12.**5** CT scan. This coronal view shows the middle ear completely filled by the tumor.

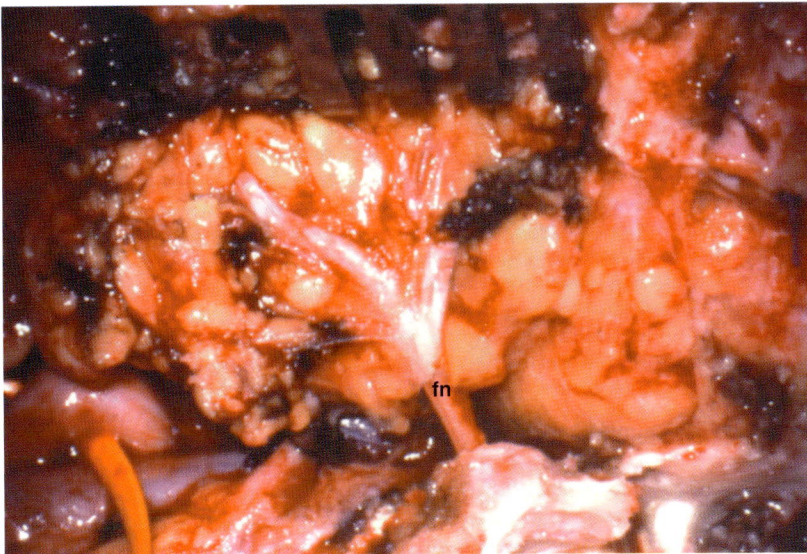

Figure 12.**6** An infratemporal fossa approach type A has been carried out (see page 148). The facial nerve at the stylomastoid foramen and its extramastoid portion, with the bifurcation in the parotid gland, are clearly seen here.

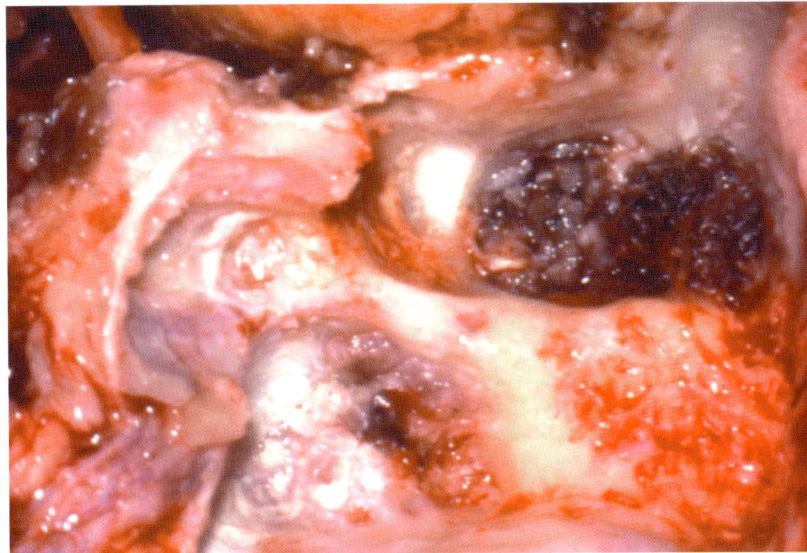

Figure 12.**7** A subtotal petrosectomy has been carried out, and the tumor in the middle ear has been coagulated. A new fallopian canal has been drilled in the anterior superior wall of the external auditory canal.

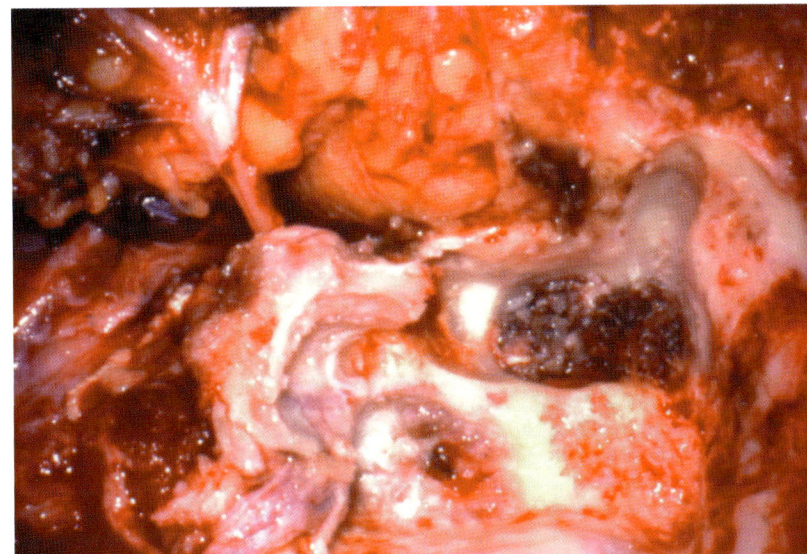

Figure 12.**8** The surgical field, with the extramastoid facial nerve, parotid gland, new fallopian canal, and mastoid tip (still in place).

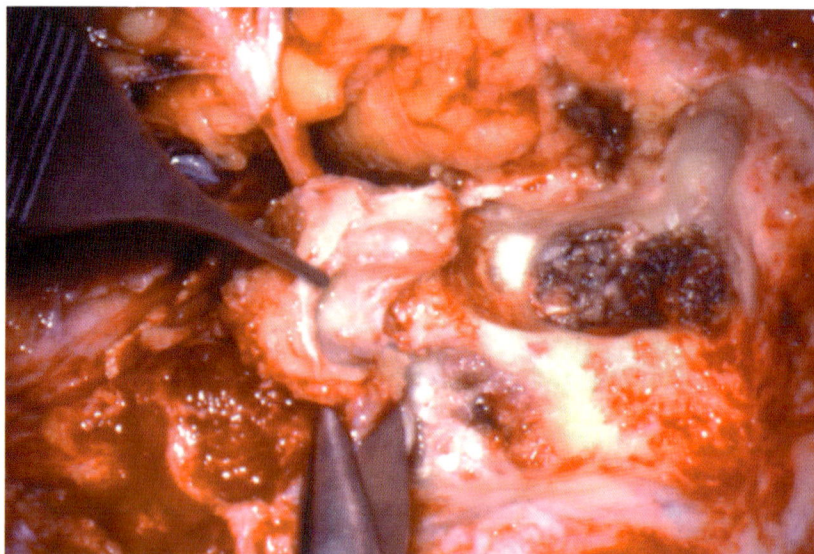

Figure 12.**9**   Removal of the mastoid tip.

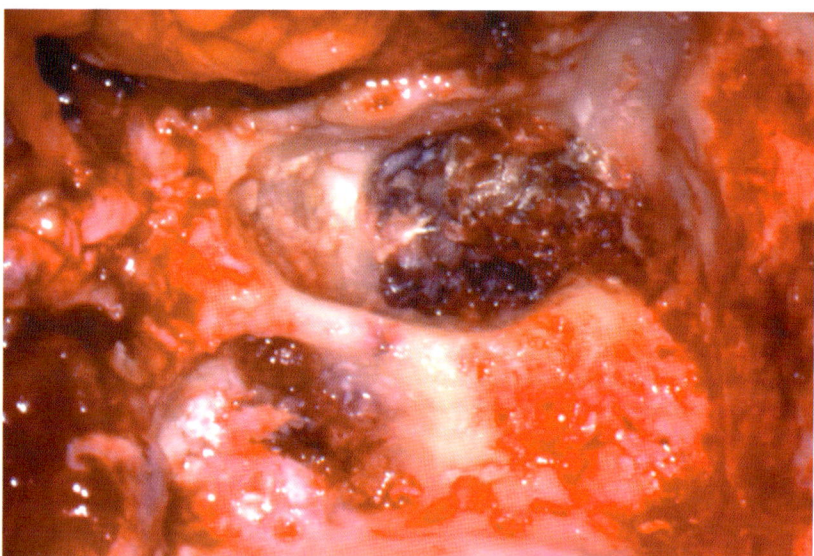

Figure 12.**10**   The mastoid tip has been removed.

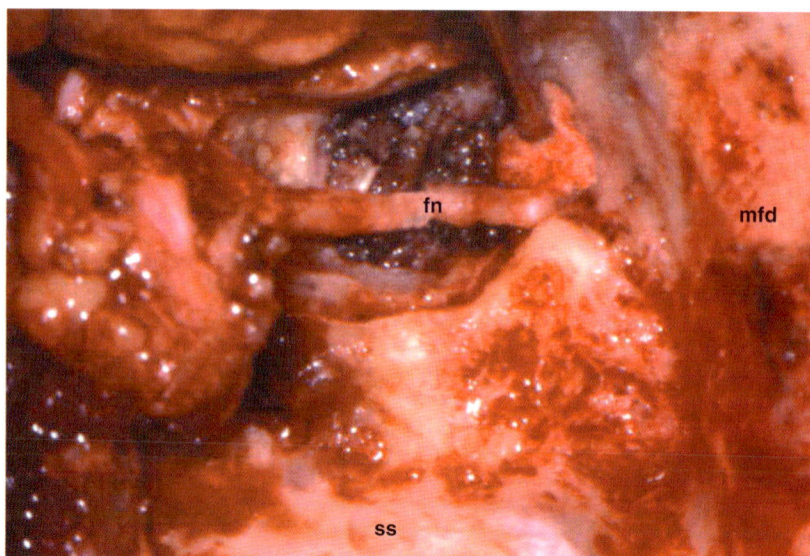

Figure 12.**11**   The facial nerve has been detached from the third and second portion of the fallopian canal, together with the tissue of the stylomastoid foramen.

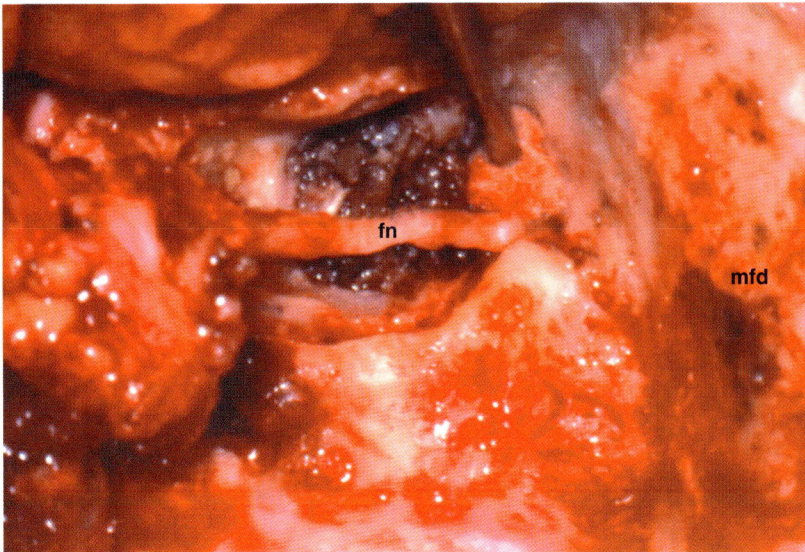

Figure 12.**12** A larger magnification of the previous picture. The bleeding in the area of the geniculate ganglion is controlled with a cottonoid pressed with the tip of the suction probe. The facial nerve has been almost completely rerouted anteriorly, and it will be placed in a new bony fallopian canal and protected inside the parotid gland.

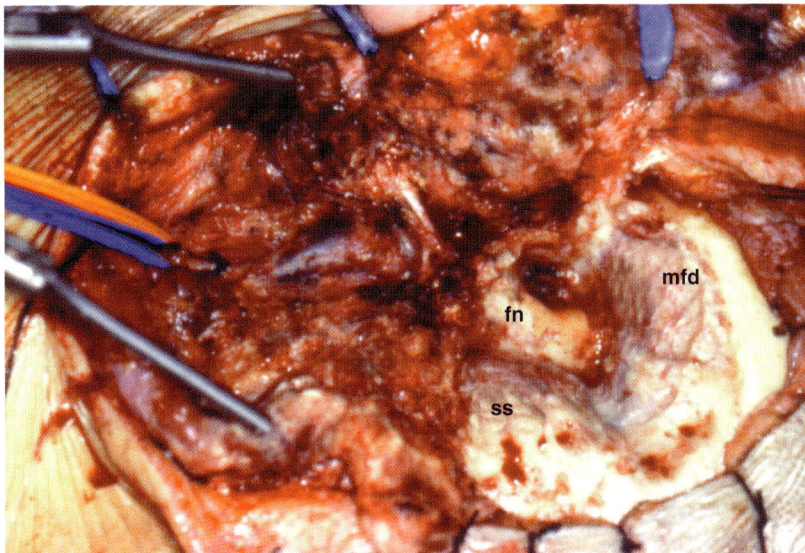

Figure 12.**13** The carotid and jugular vein have been dissected during a subtotal petrosectomy.

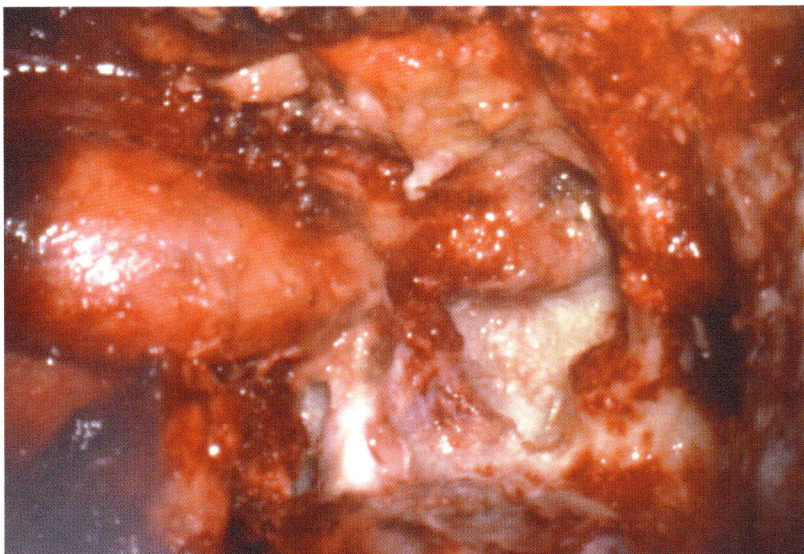

Figure 12.**14** The meningioma had infiltrated the jugular vein and jugular bulb, engulfing the vertical and horizontal portions of the carotid artery. The petrous apical compartment and the middle clivus are being drilled.

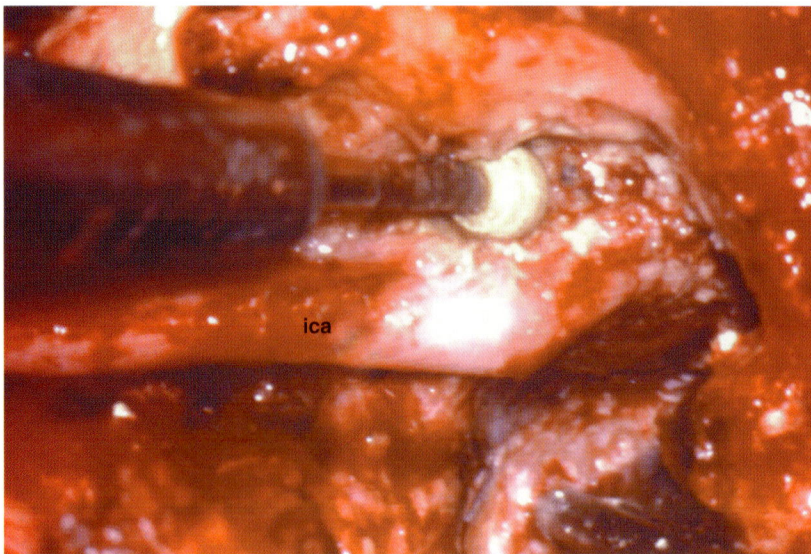

Figure 12.**15**   The carotid artery in the neck and its vertical portion in the temporal bone are dissected. A diamond burr is used to remove tumor anterior to the vertical portion of the artery.

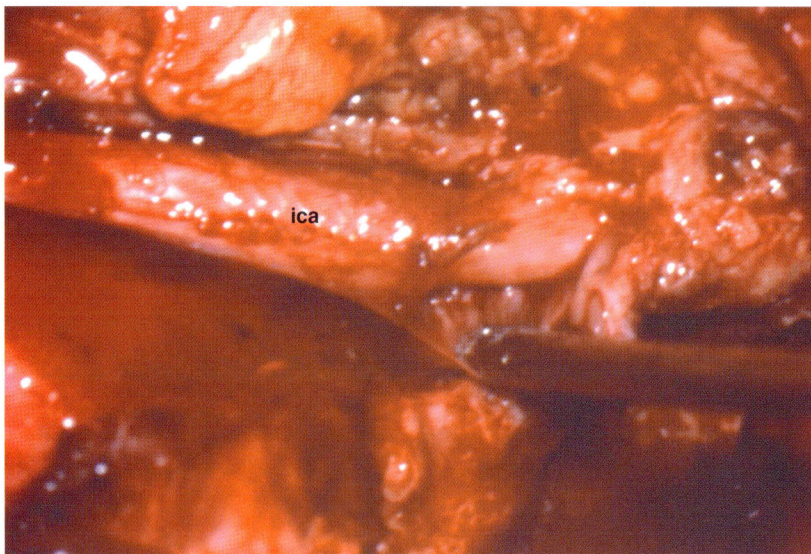

Figure 12.**16**   A subadventitial dissection of the meningioma.

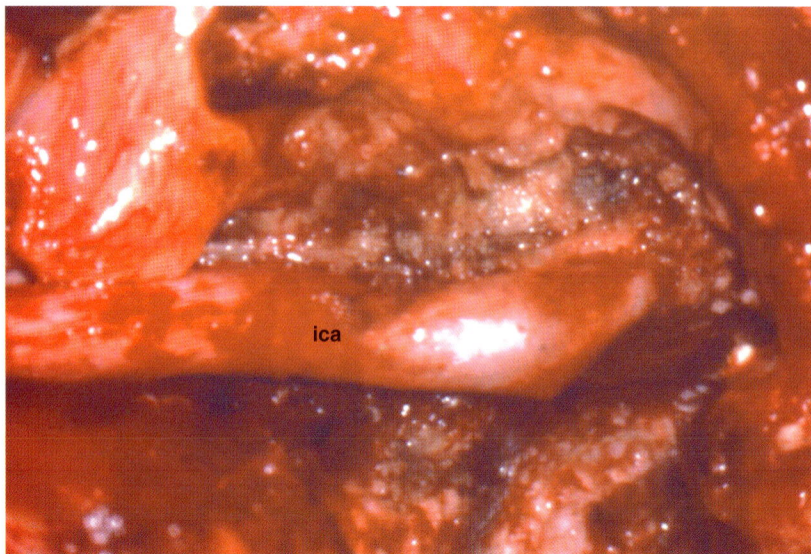

Figure 12.**17**   The carotid artery is completely free from the tumor.

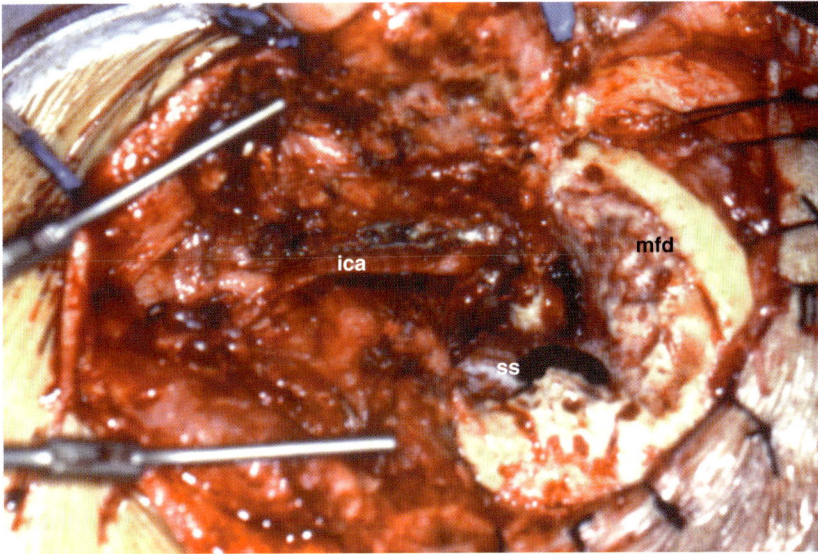

Figure 12.**18** The surgical field at the end of the procedure, with the carotid artery and the facial nerve transposed anteriorly.

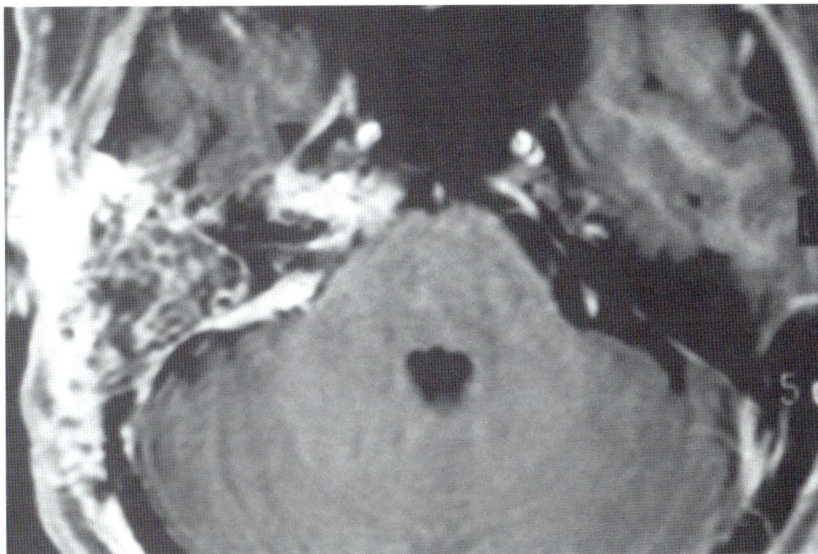

Figure 12.**19** Postoperative MRI. Only a small piece of tumor has been left at the level of the posterior fossa dura, which will be removed in the second-stage operation. The staged procedure was used in order to avoid a cerebrospinal fluid leak.

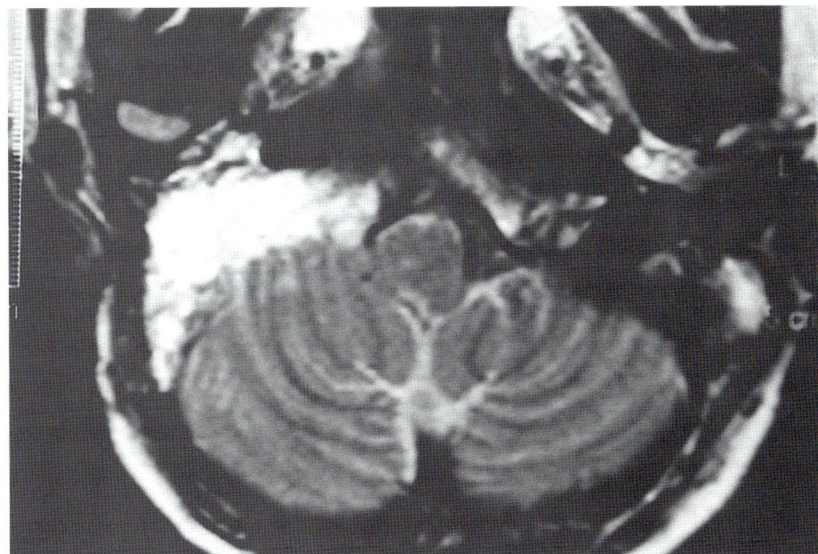

Figure 12.**20** Axial MRI after the second-stage. The surgical cavity is filled with abdominal fat.

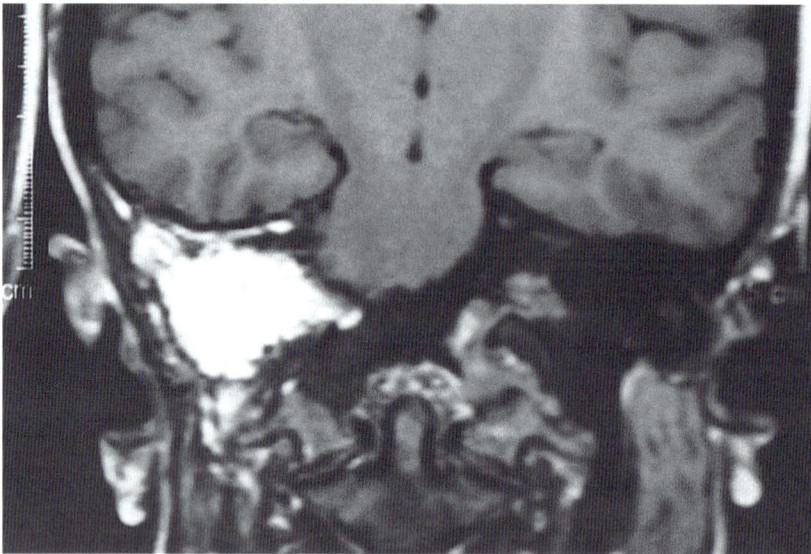

Figure 12.**21**   Coronal MRI after the second-stage. The surgical cavity is obliterated with abdominal fat.

Facial Nerve Neurinoma

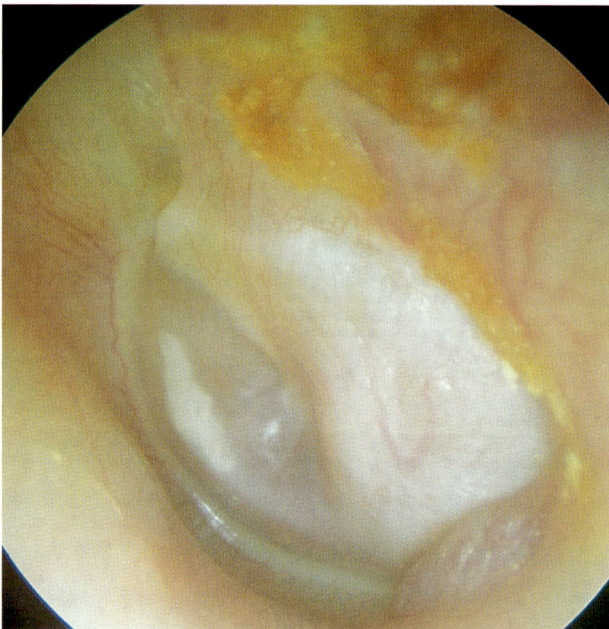

Figure 12.**22**   Left ear. Otoscopic view similar to the case, presented in Figure 12.**1**. A whitish retrotympanic mass is seen causing bulging of the posterior quadrants of the tympanic membrane. A small reddish mass is visible in the posterior inferior regions of the external auditory canal (i.e., lateral to the annulus). The patient complained of left hearing loss and non- pulsating tinnitus of 2 years' duration. In the last 3 months before presentation, left facial nerve paresis started to appear (see following figures).

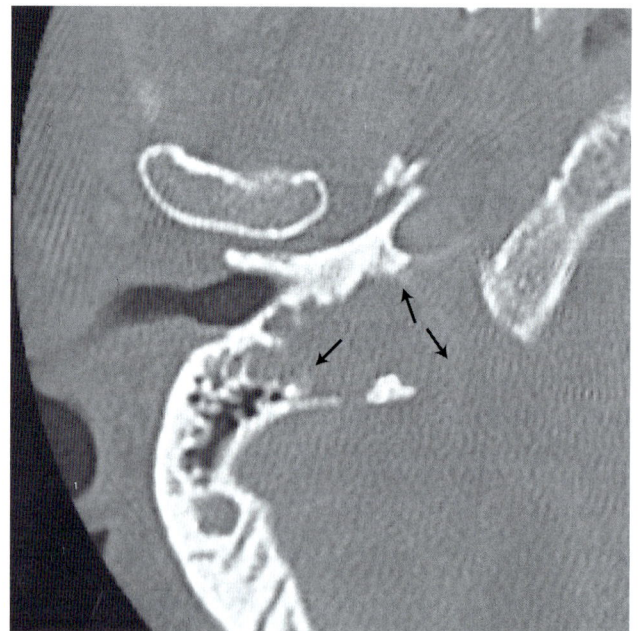

Figure 12.**23**   CT scan, axial view, of the case presented in Figure 12.**22**. The tumor is centered on the left jugular foramen.

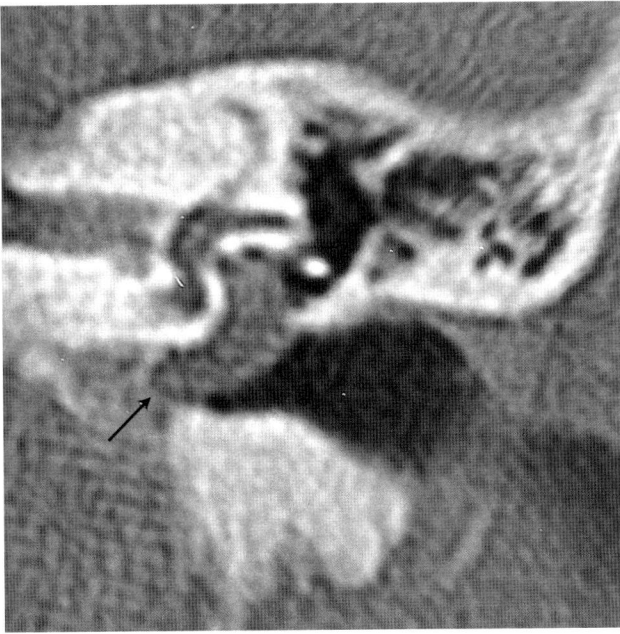

Figur 12.**24**   CT scan, coronal view. The mass eroded the bony plate over the jugular bulb extending into the hypotympanum.

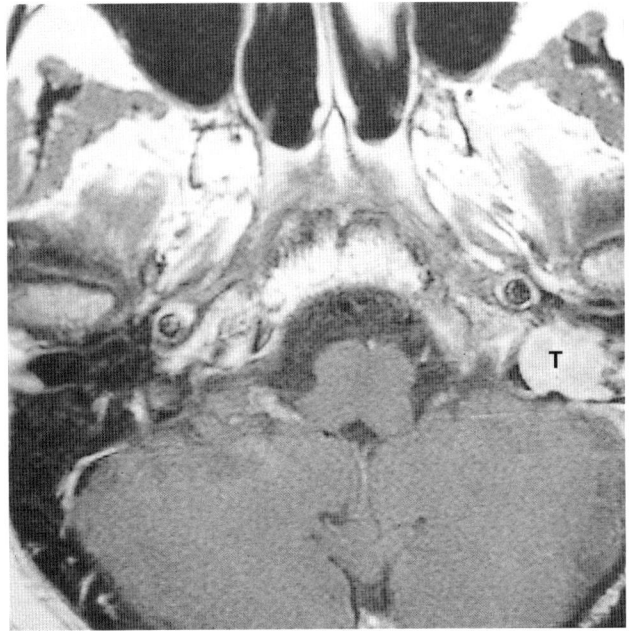

Figure 12.**25**   MRI, axial view, shows a mass centered on the jugular foramen (T= tumor).

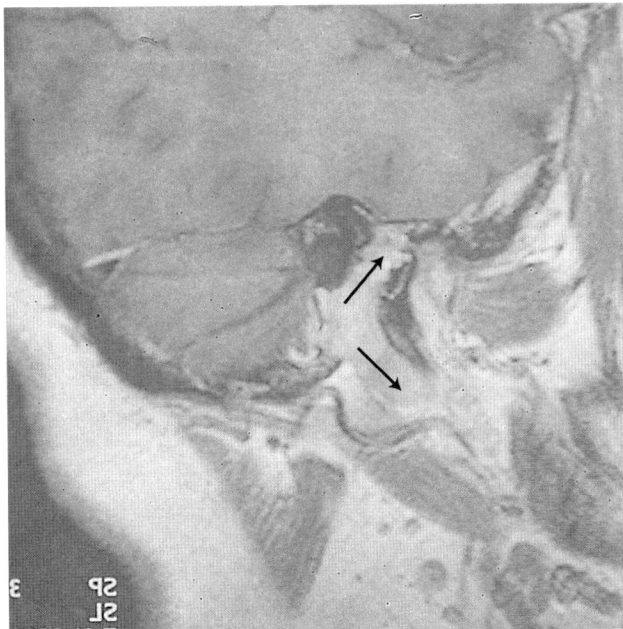

Figure 12.**26**   MRI, sagittal view, of the case in Figure 12.**22**.

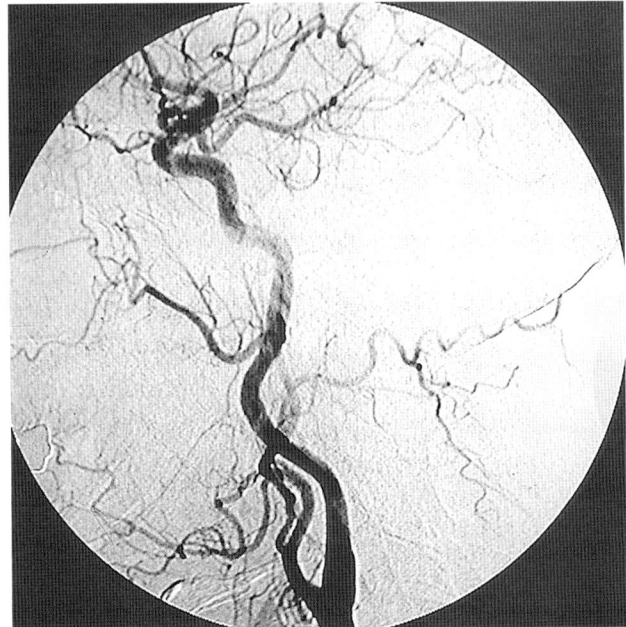

Figure 12.**27**   Angiography did not show the characteristic tumor blush of glomus tumors. During surgery, the tumor proved to be a facial nerve neurinoma, as confirmed later by histopathological examination. The tumor was arising from the mastoid segment of the nerve and extended to the jugular bulb.

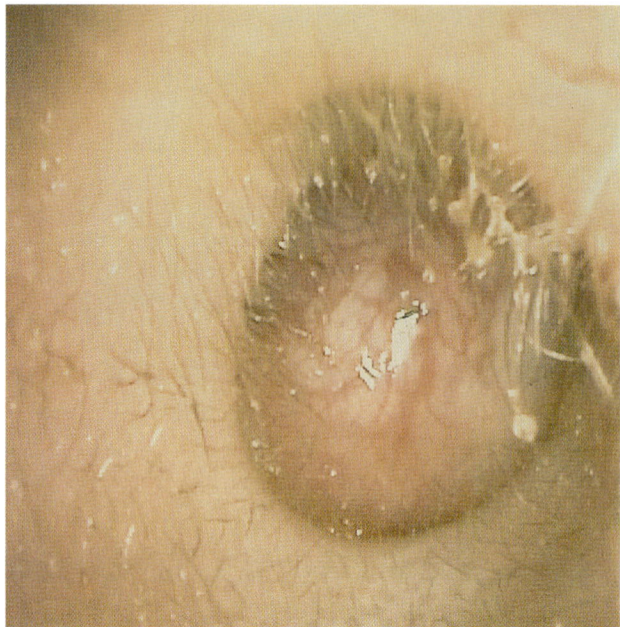

Figure 12.**28**   Left ear. The patient complained of left facial twitches of 8 months' duration, sensation of ear fullness associated with pulsating tinnitus of 6 months' duration, and progressive conductive hearing loss of 3 months' duration.

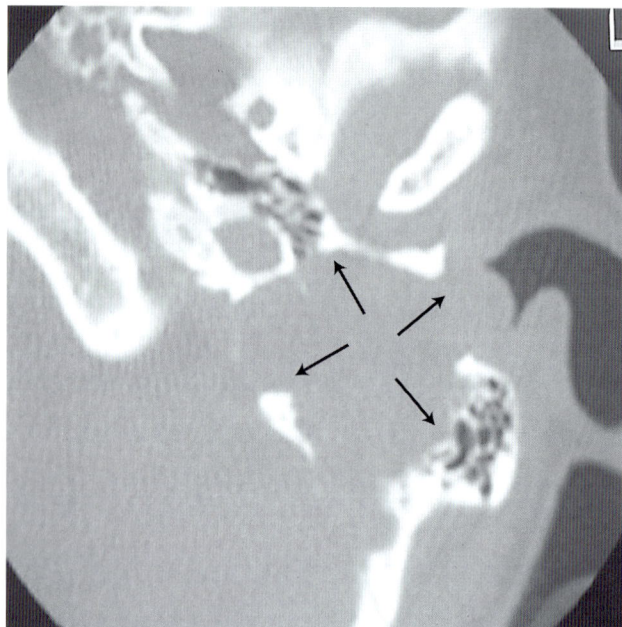

Figure 12.**29**   CT scan, axial view, showing the presence of a tumor involving the mastoid, middle ear, and hypotympanum without extension to the carotid canal.

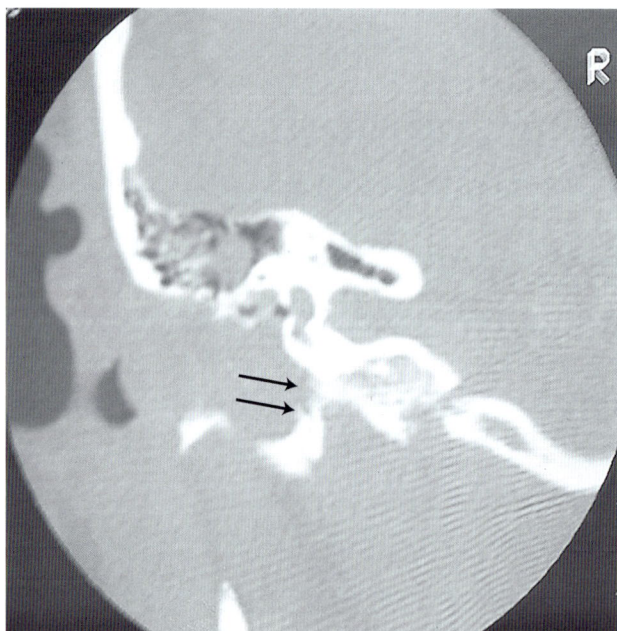

Figure 12.**30**   CT scan, coronal view. The bony plate over the jugular bulb is not eroded.

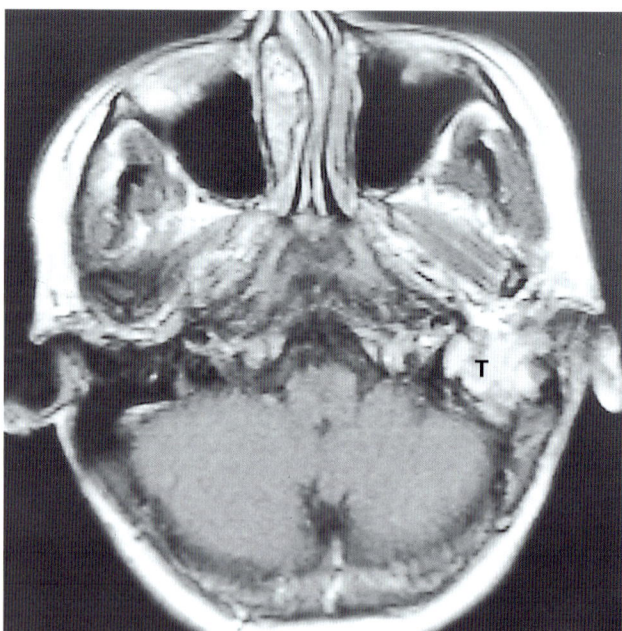

Figure 12.**31**   MRI with gadolinium of the previous case. The tumor shows nonhomogeneous enhancement with contrast. Histopathological examination following tumor removal revealed a facial nerve neurinoma (T= tumor).

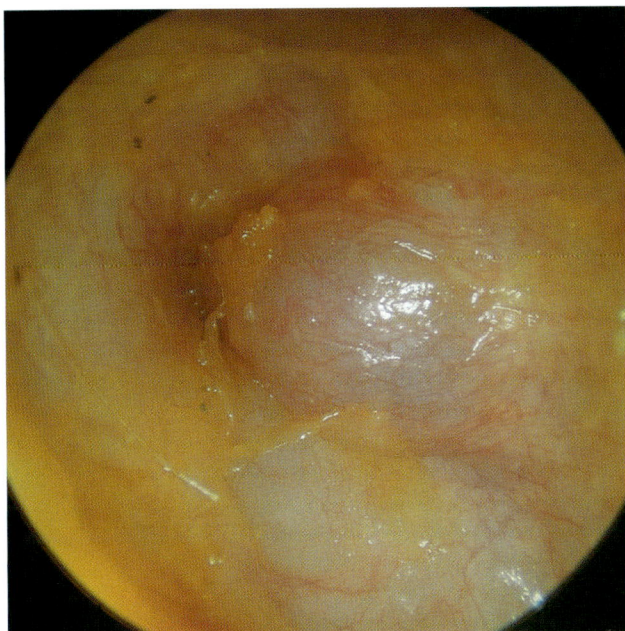

Figure 12.**32** Left ear. Mass protruding into the posterior auditory canal. The patient complained of left mild hearing loss and left facial nerve palsy H.B. grade III of 6 months' duration (H.B.: House–Brackmann [see references]).

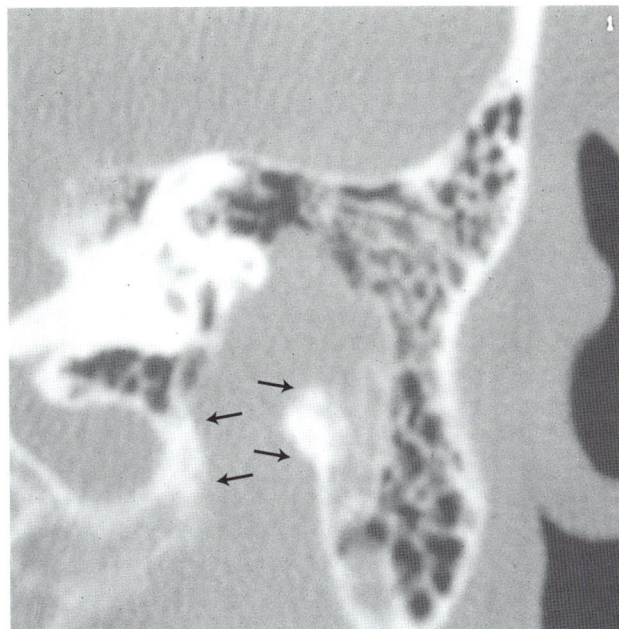

Figure 12.**33** CT scan demonstrated the presence of tumor involving the vertical portion of the facial nerve.

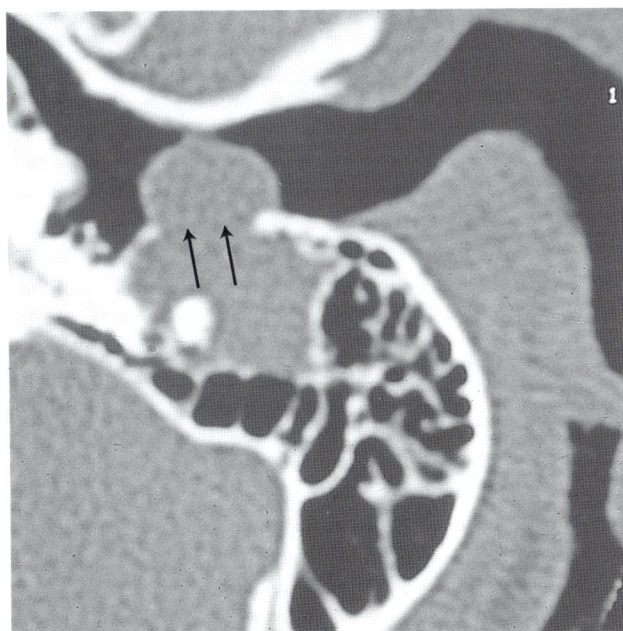

Figure 12.**34** CT scan showed also erosion of the posterior wall of the external canal.

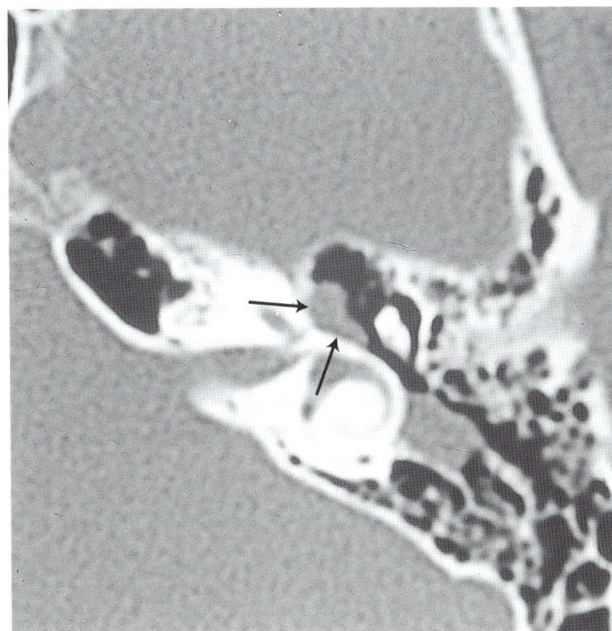

Figure 12.**35** CT scan. The tumor extended to the geniculate ganglion.

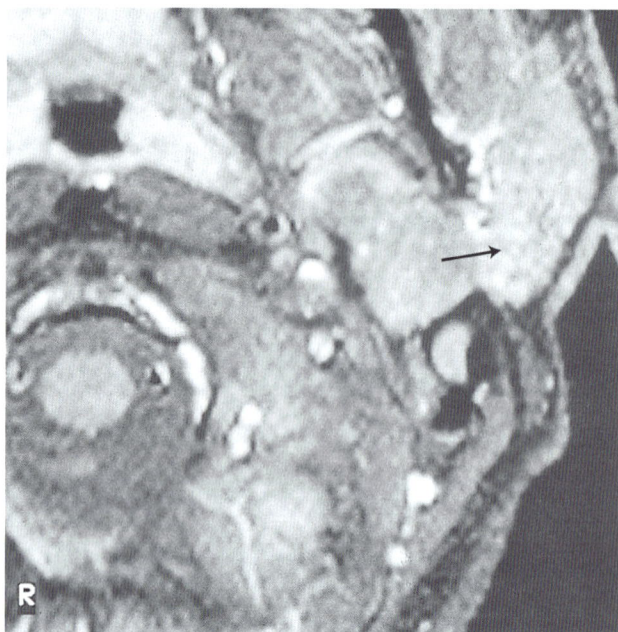

Figure 12.**36**   MRI showed a mass extending to the parotid gland area.

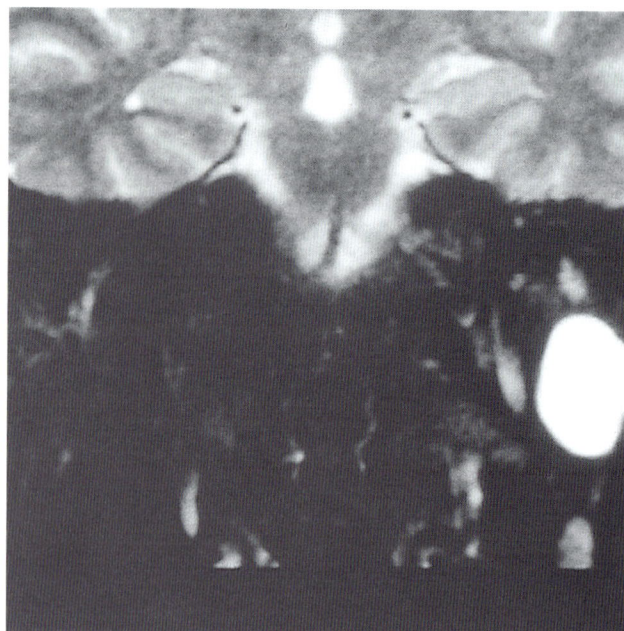

Figure 12.**37**   Another MRI of the same case. A combined middle fossa–transmastoid approach with parotid extension was performed. During surgery the tumor (T) proved to be a facial nerve neurinoma extended from the parotid to the intralabyrinthine segment of the facial nerve. The nerve was reconstructed with sural graft.

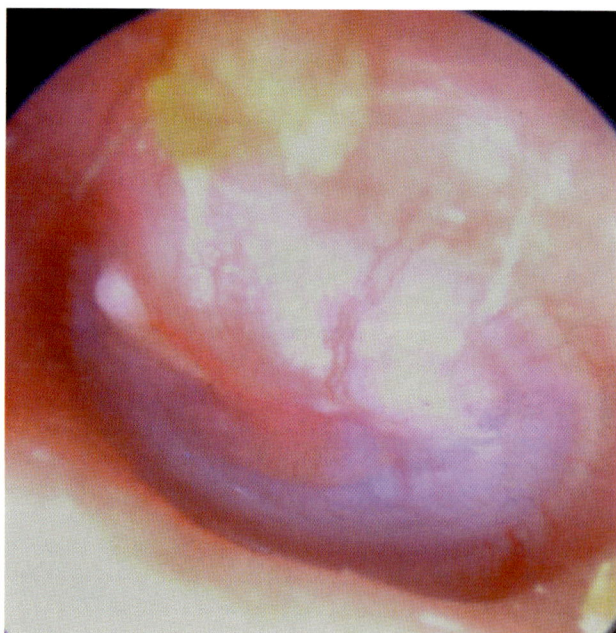

Figure 12.**38a**   A reddish mass is seen behind the posterior quadrants of the tympanic membrane. The patient complained of facial nerve palsy since 8 years. Grade III facial nerve palsy and conductive hearing loss were noted at the consultation.

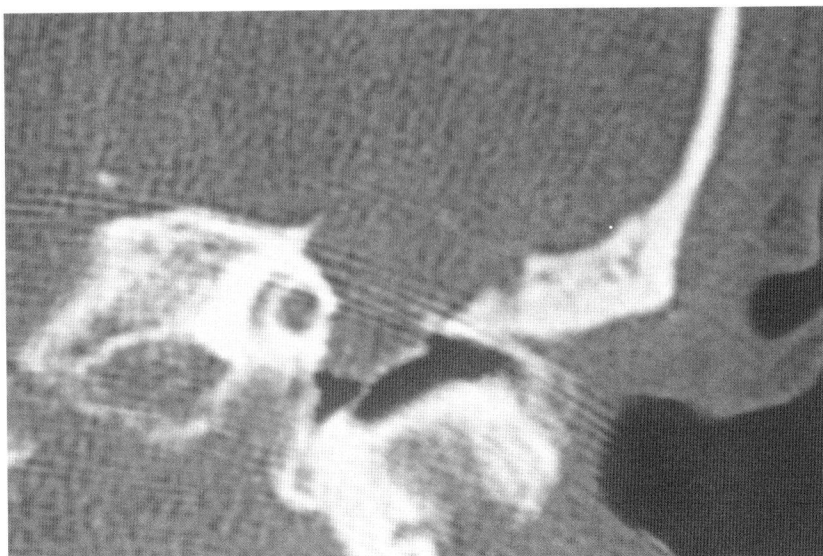

Figure 12.**38b** Coronal CT, showing a large mass extending from the middle fossa to the middle ear space. The middle fossa bony plate is absent.

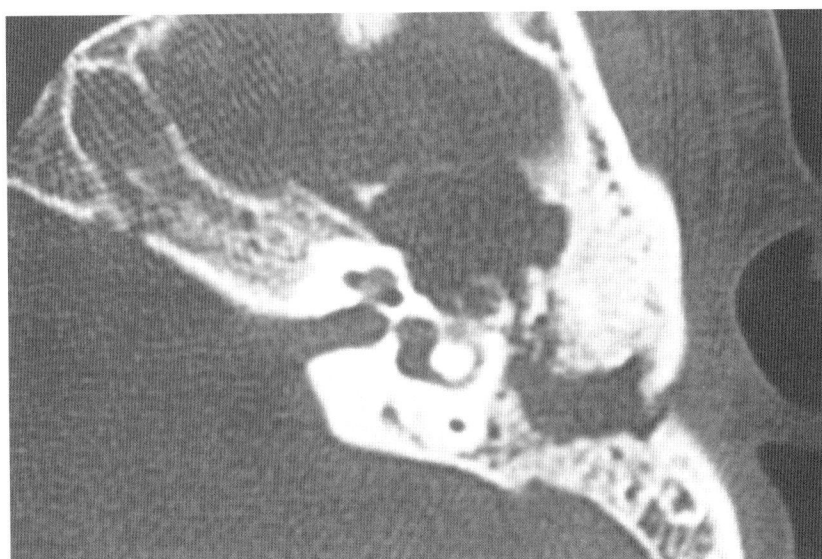

Figure 12.**38c** Axial view. A large mass is present at the level of the middle fossa and mastoid. There is bony erosion.

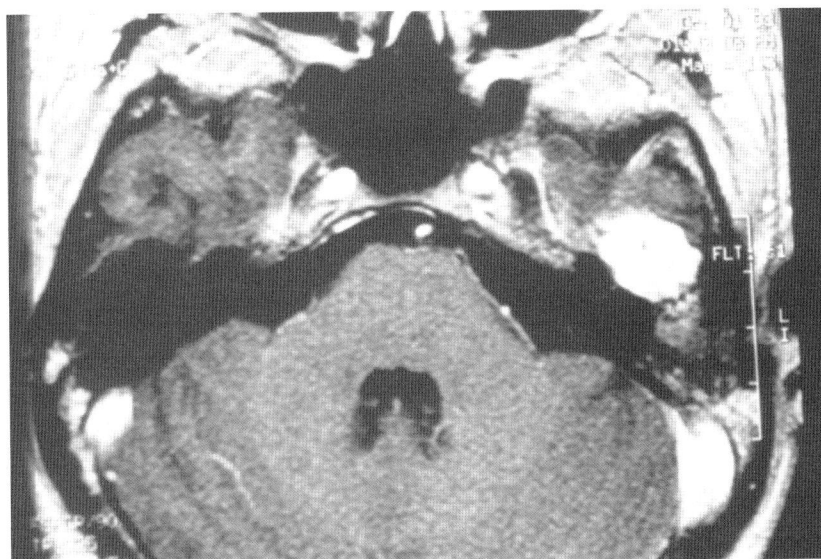

Figure 12.**38d** Axial MRI. A new formation is seen, with irregular margins protruding into the middle cranial fossa. After gadolinium administration, the mass enhances.

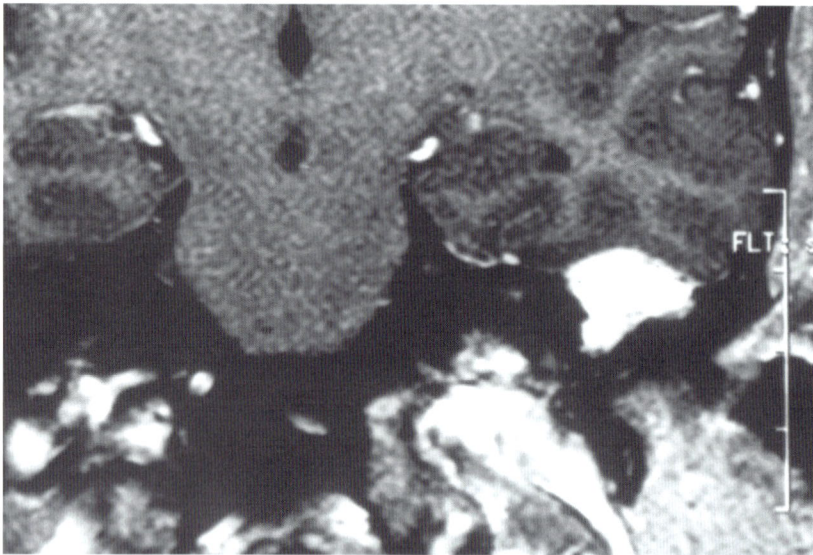

Figure 12.**38e**   Coronal MRI in the same patient. The mass is located under the temporal lobe.

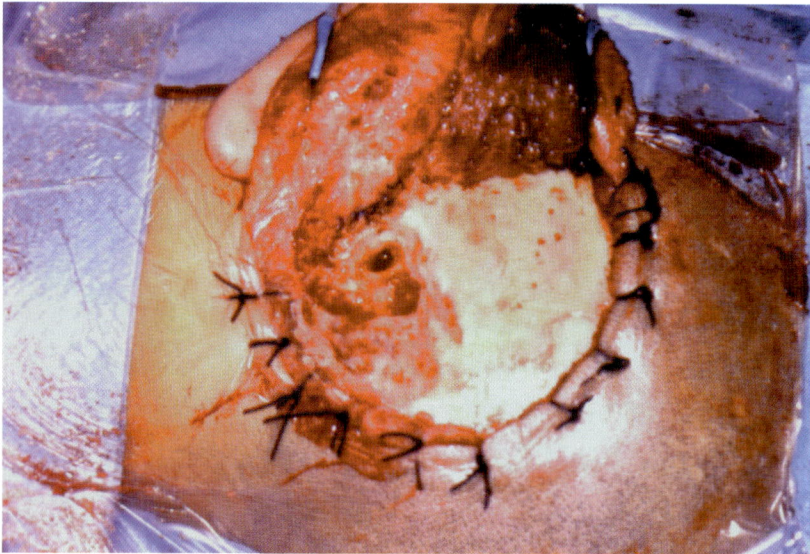

Figure 12.**39**   A combined transmastoid approach and middle fossa approach has been used.

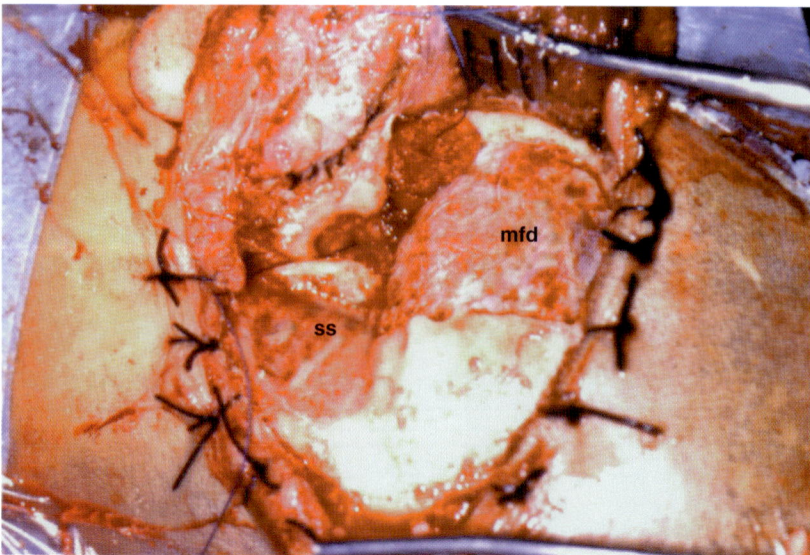

Figure 12.**40**   A large craniotomy has been made to remove the tumor.

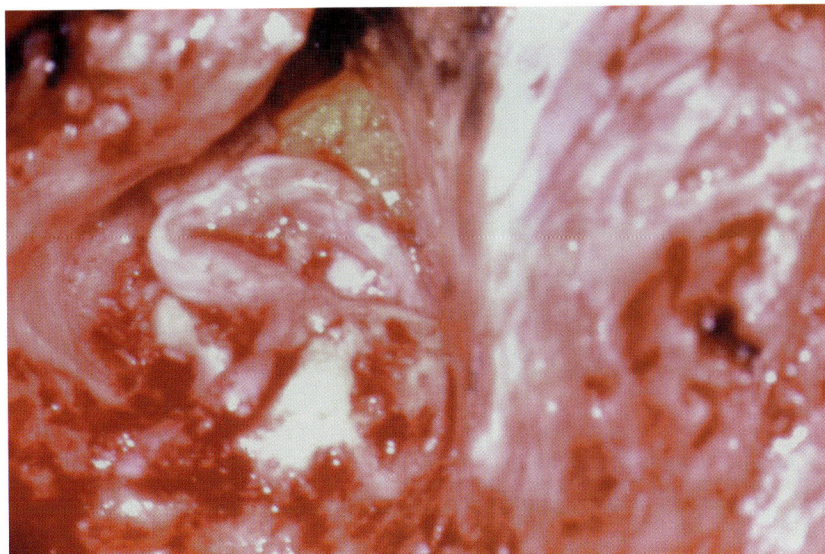

Figure 12.**41** Reconstruction of the nerve with sural graft from the third portion to the geniculate ganglion. The histologic examination revealed a transitional-type meningioma.

Ectopic Internal Carotid Artery

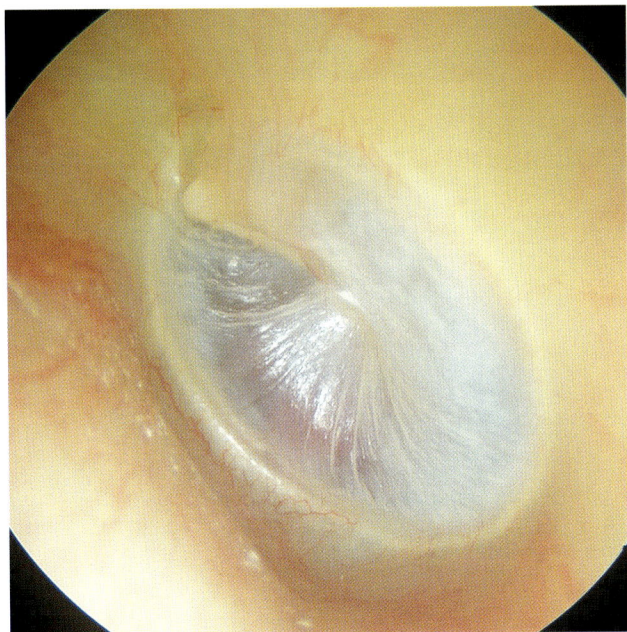

Figure 12.**42** Left ear. A small pulsating reddish area in the anteroinferior quadrant of the tympanic membrane. This picture may be confused with a glomus tympanicum tumor.

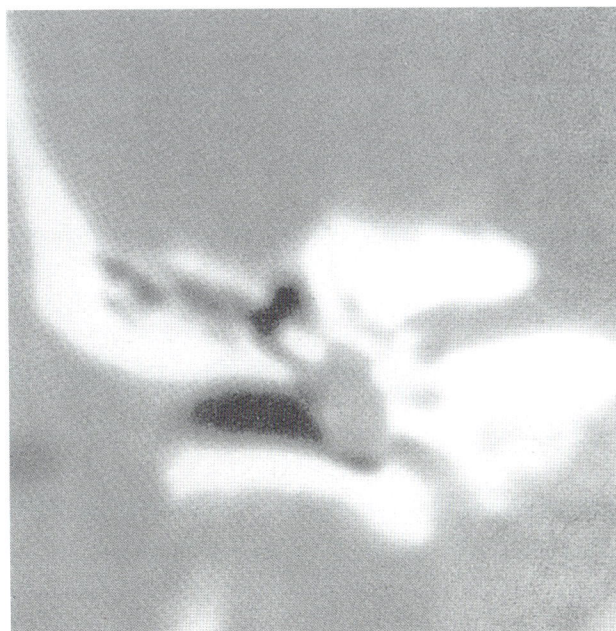

Figure 12.**43** A high-resolution CT scan established the diagnosis of an ectopic internal carotid artery.

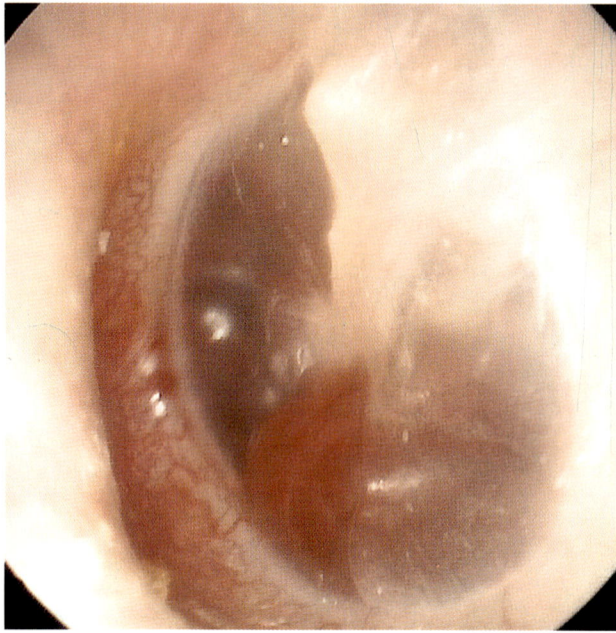

Figure 12.**44a**   A retrotympanic mass is seen at the level of the inferior quadrant. The patient complained of total deafness since 5 years.

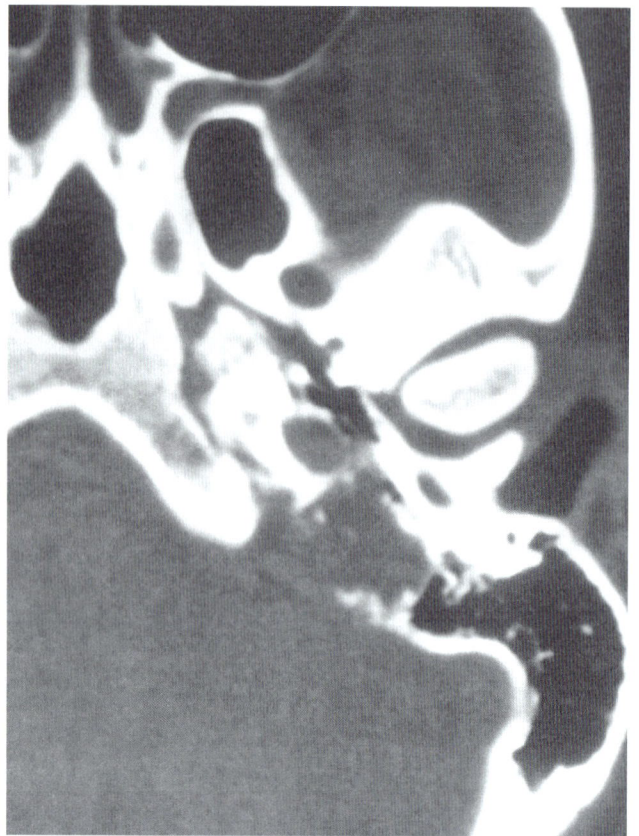

Figure 12.**44b**   Axial CT in the same patient. There is bone erosion at the level of the jugular foramen.

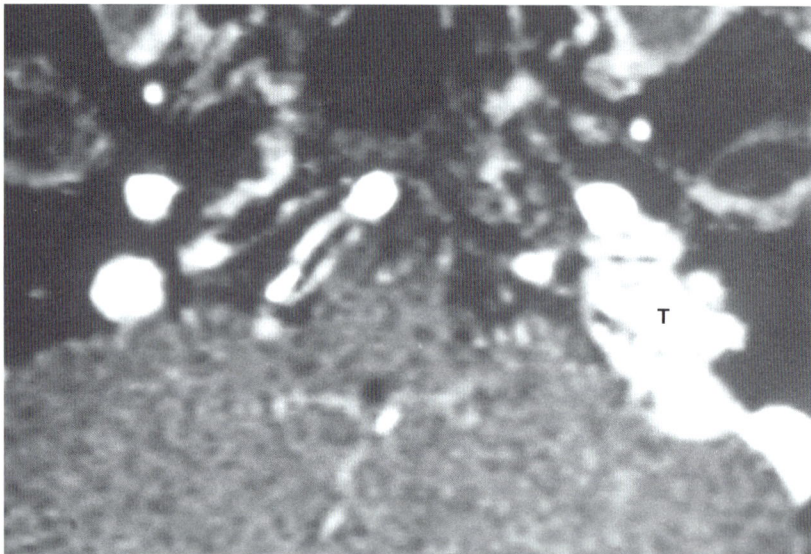

Figure 12.**44c**   MRI in the same patient. The tumor (T) is positioned between the vertical portion of the carotid artery and the lateral sinus.

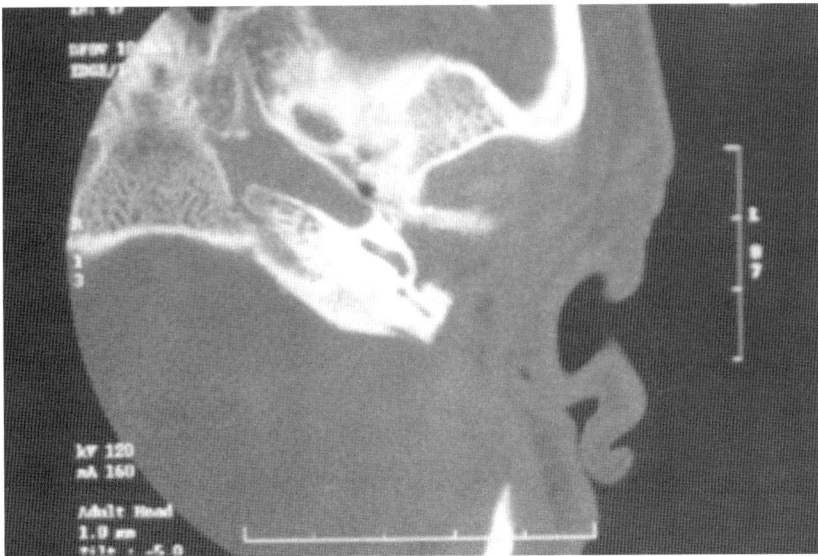

Figure 12.**44d**   Axial CT, demonstrating tumor removal using the type A infratemporal fossa approach, combined with a translabyrinthine approach. The cavity has been obliterated with abdominal fat, and the external auditory canal has been closed as a cul-de-sac.

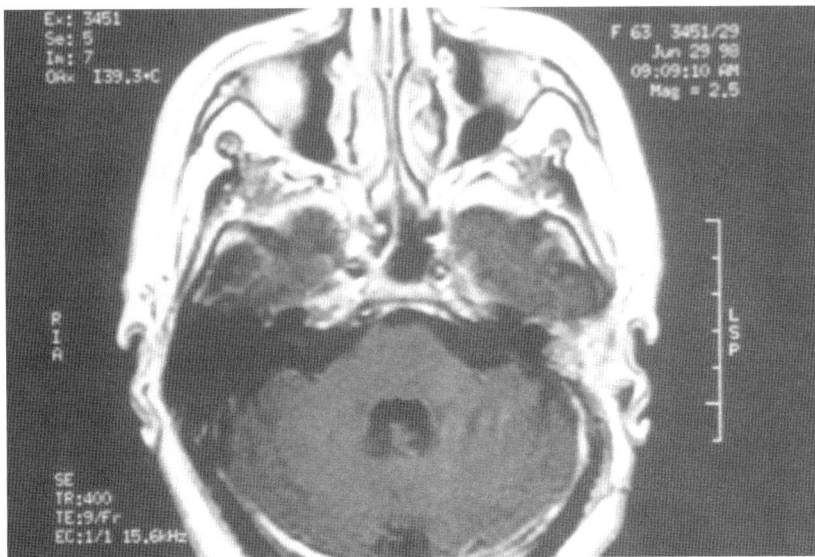

Figure 12.**44e**   Postoperative MRI in the same patient. Fat is seen obliterating the cavity. The histologic examination revealed an endolymphatic sac tumor.

High Jugular Bulb

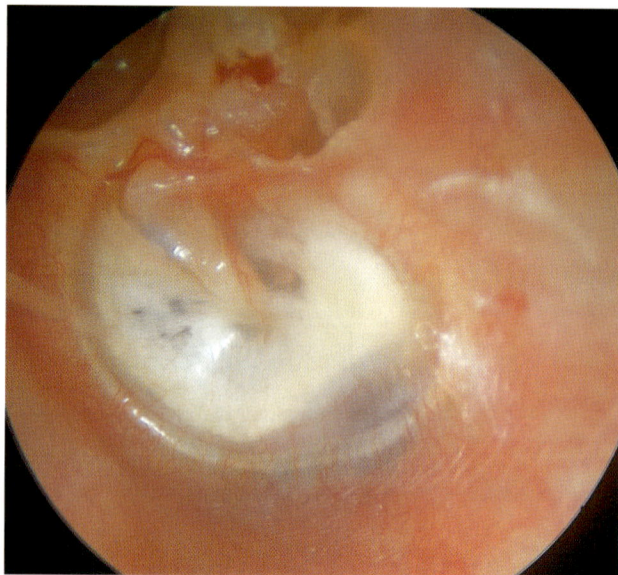

Figure 12.**45**   Left ear. Tympanosclerosis involving the whole tympanic membrane. An epitympanic erosion with cholesteatoma is also visible. At the level of the posteroinferior quadrant, a bluish mass is observed. A CT scan (see Fig. 12.**46**) proved this mass to be a high jugular bulb.

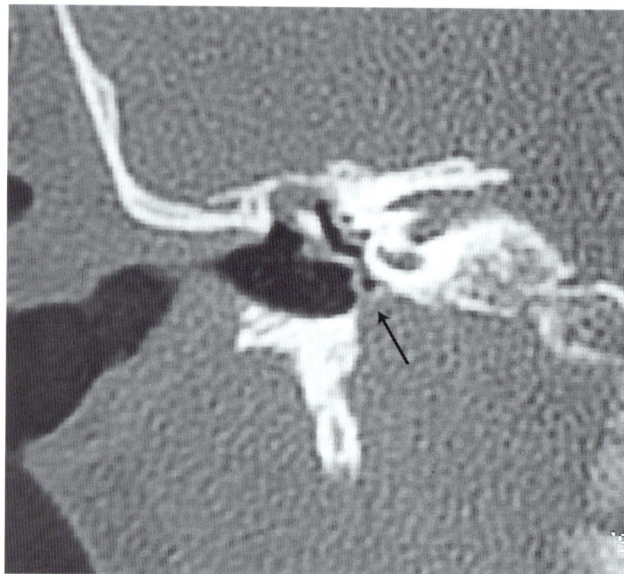

Figure 12.**46**   CT scan of the previous case. The uncovered jugular bulb is seen protruding into the middle ear.

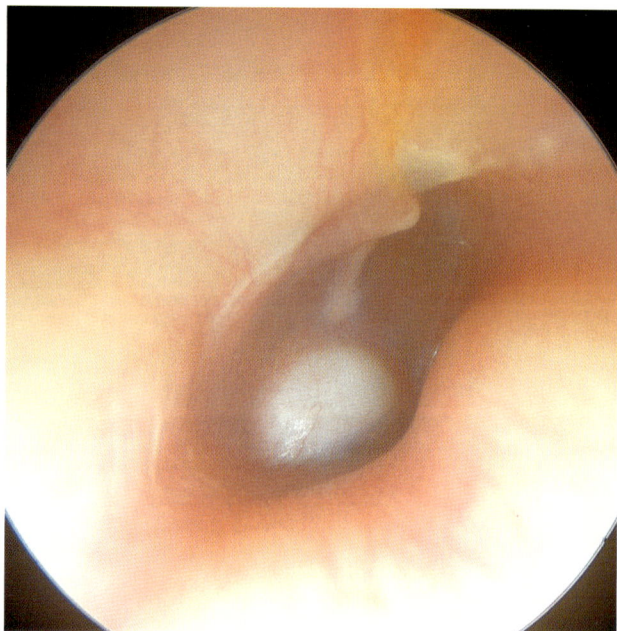

Figure 12.**47**   Right ear. Another example of a high jugular bulb covered by a thin bony shell in a young male patient with a skull-base malformation (see following figures).

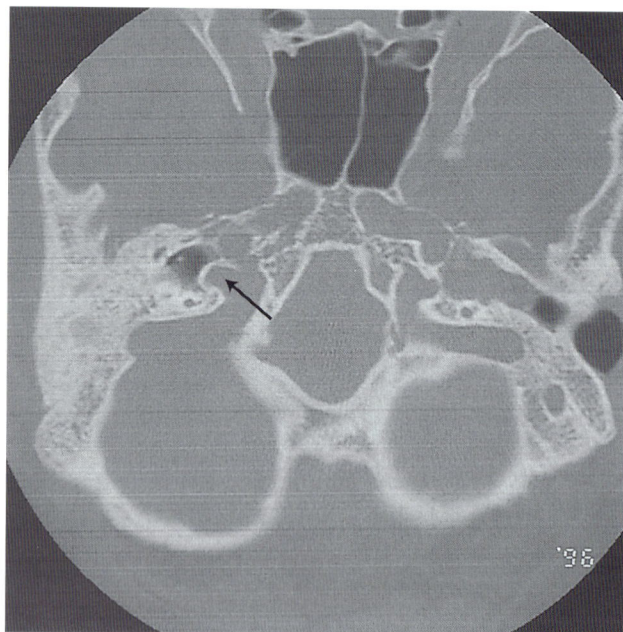

Figure 12.**48**   CT scan, axial view. The jugular bulb protrudes into the middle ear.

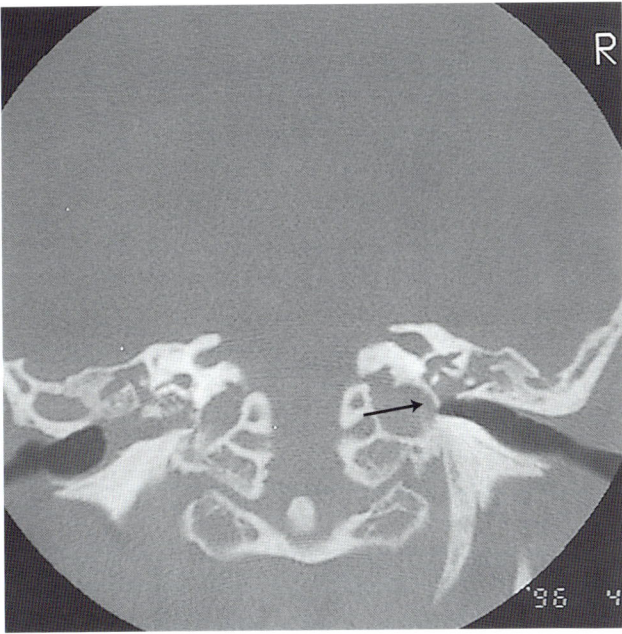

Figure 12.**49**   CT scan, coronal view. The high jugular bulb can be observed.

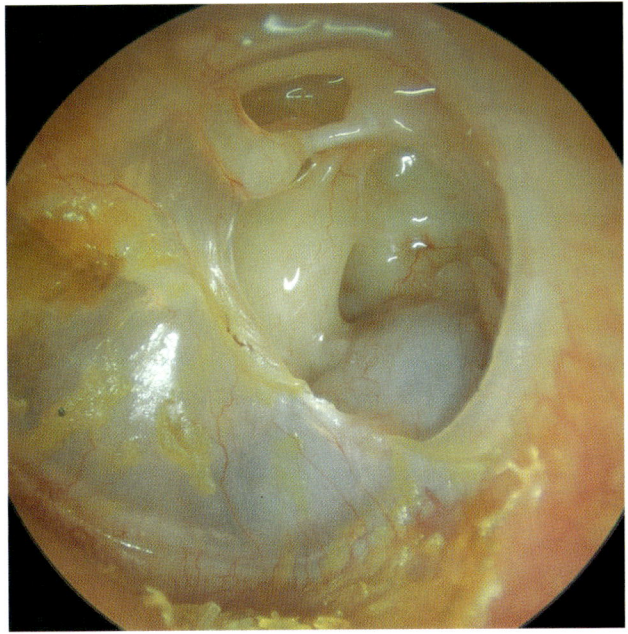

Figure 12.**50**   Left ear. A high and uncovered jugular bulb reaching up to the level of the round window is visible through a posterior tympanic membrane perforation.

Polypoidal Pulsating Mass

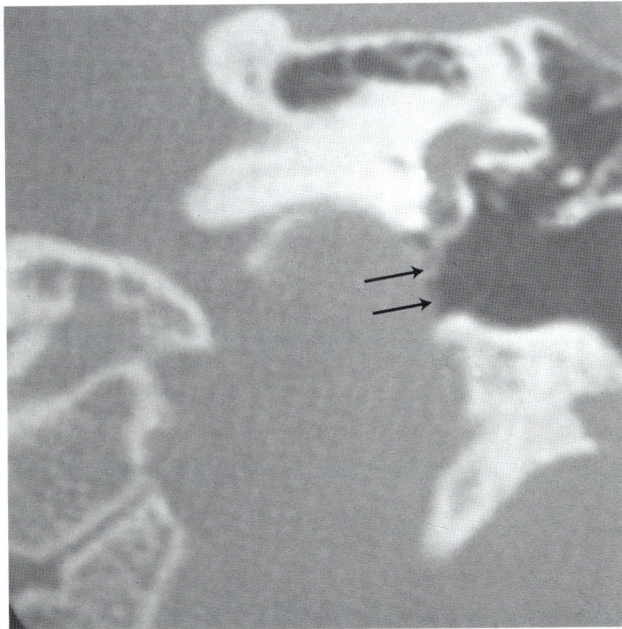

Figure 12.**51**   CT scan of the case in Figure 12.**50**.

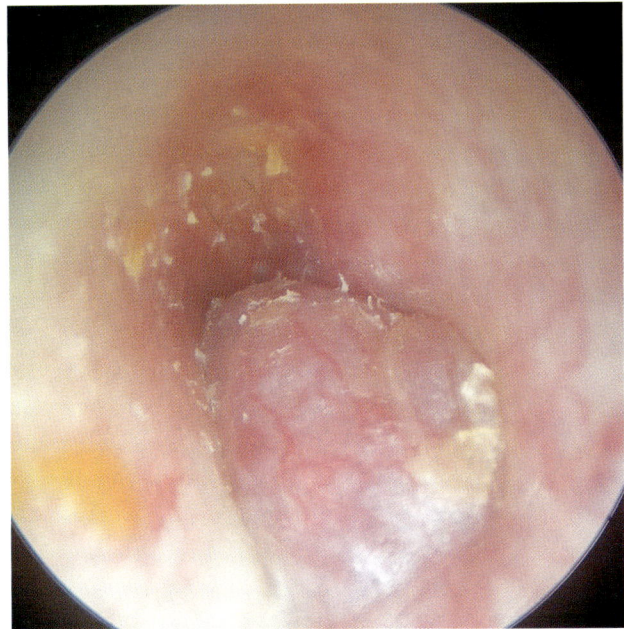

Figure 12.**52**   Left ear. A polypoidal pulsating red mass is seen in the external auditory canal. This example has been included to emphasize the fact that biopsy of external auditory canal polypi should never be taken without radiological investigations.

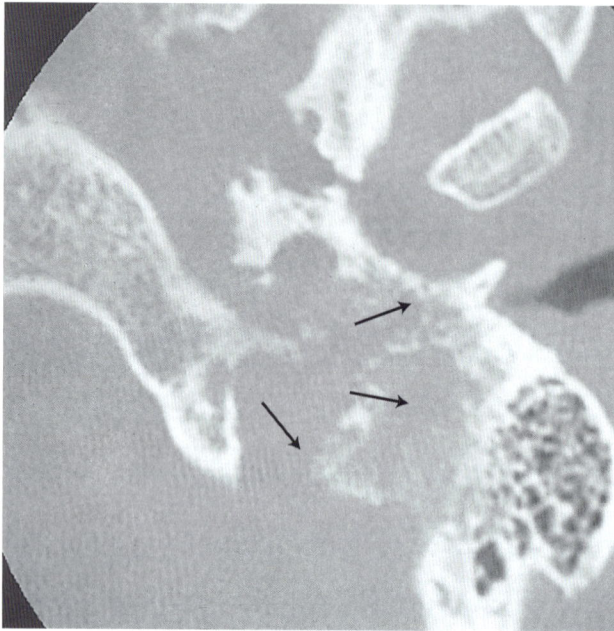

Figure 12.**53** CT scan, in this case, demonstrated the presence of a glomus tumor eroding the surrounding bone in an irregular way giving a moth-eaten appearance.

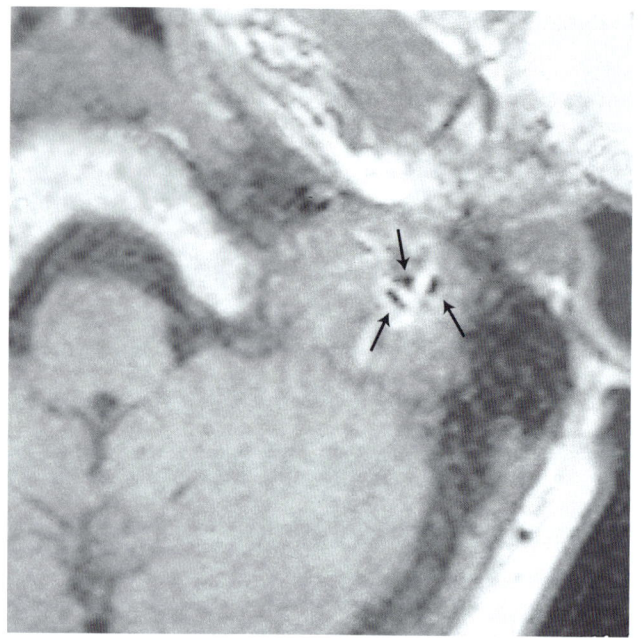

Figure 12.**54** MRI demonstrates the presence of fluid voids typical of large intratumoral vessels.

Internal Carotid Artery Aneurysm

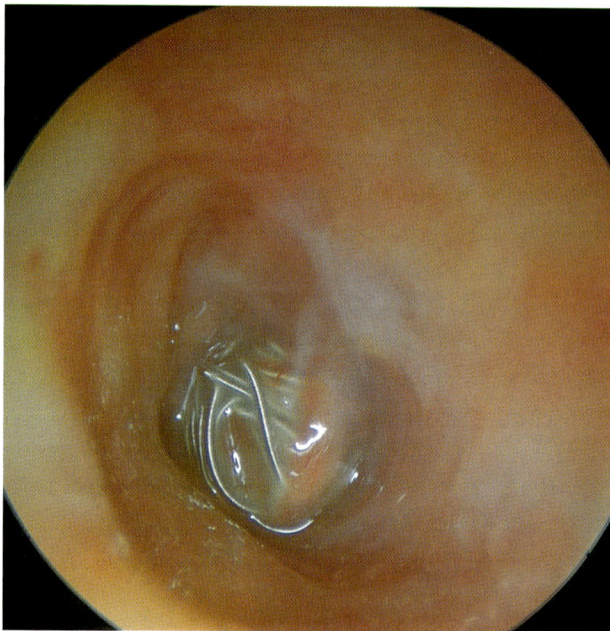

Figure 12.**55** Guglielmo coils used to occlude an intrapetrous internal carotid artery aneurysm.

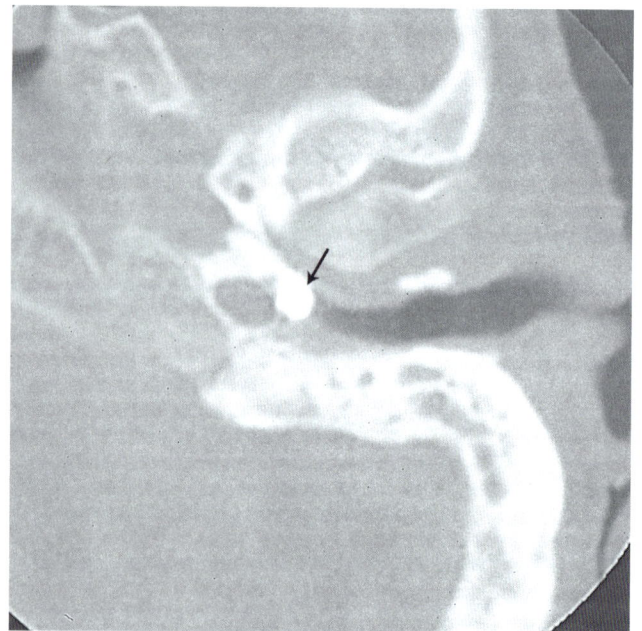

Figure 12.**56** CT scan of the case presented in Figure12.**55** demonstrating occlusion of the aneurysm with the coils.

Summary–Meningioma

Posterior fossa meningiomas are the second most common tumor of the cerebellopontine angle. These tumors are characterized by a higher morbidity and mortality than acoustic neurinoma.

Surgical removal of these lesions poses many problems because of the deep location, the involvement of vital neurovascular structures, and the large sizes these tumors usually attain before diagnosis. Moreover, they have an aggressive behavior with frequent involvement of the dura and bone. Total removal is fundamental to avoid recurrence and is better achieved in the first operation. Total removal with minimal morbidity can be obtained utilizing an array of approaches that must be adapted to each individual case.

In general, an ideal approach is that which allows total removal with minimal or no brain retraction. The site of the tumor is the most important factor for the choice of the surgical approach. The size of the tumor, the patient's age and general medical condition, and the preoperative status of the cranial nerves are other factors to consider.

Tumors localized posterior to the internal auditory canal in young patients with good preoperative hearing can be removed using a retrosigmoid approach. In the elderly, however, a translabyrinthine approach is preferred to avoid cerebellar retraction. In cases of involvement of the jugular foramen, a petro-occipital trans-sigmoid (POTS) approach is adopted.

In small tumors lying anterior to the internal auditory canal, the middle fossa transpetrous approach is utilized. In large petroclival lesions, which pose more difficulties due to their deep location, the intimate relation with the brain stem, and the involvement of vital neurovascular structures, the modified transcochlear approach should be used, irrespective of the preoperative hearing. This approach permits a wide and direct exposure, and a flat angle of vision with no cerebellar or brain stem retraction. Moreover, it allows the removal of any infiltrated dura or bone.

Though total removal can be obtained in the majority of petroclival meningiomas, it is not always necessary or even safe. Subtotal removal is decided on in the absence of an arachnoid plane of cleavage between the tumor and the brain stem or when the perforating arteries are at risk of interruption during total tumor removal.

Neuroradiologic evaluation is fundamental to plan surgery. A CT scan with contrast to evaluate the bone, MRI with gadolinium, and in some cases, digital subtraction angiography are of paramount importance in each case.

The neuroradiologist should provide the surgeon with information on the following:
- Anatomical relations of the tumor
- Tumor consistency
- Vascularity
- Peritumoral edema
- Tumor–brain stem interface
- Invasion of the dura and bone
- Relationship between the tumor and the vertebrobasilar and carotid systems
- Necessity of eventual embolization

The main blood supply of these tumors comes from large dural arteries. However, significant contributions may also come from pial arteries or from dural branches of the internal carotid and vertebral arteries. The angiographic data helps the neuroradiologist and the skull-base surgeon to determine the need for embolization. When indicated, it should be performed a few days before surgery. It not only decreases the intraoperative bleeding, but also produces a certain amount of tumor necrosis, rendering some cases easier to remove.

Close cooperation between the neuroradiologist and the skull-base surgeon offers optimal chances for successful management of these challenging tumors.

Summary–Facial Nerve Neurinoma

Tumor involvement of the facial nerve has been estimated to be the cause of facial palsy in 5% of cases. Though uncommon, facial neuromas should be considered in the differential diagnosis of facial nerve dysfunction. Unfortunately, the rarity of facial neuromas and the diversity of their clinical picture, together with the fact that their presentation may mimic other more common pathologies, renders the diagnosis of these tumors difficult.

Facial nerve dysfunction is the most common symptom. It can vary from the classic progressive palsy to sudden or recurrent facial palsy or hemifacial spasm. In limited cases the function of the nerve is normal. Therefore, all patients with progressive facial palsy must be considered to have a tumor until proved otherwise. Moreover, all patients with Bell's palsy persisting for more than 4 weeks and with recurrent facial paralysis should be investigated for the presence of a tumor.

The second most common complaint is hearing loss. Conductive hearing loss is usually associated with tumor involvement of the middle ear, with subsequent interference with the ossicular chain. Sensorineural hearing loss is attributable to inner ear erosion or extension of the tumor into the internal auditory canal.

Most diagnosed tumors are of large size. One reason is that the facial nerve can accommodate tumor expansion to some extent before significant pressure, with subsequent dysfunction, can occur. Another reason is the relatively long duration of symptoms before diagnosis is made. Because of the absence of classic symptomatology in such cases, a higher index of suspicion is needed for early diagnosis. Diagnostic work-up includes audiometric testing, vestibular testing, and auditory brain-stem evoked response. Electrophysiologic testing of facial nerve function in such cases is of little or no benefit. The usefulness of these tests in the diagnosis of facial neuromas has been challenged by other authors (Dort and Fish 1991, Neely and Alford 1974).

Advances in radiologic techniques have aided greatly in the diagnosis of these lesions. The characteristic appearance on CT is that of an enhancing soft tissue mass, usually in the perigeniculate region, with sharp bony erosion and enlargement of the fallopian canal. High resolution CT scan is the best method to assess middle and inner ear involvement by tumor. However, MRI with gadolinium is the best available method for the preoperative assessment of tumor extension, especially of those involving the internal auditory canal, cerebellopontine angle, and/or the parotid region. Both methods are believed to be complementary for the preoperative assessment and the choice of the most suitable surgical approach for removal of these tumors. However, because these tumors show intraneural spread, it is still doubtful whether MRI with gadolinium can show the full extent of the lesion. Therefore, the surgeon should be prepared to expose the whole length of the facial nerve.

Differential diagnosis of these lesions includes acoustic neuroma, congenital cholesteatoma, chemodectoma, facial nerve hemangioma, and parotid tumors. Introdural facial nerve neuromas pose a major diagnostic difficulty, usually being mistaken for acoustic neuromas. Apart from the few cases in which tumor extension to the geniculate ganglion could establish the diagnosis, most of these cases were actually diagnosed intraoperatively.

Congenital cholesteatomas of the petrous bone are uncommon lesions that usually present with hearing loss and facial weakness or paralysis and, therefore, can be mistaken for facial neuromas. Moreover, these lesions appear on CT as smoothly marginated expansile lesions, and on MRI as hypo/isointense on T1 and hyperintense on T2 images. Unlike facial neuromas, however, cholesteatomas do not show enhancement following contrast administration, a fact that helps to differentiate between the two lesions.

Treatment generally aims at total removal of the tumor, restoration or preservation of facial nerve function, and conservation of hearing. The surgical approach depends on the extent of the lesion and the preoperative hearing level. There is general agreement that surgical removal is the treatment of choice. There is some controversy, however, regarding facial neuromas and absence of or mild preoperative facial nerve paresis. Some surgeons prefer to delay surgery, because the patient is faced with the inevitable postoperative paralysis followed by some degree of recovery that will never be better than House–Brackmann grade III. Patient counseling is important in these cases.

The age at presentation is another factor to be considered. If the patient is young, early surgical resection should be done because these tumors grow inexorably with subsequent intracranial or extratemporal extension, making the approach more difficult and postoperative complications more likely. Moreover, tumor growth causes progressive degeneration and regeneration of facial nerve fibers, leading to collagenization of the distal part of the nerve with consequent poor recovery of facial function following reconstruction. Another reason is that these tumors are potentially invasive: otic capsule erosion may be present in about 20% of the cases. On the other hand, in an elderly patient with an absence of or mild facial nerve paresis, facial nerve decompression may suffice if surgery is to be performed.

When total tumor removal involves resection of a long segment of the nerve, a cable graft is usually needed for reconstruction of the facial nerve. The length of the graft and whether it is from the sural or great auricular nerve has no effect on the eventual recovery of facial function.

In summary, facial nerve neuromas are uncommon tumors requiring a high degree of suspicion for their diagnosis. Recent advances in radiological techniques are the cornerstone for the diagnosis and preoperative assessment of these cases, and early surgical resection gives the best prognosis.

13 Meningoencephalic Herniation

Meningoencephalic herniation is the herniation of meningeal and/or encephalic tissue in the middle ear or mastoid. It occurs in connection with infection, previous surgery, head trauma, or congenital tegmental defects. A patient with meningoencephalic herniation has a high risk of developing meningitis and epilepsy due to epileptogenic focus in the herniating tissues. The patient may present with a pulsatile retrotympanic mass, cerebrospinal fluid (CSF) leakage, and aphasia. However, the most common manifestation is that of a conductive or mixed hearing loss with a draining ear or serous otitis media.

Herniation of meningeal and/or encephalic tissue into the middle ear is a form of pathology that–even if rarely found by the otologist–can be life-threatening for the patient due to possible infectious intracranial complications. Four different etiological types are possible: infectious, postsurgical, traumatic, and spontaneous. From a pathogenic point of view, all of these types are characterized by a bony and dural defect located in the tegmen, through which meningeal and encephalic tissue can herniate. The symptoms are often nonspecific, so that some cases are diagnosed during surgery.

When there is strong suspicion of herniation, neuroradiological assessment procedures have to be carried out in order to establish a correct preoperative diagnosis. High-resolution computed tomography of the temporal bone, in particular, can demonstrate the exact limits and location of the bone defect, while magnetic resonance imaging (MRI) allows the nature of the tissue in the middle ear to be determined.

Surgery is the only appropriate therapy. Different approaches have been described, amongst which the transmastoid approach, with or without temporal minicraniotomy, and the middle cranial fossa (MCF) approach are the ones most frequently reported in the literature.

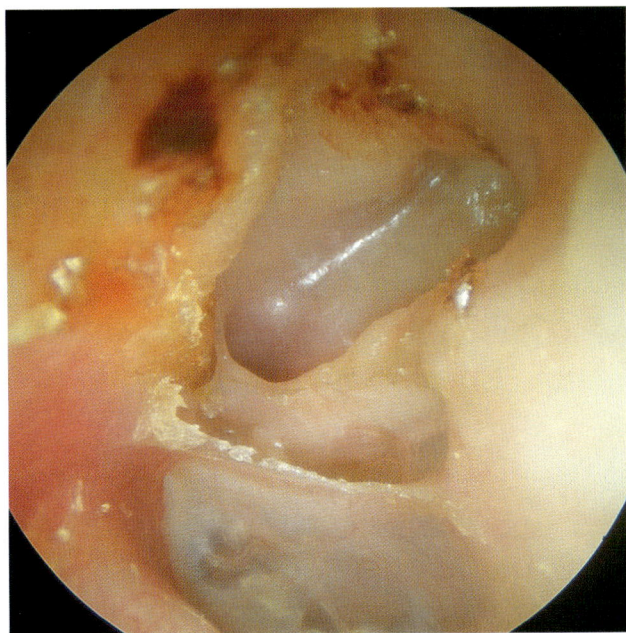

Figure 13.1 Left meningoencephalic herniation in a patient who had previously undergone open tympanoplasty. The hernia protrudes into the attic through a small tegmental defect and appears otoscopically as a pulsatile retrotympanic mass.

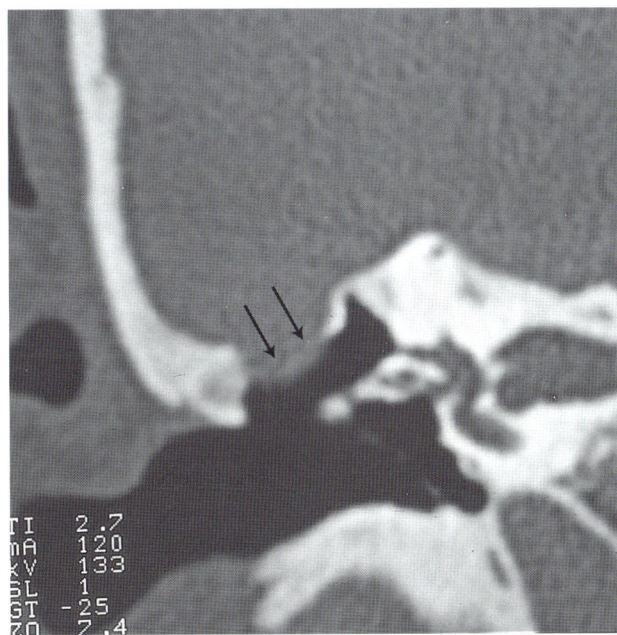

Figure 13.2 CT scan of the case described in Figure 13.1, coronal view. The osseous defect with the herniating tissue can be clearly visualized.

A new surgical technique using the MCF approach has been standardized by the Gruppo Otologico in Piacenza, Italy. The main step in this procedure consists of leaving the herniated tissue in situ in order to create a barrier between the middle ear and the subdural space. This technique is indicated in the case of large bony defects, multiple bony defects, defects with a very anterior location, or when there is infection in the middle ear.

The surgical approach is determined by the size of the defect. Other less important factors include the site of the defect and the presence or absence of middle ear infection. Hernias with small defects (< 1 cm²) are repaired through a transmastoid approach. In patients with medium-sized defects (1–2 cm²) located posteriorly in the attic or mastoid and with no active infection, the defect is repaired by combining the transmastoid approach with a minicraniotomy, which allows place-

ment of a larger piece of cartilage for reconstruction. Patients with large defects undergo surgery using a new technique employing the middle cranial fossa approach. This technique allows safe treatment of large hernias, hernias with a far anterior location, and/or hernias with active infection.

The advantage of this technique is that the herniated tissue is left in situ, where it acts as a barrier against infection. This tissue progressively atrophies, remaining as a scar in the middle ear without creating any problems. Another advantage of the middle cranial fossa technique is that it avoids an additional transmastoid approach, which would be necessary for resection of the herniated tissue under direct vision. If necessary, a second operation is carried out to manage the middle ear condition. Based on the authors' experience, the use of both fascia and cartilage is recommended for repair of the defect.

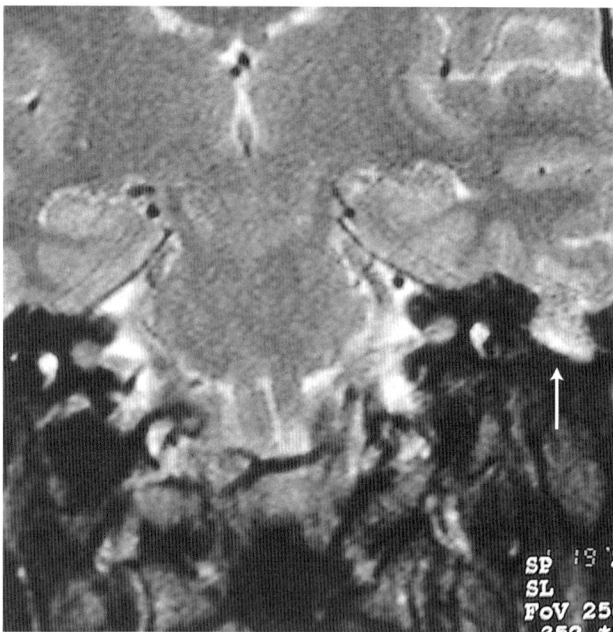

Figure 13.**3** MRI of the previous case. The protrusion of the cerebral tissue into the middle ear is visible.

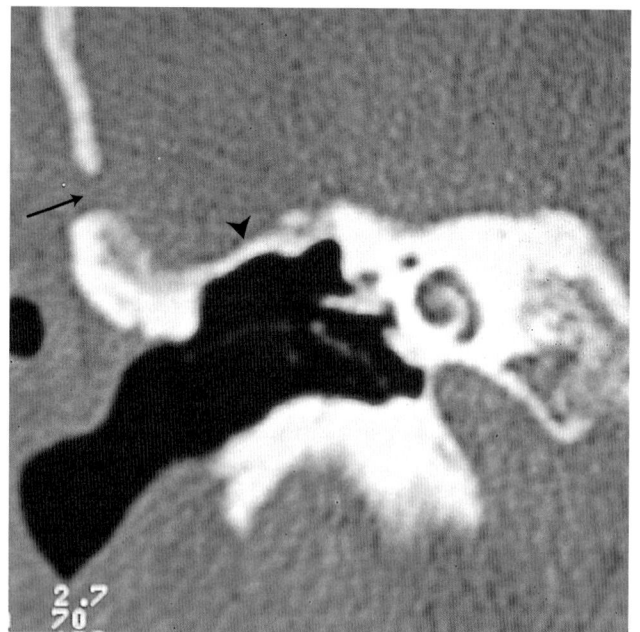

Figure 13.**4** Postoperative CT scan. The hernia was managed using a middle fossa approach. The bony defect was repaired using cartilage. The temporal craniotomy (arrow) and the cartilage (arrowhead) are clearly visible.

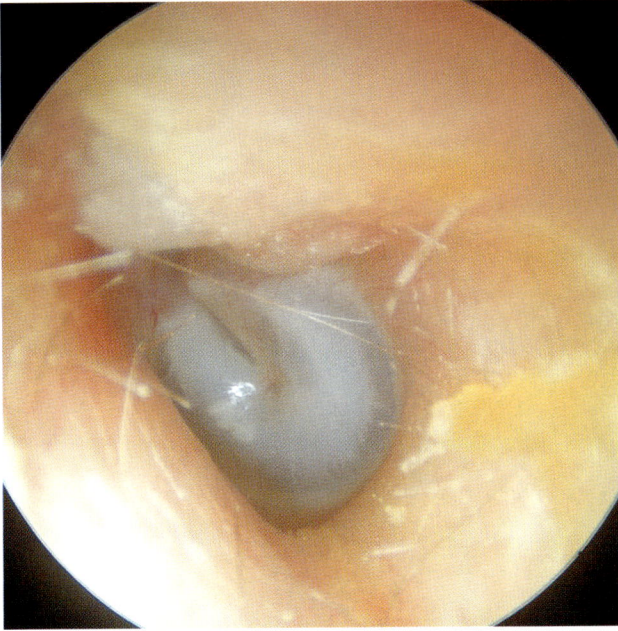

Figure 13.**5** Left meningoencephalic hernia. The superior wall of the external auditory canal is dehiscent. A soft, reducible, non-pulsating mass is observed. The patient had a history of head trauma with transverse fracture of the temporal bone that occurred 3 years before presentation. He complained of left hearing loss and the sensation of ear fullness.

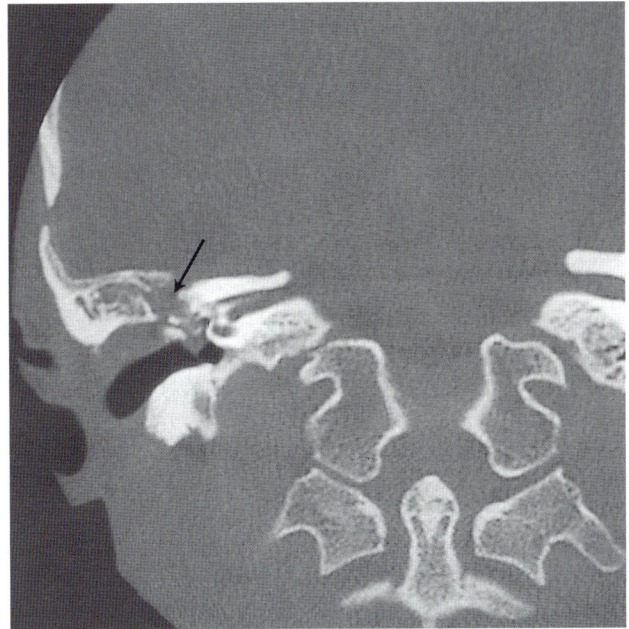

Figure 13.**6** Preoperative CT scan of the case in Figure 13.**5** demonstrating the herniation of cerebral tissue into the middle ear.

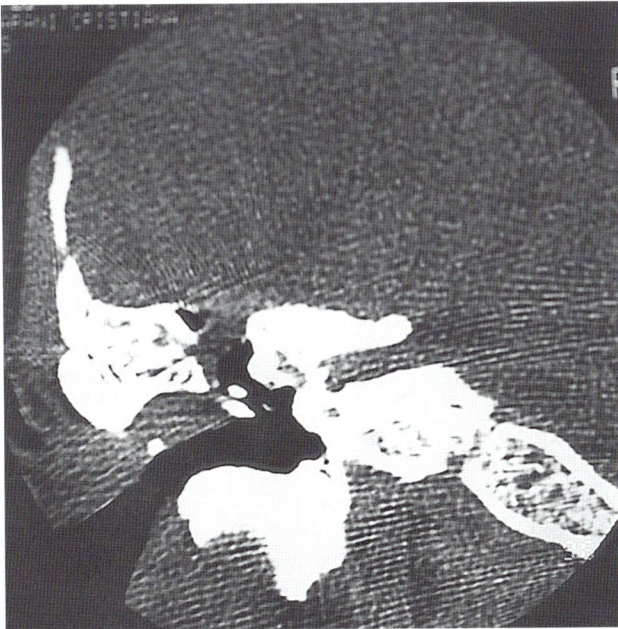

Figure 13.**7** CT scan of the previous case 1 year postoperatively. The hernia was managed using a middle fossa approach, placing a cartilaginous plate to reconstruct the bony defect after having sectioned the neck of the herniating tissue. The cerebral tissue, which is left in the ear during the operation, is resorbed with time as seen in the CT scan.

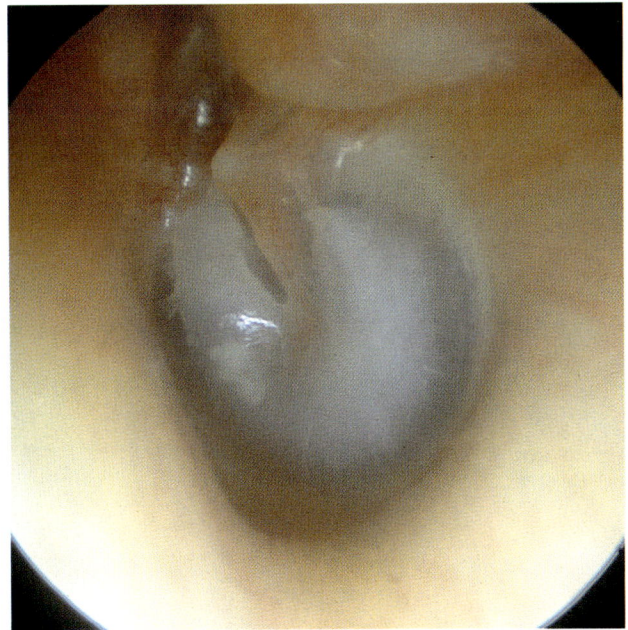

Figure 13.**8** Left ear. Otoscopy 6 months postoperatively in the same patient. The soft mass protruding from above into the external auditory canal has shrinked, indicating progressive atrophy of the herniated tissue left in the attic.

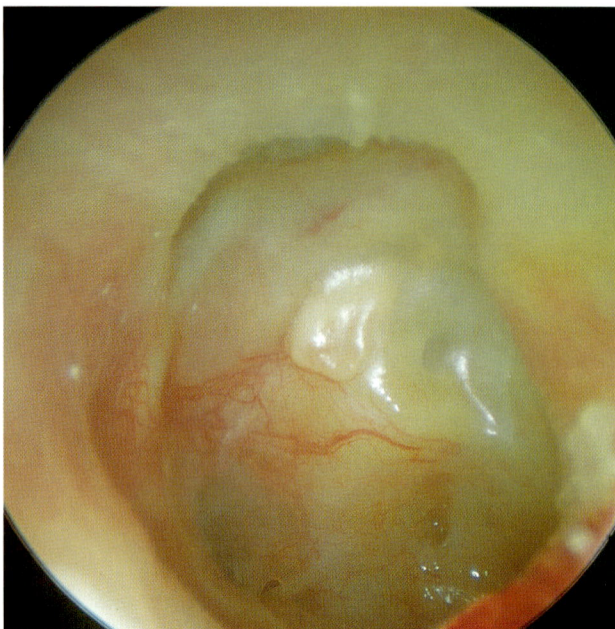

Figure 13.**9**   Left meningoencephalic herniation in a patient who had previously undergone multiple ear surgeries. The only manifestation was conductive hearing loss.

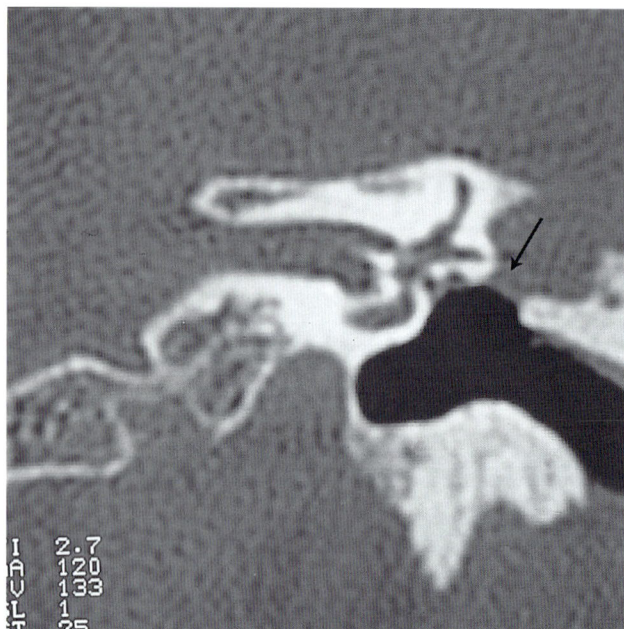

Figure 13.**10**   CT scan of the case presented in Figure 13.**9**.

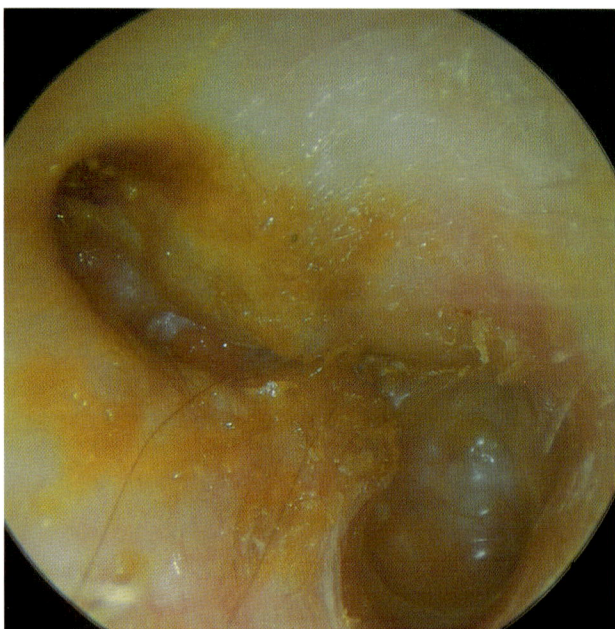

Figure 13.**11**   Another example of a right meningoence-phalic herniation in a patient who had undergone open tympanoplasty. Otoscopically, a large pulsatile mass is visible in the attic.

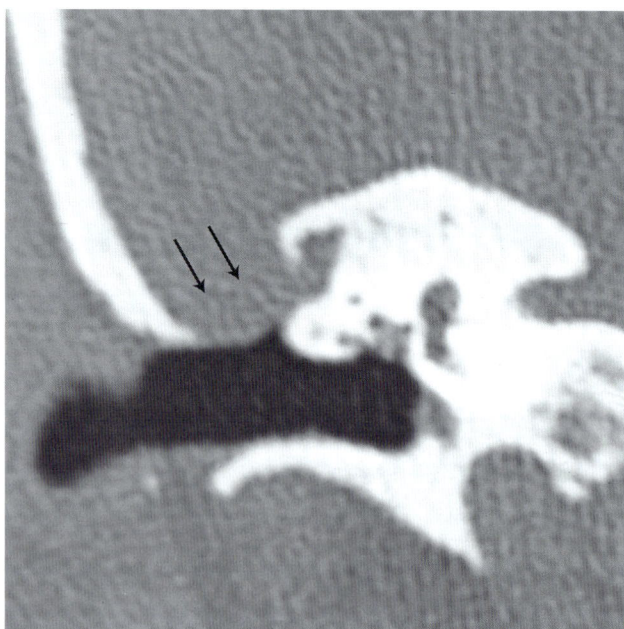

Figure 13.**12**   CT scan of the case presented in Figure 13.**11**, coronal view. The tegmen antri is absent and the herniation of the temporal lobe in the mastoid cavity and external auditory canal is demonstrated.

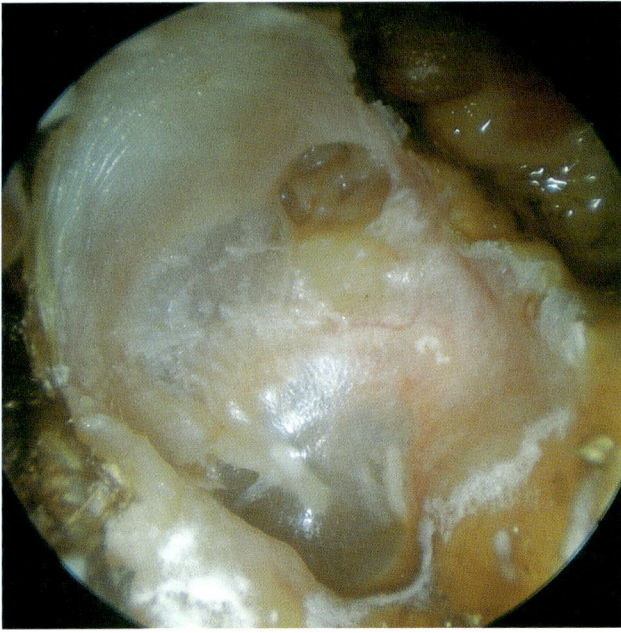

Figure 13.**13** A patient with a history of left open tympanoplasty presenting with conductive hearing loss. Otoscopy demonstrates a badly performed cavity with high facial ridge, secretions, granulations in the posterior wall of the cavity and an attic defect through which a soft-tissue mass protrudes into the middle ear. A CT scan was performed that confirmed the presence of a meningoencephalic hernia (see following figures).

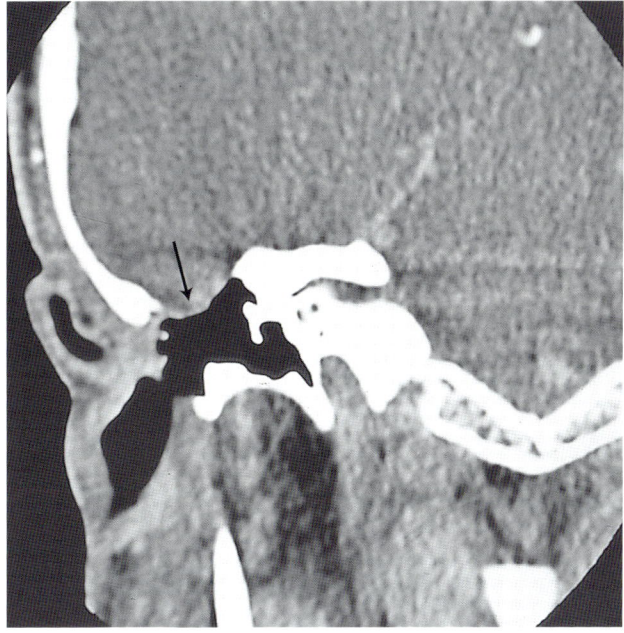

Figure 13.**14** CT scan, coronal view, soft-tissue window of the case presented in Figure 13.**13**, demonstrating the cerebral tissue herniating into the cavity.

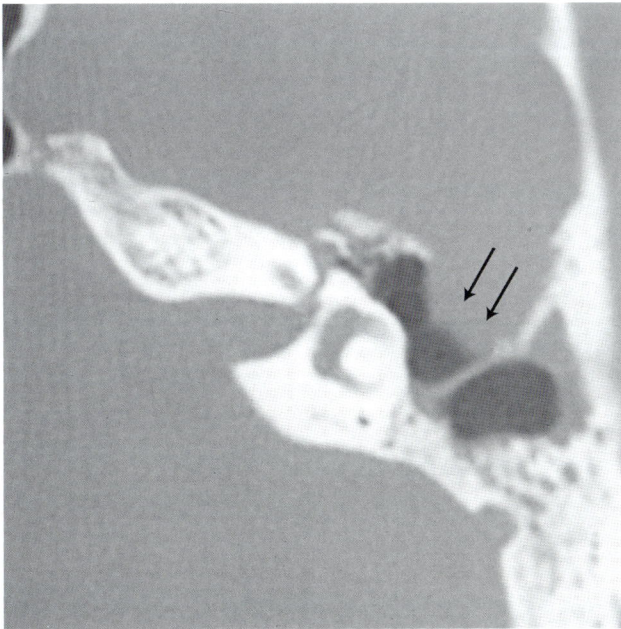

Figure 13.**15** CT scan, axial view. Arrows show the herniating cerebral tissue.

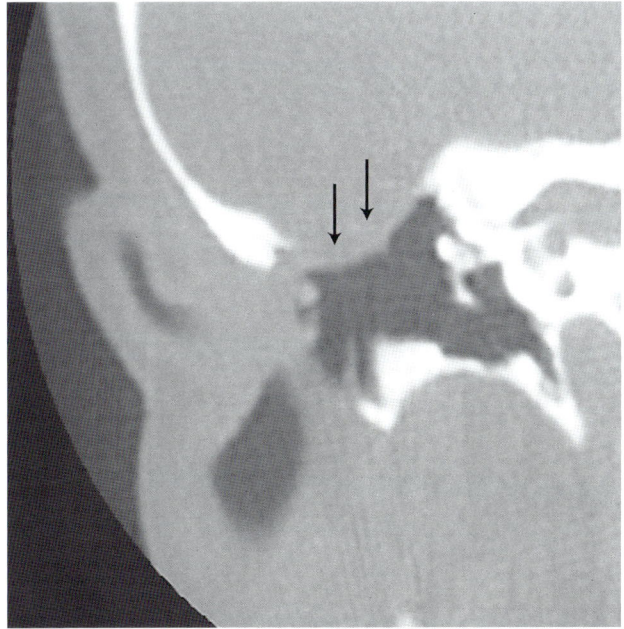

Figure 13.**16** CT scan, coronal view, bone window.

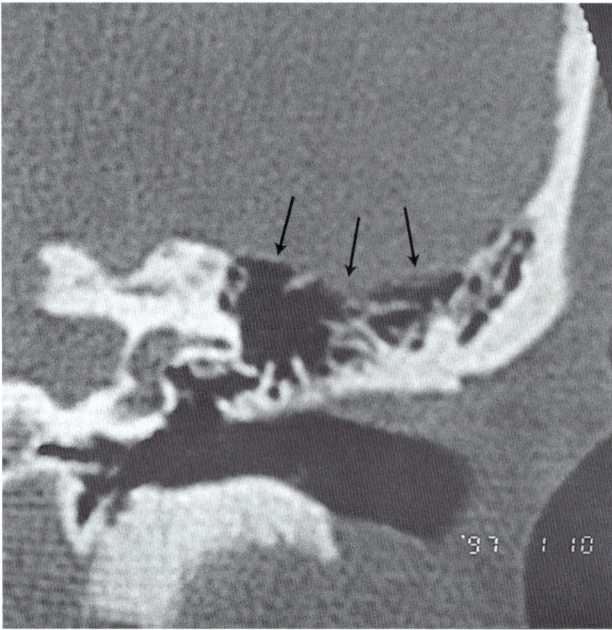

Figure 13.**17**   CT scan of a patient with a congenital tegmental defect. This patient has a higher risk of meningitis following an episode of otitis.

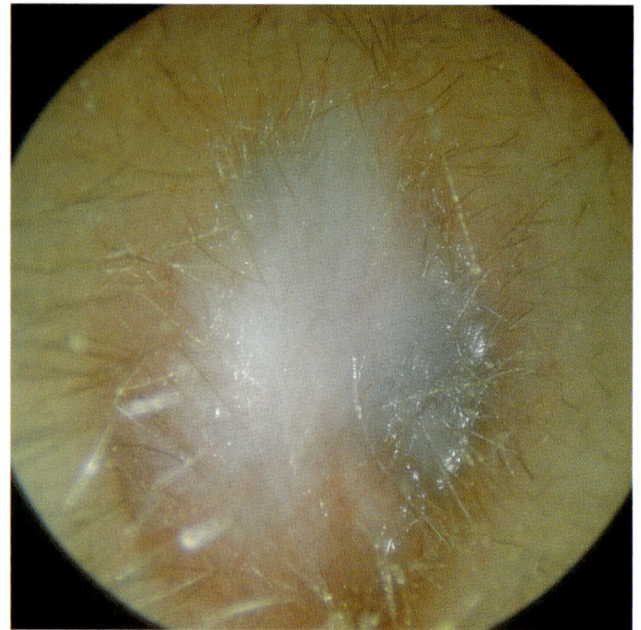

Figure 13.**18**   Right ear. Meningoencephalic herniation in a patient who had undergone several previous operations. The otoscopy shows a new tympanic membrane lateralized by a retrotympanic whitish mass. The patient complained of right ear anacusis and House–Brackmann grade III facial nerve palsy of 1 year's duration.

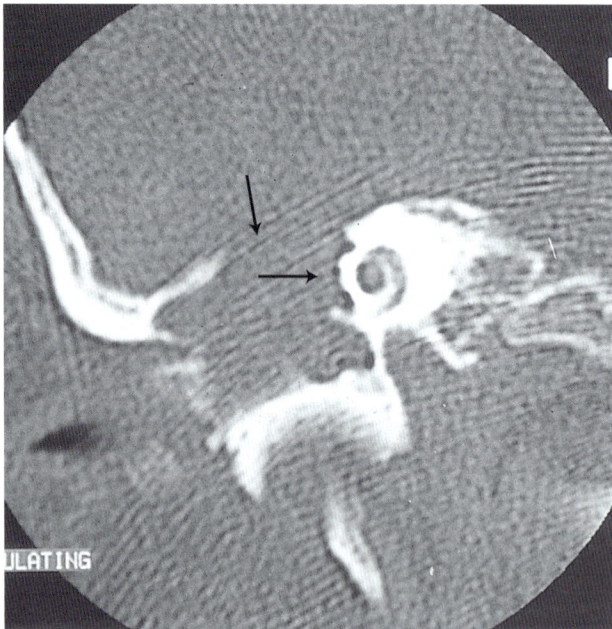

Figure 13.**19**   CT scan revealed the presence of a mass occupying the surgical cavity with erosion of the cochlea and absence of the tegmen.

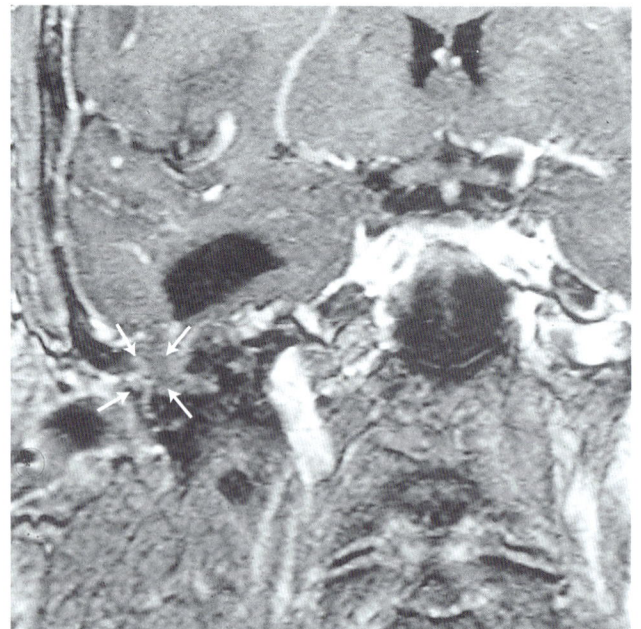

Figure 13.**20**   MRI also demonstrated the presence of meningoencephalic herniation (arrows). During surgery, the cholesteatoma was confirmed, together with a large encephalic herniation.

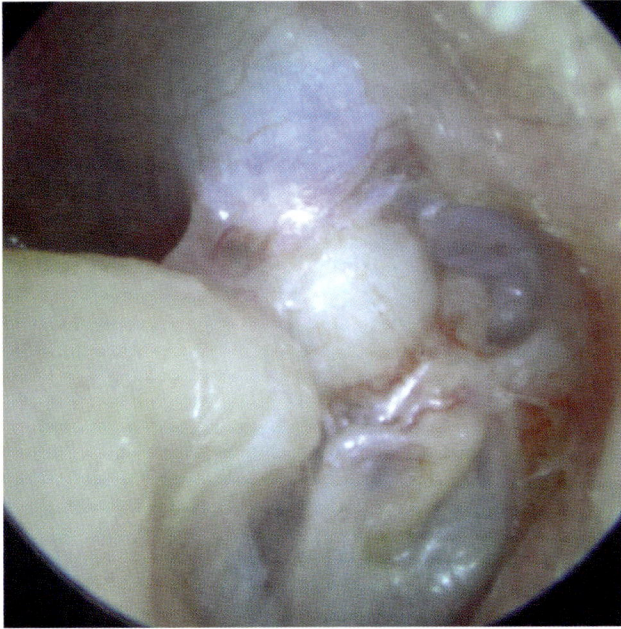

Figure 13.**21** Left ear. Open tympanoplasty. The tympanic membrane is normal, and slightly retracted. A residual cholesteatoma is present between the malleus and the lateral semicircular canal. A blue bulging area over the residual cholesteatoma is clearly seen. Iatrogenic meningoencephalic herniation was diagnosed.

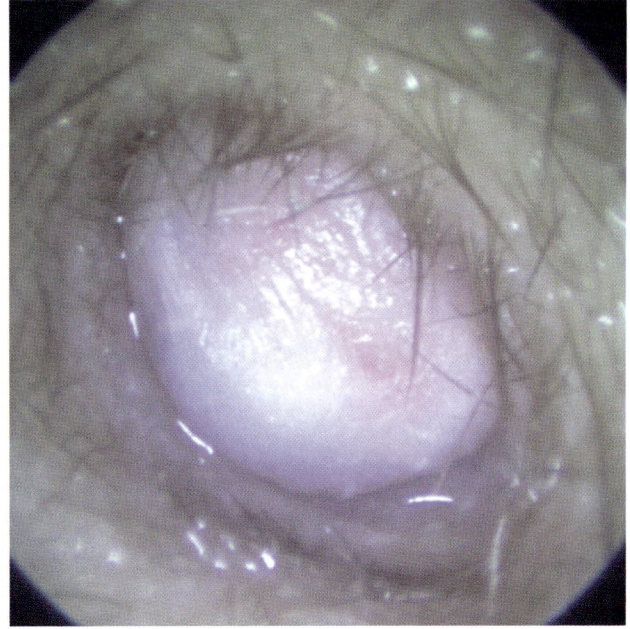

Figure 13.**22** Right ear. There is a pulsating polypoid mass protruding out of the external auditory canal. The patient went under open tympanoplasty many years previously. The cerebrospinal fluid leak (otoliquorrea) was present at the time of the consultation, and a meningoencephalic herniation was found on the CT scan. A middle fossa approach was adopted to reduce the herniation.

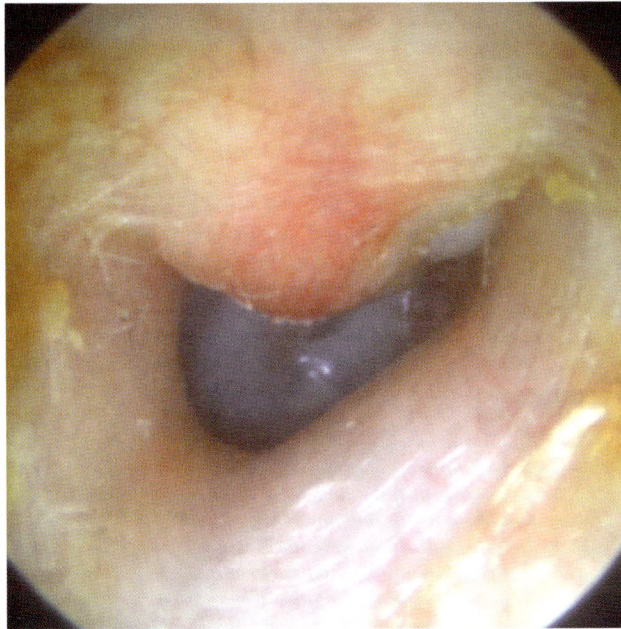

Figure 13.**23** Right post-traumatic meningoencephalic herniation. The superior wall of the external auditory canal is dehiscent. The CT scan showed a transverse fracture of the temporal bone. The patient also had sensorineural hearing loss.

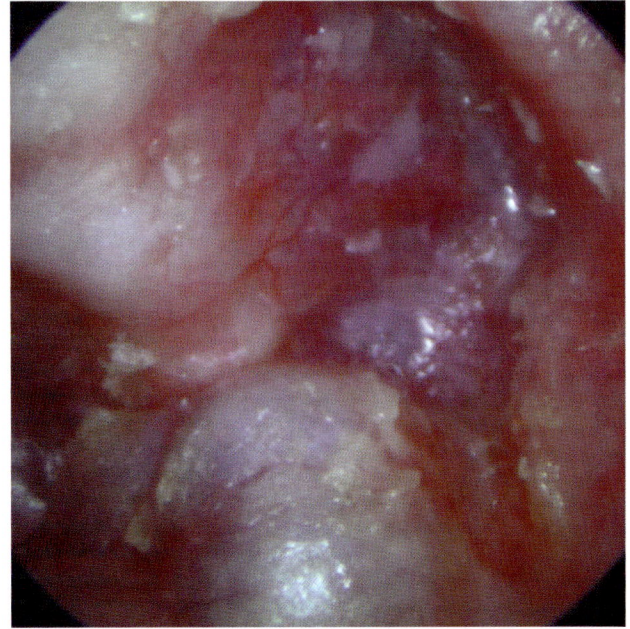

Figure 13.**24** A right modified radical mastoidectomy, with a pulsatile mass (meningoencephalic herniation) visible in upper part of the cavity. A middle fossa approach is indicated.

Transmastoid Approach with Minicraniotomy

Surgical Technique

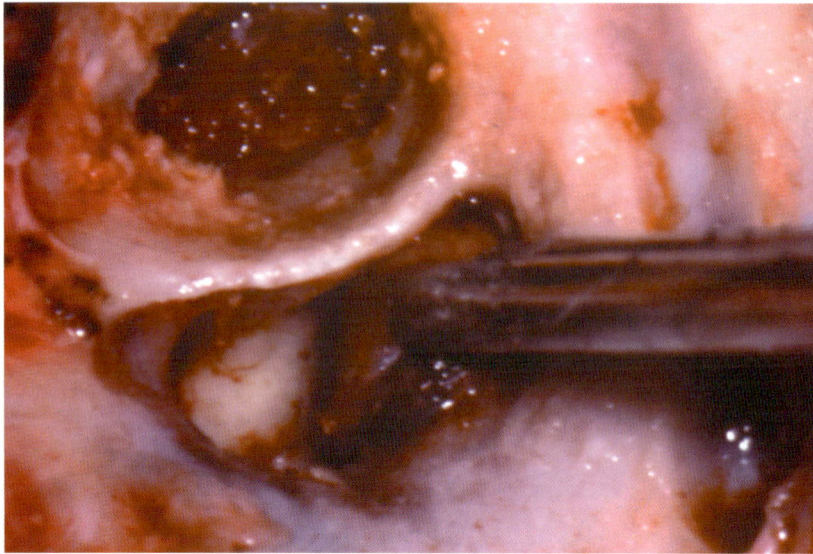

Figure 13.**25**   Left ear. A mastoidectomy has been completed. There is a large brain herniation occupying the mastoid cavity.

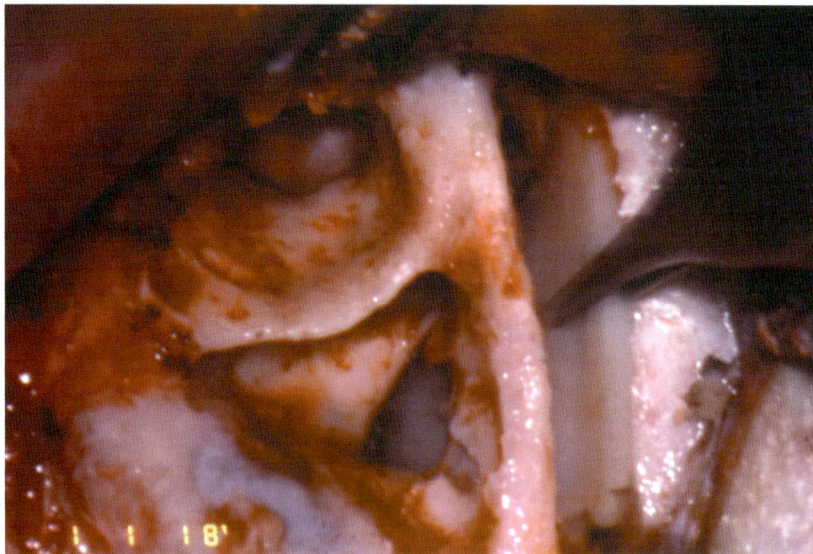

Figure 13.**26**   After the brain herniation has been reduced, a large piece of homologous septal cartilage is inserted through a minicraniotomy. The defect causing the brain herniation is clearly seen in the tegmen antri.

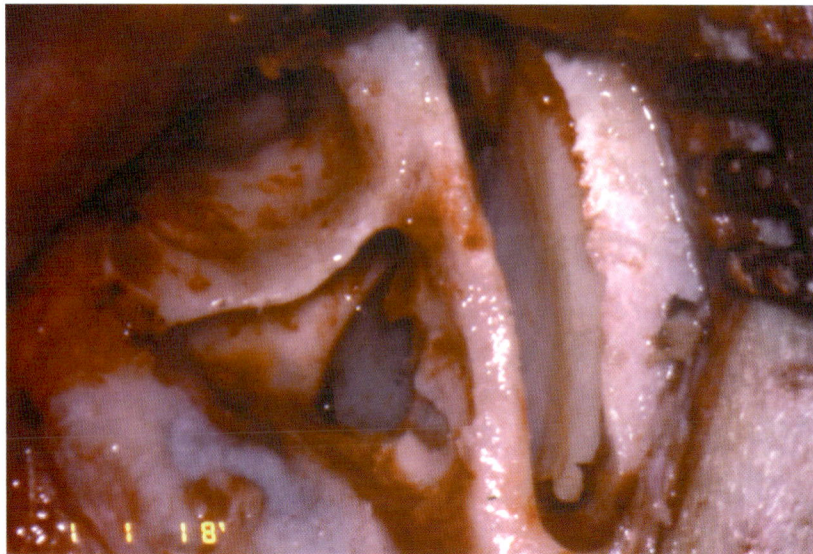

Figure 13.**27**   The final position of the septal cartilage reconstructing the bony defect.

Middle Cranial Fossa Approach

Surgical Technique

A temporal preauricular S-shaped skin incision is made, and the temporal muscle is divided in an inverted S fashion to avoid overlapping of the two incisions. A conventional temporal craniotomy is made, centered on the zygomatic root or on the external auditory canal, depending on the location of the hernia. The dura of the temporal lobe is carefully elevated until the neck of the herniated tissue is identified.

The neck of the hernia is coagulated with bipolar coagulation, and if necessary divided with microscissors. The herniated part is left inside the middle ear, where until it atrophies it acts as a barrier against infection of the intracranial spaces. A piece of fascia is placed intradurally between the cerebral tissue and the dura, and another piece of fascia is placed extradurally. Both pieces of fascia are kept in place with fibrin glue. A piece of homologous cartilage is then positioned between the bony defect and the extradurally placed fascia. In some cases, a piece of free muscle can be placed between the bony defect and the cartilage to reinforce the sealing. This reinforcement creates a stable and safe barrier that prevents recurrence of the defect and eliminates the possibility of infection of the intercranial spaces, especially in patients with middle ear cholesteatoma or middle ear infection.

The bone of the craniotomy is replaced, and the wound is closed in layers. Careful hemostasis is carried out, and no drainage is applied. After 3–6 months, when the defect has healed and the risk of intracranial infection is excluded, middle ear disease is managed with an additional procedure.

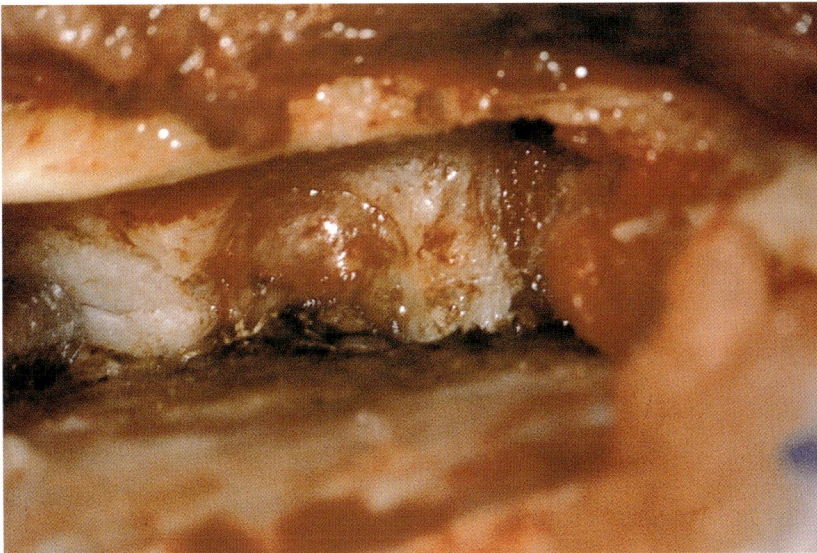

Figure 13.**28** A large brain herniation is seen protruding into the temporal bone.

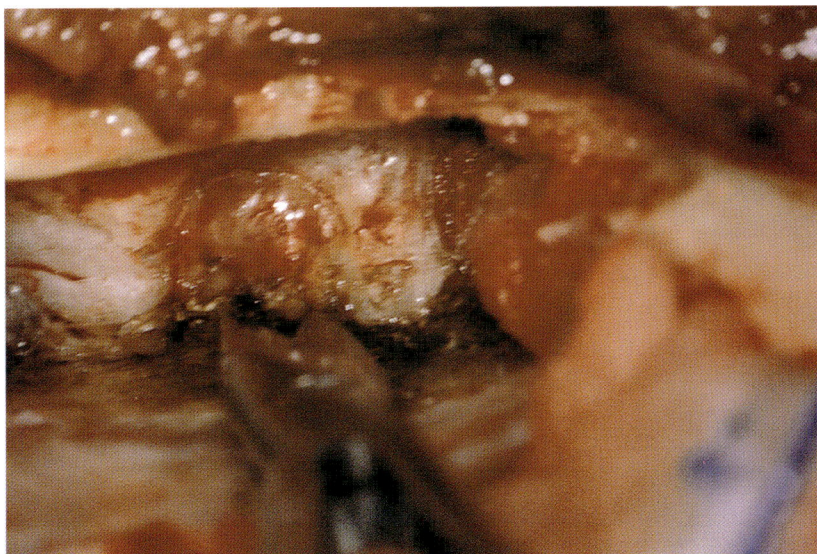

Figure 13.**29** The neck of the brain herniation is incised with scissors after bipolar coagulation.

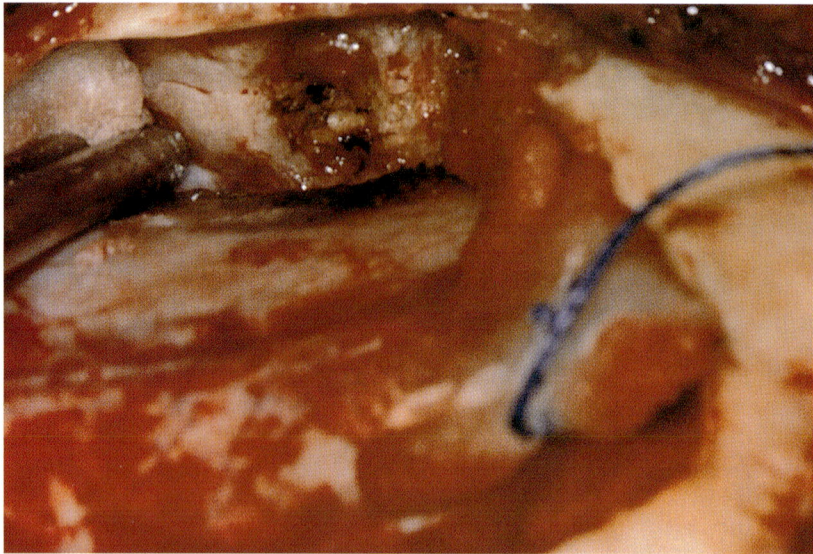

Figure 13.**30**   The brain herniation, divided from the dura, is left in place.

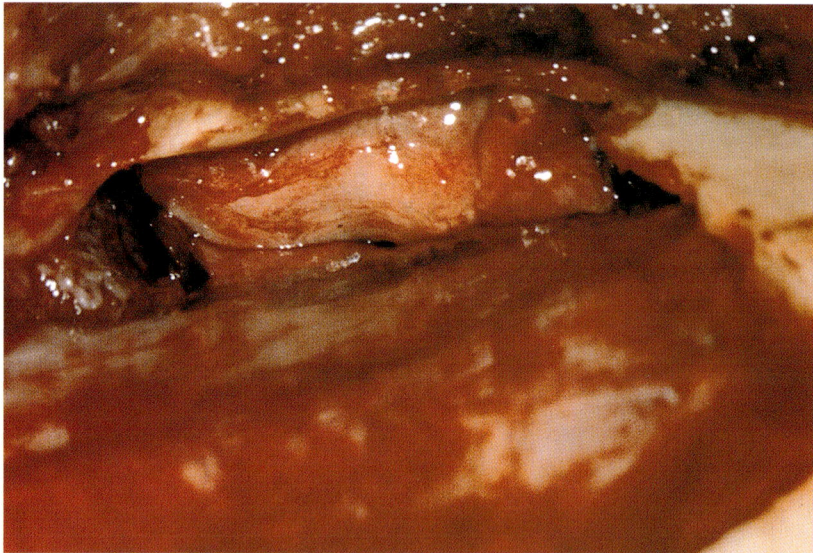

Figure 13.**31**   Temporalis fascia is used to separate the temporal bone opening from the middle fossa dura.

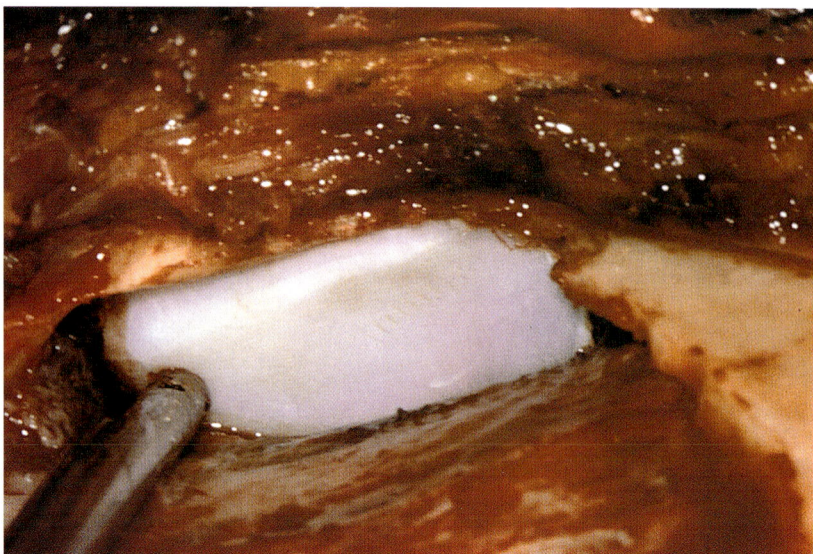

Figure 13.**32**   A large septal homologous cartilage is used over the fascia to reinforce the bony erosion and to prevent a secondary herniation.

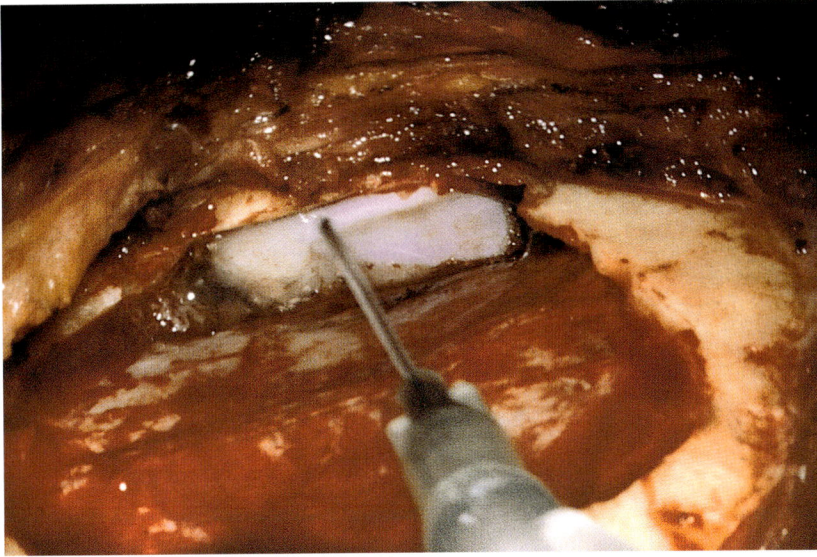

Figure 13.**33** Fibrin glue is used to secure the cartilage.

Summary

Herniation of the meningeal and/or encephalic tissue into the middle ear space is a rare condition occurring most frequently postsurgically, spontaneously due to congenital defects, post infection, and post trauma. For herniation to occur, a bony defect should be present. Through this dehiscence, a meningocele, an encephalocele, or both can occur. The most appropriate term seems to be *meningoencephalic herniation*.

The condition can lead to serious sequelae such as CSF leak, meningitis, epilepsy, and aphasia. Therefore, once diagnosed, surgical correction should be performed. The herniated tissue is usually resected and the defect is reconstructed. The surgical approach is determined by the size of the defect. Small defects are managed using a transmastoid approach. In hernias with middle-sized defects, the transmastoid approach is combined with a minicraniotomy, which allows the placement of a larger piece of septal cartilage for reconstruction of the defect. In large defects, however, a middle cranial fossa approach is adopted. In this approach, the dura of the temporal lobe is carefully elevated until the neck of the hernia is identified and bipolarly coagulated. The herniated part is left inside the middle ear or mastoid where it acts as a barrier against infection of the intracranial spaces. The defect is reconstructed by placing a piece of temporalis fascia between the cerebral tissue and the dura; another piece of fascia is placed extradurally. Next, a piece of cartilage is placed between the bony defect and the dura to reinforce the sealing. In other cases, a piece of muscle can also be placed between the bony defect and the cartilage for further reinforcement.

14 Postsurgical Conditions

As seen in the previous chapters, some otoscopic views may be difficult to interpret. This difficulty increases in cases involving previous surgery, because of the distortion of the normal anatomy. The examiner should be competent and experienced enough to distinguish between cases with normal postoperative healing and those with recurring pathology and/or immediate and late postoperative complications.

In this chapter, postoperative otoscopic views with and without complications and/or recurrence are presented.

Myringotomy and Insertion of a Ventilation Tube

The indications for myringotomy and ventilation tube insertion have been discussed previously. Myringo-tomy is usually performed in the anteroinferior quadrant of the tympanic membrane in the region of the cone of light. The incision is made in a radial direction using a myringotomy knife. In cases with a hump on the anterior wall of the external auditory canal, myringotomy can be performed immediately inferior to the umbo in the posteroinferior quadrant. The incision should never be made in the posterosuperior quadrant, to avoid injury to the ossicular chain. The operation is performed under general anesthesia in children. In adults, however, local anesthesia is sufficient. After making a radial incision in the tympanic membrane, the middle ear effusion is aspirated and the ventilation tube is inserted. In the majority of cases, hearing improves immediately.

The patient is instructed to avoid water entering the ear by blocking it with cotton daubed with petrolatum when taking a shower, or with rubber earplugs when swimming. Infection could occur if water were to enter the middle ear through the ventilation tube. Should this occur, ear lavage with a disinfectant solution consisting of 2% boric acid in 70% alcohol is indicated. When the tube is obstructed by cerumen or crusts, the administration of hydrogen peroxide drops is usually sufficient to restore its patency.

There are many types of commercially available ventilation tubes, but they can be generally grouped into short- and long-term tubes. Tubes with a larger inner flange usually remain in place longer. Once extruded, the myringotomy site closes spontaneously in about 98% of cases.

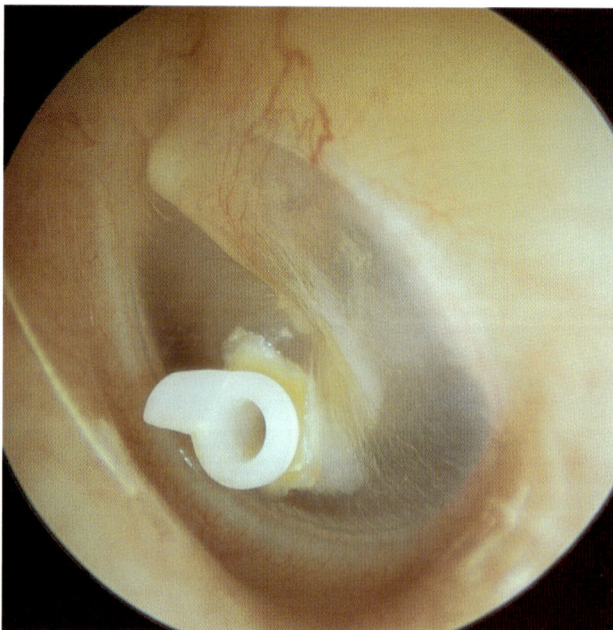

Figure 14.**1**   Left ear. The Sultan ventilation tube. This type has two small wings: an outer one with which the tube can be held using the ear forceps and an inner one, viewed through the tympanic membrane, which facilitates tube insertion and prevents rapid extrusion. If properly inserted, the Sultan ventilation tube can remain for about 6 to 18 months before extrusion.

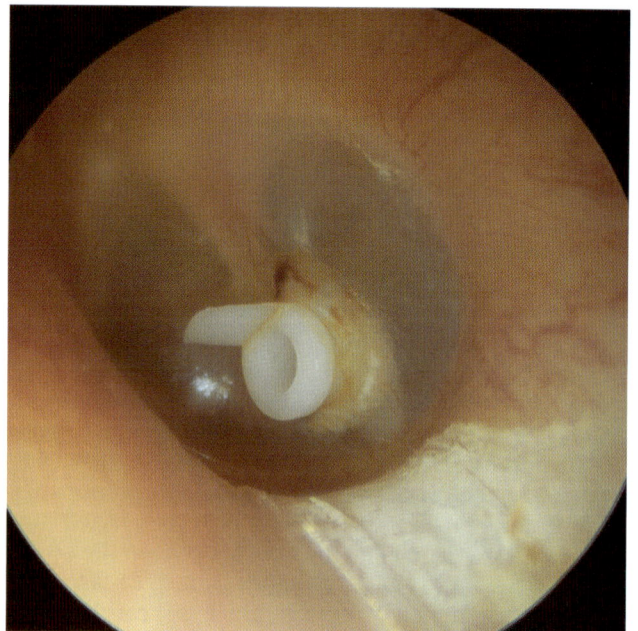

Figure 14.**2**   Left ear. In this case, the tube has been placed inferior to the umbo due to the presence of an anterior hump in the anterior canal wall.

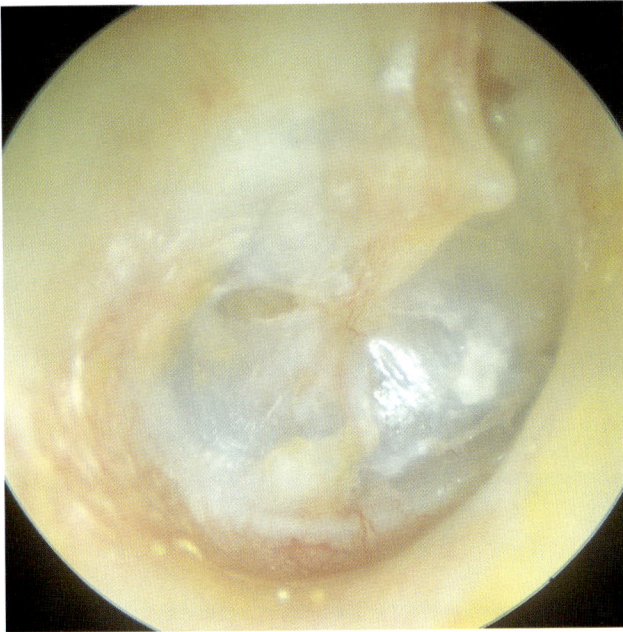

Figure 14.**3** Right ear. The consequences of a misplaced venti-lation tube is shown. A healed myringotomy is seen in the pos-terosuperior quadrant (at 9 o'clock). Two months later the tube was extruded. During tube insertion, however, dislocation of the incus occurred. The dislocated incus fell to the hypotympanum, where its body and short process can be clearly seen. In the anteroinferior quadrant, immediately under the umbo, another healed myringotomy site (this time correctly placed) is visible. In the latter, tube extrusion occurred 1 year later.

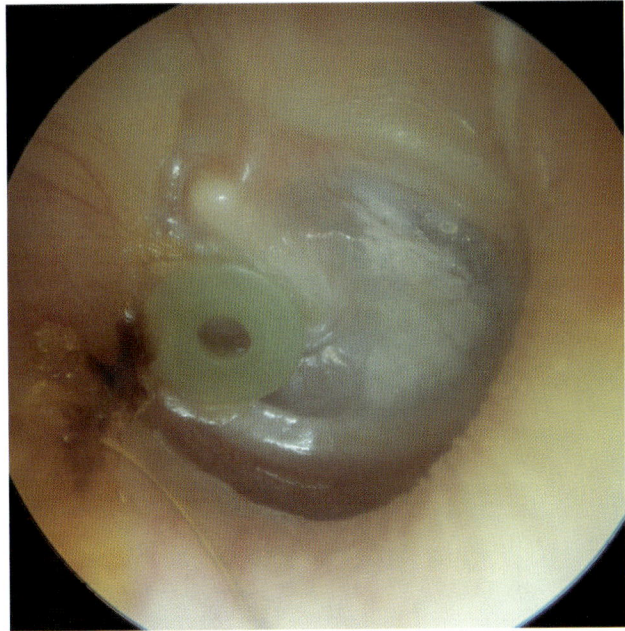

Figure 14.**4** Left ear. A long-term ventilation tube inserted 6 months after tympanoplasty because of an observed tendency for graft retraction. The graft is seen in an optimal condition with no evidence of retraction, indicating patency of the ventilation tube. This tube has been in situ for more than 10 years.

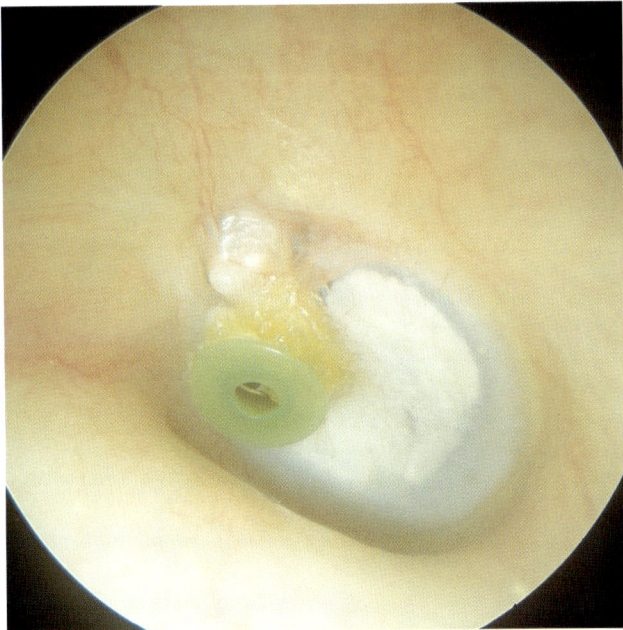

Figure 14.**5** Left ear. Long-term ventilation tube. A large tym-panosclerotic plaque that formed 1 year after the tube insertion can be clearly seen. Such plaques result from hemorrhagic infil-trate between the epidermal and fibrous layers of the tympanic membrane secondary to the myringotomy, and are asympto-matic.

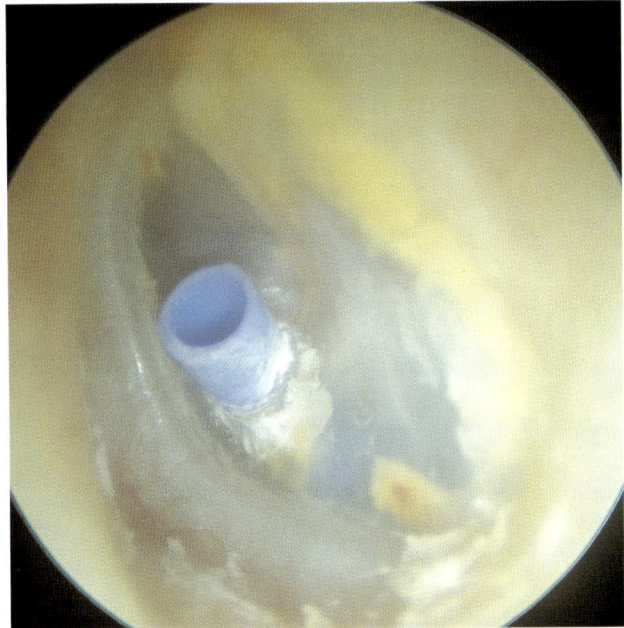

Figure 14.**6** Left ear. Example of a long-term T tube inserted in the anteroinferior quadrant of the tympanic membrane. After its insertion the two wings of the tube open by virtue of their retained "memory," thereby preventing tube extrusion.

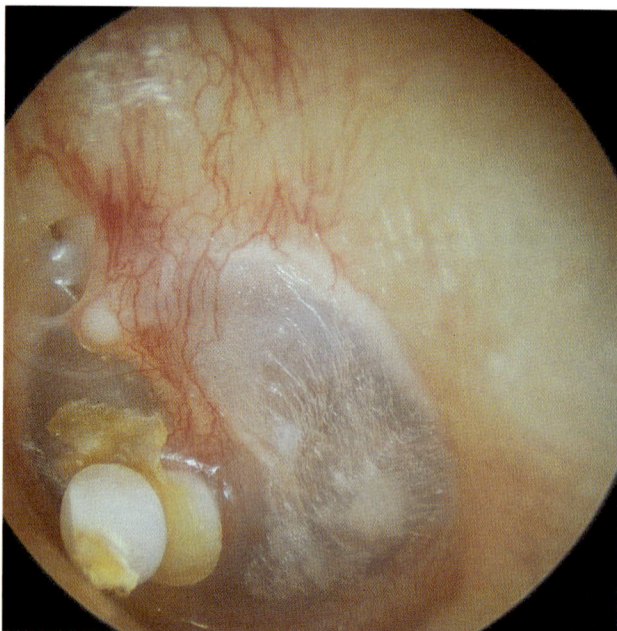

Figure 14.**7**   Left ear. A ventilation tube in the process of extrusion. It is preferable not to take out the tube but rather wait for self-extrusion to occur. Closure of the myringotomy site occurs in about 98% of cases.

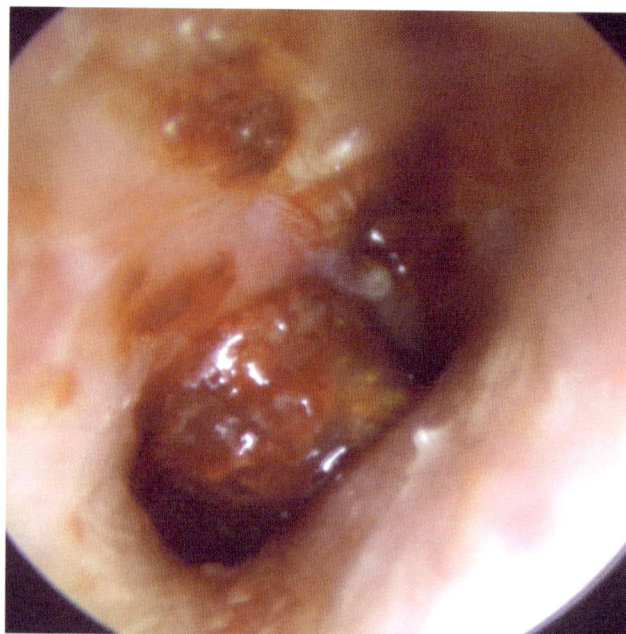

Figure 14.**8**   Right ear. Granulation tissue after ventilation tube insertion. This complication is generally resolved with removal of the tube.

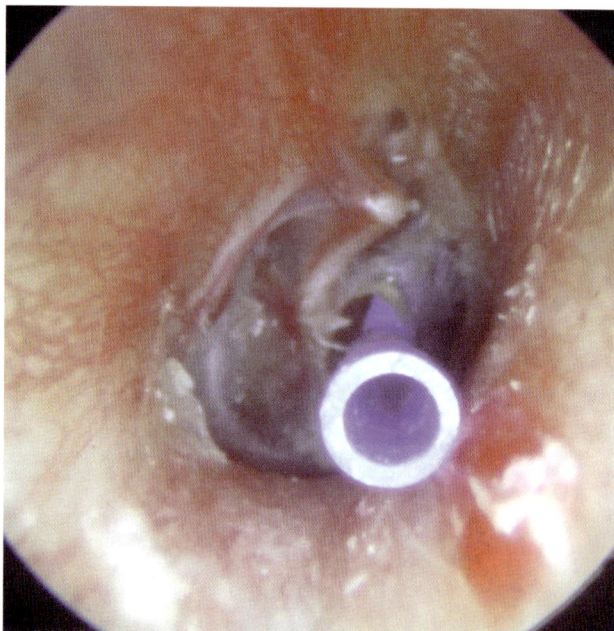

Figure 14.**9**   Right ear. Another example of a long-term T tube. This type of tube unfortunately very often causes perforation of the tympanic membrane.

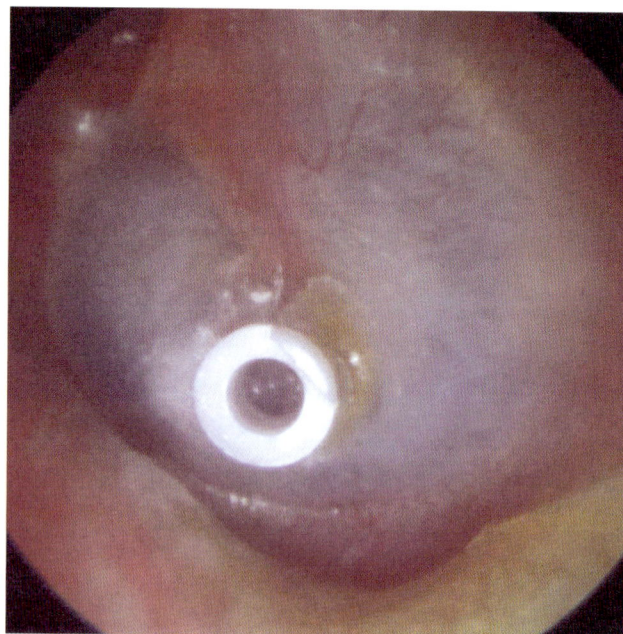

Figure 14.**10**   Left ear. A short-term ventilation tube. The lumen is closed with glue. The tube can be reopened using drops of H_2O_2.

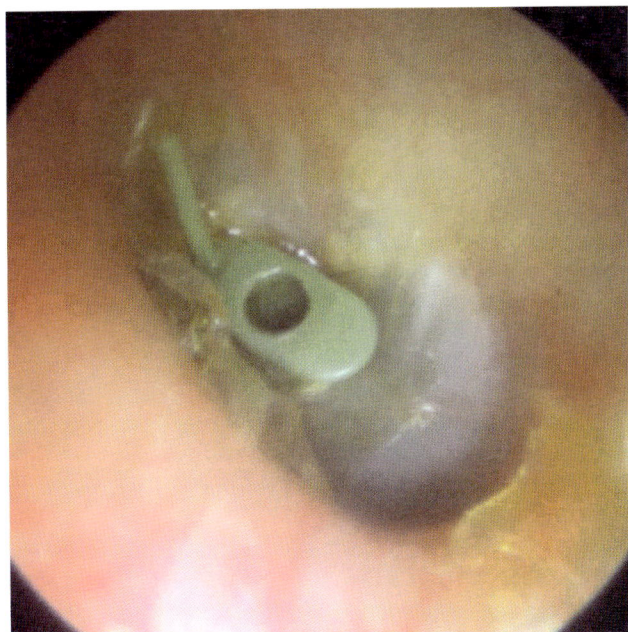

Figure 14.**11**   Left ear, with a T tube positioned in the anterosuperior quadrant.

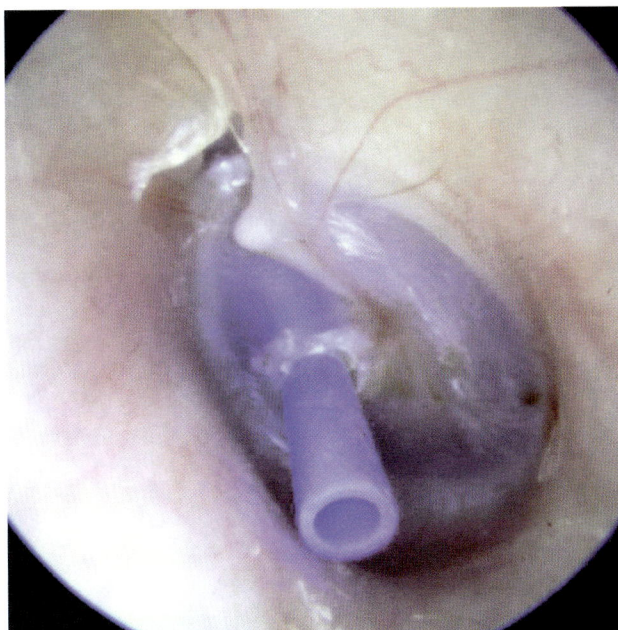

Figure 14.**12**   Left ear. Another example of a long-term ventilation tube.

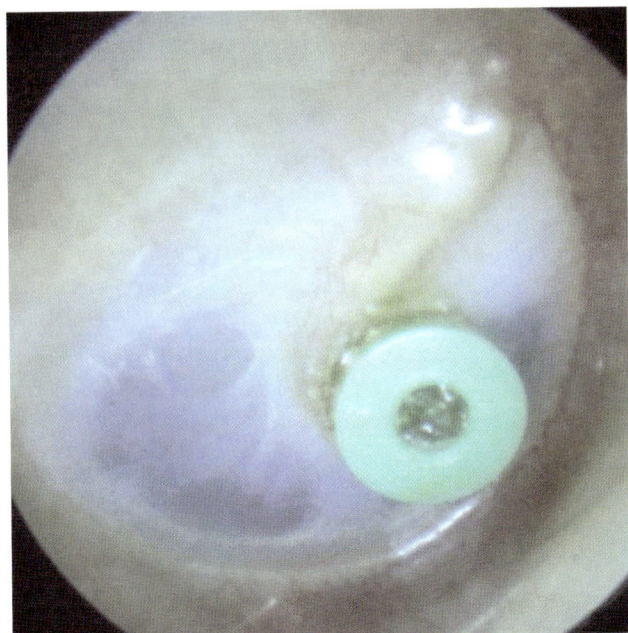

Figure 14.**13**   Right ear. A short ventilation tube, with closure of the lumen with glue.

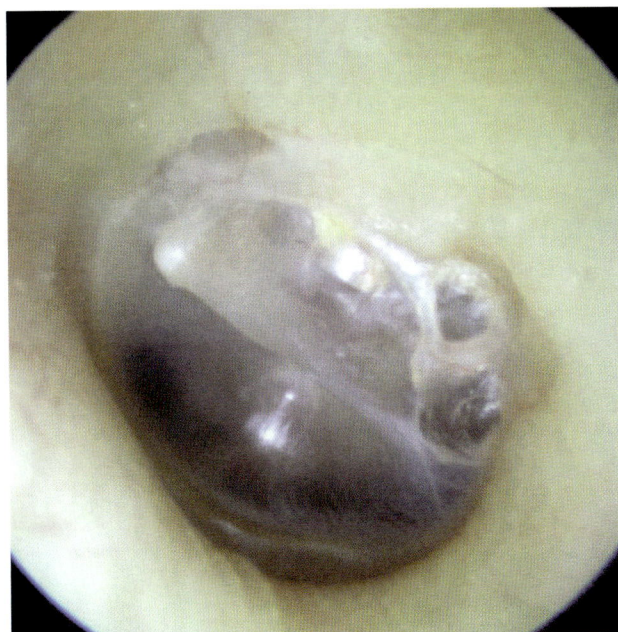

Figure 14.**14**   Left ear. Otoscopy view after stapedectomy. The atticotomy is visible; the prosthesis, dislocated from the incus, has adhered to the tympanic membrane.

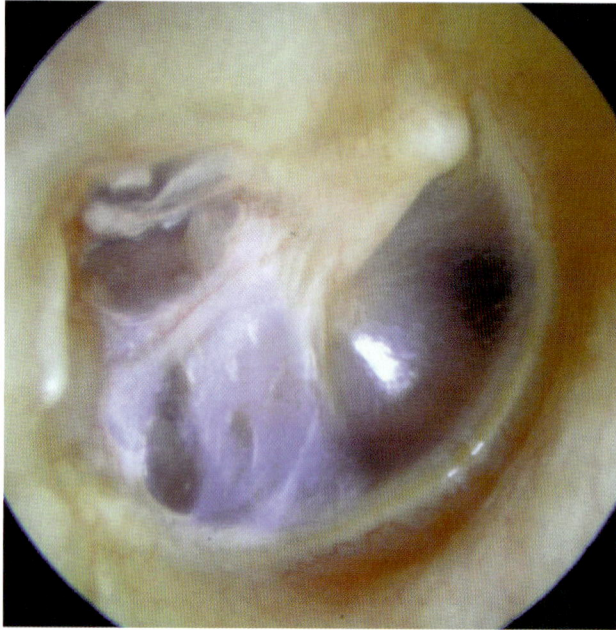

Figure 14.**15** The atticotomy is clearly seen, and the chorda tympani is attached to the tympanic membrane.

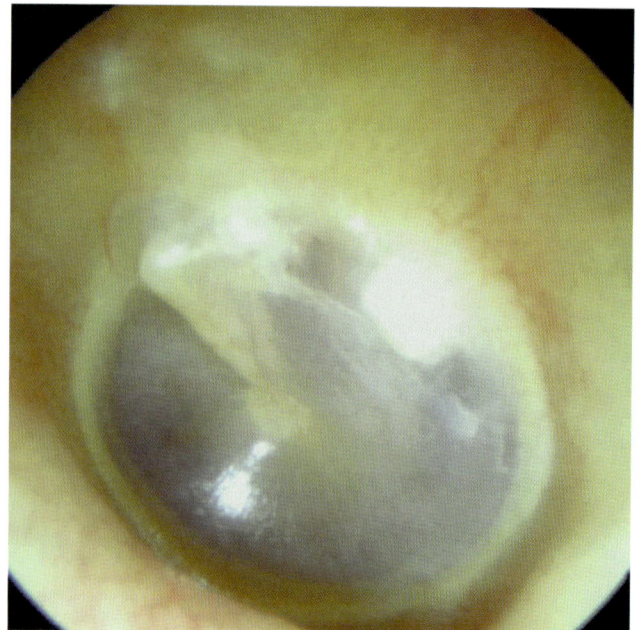

Figure 14.**16** Left ear. A small piece of retrotympanic bone from the atticotomy is clearly seen.

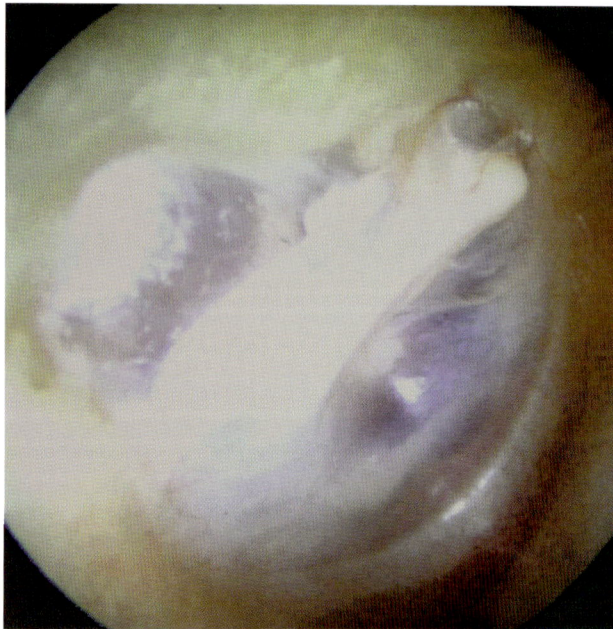

Figure 14.**17** Right ear. An example of a large atticotomy.

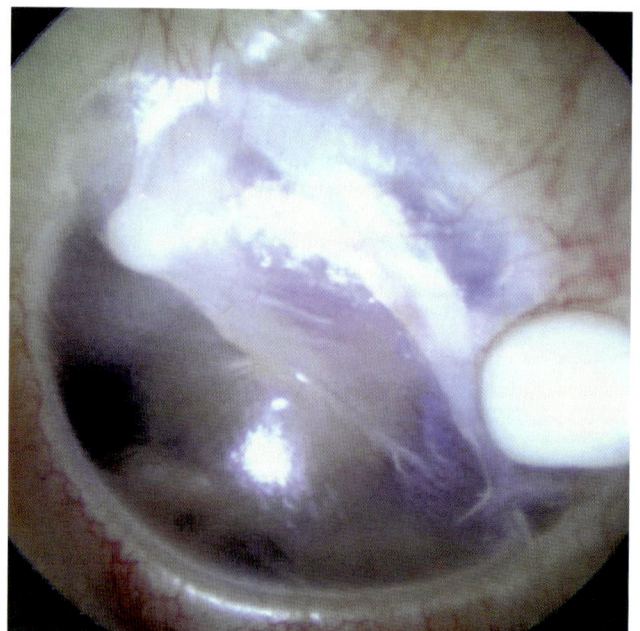

Figure 14.**18** Left ear. A small pearl of iatrogenic cholesteatoma is present in the external auditory canal, attached to the posterior quadrant of the tympanic membrane.

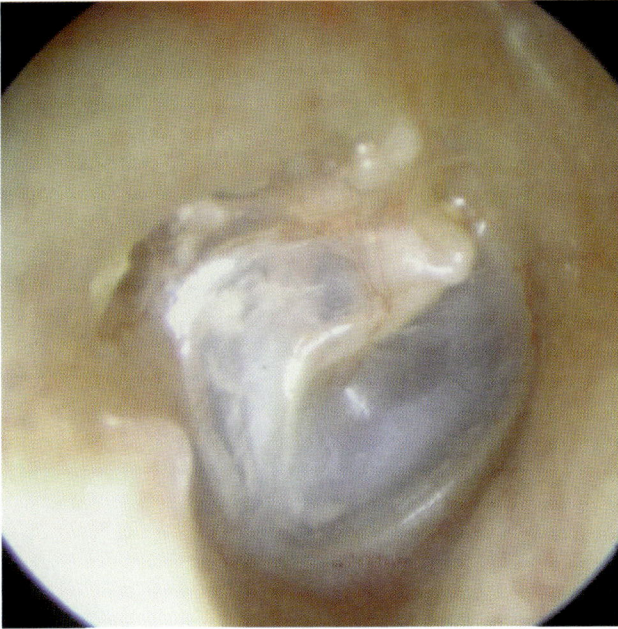

Figure 14.**19** Right ear. A small retraction pocket is present at the level of the atticotomy. The posterior annular ring is clearly seen.

Myringoplasty

The aim of reconstructing a tympanic membrane perforation is twofold: first, to allow the patient to have a normal social life with no restrictions, even regarding water entry into the ear, and second, to correct the hearing loss resulting from the perforation.

There are essentially two techniques for myringoplasty. The underlay technique is utilized in the presence of an anterior residue (at least the annulus) of the tympanic membrane, under which the graft can be placed. In the absence of any anterior residue of the membrane, the overlay technique is used. In such cases, the graft is positioned against the anterior wall of the external auditory canal.

Normally, the tympanic membrane forms an acute angle with the anterior wall of the external auditory canal. While performing myringoplasty, it is generally possible to respect this angulation when the annulus is present anteriorly.

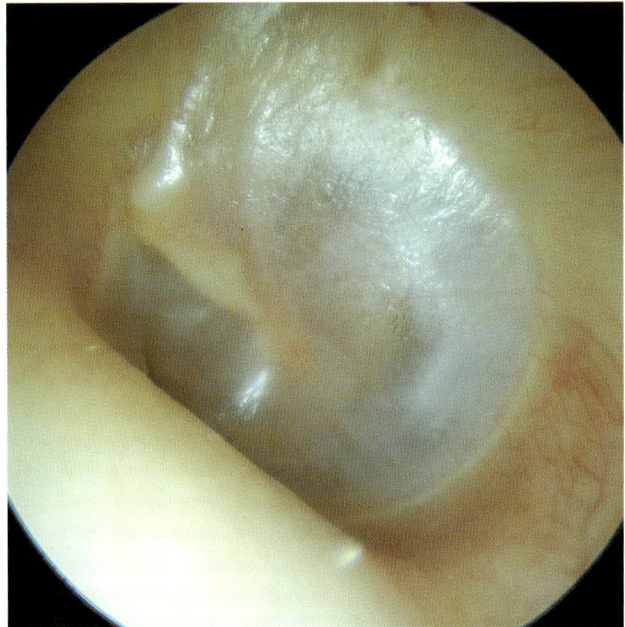

Figure 14.**20** Left ear. Normal aspect of the reconstructed tympanic membrane. The posterior quadrant is slightly elevated. In this case, a posterior perforation was grafted with temporalis fascia using an underlay technique.

The myringoplasty operation is considered a success when the reconstructed tympanic membrane is intact, well epithelialized, and has normal angulation with the external auditory canal. These characteristics allow the patient to have a normal social life (hearing improvement and possibility of water entry into the ear). Reperforation is a frequent complication of myringoplasty that occurs in about 5 to 10% of cases in the best series. Reperforation occurs more commonly in the underlay technique, particularly in the anterior quadrant when the graft is detached from the anterior residues of the tympanic membrane and falls into the middle ear. When an overlay technique is utilized, blunting of the anterior angle can occur, with resultant conductive hearing loss. Lateralization, in which the graft is detached from the handle of the malleus, is another possible complication that leads to conductive hearing loss. It occurs mostly when the graft is placed lateral rather than medial to the handle of the malleus. Stenosis of the external auditory canal, due either to inflammatory reaction or as a result of bad repositioning of the meatal flaps, can also occur.

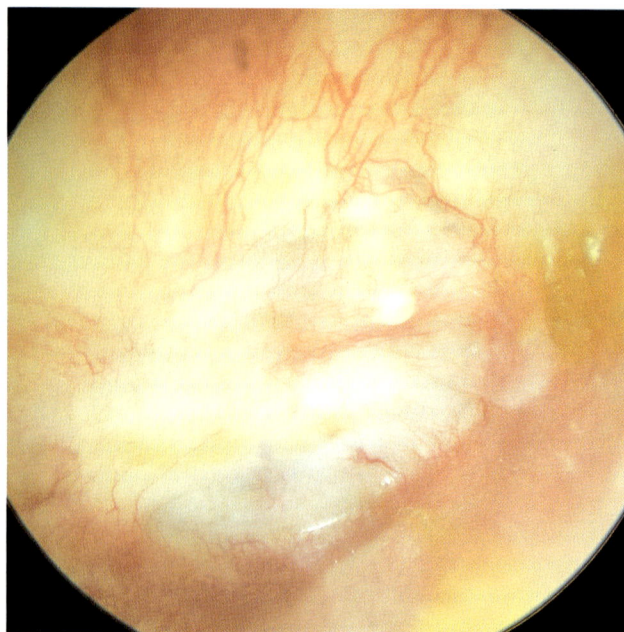

Figure 14.**21**   Right ear. Myringoplasty with an underlay technique. The reconstructed tympanic membrane is thicker than normal. The anterior angle is maintained. The handle of the malleus is clearly visible except for the umbo, which is detached from the membrane. Tympanosclerotic plaques are also visible.

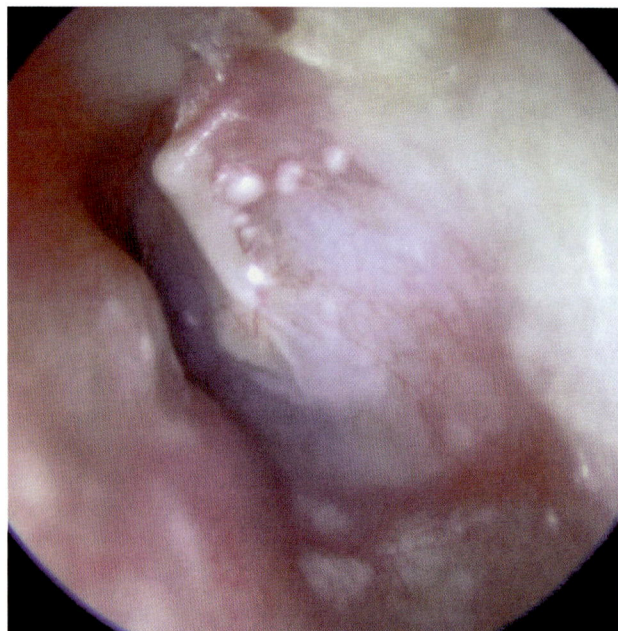

Figure 14.**22**   Left ear. The repaired tympanic membrane retains its normal position, with a perfect anterior angle. There are small pearls posterior to the handle of the malleus, which can be removed under microscopic vision during the consultation.

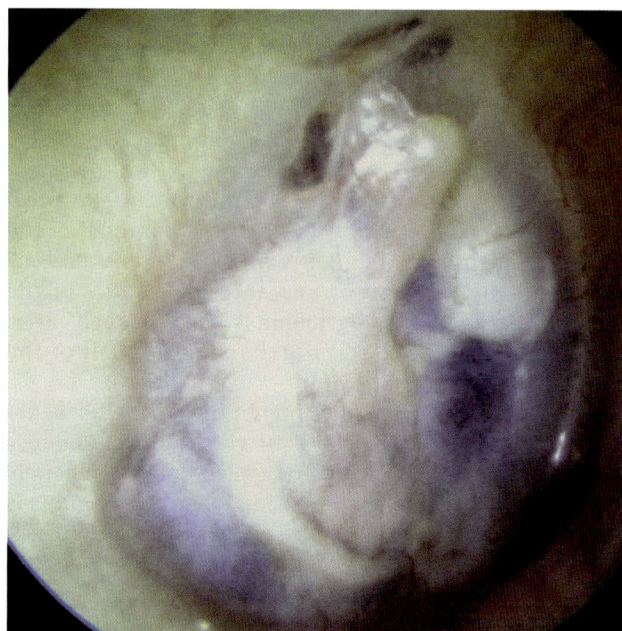

Figure 14.**23**   Right ear. Underlay myringoplasty. The anterior angle is perfectly normal, as is the thickness of the membrane. There is a whitish tympanosclerotic mass in the anterosuperior quadrant.

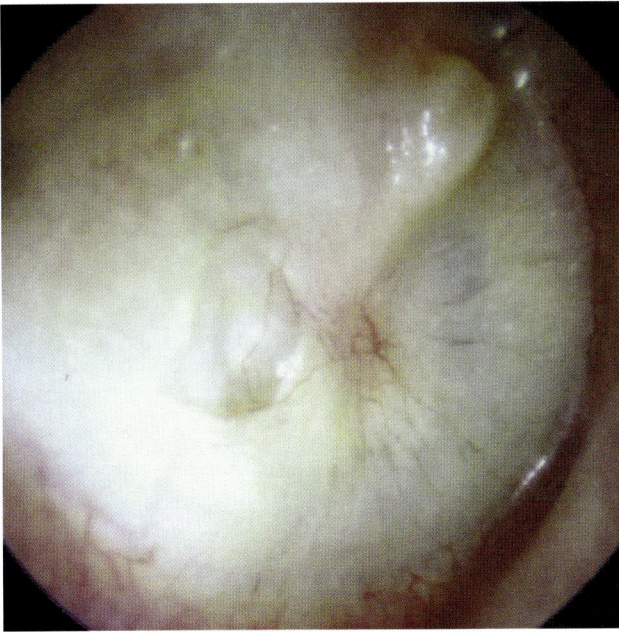

Figure 14.**24** Right ear. Myringoplasty with an underlay technique. The reconstructed membrane is thicker than normal, with a tympanosclerotic appearance. The anterior angle is maintained.

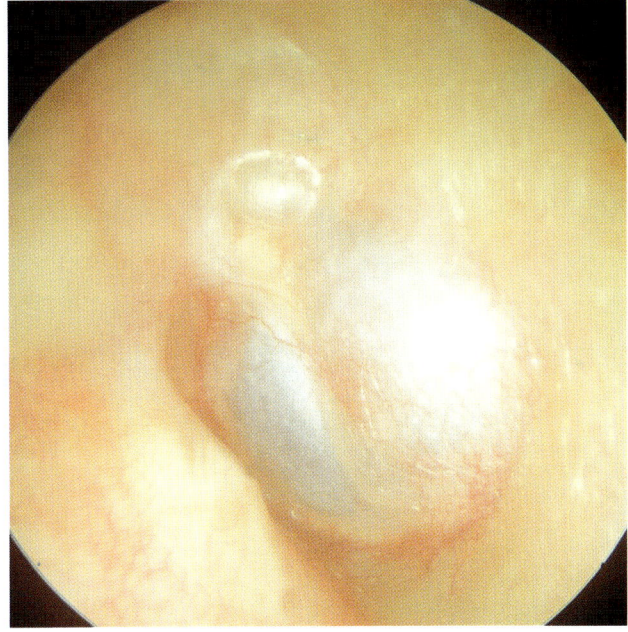

Figure 14.**25** Left ear. Another example of a tympanic membrane perforation that was repaired using an underlay technique with preservation of the anterior residue. The posterior quadrants are slightly lateralized, making it difficult to see the handle of the malleus.

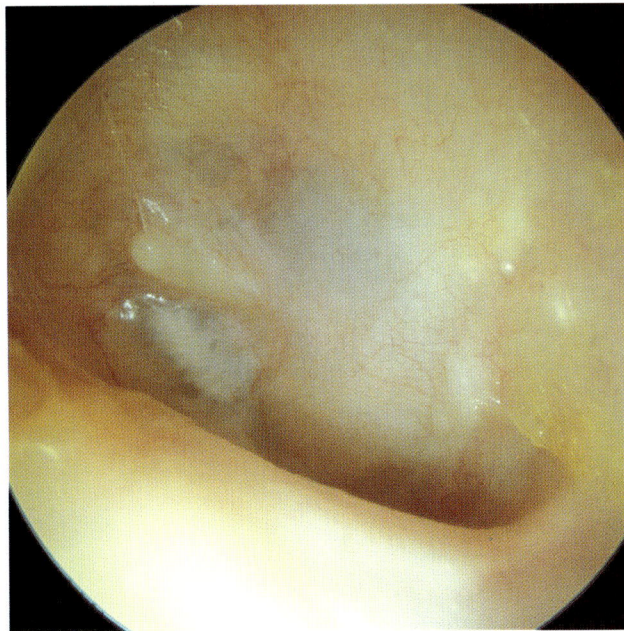

Figure 14.**26** Left ear. Similar case. The repaired tympanic membrane is well attached to the malleus except for the area of the umbo due to lateralization of the posteroinferior quadrant.

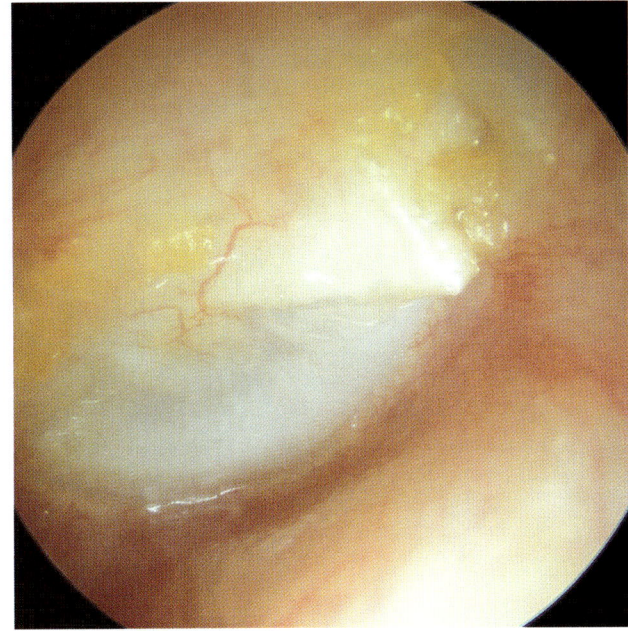

Figure 14.**27** Right ear. Underlay myringoplasty. The malleus is slightly medialized. The repaired tympanic membrane is whitish in its anterior quadrants and vascularized in the posterior ones. The anterior angle is normal.

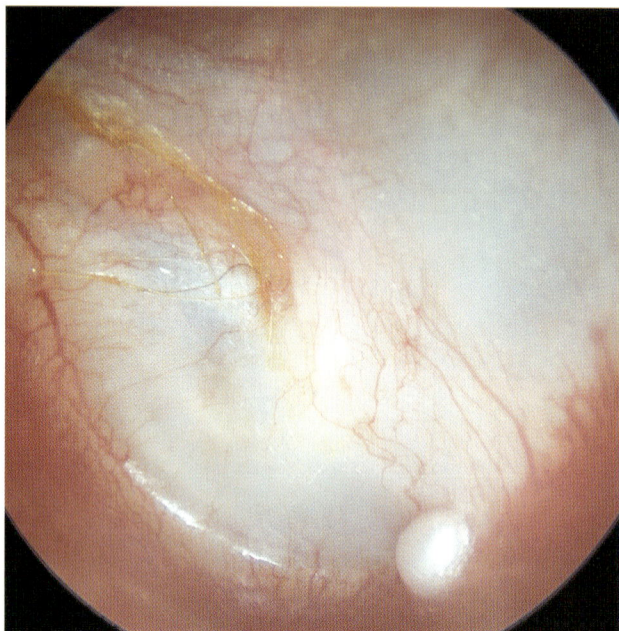

Figure 14.**28**   Left ear. The repaired tympanic membrane retains a normal anterior angle and is well vascularized, though thicker than normal. A small cholesteatomatous pearl is observed. This pearl can be easily removed in the outpatient clinic under the microscope.

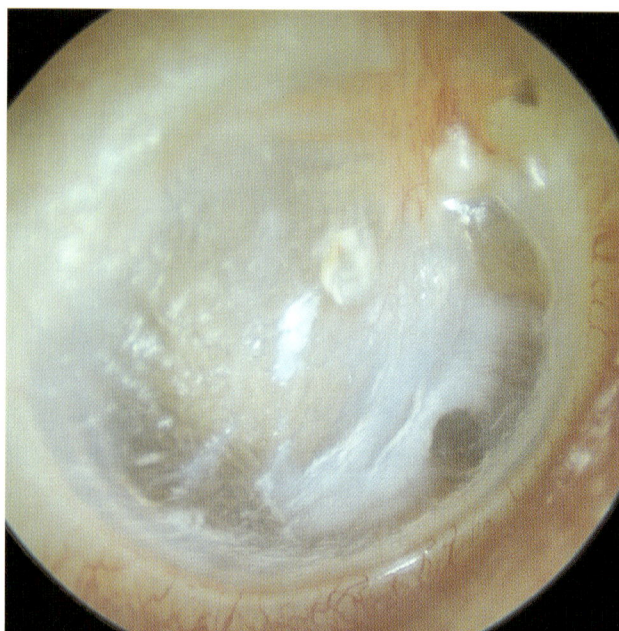

Figure 14.**29**   Right ear. The repaired tympanic membrane has normal thickness. The short process of the malleus can be observed, although the handle is not visible due to lateralization.

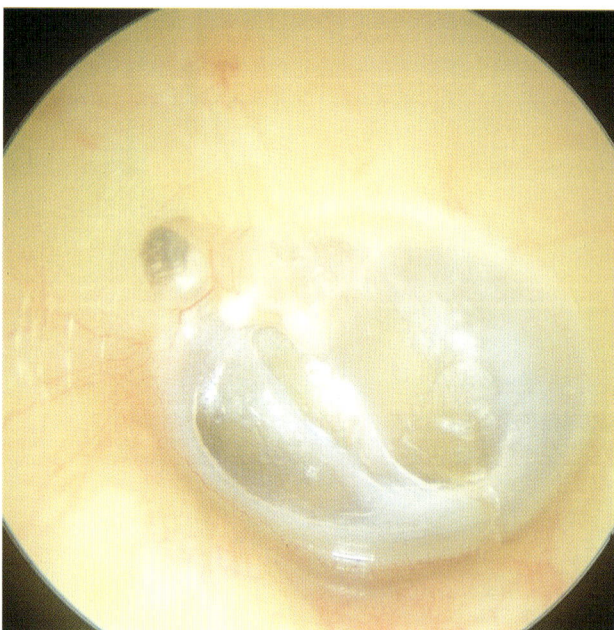

Figure 14.**30**   Left ear. Another example of a graft that is detached from the handle of the malleus using an underlay technique.

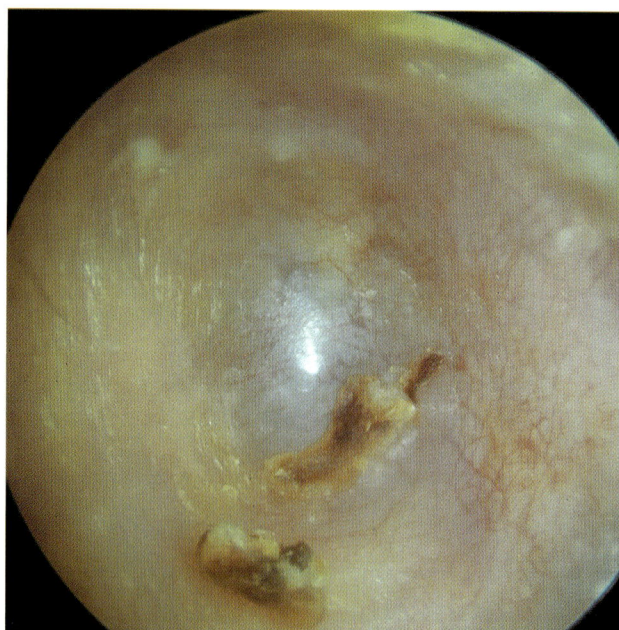

Figure 14.**31**   A lateralized reconstructed tympanic membrane with blunting of the anterior angle following an overlay technique. Both complications lead to altered mobility of the tympanic membrane with consequent conductive hearing loss.

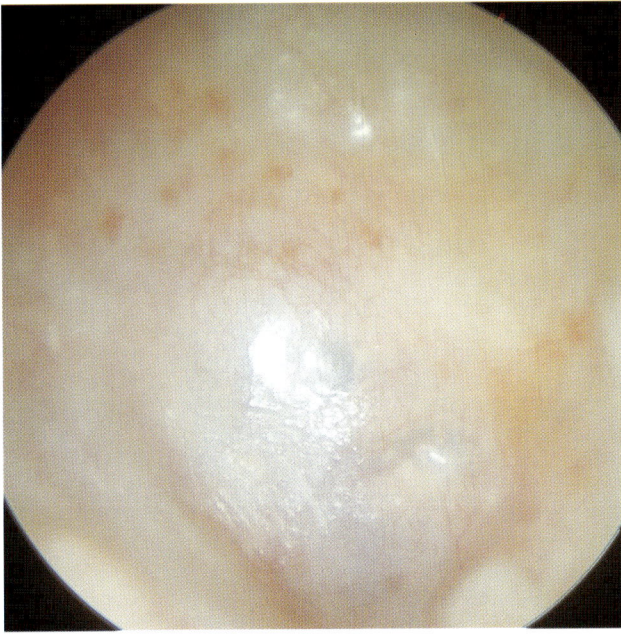

Figure 14.**32** The external auditory canal is wide but the repaired tympanic membrane is lateralized and shows blunting.

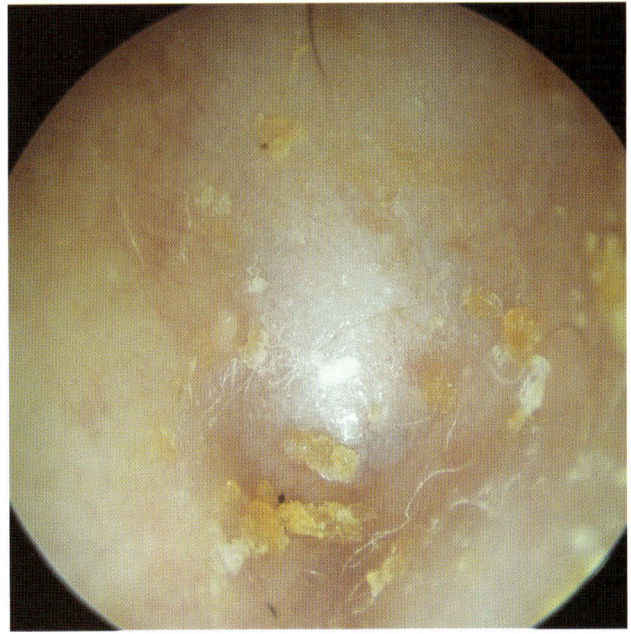

Figure 14.**33** Similar case. The reconstructed tympanic membrane is lateralized with marked blunting of the anterior angle.

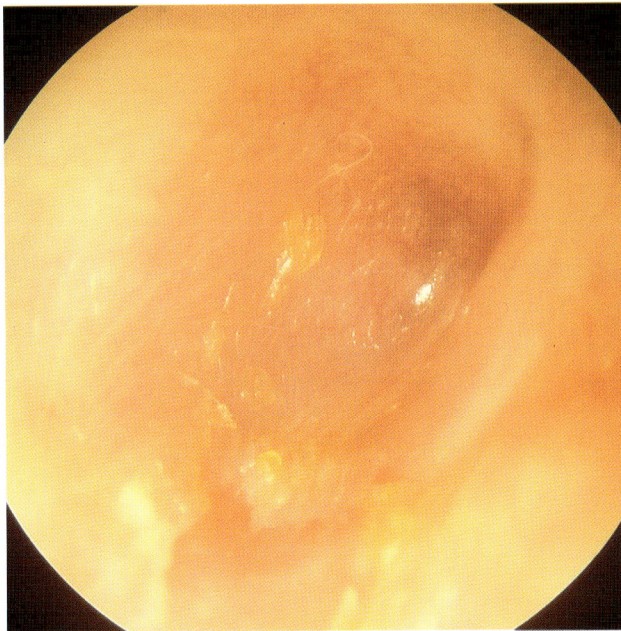

Figure 14.**34** Postoperative myringitis. The tympanic membrane is hyperemic, thickened, and lateralized following a tympanoplasty. The epidermal layer is substituted by granulation tissue. Myringitis is a rare complication that usually resolves with local steroid applications. In very rare cases, re-operation is necessary. The pathological tympanic membrane is removed followed by grafting.

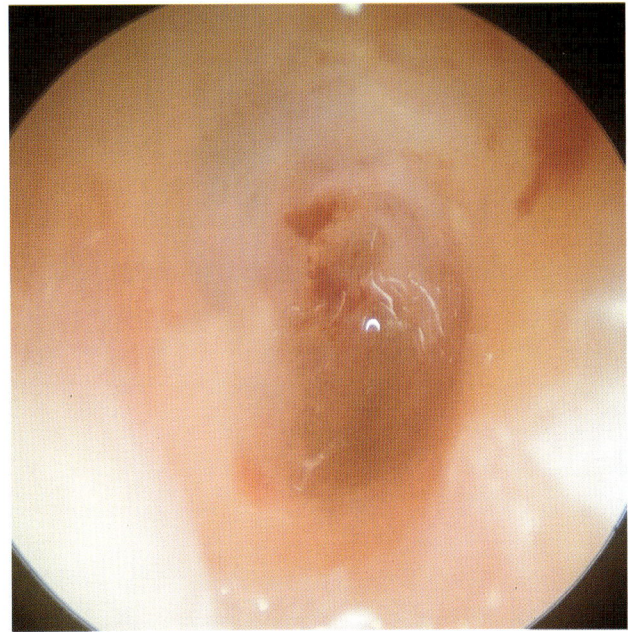

Figure 14.**35** A patient who had undergone quadruple myringoplasty. In these cases, myringitis and canal stenosis are frequent; therefore, it is necessary to remove the pathological tissues, perform canalplasty, and use free skin flaps.

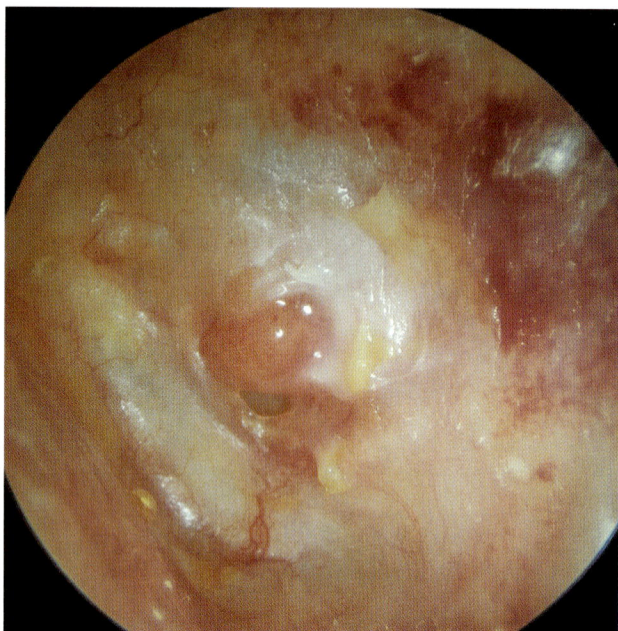

Figure 14.**36** Left ear. Reperforation of the tympanic membrane with granulations near the perforation. In such cases, curettage of the granulation and freshening of the edges under the microscope may lead to spontaneous closure of the perforation.

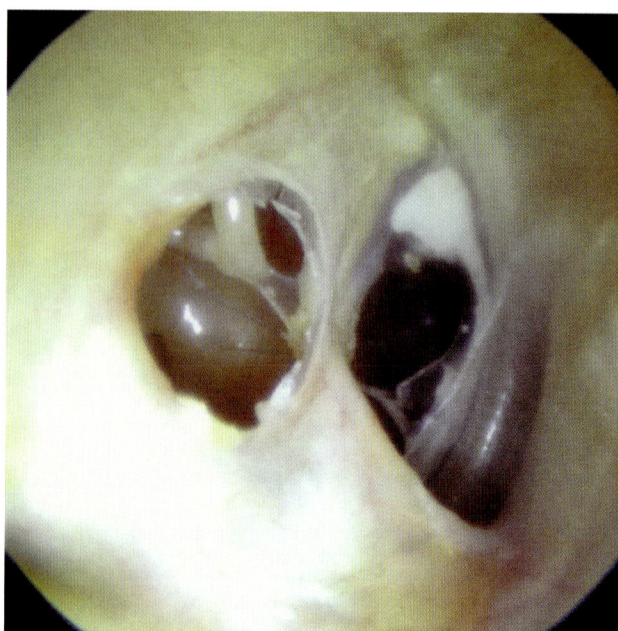

Figure 14.**37** Right ear. Recurrent perforation of the tympanic membrane, anterior and posterior to the malleus handle, with abnormal scar tissue between the umbo and the anteroinferior wall of the external auditory canal.

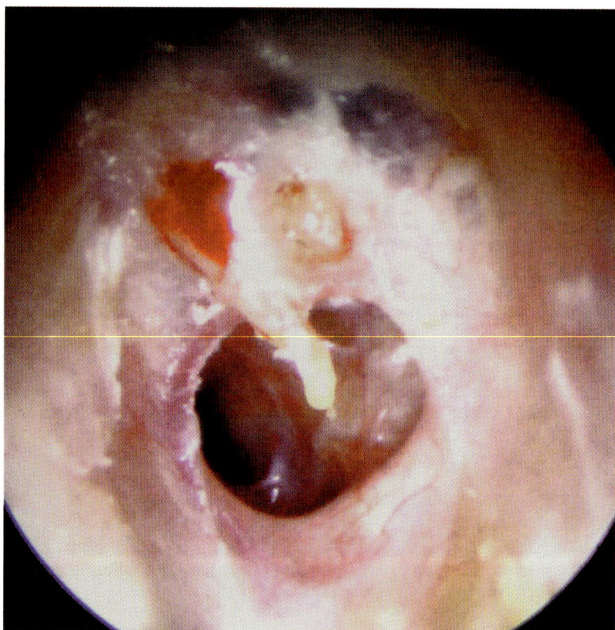

Figure 14.**38** Left ear. Central reperforation of the tympanic membrane.

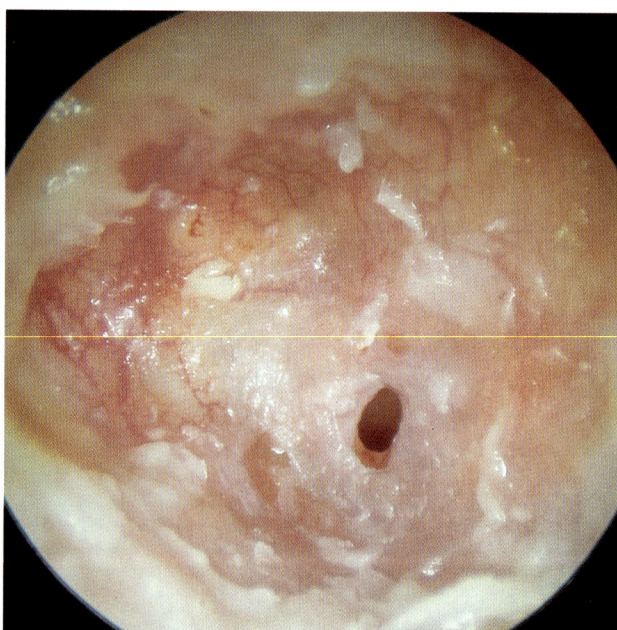

Figure 14.**39** Reperforation of the tympanic membrane. Myringitis with otorrhea can be observed. Lavage and freshening of the perforation edges as well as insertion of Gelfoam (in the middle ear) can favor spontaneous closure of the perforation.

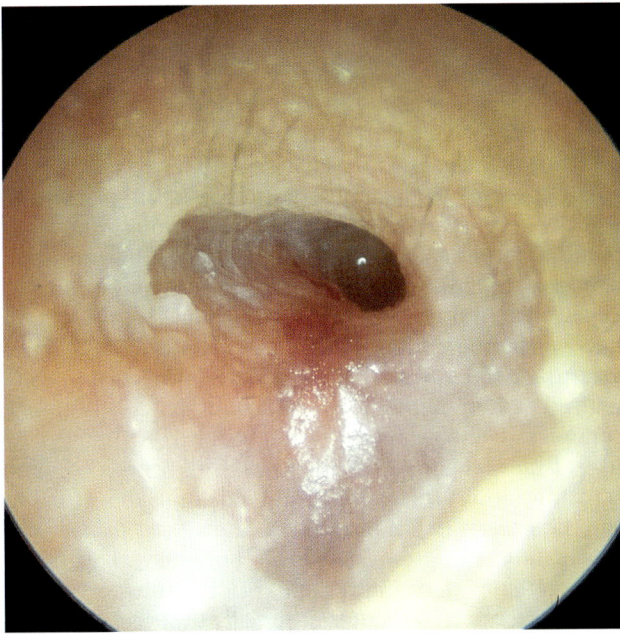

Figure 14.**40** Left ear. Stenosis of the external auditory canal following myringoplasty.

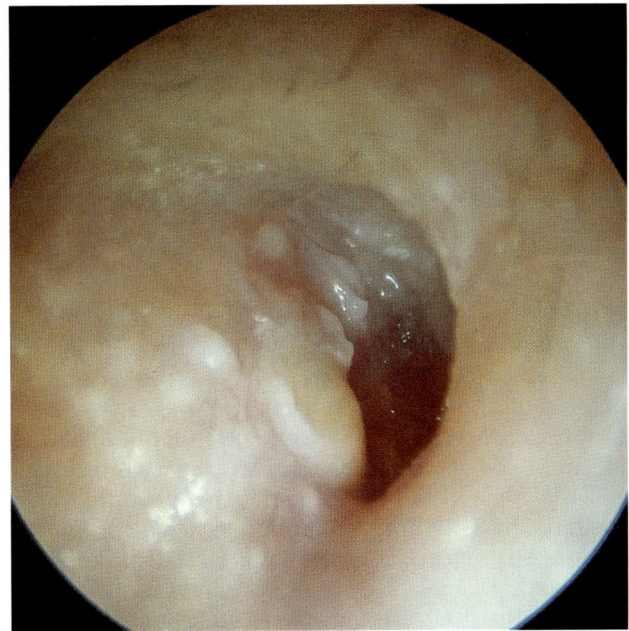

Figure 14.**41** Right ear. Partial stenosis of the external auditory canal following myringoplasty. For the management of this complication, it is usually sufficient to incise the skin of the canal and insert a plastic sheet for about 20 days, while using local medication with steroid lotion.

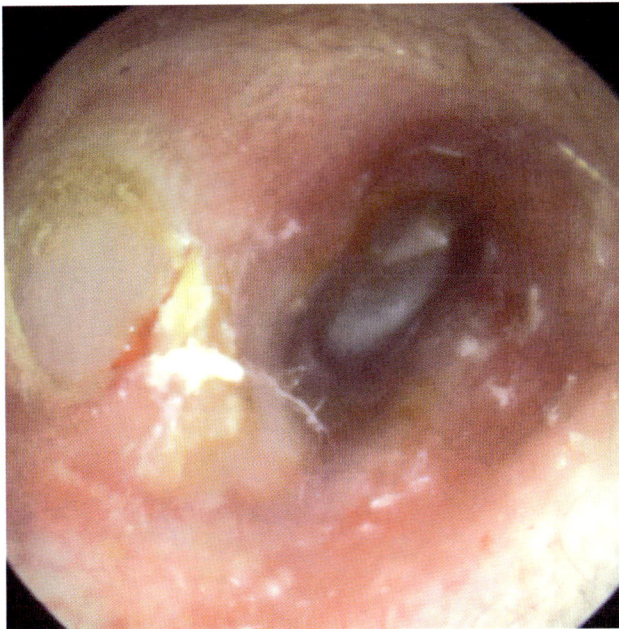

Figure 14.**42** Right ear. The skin of the external auditory canal is thick and infiltrated. In the posterosuperior part of the canal, the skin is absent and the bone is denuded.

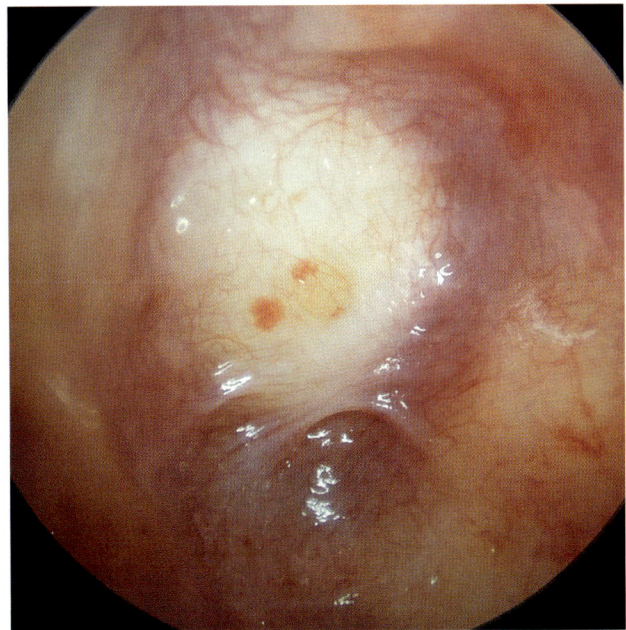

Figure 14.**43** Retrotympanic cholesteatoma following myringoplasty. This iatrogenic cholesteatoma can be explained by the entrapment of epidermal residues in the middle ear or malpositioning of the meatal flap at the level of the anterior angle. It can be managed by incision of the cholesteatoma sac, aspiration of its contents, and insertion of a plastic sheet into the external auditory canal for about 20 days to favor healing.

Tympanoplasty

Tympanoplasty operations can be classified into those without mastoidectomy, performed with chronic otitis media in which the tympanic membrane perforation is associated with necrosis of the ossicular chain, and those with mastoidectomy, performed in chronic suppurative otitis media with cholesteatoma. As mentioned previously, tympanoplasty with mastoidectomy can be either closed or open.

In closed tympanoplasty, the posterior wall of the external auditory canal is kept intact. This technique is employed in children and in patients with very pneumatized mastoids, to avoid having a large cavity. Regular otoscopic follow-up is essential to identify the formation of a retraction pocket or a recurrent cholesteatoma. Should these occur, there should be no hesitation in switching to an open technique.

In open tympanoplasty, the posterior wall of the external auditory canal is removed. The indications of this technique in the treatment of cholesteatoma include: a wide erosion of the posterosuperior wall, cholesteatoma in the only hearing ear, bilateral cholesteatoma, cholesteatoma in patients with Down's syndrome, the presence of a contracted mastoid, a large labyrinthine fistula, and recurrent cholesteatoma following a closed tympanoplasty. Because the posterior canal wall is removed, the mastoid cavity is exteriorized and on otoscopy the external auditory canal and the mastoid appear as one communicating cavity. If properly performed, the cavity appears rounded in shape, dry, and well epithelialized. On the other hand, a badly performed cavity may appear wet, irregular, and be lined with granulation tissue in addition to accumulated debris. There may also be the possibility of a residual cholesteatoma.

In cases of tympanoplasty, it is usually possible to see the reconstructed ossicular chain through the tympanic membrane. We generally prefer to utilize an autologous or homologous incus for reconstruction. In our experience (more than 1000 tympanoplasties) we have never encountered any case of extrusion when the incus was used. In contrast, variable rates of extrusion were noticed when biological materials (e.g., plastipore, ceramics, hydroxyapatite) were utilized. Although the use of homologous ossicles has never been proven to transmit slow viruses (e.g., Creutzfeldt–Jakob disease), the theoretical risk makes it more prudent to use predominantly autologous tissue or biomaterial of better characteristics that might appear in the future.

Later on in this chapter, some otoscopic views of cases managed by the modified Bondy technique are shown. This is an open technique indicated in epitympanic cholesteatoma with a good preoperative hearing in which the tympanic membrane and the ossicular chain are intact. Some cases of radical mastoidectomy are also shown. This technique is used mainly in elderly patients with sensorineural hearing loss, in whom the only goal of surgery is to have a dry and safe ear.

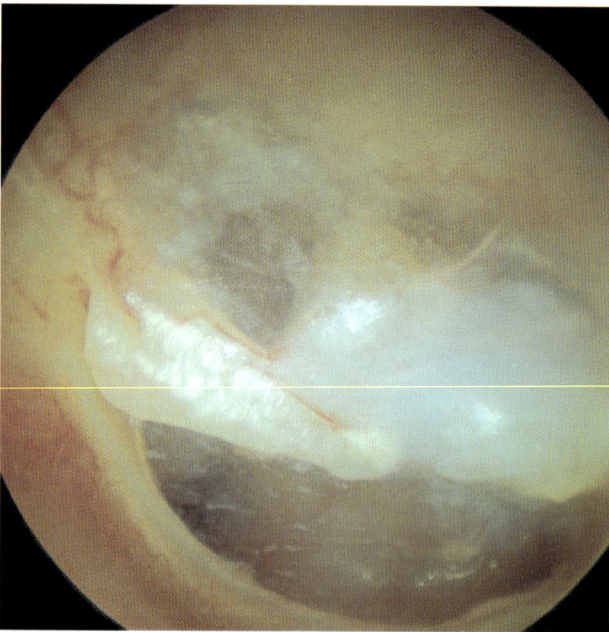

Figure 14.**44** Left ear. The sculptured incus is visible under the handle of the malleus. The reconstructed tympanic membrane appears very thin but intact. The anterior angle is perfect. A piece of cartilage placed over the incus is clearly visible.

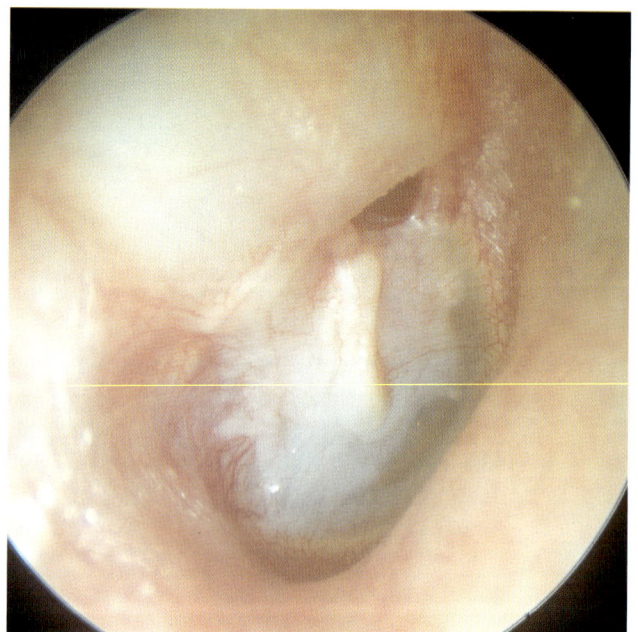

Figure 14.**45** Right ear. Staged closed tympanoplasty. The tympanic membrane has a normal angle and is well attached to the handle of the malleus. The cartilage used for reconstructing the attic is visible. In this region, a small self-cleaning retraction pocket can be seen.

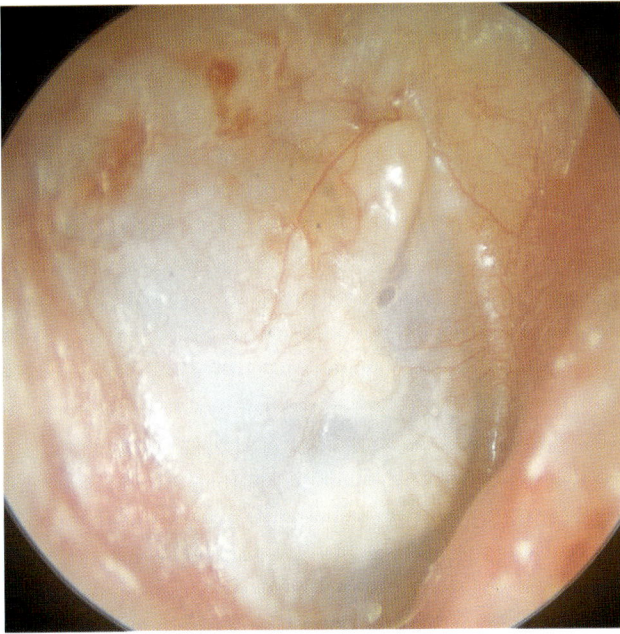

Figure 14.**46** Right ear. Staged closed tympanoplasty performed 10 years previously for the management of a cholesteatoma. The tympanic membrane is whitish, slightly thicker than normal, but retains a good anterior angle. The annulus is well seen anteriorly. The handle of the malleus is in a good position. There are no signs of resorption of the posterior canal wall.

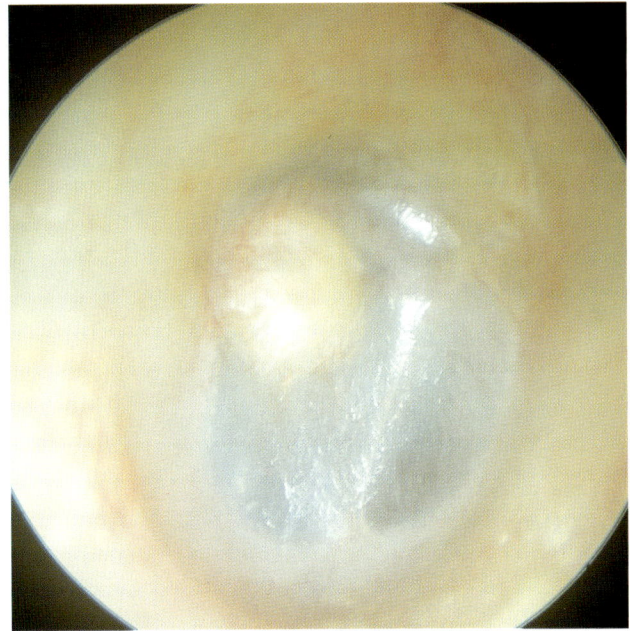

Figure 14.**47** Right ear with a previous tympanoplasty. The tympanic membrane is thin with mild blunting. The sculptured incus is visible.

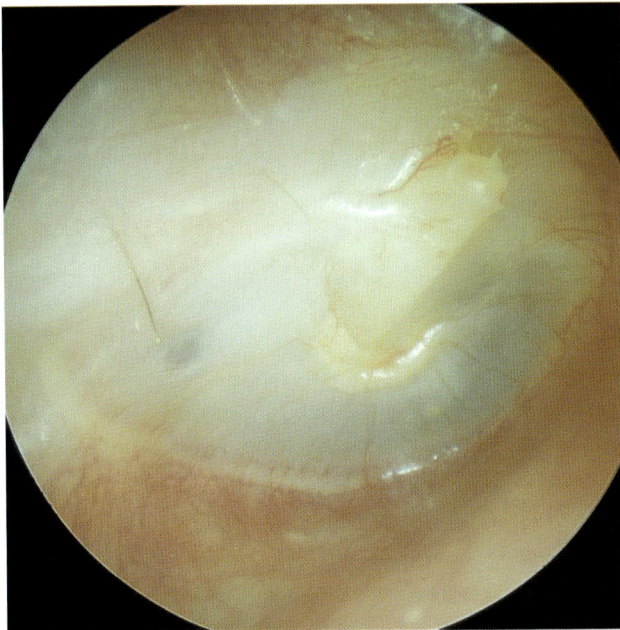

Figure 14.**48** Right ear. Otoscopic view after a second-stage tympanoplasty in which the incus was used for ossiculoplasty. The tympanic membrane and the handle of the malleus are excellently positioned.

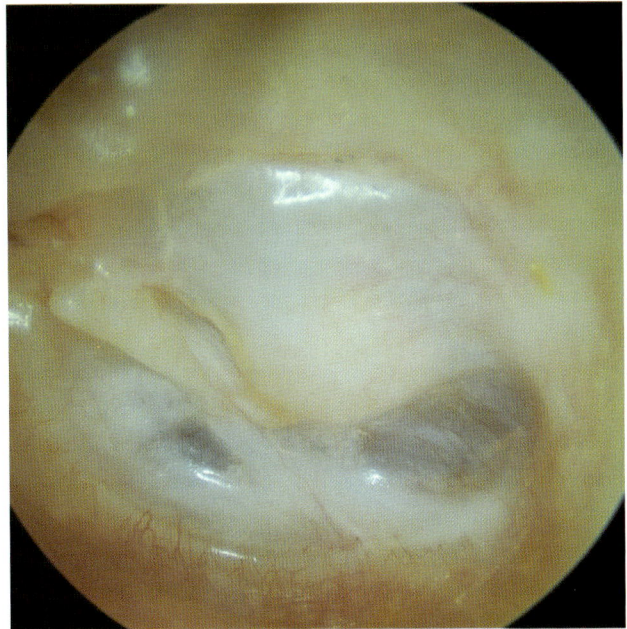

Figure 14.**49** Left ear. Perfect reconstructed tympanic membrane with optimal thickness and no blunting. The sculptured incus is in contact with the handle of the malleus. It is slightly elevated with respect to the level of the tympanic membrane.

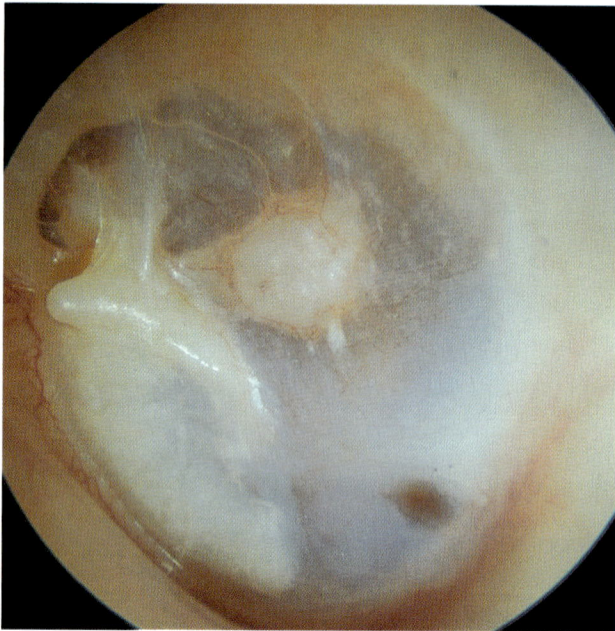

Figure 14.**50**   Left ear. Another example of the incus positioned under the handle of the malleus.

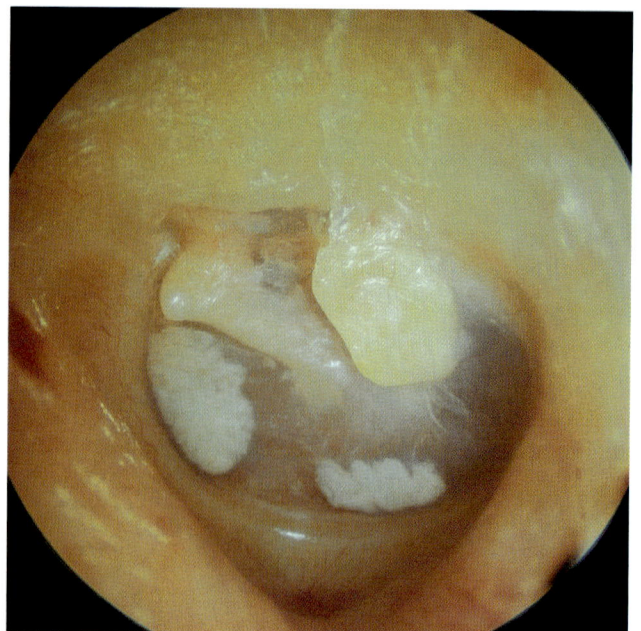

Figure 14.**51**   Left ear. Ossiculoplasty. The tympanic membrane is retracted and the malleus is medialized. The sculptured incus is displaced posteriorly and is adherent to the posterior mesotympanum. Two tympanosclerotic plaques are noted anteriorly and inferiorly.

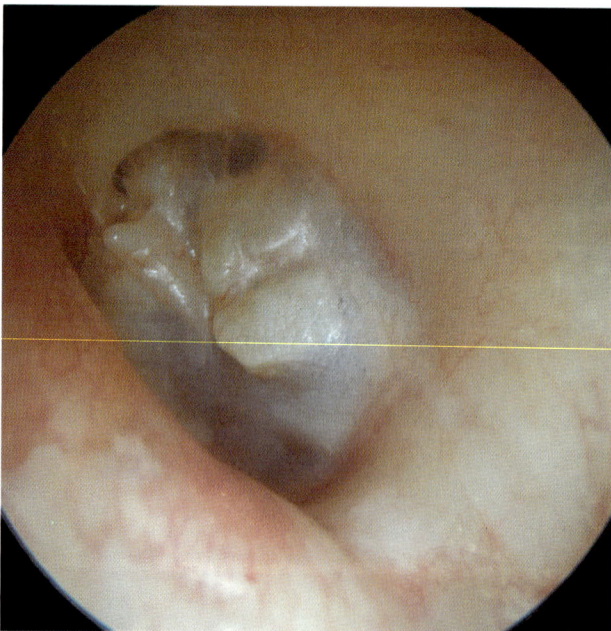

Figure 14.**52**   Left ear. Posteriorly displaced incus that was used for ossiculoplasty. The trough created on the incus to fit the handle of the malleus is clearly seen. Revision surgery is necessary to reposition the displaced incus and improve the patient's hearing.

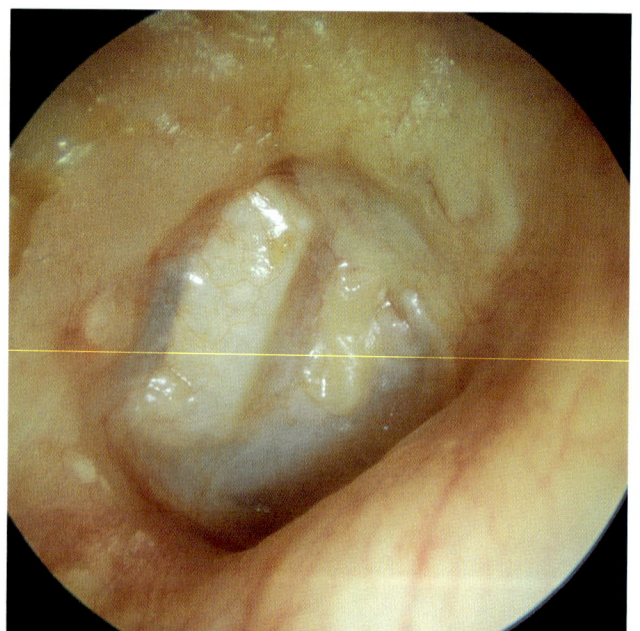

Figure 14.**53**   Right ear. Slightly retracted reconstructed tympanic membrane. A T-shaped columella from homologous cartilage is visible. The columella has been placed between the tympanic membrane and the footplate of the stapes.

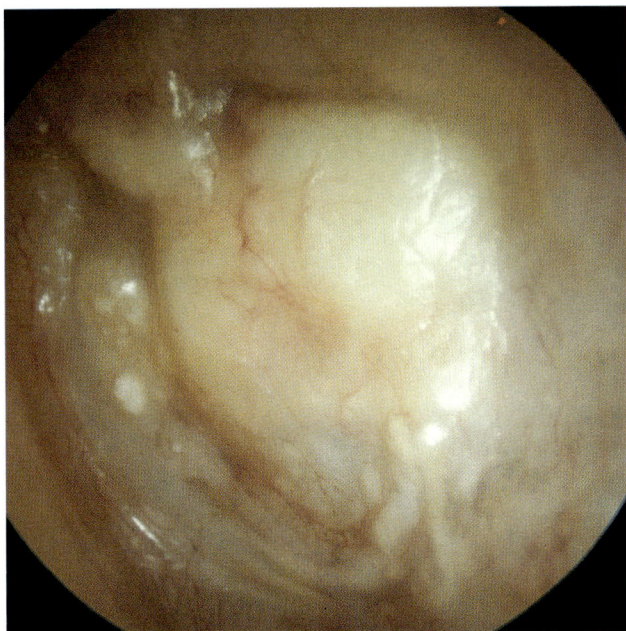

Figure 14.**54** Left ear. Ossiculoplasty. A piece of cartilage that was interposed between the reconstructed ossicular chain and the tympanic membrane can be visualized. It appears as a whitish thick mass that causes elevation of the posterior quadrants of the tympanic membrane.

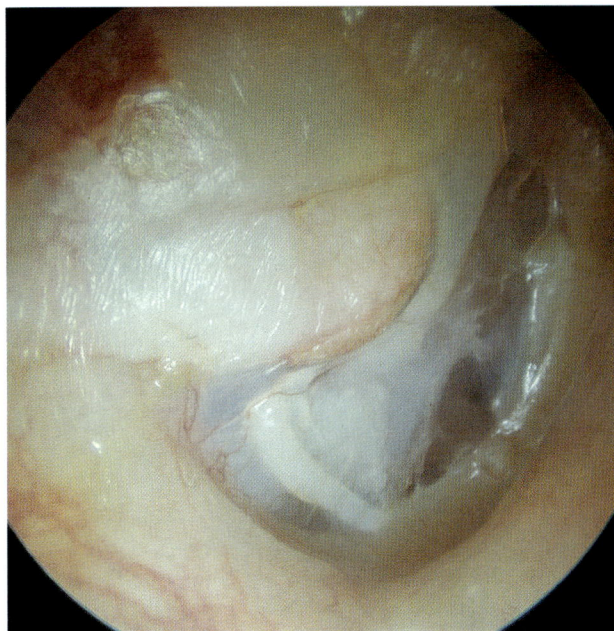

Figure 14.**55** Right ear. Closed tympanoplasty. Sculptured incus in a perfect position under the reconstructed tympanic membrane. The cartilage used to reconstruct the postero-superior wall of the external auditory canal is also visible.

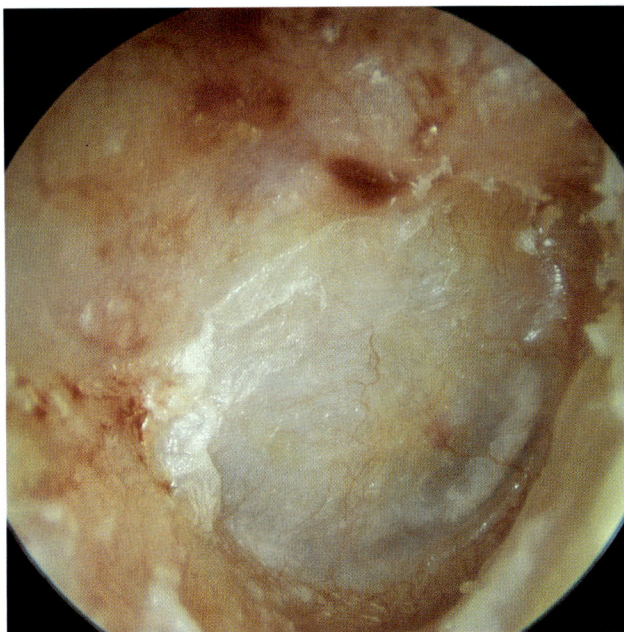

Figure 14.**56** Right ear. Post tympanoplasty. Good position of the tympanic membrane. In this case, it is difficult to identify the type of ossicular chain reconstruction due to the thickness of the tympanic membrane, particularly noted at its posterior quadrants.

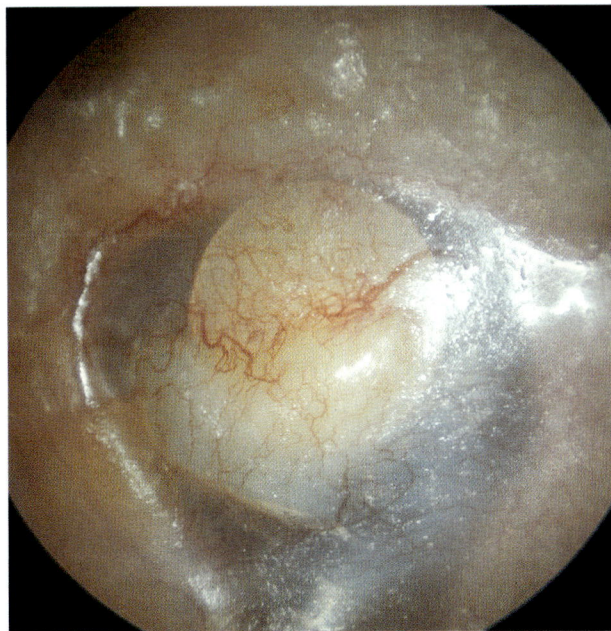

Figure 14.**57** Left ear. In the posterosuperior quadrant a TORP (total ossicular replacement prosthesis) with its circular head is noted. The overlying cartilage is partially resorbed. There are no signs of extrusion.

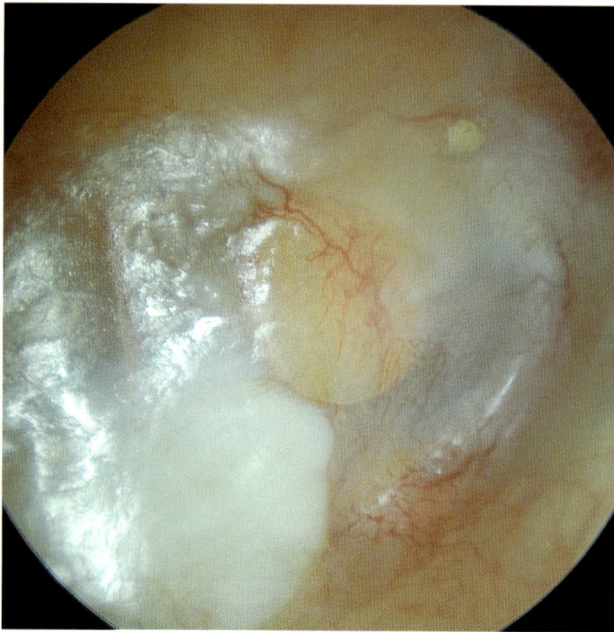

Figure 14.**58**   Right ear. Another example of a TORP that is visible through the tympanic membrane. The overlying cartilage, which is whitish in color, has been displaced into the posteroinferior quadrant. There are no signs of extrusion.

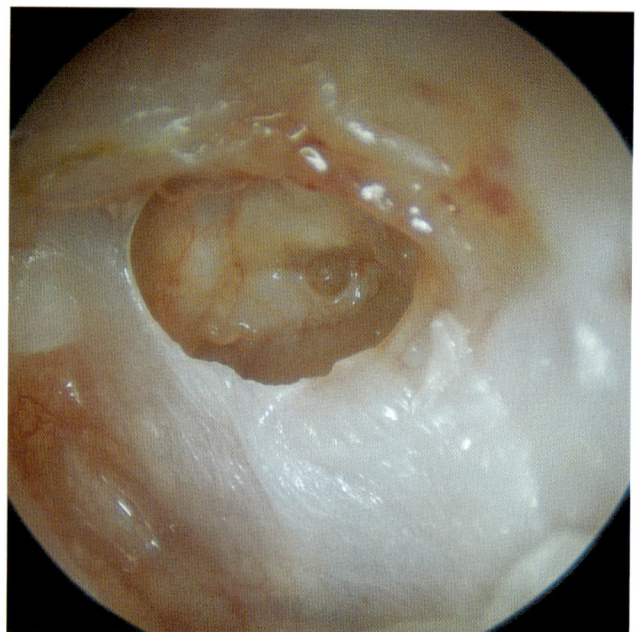

Figure 14.**59**   Left ear. Posterosuperior perforation of the reconstructed tympanic membrane with extrusion of the TORP. The shaft of the prosthesis has caused an erosion of the footplate of the stapes (which appears through the perforation as a rounded dark area).

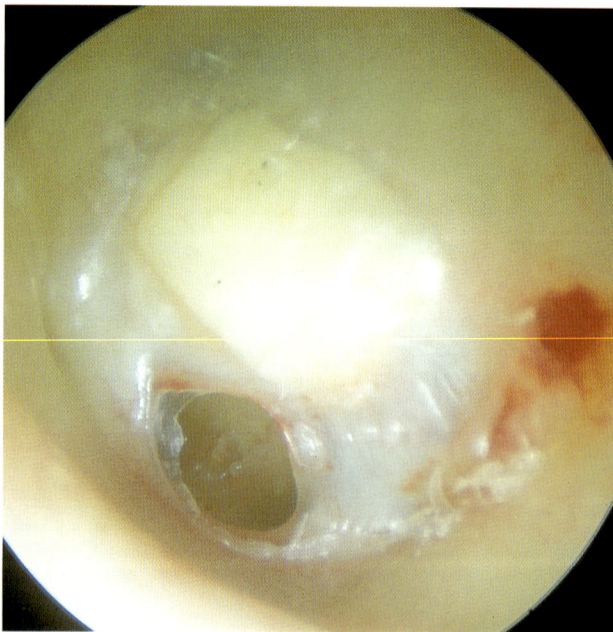

Figure 14.**60**   Left ear. Anteroinferior reperforation due to an acute otitis media, occurring 3 years after a staged closed tympanoplasty. A rectangular cartilage used for ossiculoplasty is visible. The cartilage is well integrated in the tympanic membrane residue.

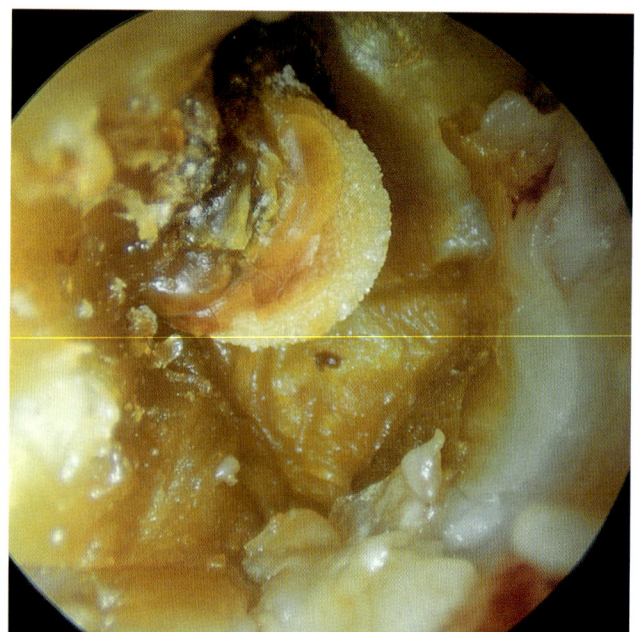

Figure 14.**61**   Right ear. An example of TORP extrusion that occurred 1 year after a second-stage tympanoplasty. The head of the prosthesis can be seen despite the surrounding wax. The tympanic membrane residue is atelectatic.

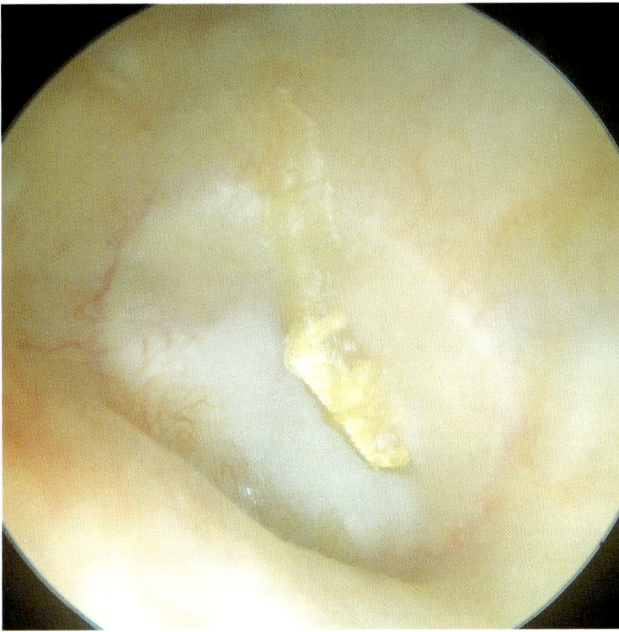

Figure 14.**62** Left ear. Gold prosthesis in the process of extrusion in a staged closed tympanoplasty.

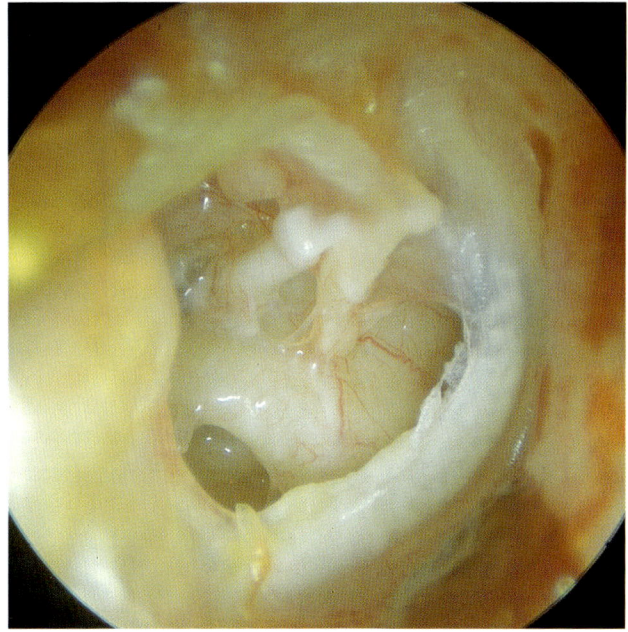

Figure 14.**63** Right ear. Post tympanoplasty. Large reperforation. In the posterosuperior quadrant a Teflon prosthesis is interposed between the medialized malleus and the footplate of the stapes. The round window is visible in the postero- inferior quadrant. The anterior residue of the tympanic membrane is tympanosclerotic.

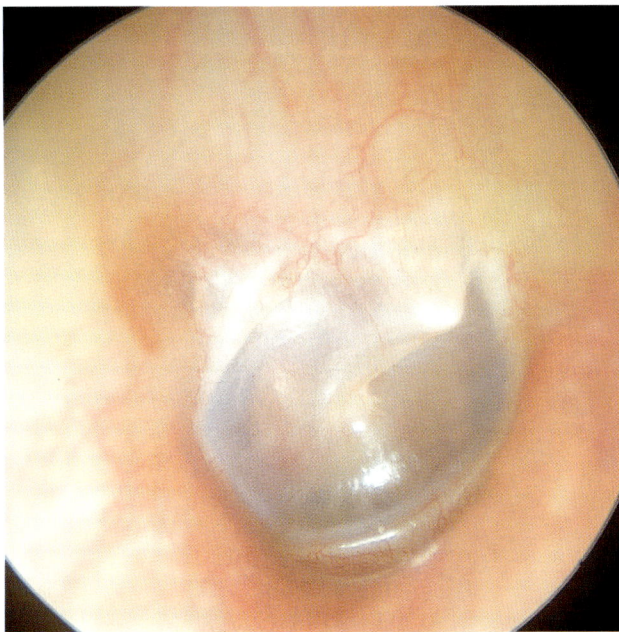

Figure 14.**64** Right ear. Post stapedectomy. The atticotomy is seen in the posterosuperior quadrant. The preserved chorda tympani is well visualized.

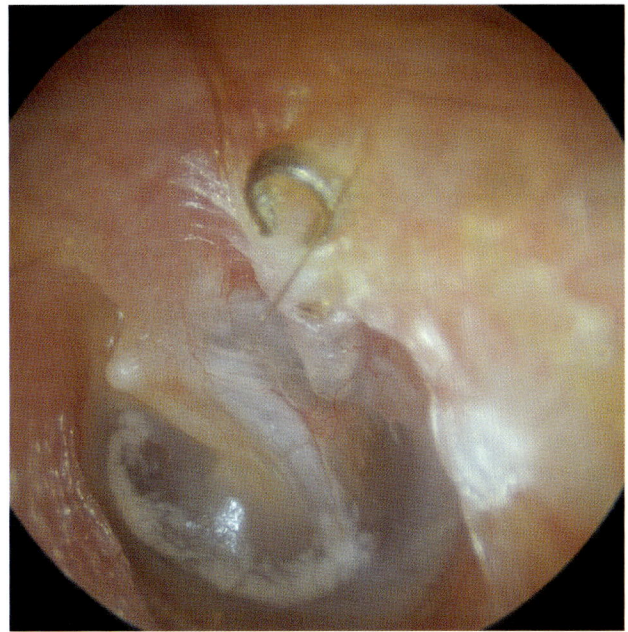

Figure 14.**65** Left ear. A rare case of extrusion of a stapes prosthesis. The metallic ring is seen extruding through a microperforation covered with epidermal squames. The Teflon shaft of the prosthesis can be visualized through the tympanic membrane.

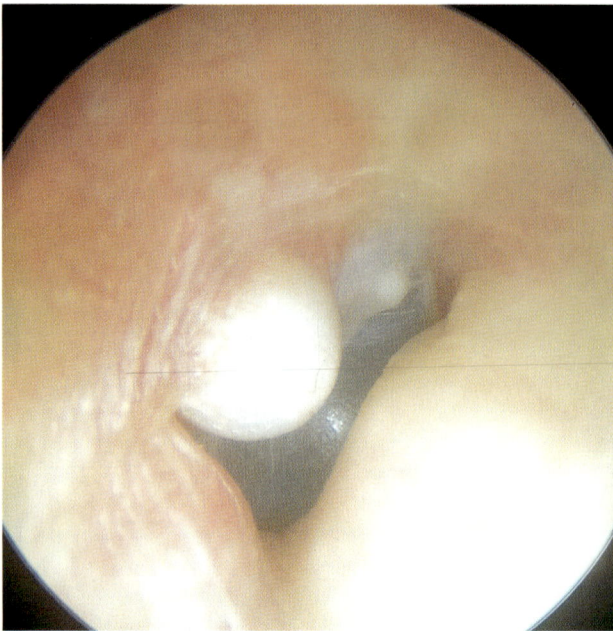

Figure 14.**66**   Right ear. A cholesteatomatous pearl in the external auditory canal in a patient who had previously undergone a stapedectomy. The tympanomeatal flap was not correctly repositioned. This skin was thus folded in on itself and the entrapped epithelium gave rise to this pearl. This complication was easily resolved in the outpatient clinic by incising the skin (see Fig. 14.**67**) and removing the cholesteatomatous cyst (see Fig. 14.**68**).

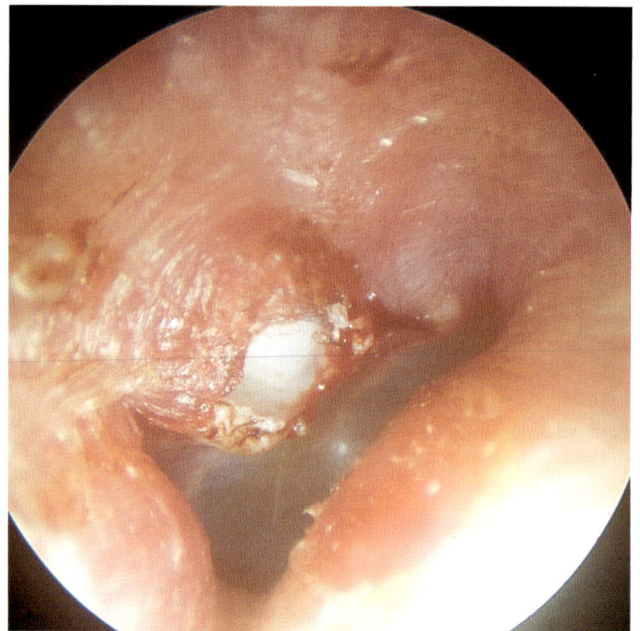

Figure 14.**67**   Incision of the skin over the cyst.

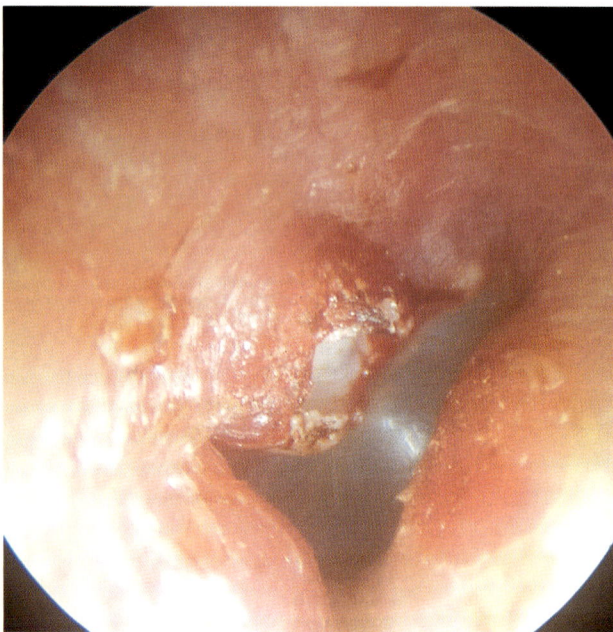

Figure 14.**68**   Removal of the cholesteatomatous cyst.

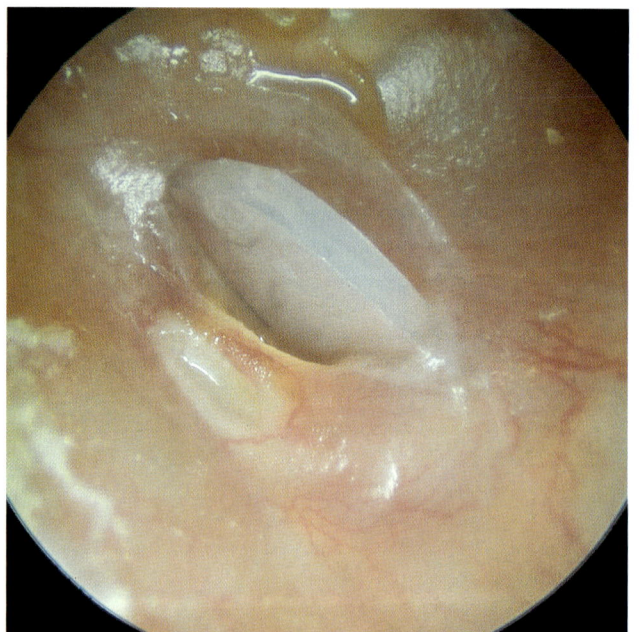

Figure 14.**69**   Left ear. Silastic sheet in extrusion through a posterosuperior perforation. The handle of the malleus is clearly visible anteriorly. In general, Silastic is inserted in first-stage tympanoplasty. This material is usually placed in the middle ear to favor the restoration of the normal mucosal lining of the middle ear and to avoid the formation of adhesions in the meantime. It is removed during the second-stage tympanoplasty, except in cases showing a tendency towards atelectasis.

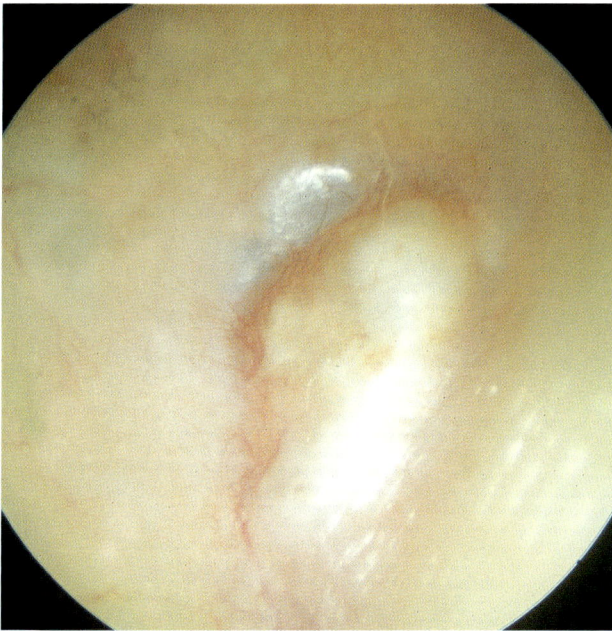

Figure 14.**70**   Right ear. Post tympanoplasty. A white retrotympanic mass (cholesteatoma of the anterior angle) is noted, causing bulging of the tympanic membrane. The cholesteatoma is probably the result of inadequate removal of the epithelium in an overlay technique. The entrapped skin led to the formation of the cholesteatoma.

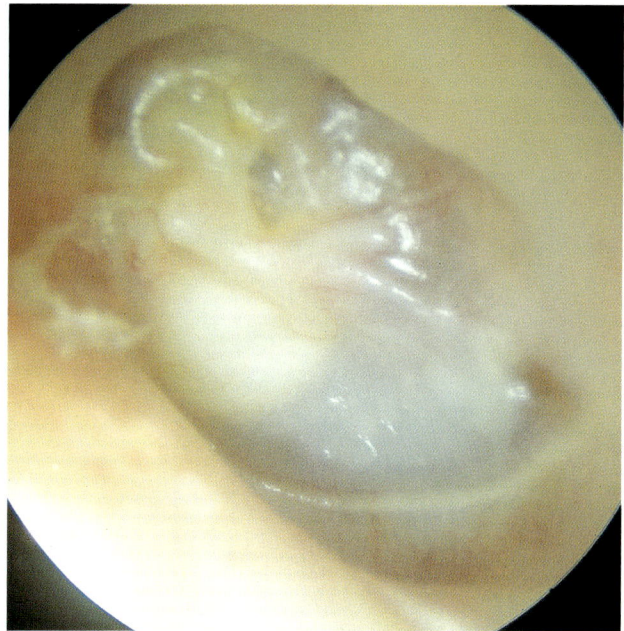

Figure 14.**71**   Left ear. Good anterior angle of the reconstructed tympanic membrane. An anteromalleolar choleste-atomatous cyst is seen. An epitympanic retraction pocket that is adherent to the head of the malleus and body of the incus is also observed.

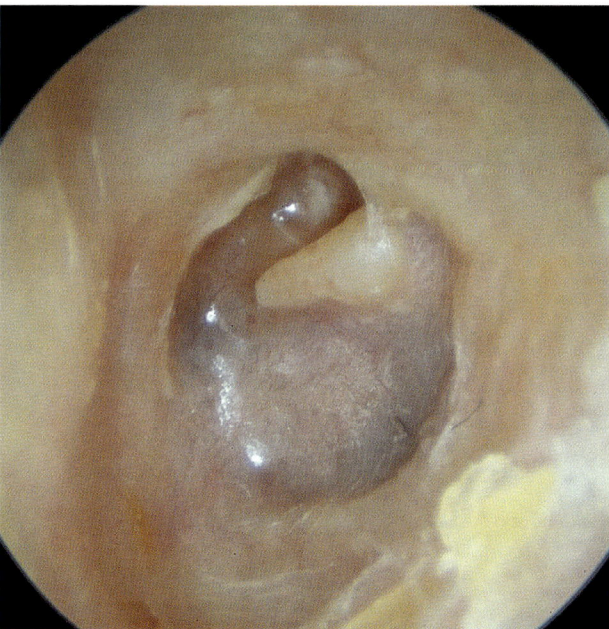

Figure 14.**72**   Left ear. In the posterosuperior quadrant, the sculptured incus with the short process pointing anteriorly is seen through the retracted tympanic membrane. In patients with hearing loss, repeat surgery is indicated to reinforce the tympanic membrane and improve the hearing. Surgery entails dissection of the retraction pocket from the incus, and the placement of cartilage between the sculptured incus and the tympanic membrane. This cartilage prevents (or delays) the reformation of a retraction pocket and corrects the hearing deficit.

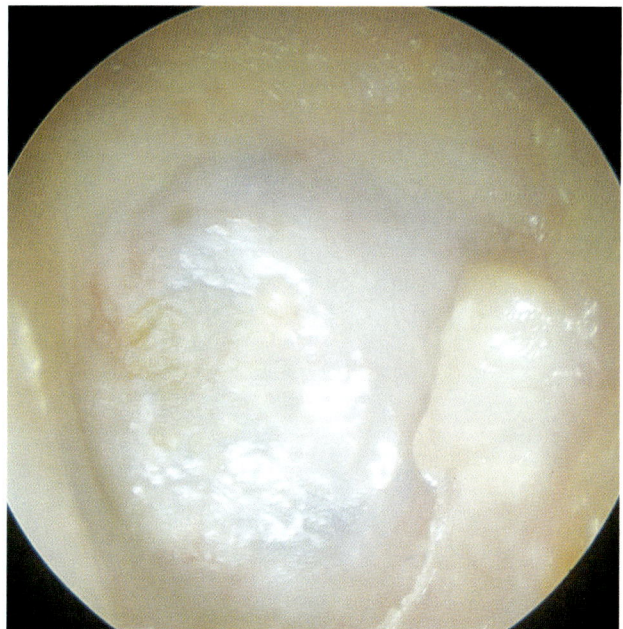

Figure 14.**73**   Left ear. Another example of retraction of the tympanic membrane leading to inclination of the sculptured incus. The dislocated incus becomes fixed to the posterior mesotympanum, resulting in hearing loss.

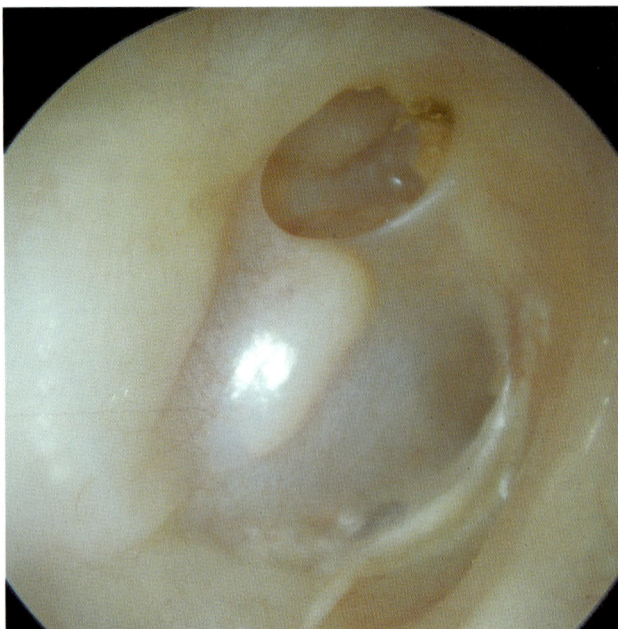

Figure 14.**74** Right ear. Sculptured incus seen through the tympanic membrane in a case of closed tympanoplasty. An epitympanic retraction pocket is seen. This pocket should be followed up regularly to guard against the formation of a recurrent cholesteatoma. Should this occur, the closed technique must be transformed into an open one to avoid further recurrence of the cholesteatoma.

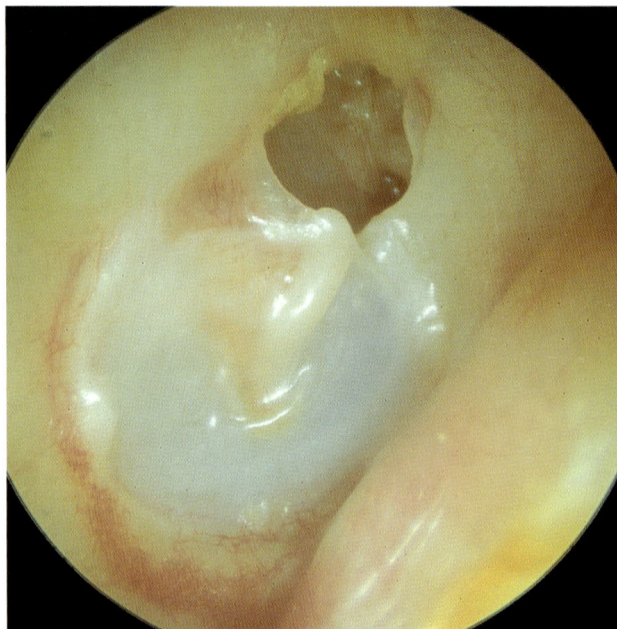

Figure 14.**75** Right ear. Recurrent epitympanic cholestea-toma following closed tympanoplasty. The reconstructed tympanic membrane (pars tensa) shows an optimal anterior angle and is perfectly attached to the handle of the malleus. In this case, transformation to an open technique is indicated, while conserving the tympanic membrane and ossicular chain if there is no hearing loss.

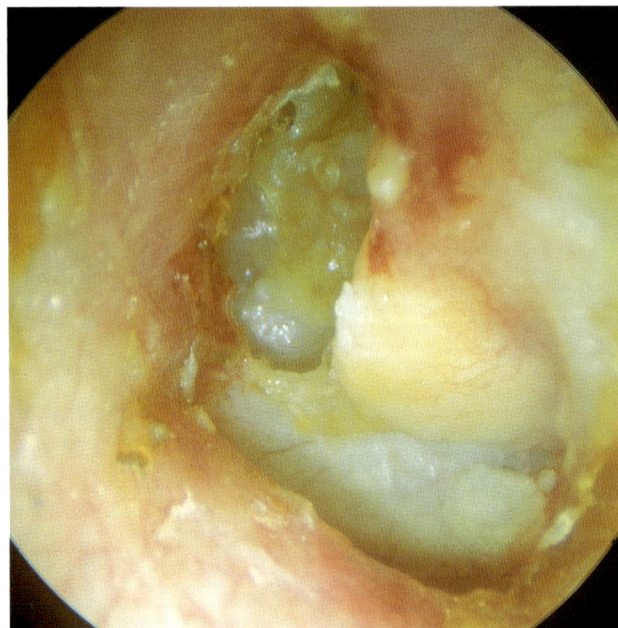

Figure 14.**76** Left ear. Another example of a staged closed tympanoplasty 6 years after the second stage. A large resorption of the posterosuperior wall of the external auditory canal associated with recurrent cholesteatoma is observed. In the posterosuperior quadrant, the cartilage used for ossiculoplasty is seen. Revision surgery was performed with transformation into an open technique.

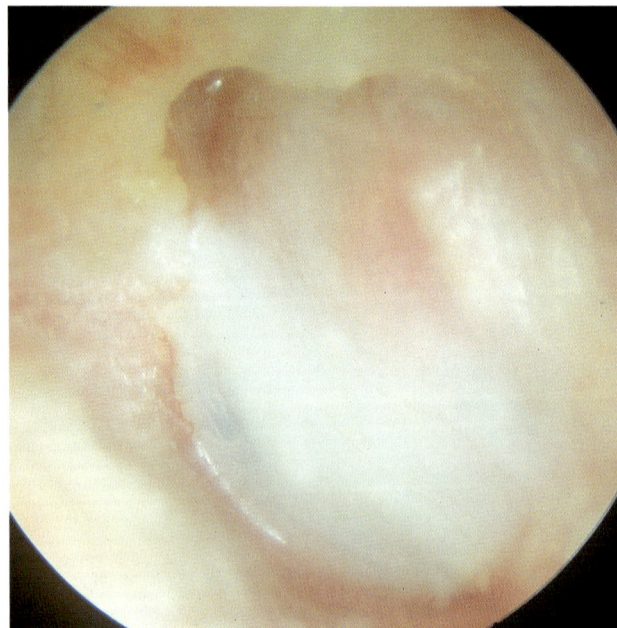

Figure 14.**77** Left ear. A small epitympanic retraction pocket is observed. Though small and shallow, this pocket should be followed up regularly as it may become deeper with time, leading to the formation of a recurrent cholesteatoma.

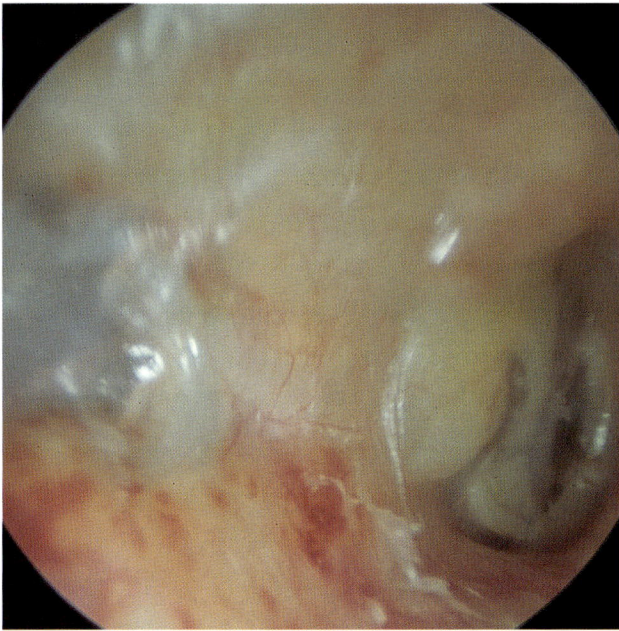

Figure 14.**78**   Right ear. Partial resorption of the posterior wall of the external auditory canal about 7 to 8 mm from the annulus following a closed tympanoplasty. The atrophic area appears bluish due to lack of underlying bone. No cutaneous retraction is seen. However, due to the lack of bone, the skin can invaginate into the mastoid cavity giving rise to recurrent cholesteatoma. In such cases, regular long-term follow-up is indicated.

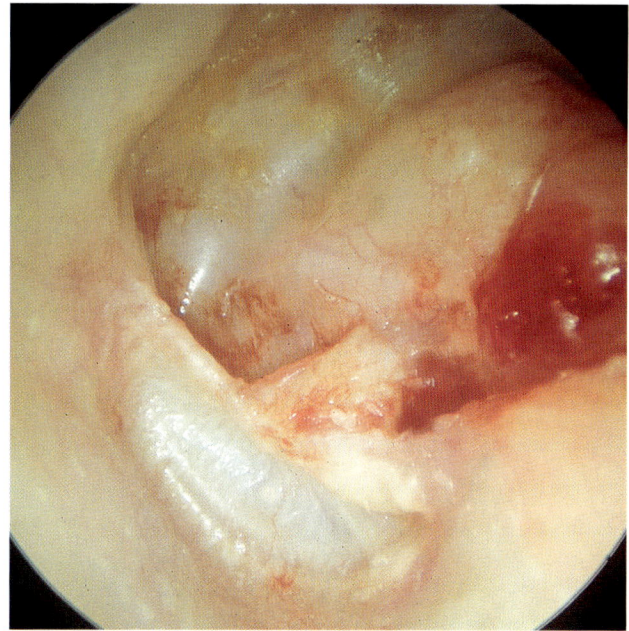

Figure 14.**79**   Left ear. Total resorption of the posterior wall of the external auditory canal 3 years after a closed tympanoplasty. The otoscopic view is similar to that observed after an open tympanoplasty. Repeat surgery was necessary. The facial ridge was lowered and all bony irregularities were smoothed to avoid the retention of squamous debris with subsequent otorrhea. An adequate meatoplasty was also performed.

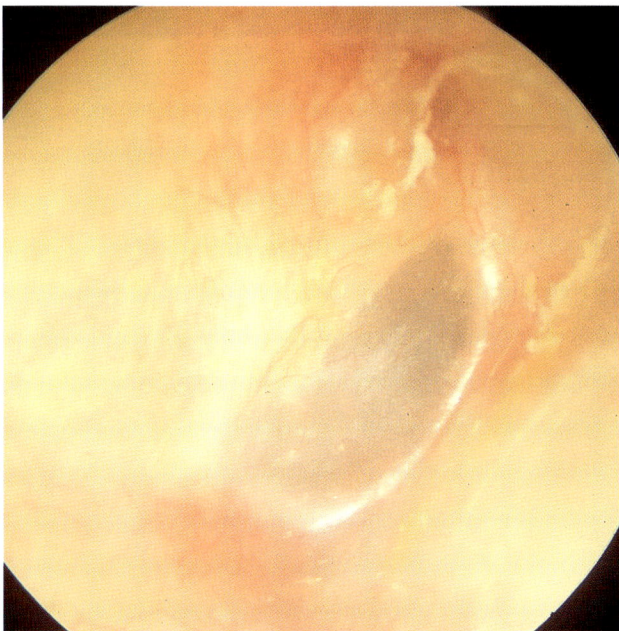

Figure 14.**80**   Right ear. An example of a successful closed tympanoplasty 11 years postoperatively. The tympanic membrane is in perfect position and angulation. The posterior canal wall is intact, and there is no evidence of recurrent cholesteatoma (see previous cases in Figs. 14.**78** and 14.**79**).

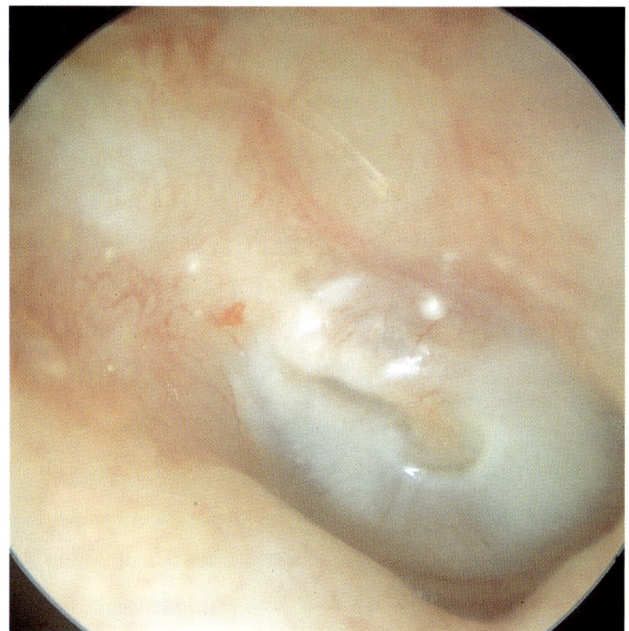

Figure 14.**81**   Left ear. Another example of a closed tympanoplasty 2 years postoperatively. The attic was reconstructed using cartilage and bone paste and shows no signs of erosion. A small cholesteatomatous pearl is seen in the posterosuperior quadrant. It can be easily removed in the outpatient clinic under microscopic control.

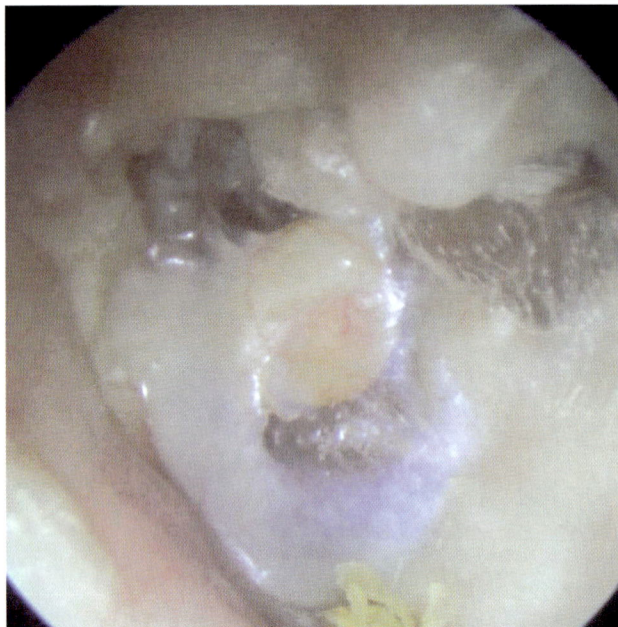

Figure 14.**82** Left ear. A staged closed tympanoplasty after 10 years. A total ossicular replacement prosthesis (TORP) is seen. The overlying cartilage has been partially resorbed. There is no sign of extrusion.

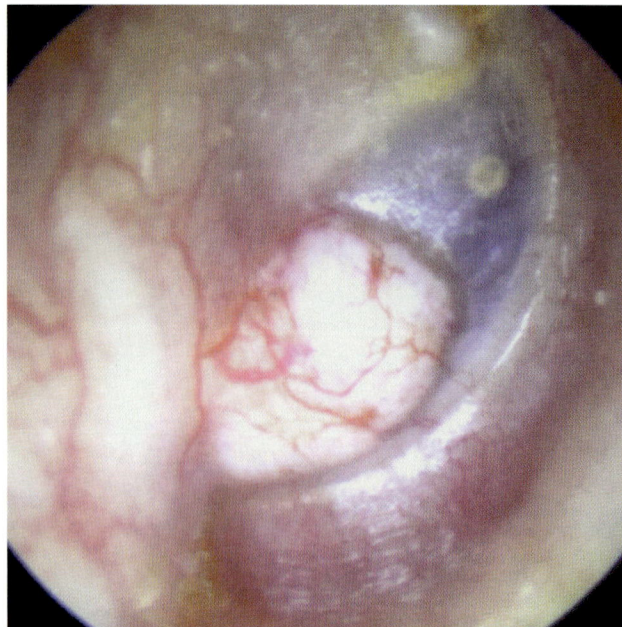

Figure 14.**83** Right ear. Closed tympanoplasty. A bulging residual pearl of cholesteatoma is present.

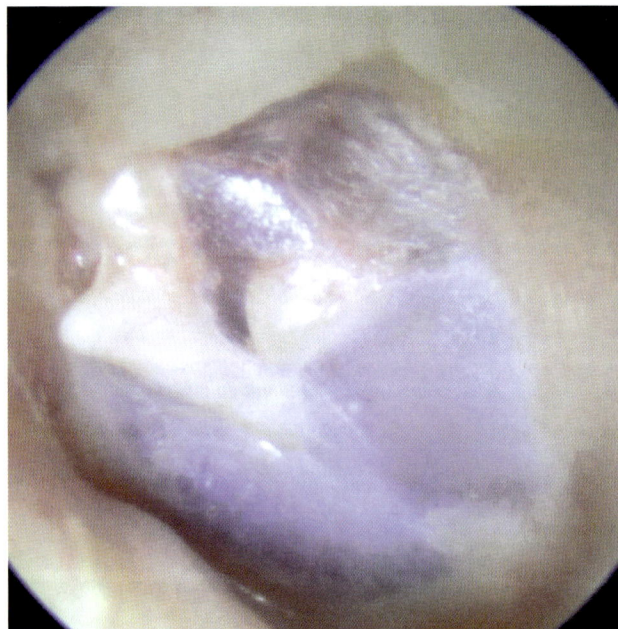

Figure 14.**84** Left ear. A staged closed tympanoplasty with underlay reconstruction of tympanic membrane. An autologous molded incus, positioned between the handle of the malleus and the head of the stapes, has been used.

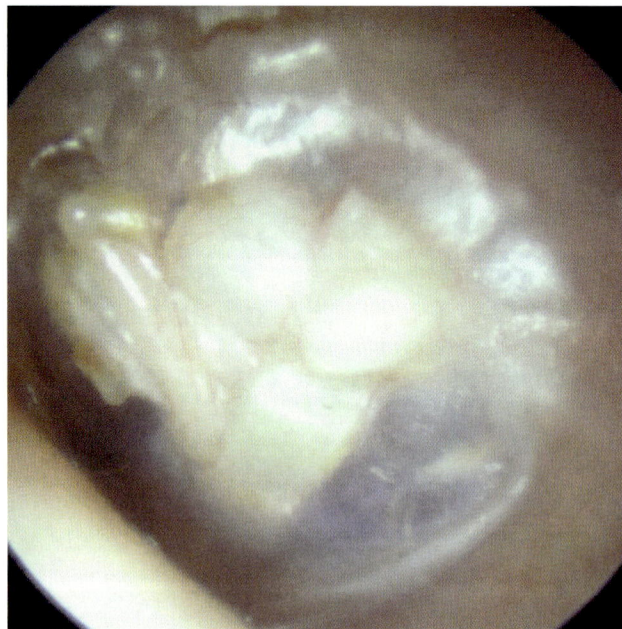

Figure 14.**85** Left ear. Staged closed tympanoplasty. Homologous cartilage has been used to reconstruct the ossicular chain. The new chain is dislocated, and a residual pearl is seen anterior to the malleus. In this case, revision surgery is required to remove the residual pearl.

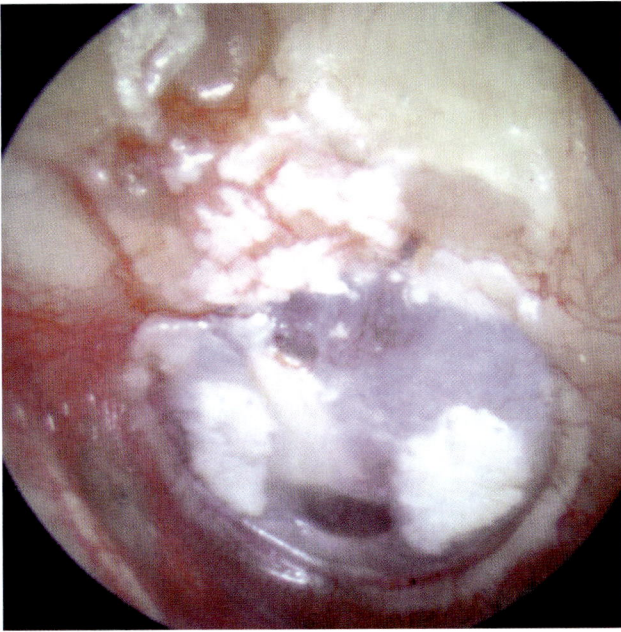

Figure 14.**86** Left ear. An example of closed tympanoplasty, with a very well-positioned tympanic membrane. The attic was reconstructed with cartilage and bone paste.

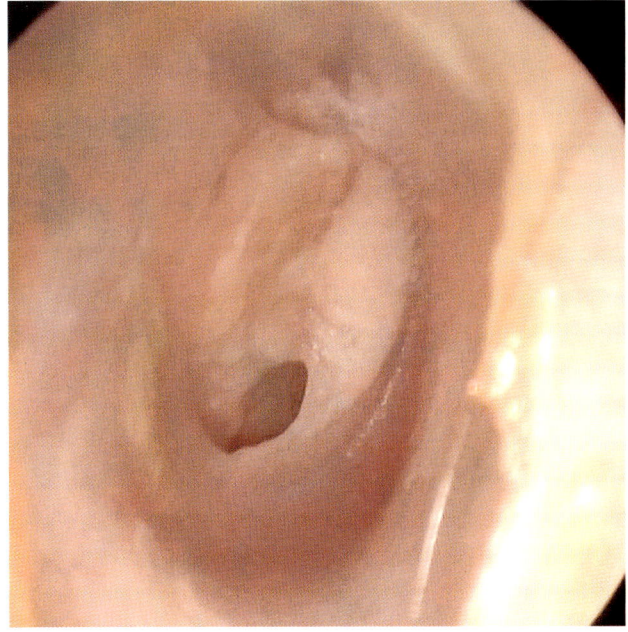

Figure 14.**87** Preoperative image in a patient with an inferior perforation and tympanosclerotic pearl in the anterior quadrants.

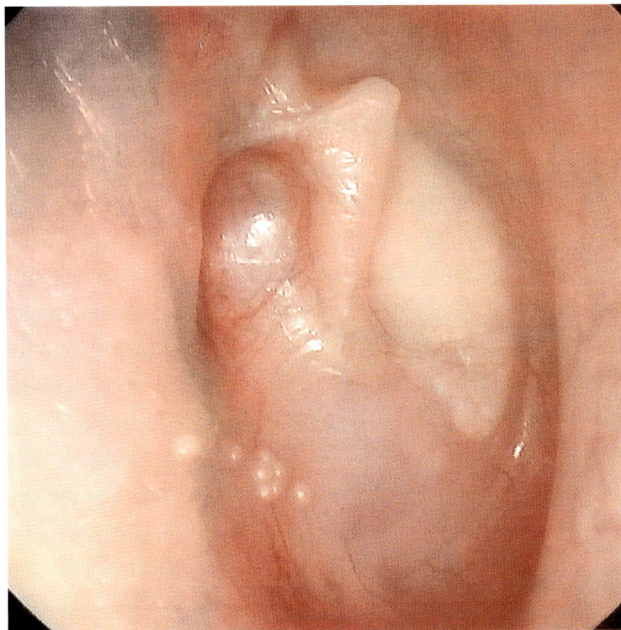

Figure 14.**88** The same patient, 1 year postoperatively. A small retraction pocket is present.

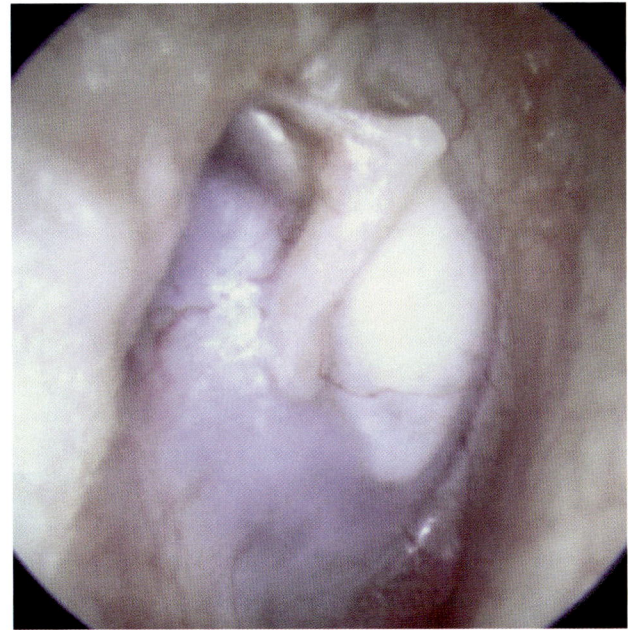

Figure 14.**89** The same patient, 2 years postoperatively. There is a retromalleolar residual cholesteatoma pearl.

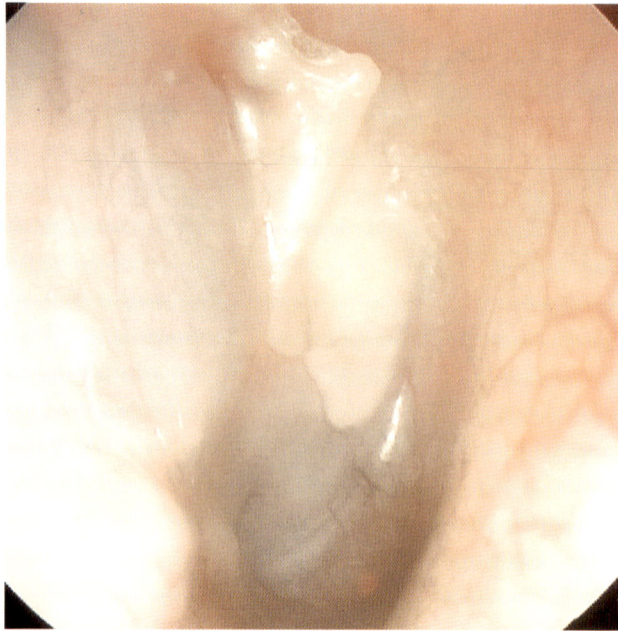

Figure 14.**90** After removal of the cholesteatoma, the posterior quadrants have been reinforced with cartilage.

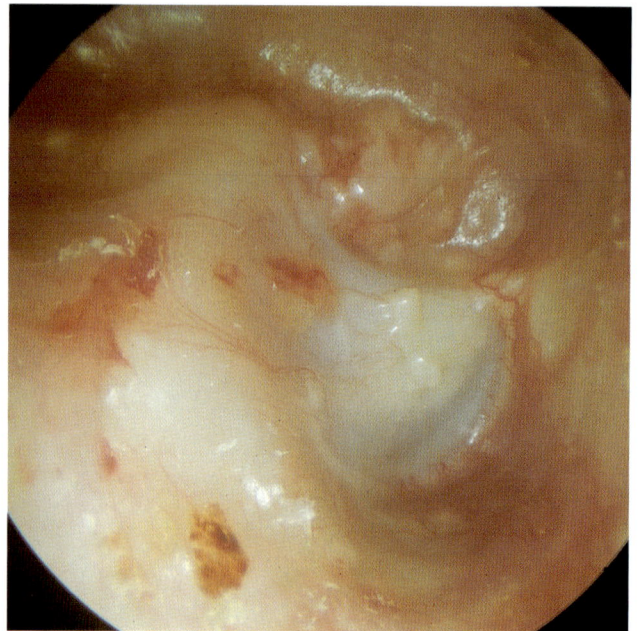

Figure 14.**91** Right ear. A well performed open tympanoplasty. The cavity is epithelialized and the facial ridge is adequately lowered. In the attic region, the material used for obliteration can be noted.

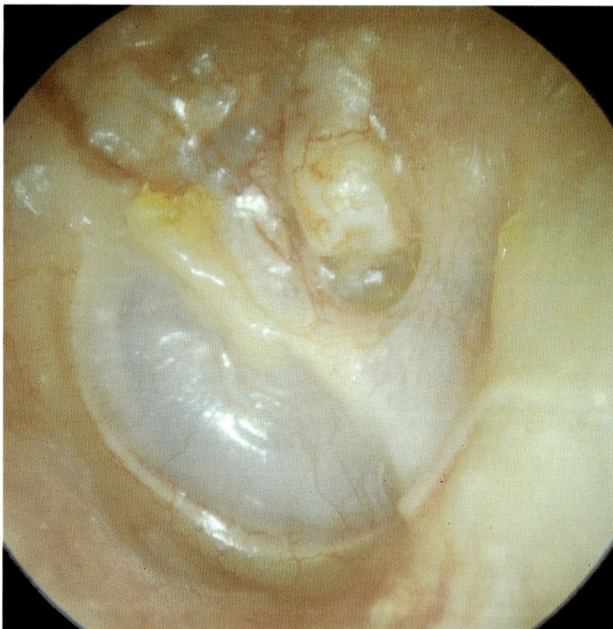

Figure 14.**92** Left ear. Open tympanoplasty. Attic obliteration with autologous bone.

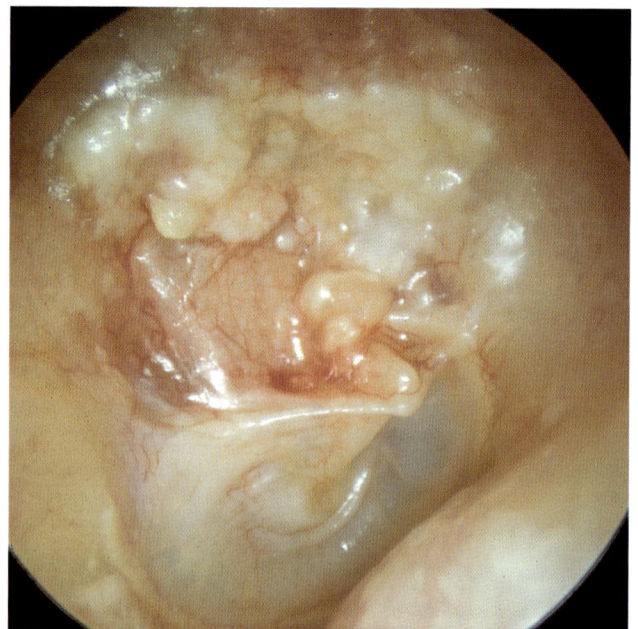

Figure 14.**93** Right ear. Open tympanoplasty. Partial obliteration of the attic with bone paste.

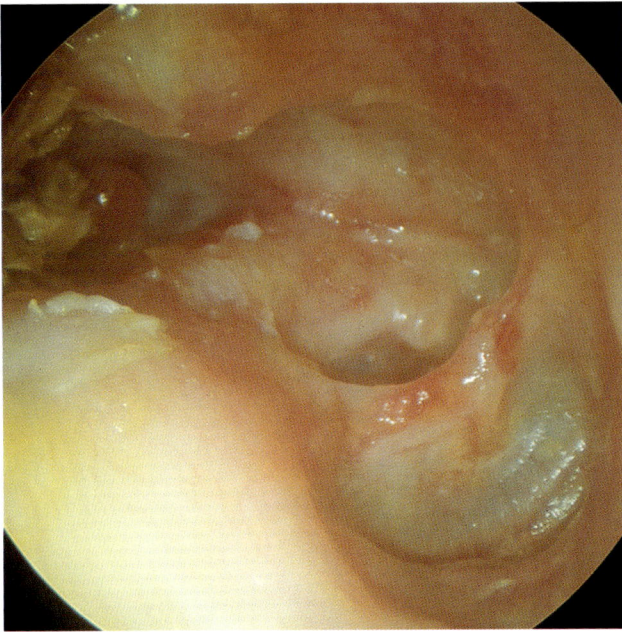

Figure 14.**94**　Right ear. A patient with bilateral cholesteatoma. An open tympanoplasty with obliteration was performed. The material used for obliteration of the attic (cartilage and bone paste) has nearly totally resorbed. The cavity is humid, granulating, and wet. Hearing is poorer than that of the other side, in which an open technique without obliteration was performed (see next figure).

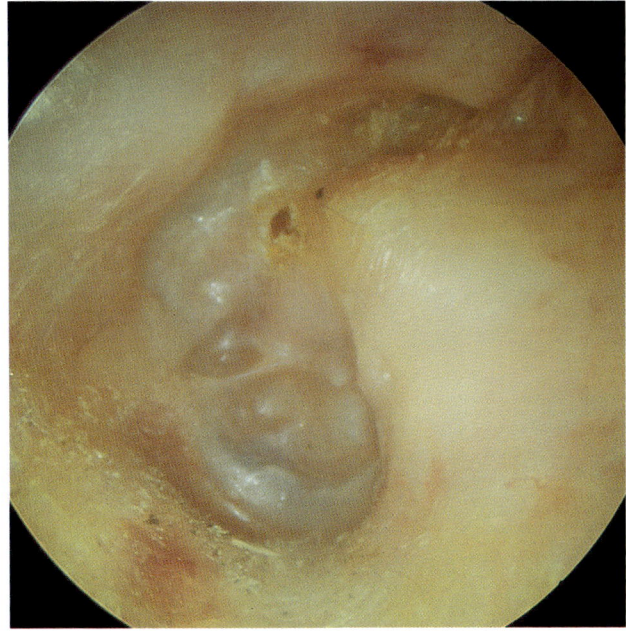

Figure 14.**95**　Same patient, left ear. The cavity is dry, smooth, well epithelialized, and the facial ridge is low.

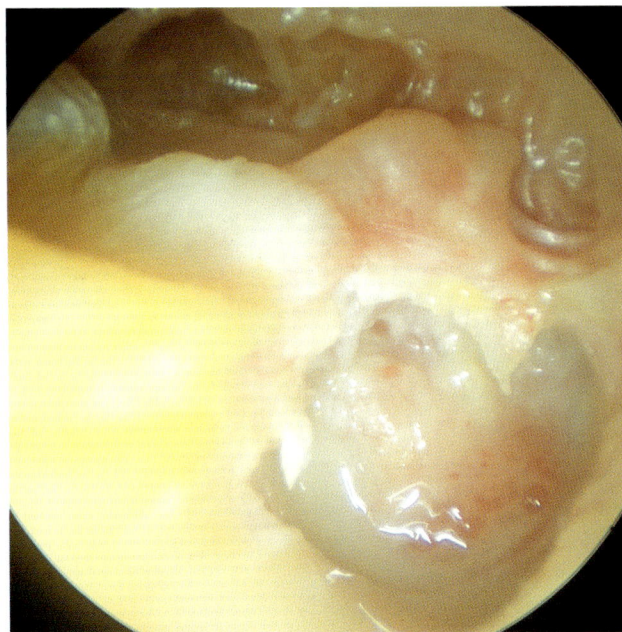

Figure 14.**96**　Right ear. A badly performed open tympanoplasty. The cavity is irregular, with undermined borders, and a very high facial ridge. Purulent secretion is present in the middle ear and the rest of the cavity.

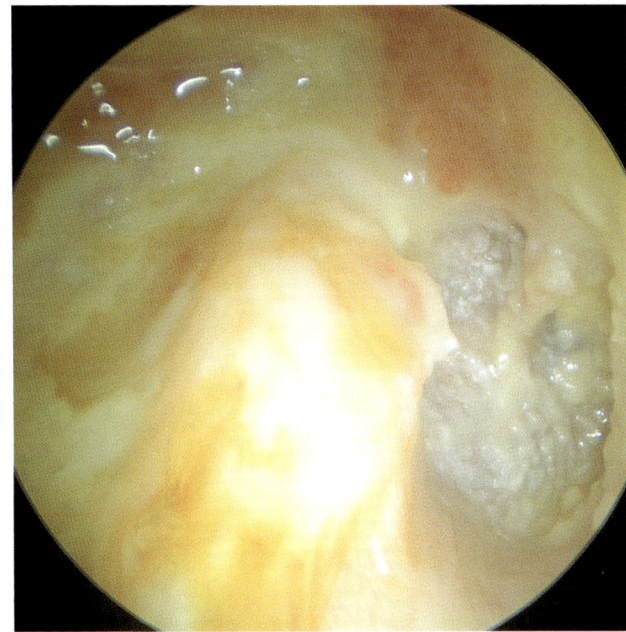

Figure 14.**97**　Right ear. Another example of a badly performed open tympanoplasty. Purulent secretions and a high facial ridge are observed.

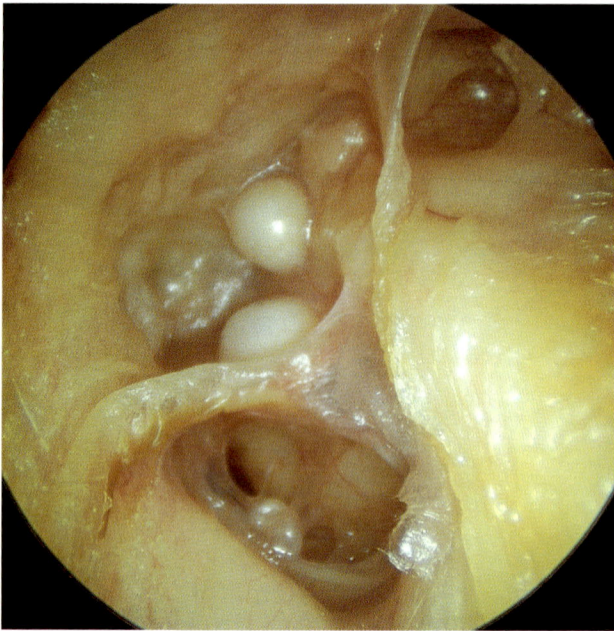

Figure 14.**98**   Left ear. Open tympanoplasty. A large perforation of the reconstructed tympanic membrane is seen. Cholesteatomatous pearls are observed in the attic.

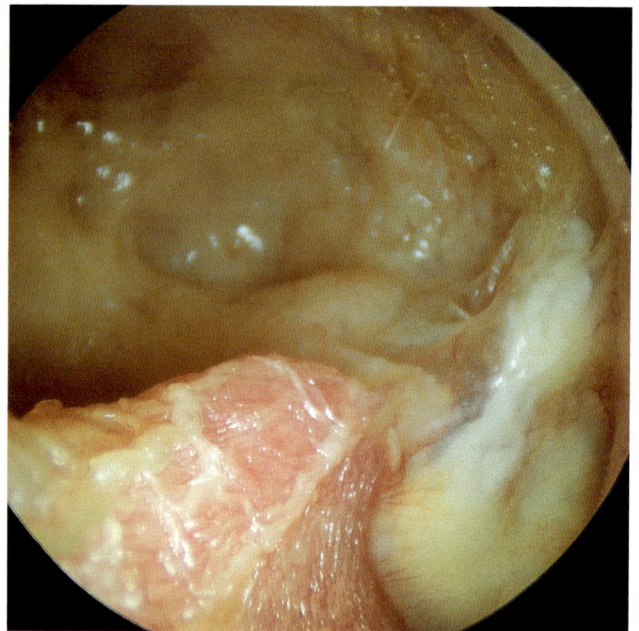

Figure 14.**99**   Right ear. Open tympanoplasty. The facial ridge has not been sufficiently lowered in this case. This leads to accumulation of cerumen and cellular debris in the cavity, with subsequent infection, secretion, and maceration of the skin lining the cavity.

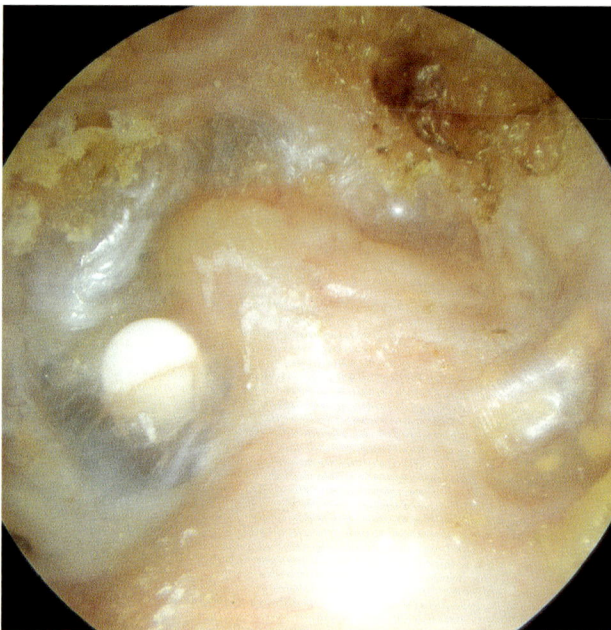

Figure 14.**100**   Left ear. TORP in extrusion following a second-stage open tympanoplasty. In the first stage, a cholesteatoma involving the attic and mesotympanum and causing erosion of the ossicular chain was removed. In the second stage, a TORP was used for reconstruction. It was placed between the footplate of the stapes and the tympanic membrane. One year postoperatively, early extrusion of the prosthesis is observed. To avoid this complication, a tragal cartilage has to be placed between the prosthesis and the tympanic membrane.

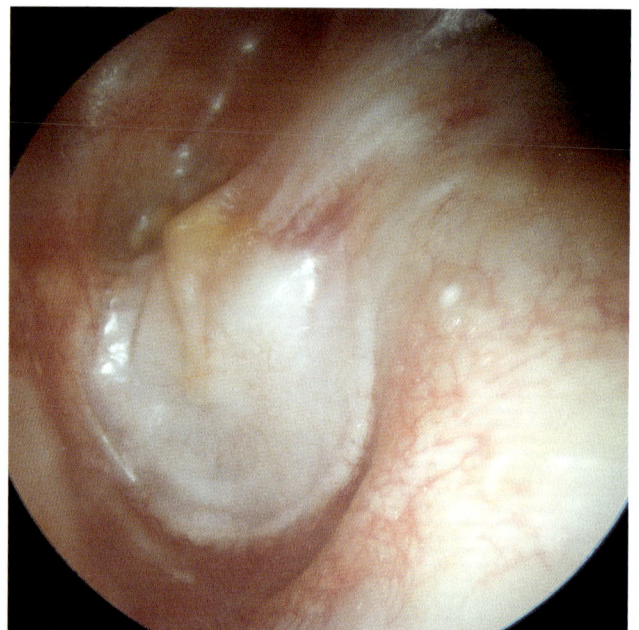

Figure 14.**101**   Left ear. An example of a correctly performed open tympanoplasty. The cavity shows perfect epithelialization. The facial ridge is low. The tympanic membrane is well positioned with excellent contact with the handle of the malleus.

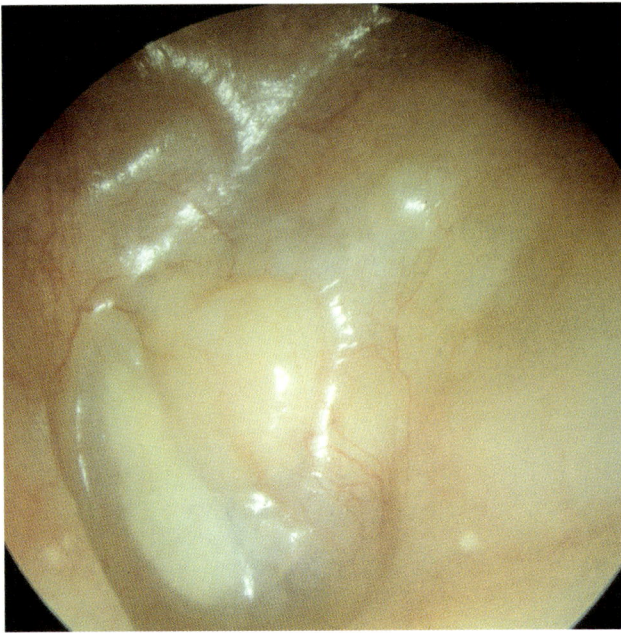

Figure 14.**102**   Left ear. Open tympanoplasty with a well epithe-lialized cavity. The tympanic membrane shows a tympanosclerot-ic plaque anteriorly; posteriorly, the ossicular chain reconstruction is observed.

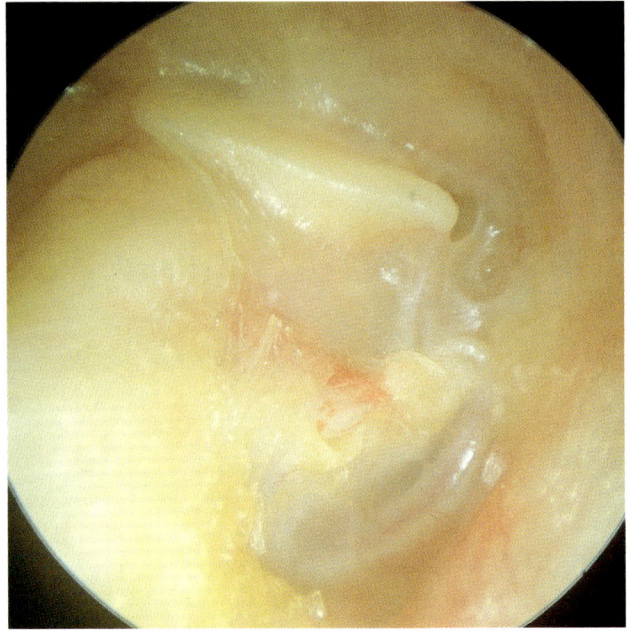

Figure 14.**103**   Right ear. Open tympanoplasty. The cartilage used for obliteration of the attic is seen in the superior part.

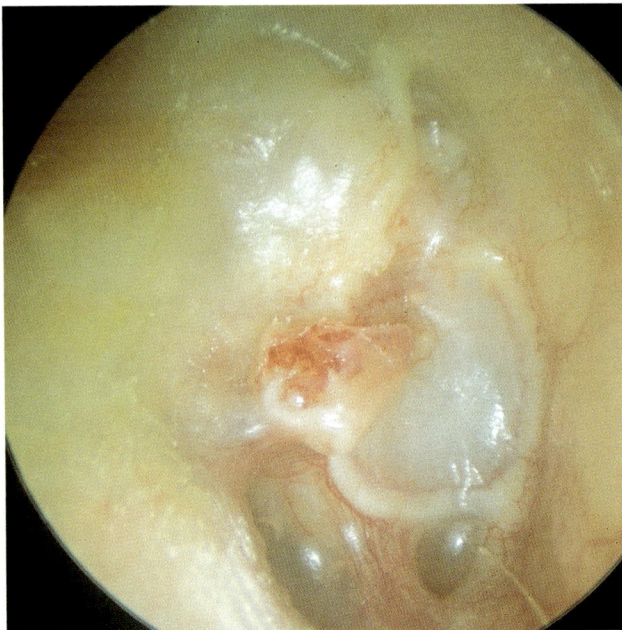

Figure 14.**104**   Right ear. Open tympanoplasty. The tympanic bone was drilled in this case because it was involved with the cholesteatoma. The inferior annulus is visible. Superiorly, the chorda tympani is observed close to the incus used for recon-struction of the ossicular chain.

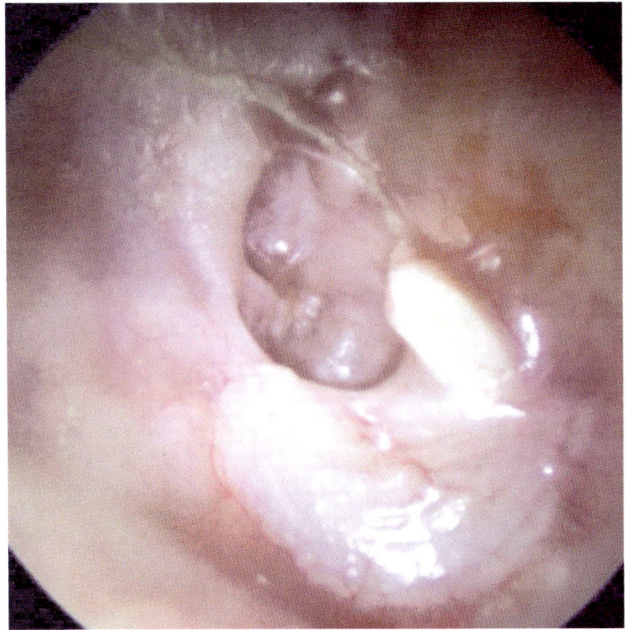

Figure 14.**105**   Left ear. Open tympanoplasty. There is a large epitympanic retraction pocket adherent to the attic wall. In the posterosuperior quadrant, the ossicle used for ossicular recon-struction is present. Revision surgery is not indicated in this case, due to the atelectasis.

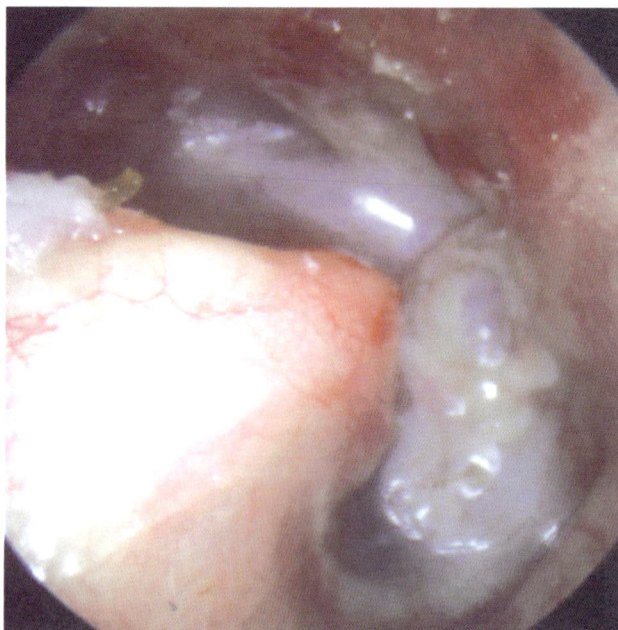

Figure 14.**106** Right ear. A badly performed open tympanoplasty. The cavity is irregular and the facial ridge is too high. There is a purulent secretion in the posterior part of the cavity.

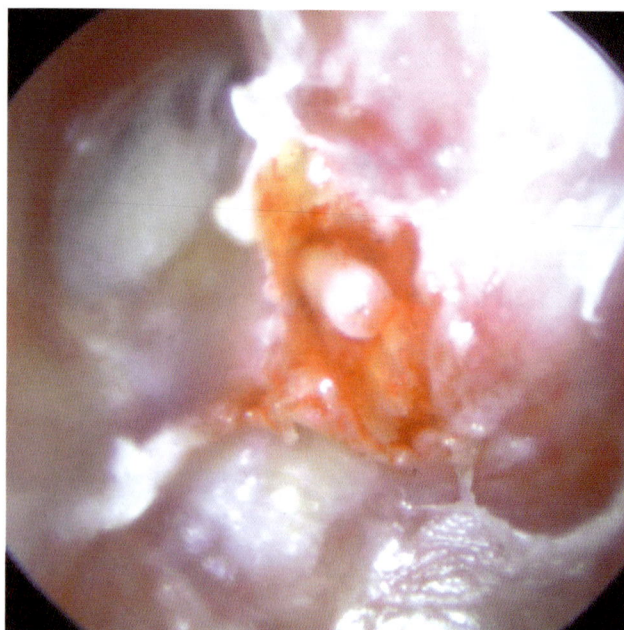

Figure 14.**107** Open tympanoplasty, with extrusion of the ossicular prosthesis.

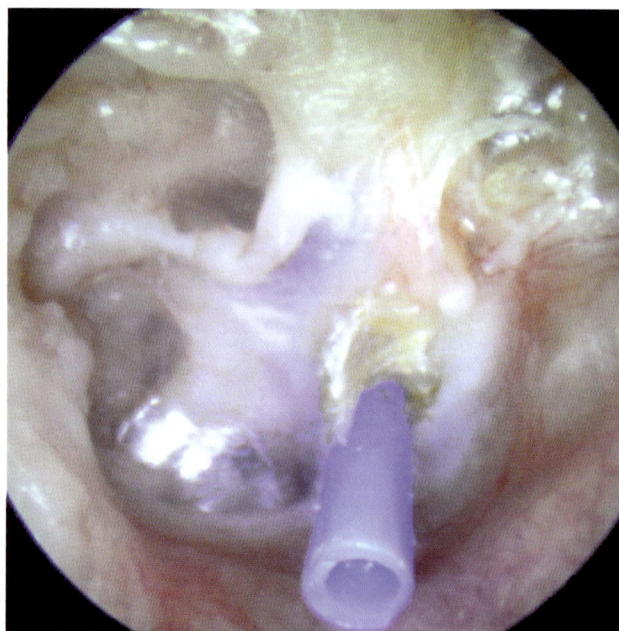

Figure 14.**108** A Bondy technique, with simultaneous insertion of a long-term T tube. The stapes, stapedius tendon, pyramidal eminence, incudostapedial joint, and facial nerve are clearly seen.

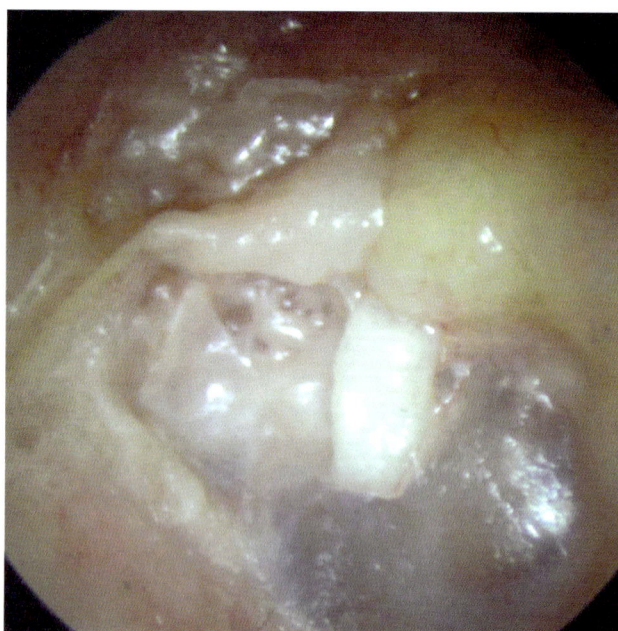

Figure 14.**109** Open tympanoplasty, with ossicular reconstruction using T cartilage.

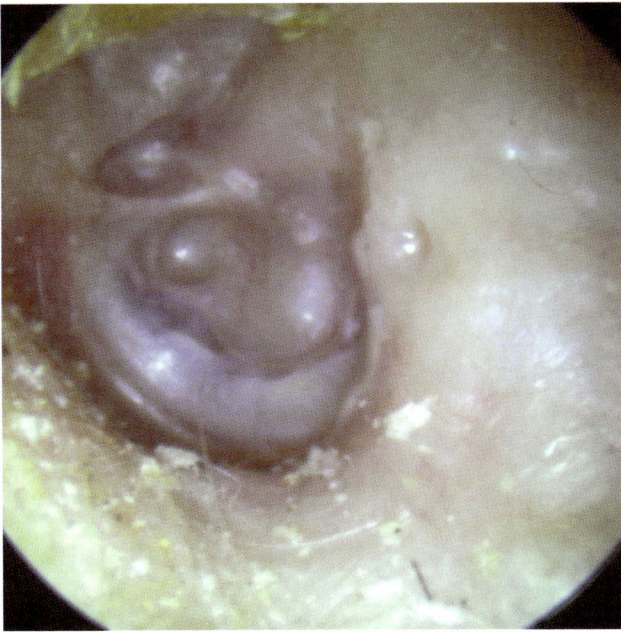

Figure 14.**110**   Left ear. Modified radical mastoidectomy. The cavity is dry and perfectly epithelialized. There is a grade IV atelectatic tympanic membrane.

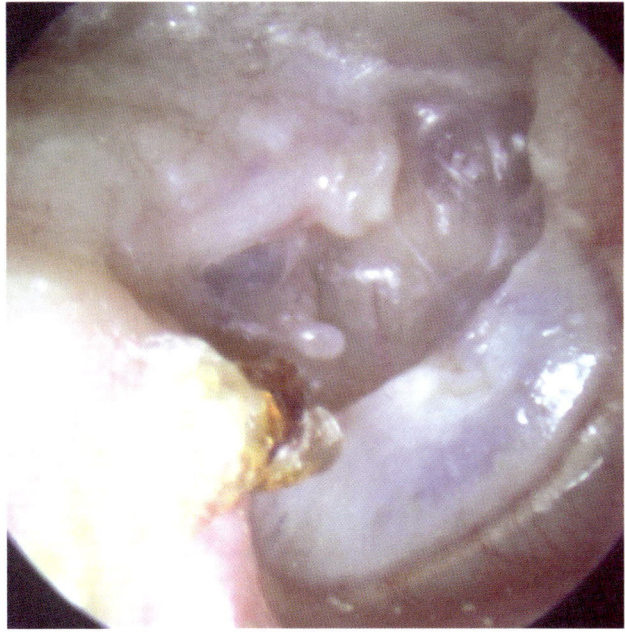

Figure 14.**111**   Right ear following a Wullstein type III open technique. The two anterior thirds of the tympanic membrane are present. There is thin epithelialization of the posterior part of the middle ear. The stapes is clearly seen, as well as the second portion of the facial nerve and the cochleariform process.

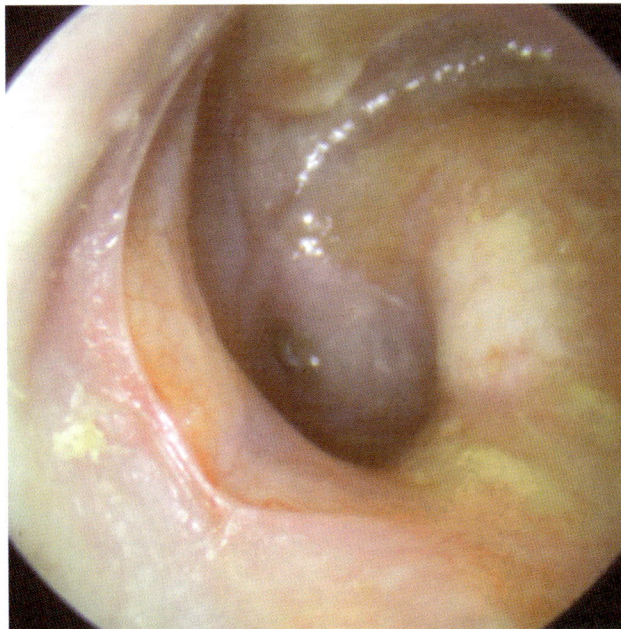

Figure 14.**112**   Left ear. Radical mastoidectomy. In this imperfectly conducted procedure, the open cavity has been completely covered by a mucosal layer. There is a central perforation, with otorrhea. It is necessary to close the perforation in this cavity.

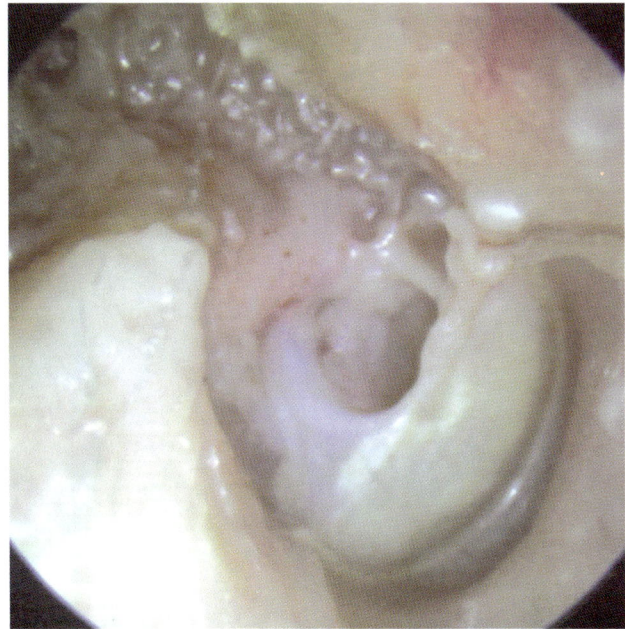

Figure 14.**113**   Right ear. Radical mastoidectomy. The facial ridge is not low enough, and the perilabyrinthine pneumatic cells and middle fossa plate have not been drilled. The eustachian tube and middle ear mucosa are connected with the cavity, leading to frequent secretion and infection. A new operation is required in order to close the eustachian tube and reconstruct the tympanic membrane.

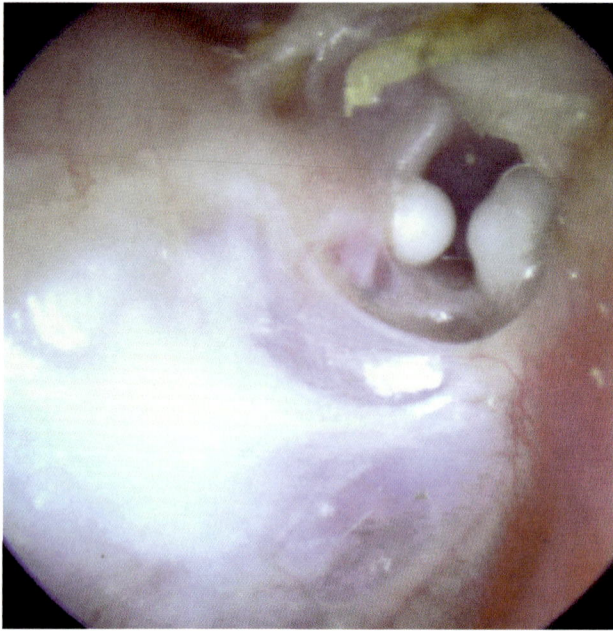

Figure 14.**114**   Right ear. Open tympanoplasty. The reconstructed tympanic membrane is seen in good position. Cholesteatomatous pearls are present in the attic, with epitympanic retraction.

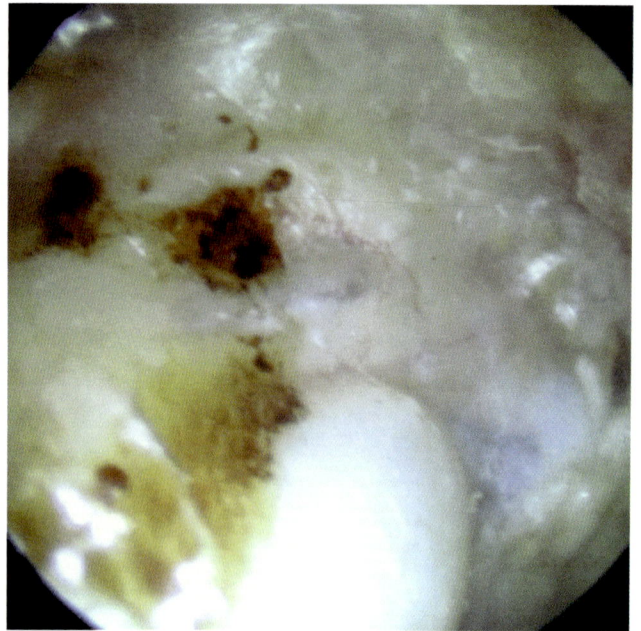

Figure 14.**115**   Right ear. Open tympanoplasty. There is a large residual cholesteatoma pearl protruding into the external auditory canal. A blue line is clearly seen superiorly to the residual cholesteatoma, which is a fistula of the lateral semicircular canal.

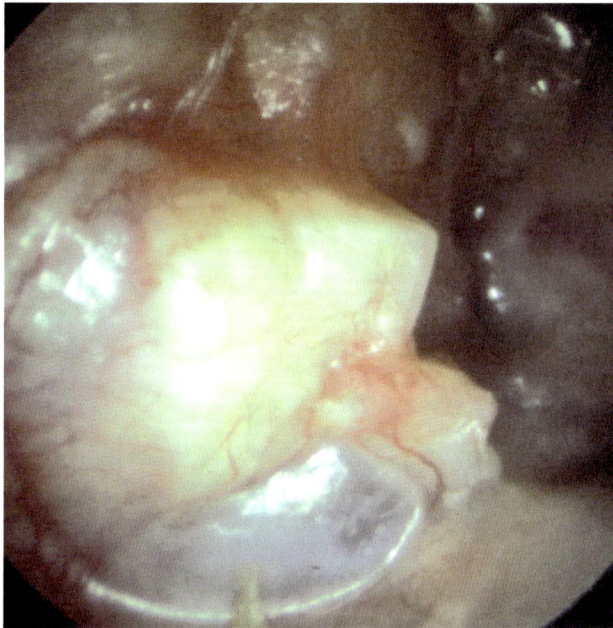

Figure 14.**116**   Left ear. One-stage open tympanoplasty. The ossicular chain has been reconstructed with homologous cartilage.

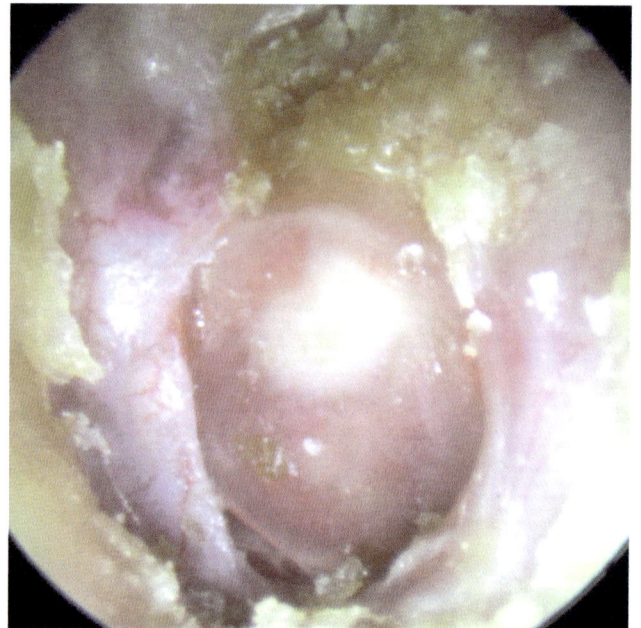

Figure 14.**117**   Left ear. An open tympanoplasty with subtotal repeat perforation of the tympanic membrane. There is a Silastic sheet in the middle ear.

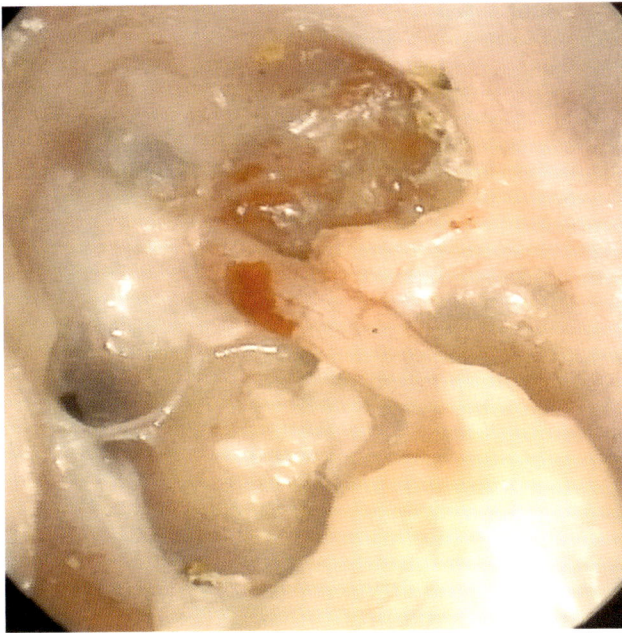

Figure 14.**118** Subtotal petrosectomy in a patient with a massive petrous bone cholesteatoma. The vertical segment of the facial nerve is uncovered, lying like a bridge in the cavity.

Figure 14.**119** Left ear. Example of a modified Bondy technique. In this case, the preoperative pure tone average was 20 dB. The patient conserved his preoperative hearing. The modified Bondy technique is indicated in epitympanic cholestea-toma with an intact tympanic membrane and ossicular chain. It is an open technique in which the attic and the mastoid are exteriorized

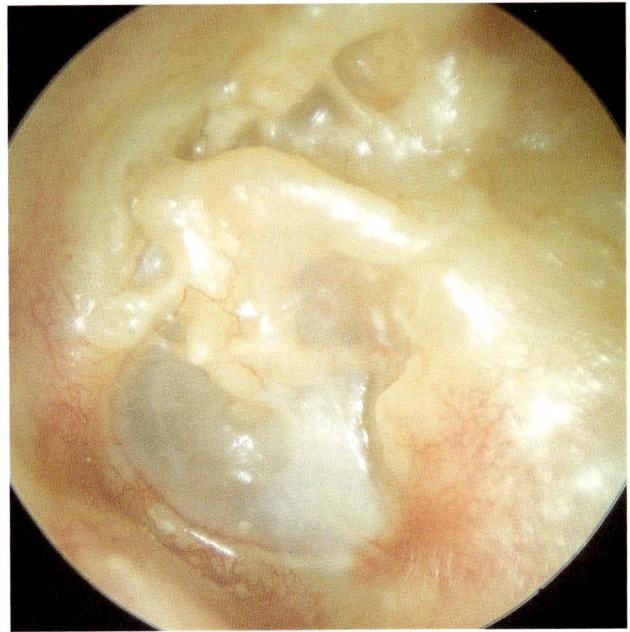

(Fig. 14.**120**) and the facial ridge is lowered until the level of the annulus. The ossicular chain and the tympanic membrane are left in situ (Fig. 14.**121**). If necessary, the attic is obliterated with a piece of cartilage; this procedure helps to reduce the risk of retractions around the ossicles (Fig. 14.**122**). Fascia is then inserted with two anterior tongues; one is positioned under the incus body, the other between the handle of the malleus and the long process of the incus (Figs. 14.**123**, 14.**124**). A meatoplasty according to the size of the cavity is performed at the end of the procedure.

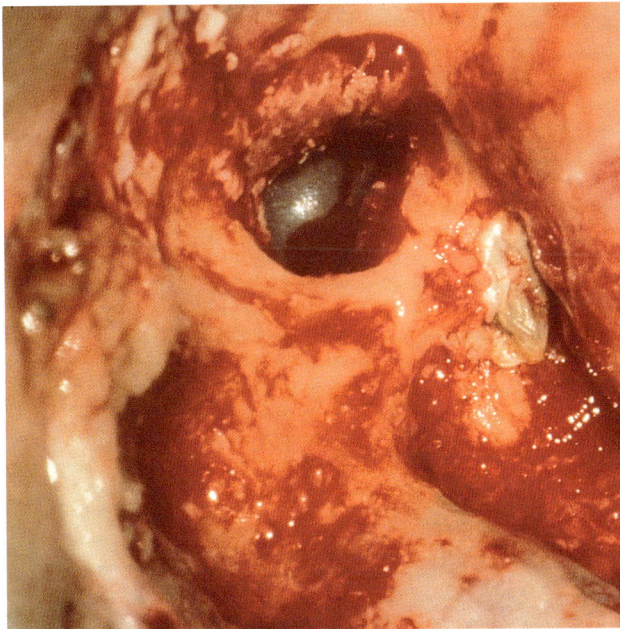

Figure 14.**120** Same case, intraoperative view. Exteriorization of the attic and the mastoid, lowering the facial ridge until the level of the annulus.

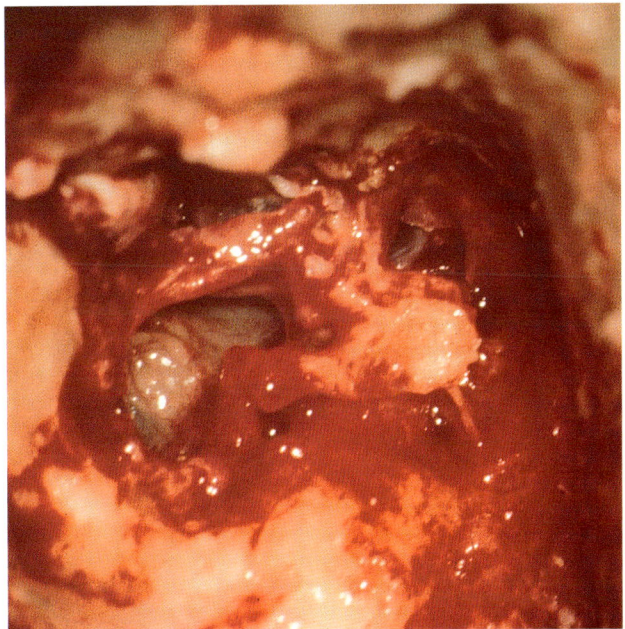

Figure 14.**121** The ossicular chain and the tympanic membrane are left in situ.

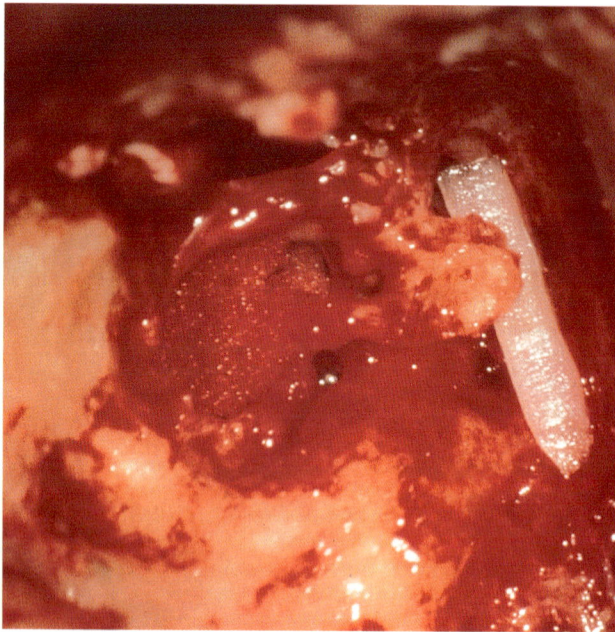

Figure 14.**122**   The attic is obliterated with a piece of cartilage.

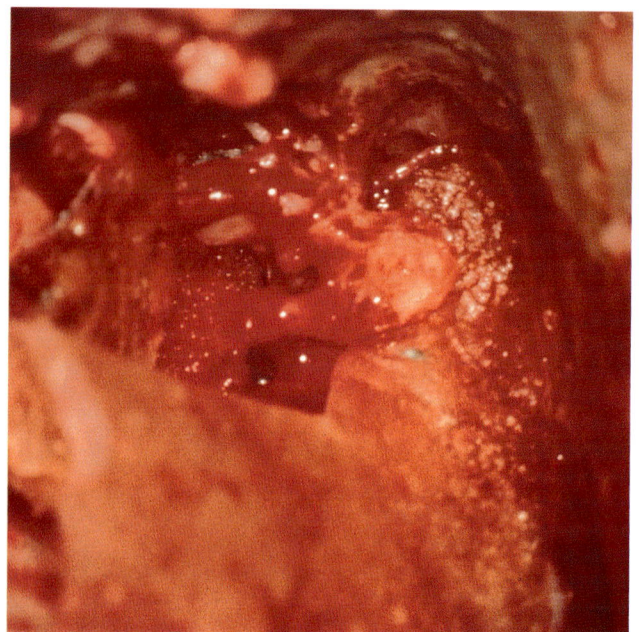

Figure 14.**123**   Fascia is inserted with two anterior tongues: one is positioned under the incus body, another between the handle of the malleus and the long process of the incus.

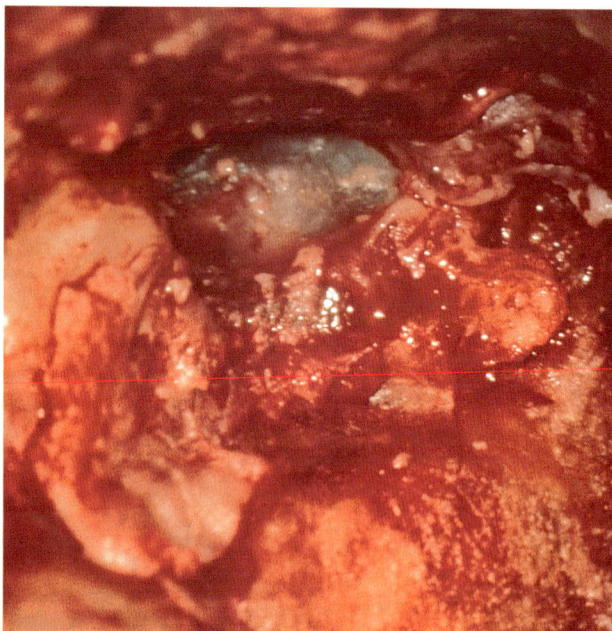

Figure 14.**124**   At the end of the procedure the skin flaps are repositioned over the fascia.

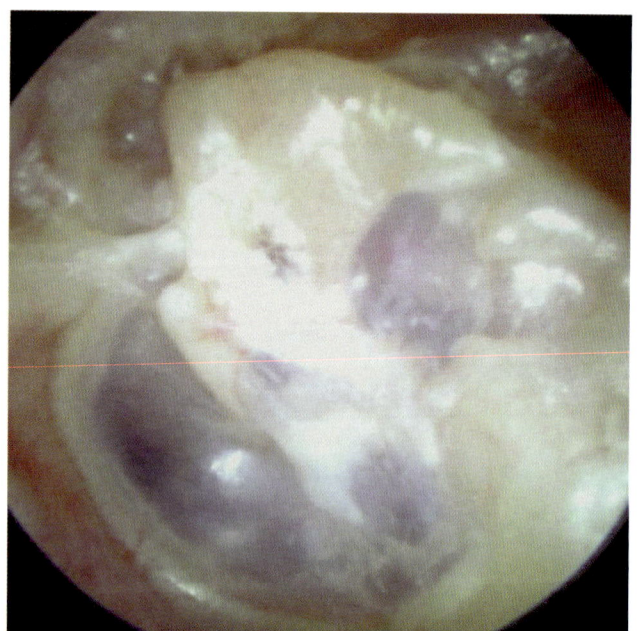

Figure 14.**125**   Left ear. Another case of modified Bondy technique. The ossicular chain, left intact during the operation, is clearly seen.

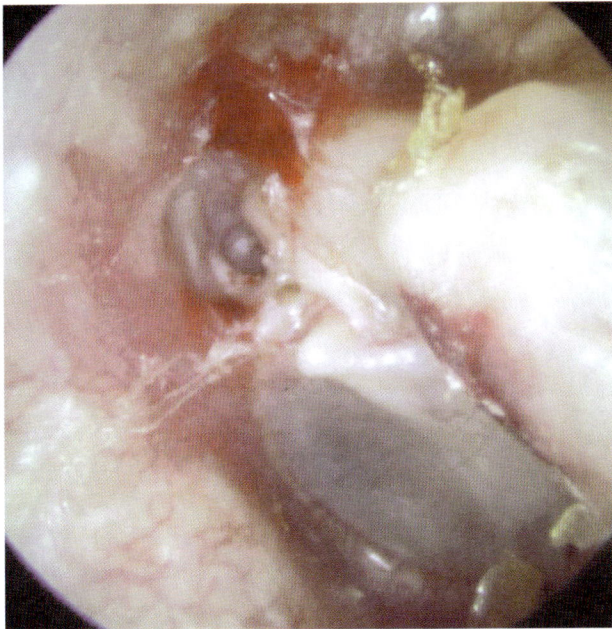

Figure 14.**126**　Left ear. Modified Bondy technique with an anteromalleolar retraction pocket. The pars tensa is in perfect position in a dry cavity.

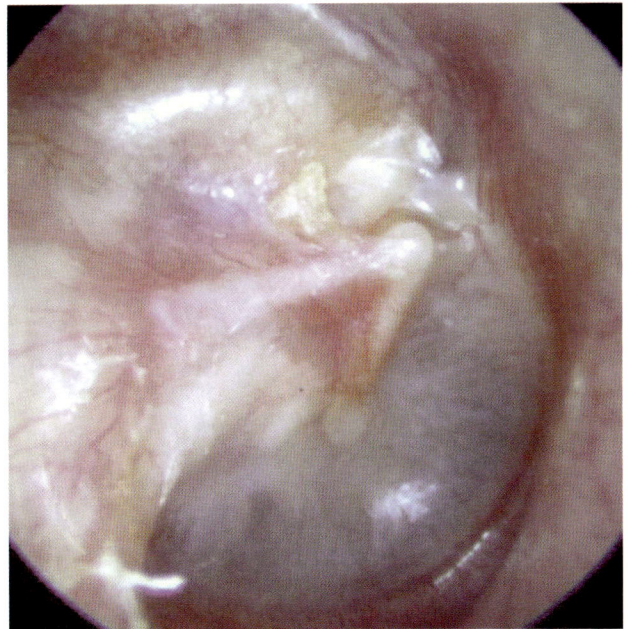

Figure 14.**127**　Right ear. An example of a well-healed cavity after a modified Bondy technique. No retraction is observed in the attic.

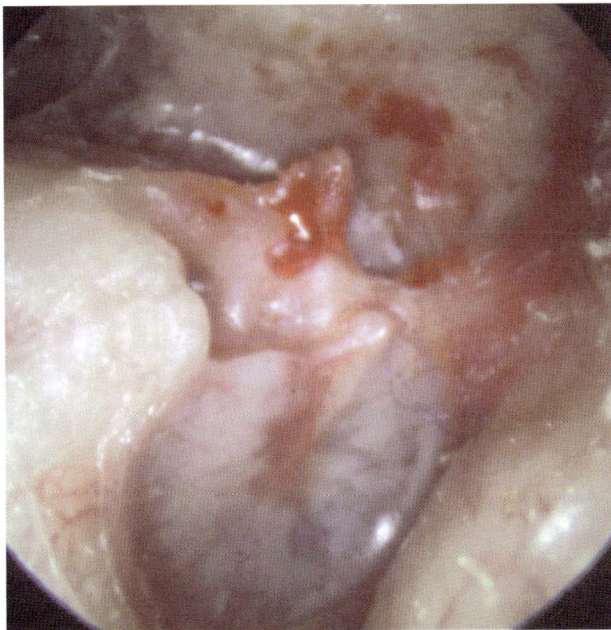

Figure 14.**128**　Right ear. Another case of modified Bondy technique.

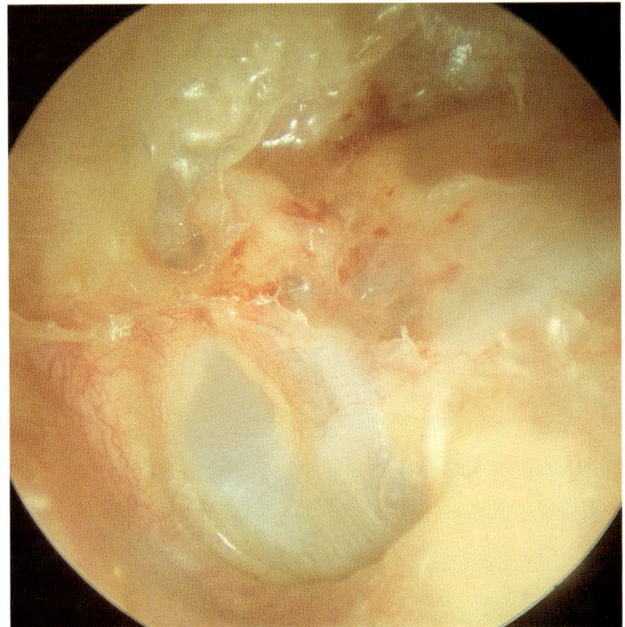

Figure 14.**129**　Left ear. Another case of the modified Bondy technique. Note the intact ossicular chain.

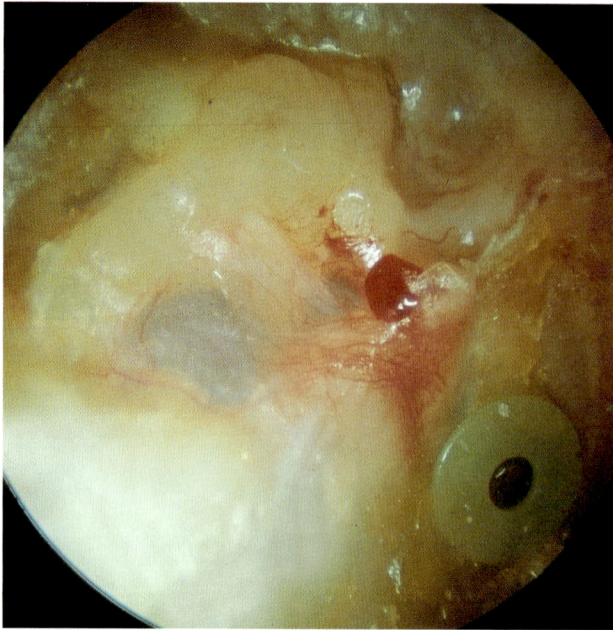

Figure 14.**130**   Right ear. The modified Bondy technique. A ventilation tube was inserted because of the presence of middle ear effusion that did not respond to medical treatment.

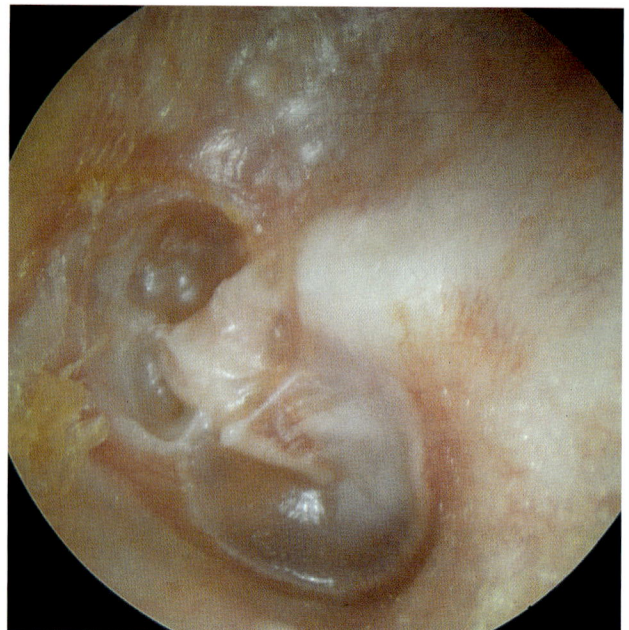

Figure 14.**131**   Left ear. The modified Bondy technique. Although an attic retraction is noted recurrent cholesteatoma is uncommon with this technique. The tympanic membrane is retracted and middle ear effusion is noted. In this case, the insertion of a ventilation tube is indicated.

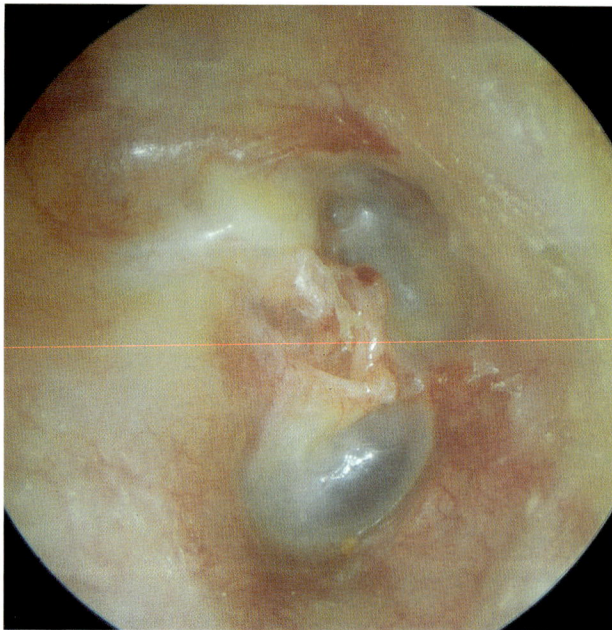

Figure 14.**132**   Right ear. The modified Bondy technique. The attic is obliterated with cartilage.

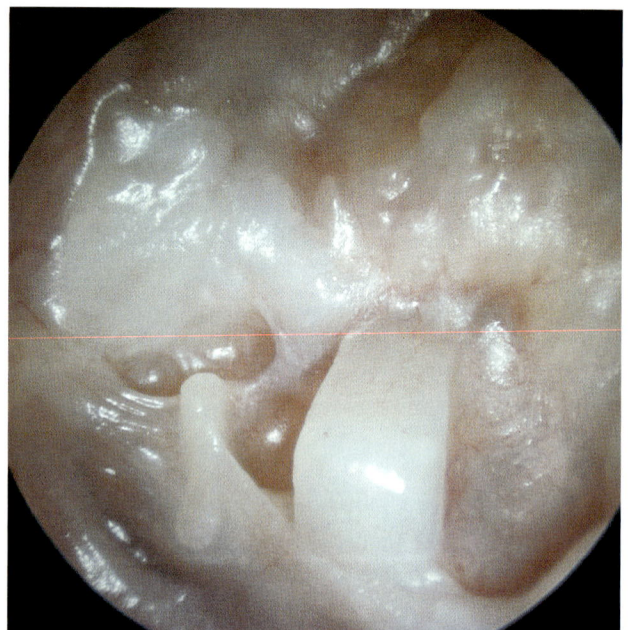

Figure 14.**133**   Left ear. Open tympanoplasty. The ossicular chain was reconstructed using an autologous cartilage that was not extruded despite the presence of atelectasis of the tympanic membrane.

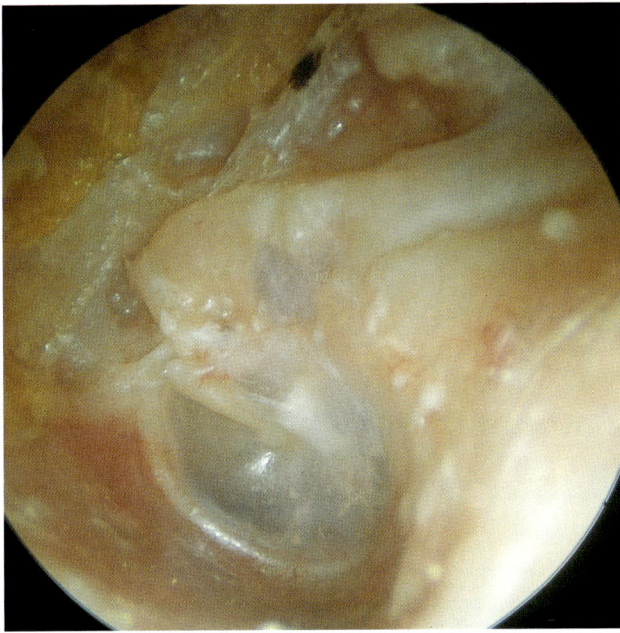

Figure 14.**134** Left ear. Another case of the modified Bondy technique. As the incus was slightly eroded, a piece of cartilage was placed between it and the malleus. The attic was obliterated with cartilage.

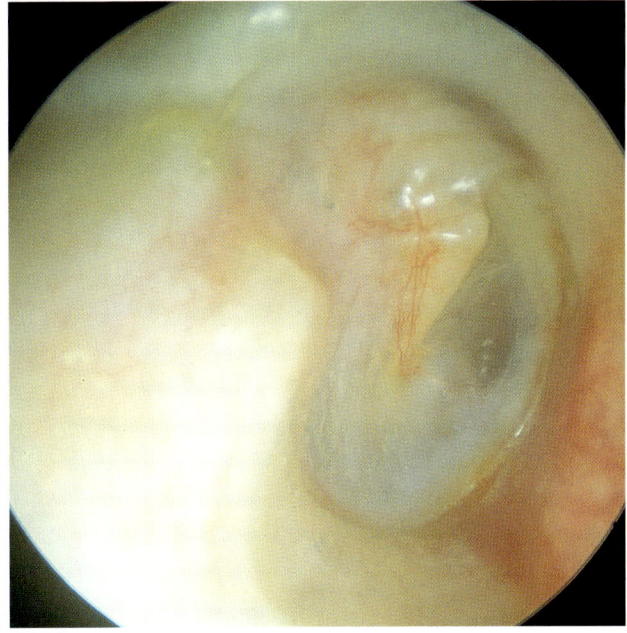

Figure 14.**135** Right ear. The modified Bondy technique. The tympanic membrane is normal and the cavity is dry and perfectly epithelialized.

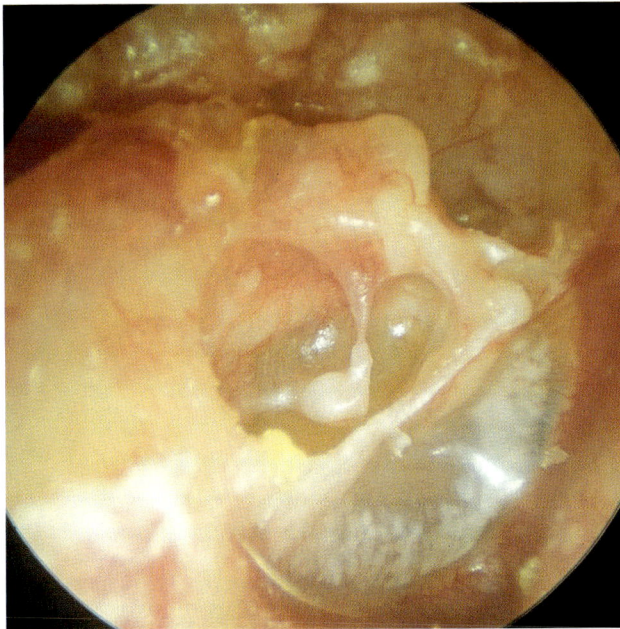

Figure 14.**136** Right ear. In this case of a modified Bondy technique, incus erosion occurred 3 years postoperatively due to the presence of a significant retraction pocket. The middle ear shows a catarrhal effusion.

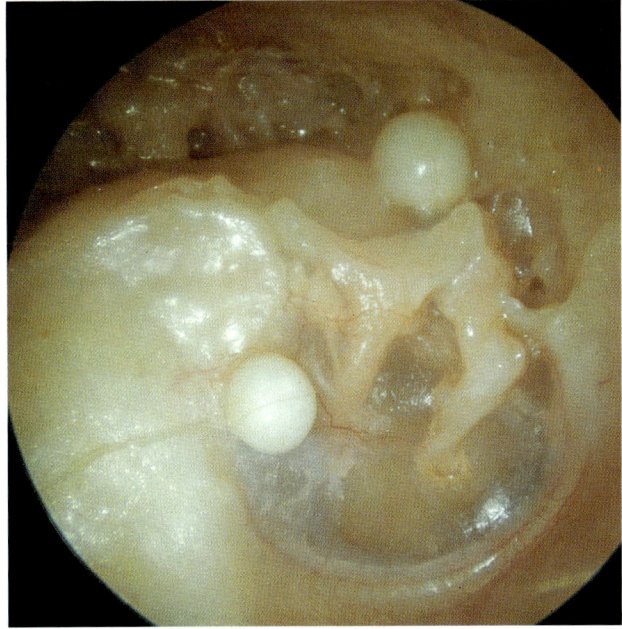

Figure 14.**137** Right ear. A modified Bondy technique. Two cholesteatomatous pearls are present in the cavity. They were easily removed in the outpatient clinic. The attic, antrum, and mastoid were exteriorized. The ossicular chain was left in situ.

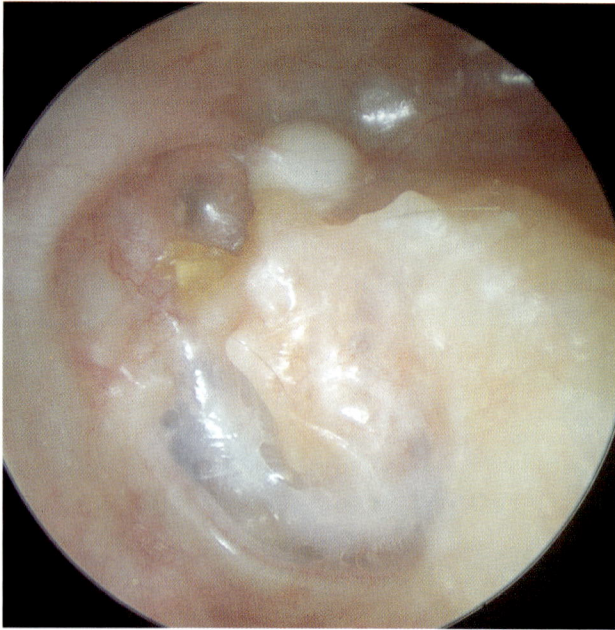

Figure 14.**138**   Left ear. A cholesteatomatous pearl seen in the attic following a modified Bondy technique.

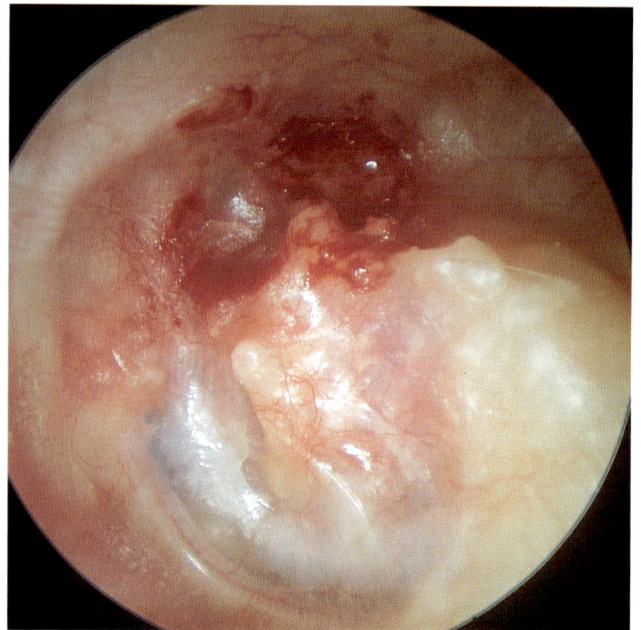

Figure 14.**139**   Same patient after removal of the pearl in the outpatient clinic.

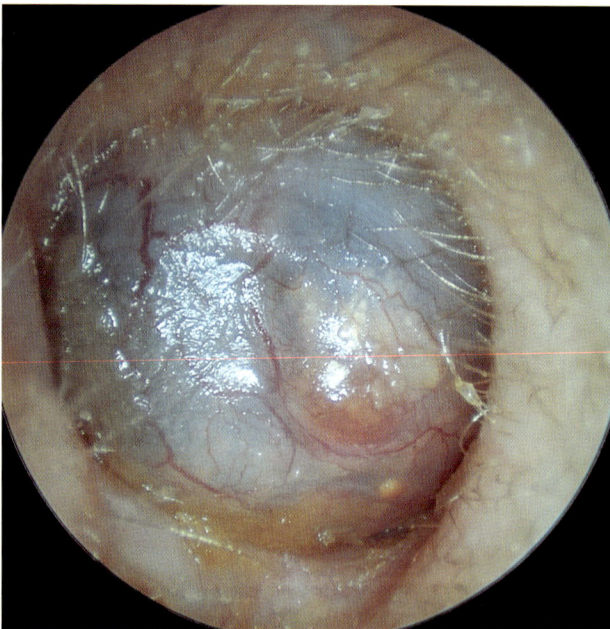

Figure 14.**140**   Radical mastoidectomy. A mucosal cyst causes complete obstruction of the external auditory canal.

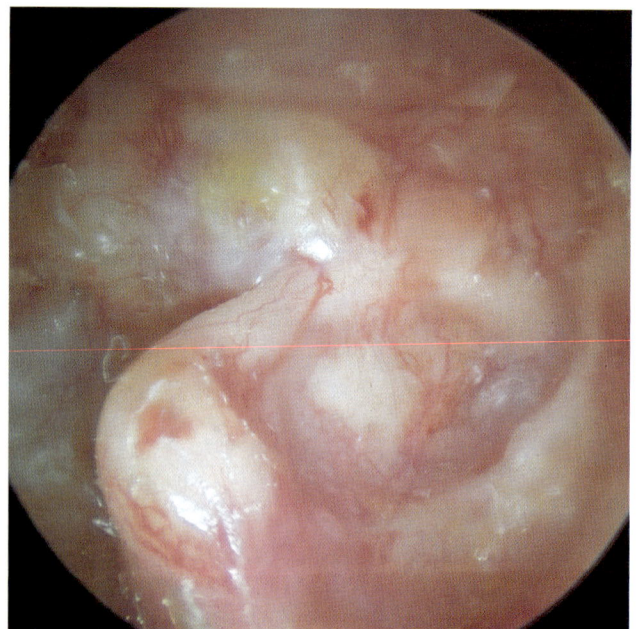

Figure 14.**141**   Right ear. Radical mastoidectomy. The second portion of the facial nerve is uncovered. Scars around the nerve produced a House–Brackmann grade III palsy.

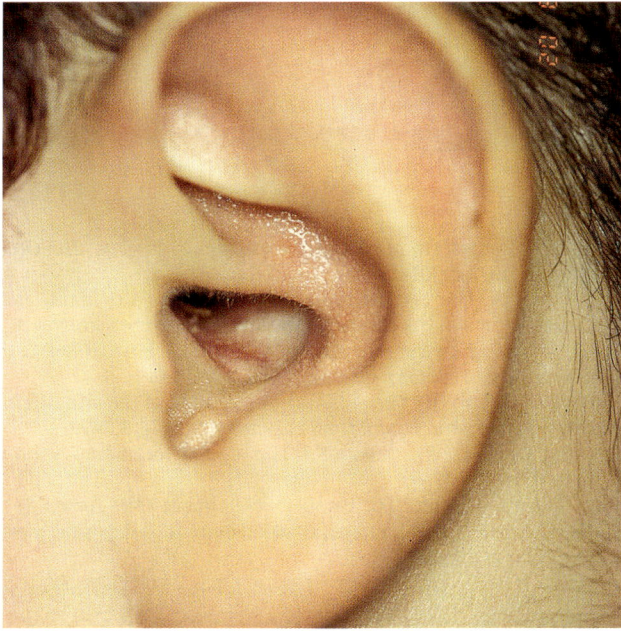

Figure 14.**142** Example of a well-performed meatoplasty in an open tympanoplasty. The performance of an adequate meatoplasty that suits the dimension of the cavity is fundamental to assure proper aeration and prevent accumulation of epithelial debris and cerumen in the cavity.

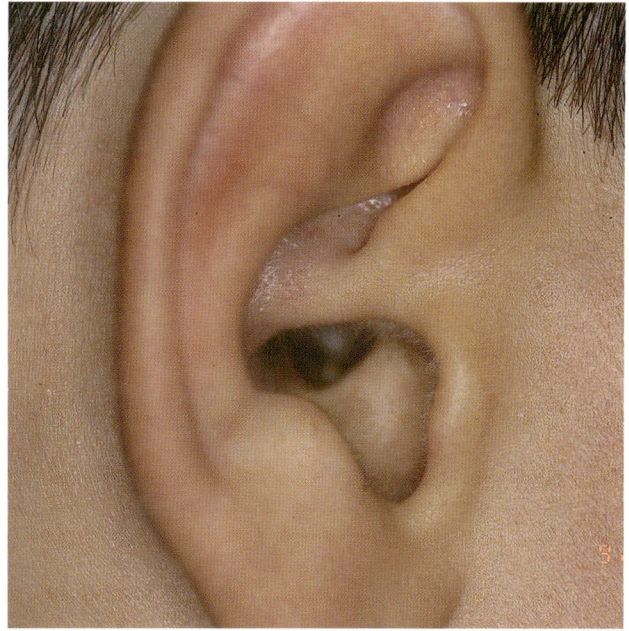

Figure 14.**143** Another example of a meatoplasty performed in a 10-year-old boy who underwent surgery for bilateral epitympanic cholesteatoma using a modified Bondy technique.

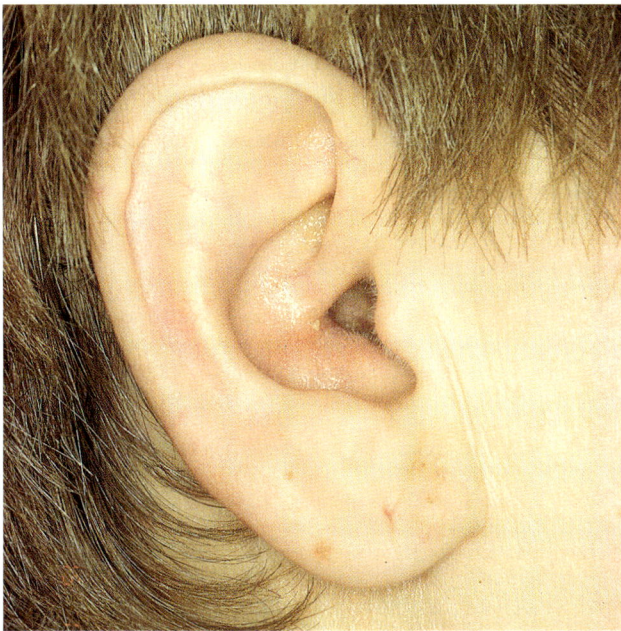

Figure 14.**144** Example of a meatoplasty that shows mild stenosis.

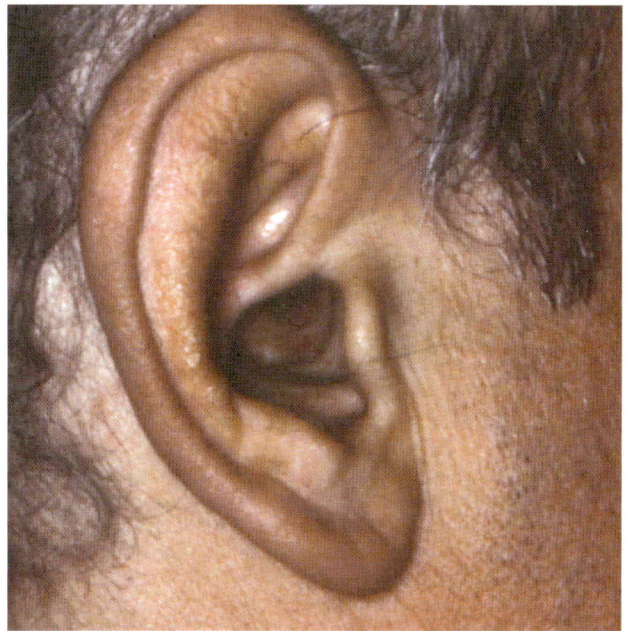

Figure 14.**145** A well-performed large meatoplasty in an open tympanoplasty, providing perfect aeration of the cavity.

References

Amendola S, Falcioni M, Caylan R, Sanna M. Recurrent cholesteatoma in open vs closed technique tympanoplasties and its surgical management. *Proceedings of the Fifth International Conference on Cholesteatoma and Mastoid Surgery.* Alghero-Sardinia, Italy, 1-6 September 1996. CIC Edizioni Internazionali.

Aristegui M, Cokkeser Y, Saleh E, Naguib M, Landolfi M, Taibah A, et al. Surgical anatomy of the extended middle cranial fossa approach. *Skull Base Surg* 1994;4:188-95.

Aristegui M, Falcioni M, Saleh E, Taibah A, Russo A, Landolfi M et al. Meingoencephalic herniation into the middle ear: A report of 27 cases. *Laryngoscope* 1995;105:513-18.

Austin DF. The significance of the retraction pockets in the treatment of cholesteatoma. In: McCabe BF, Sadè J, Abramson M, eds. *Cholesteatoma: First International Conference.* Birmingham, AL: Aesculapius, 1977;379-83.

Balyan FR, Celikkanat S, Aslan A, Taibah A, Russo A, Sanna M. Mastoidectomy in noncholesteatomatous chronic suppurative otitis media: Is it necessary? *Otolaryngol Head Neck Surg* 1997;117:592-5.

Bhatia S, Karmarkar S, De Donato G, Mutlu C, Taibah A, Russo A, Sanna M. Canal wall down mastoidectomy: causes of failure, pitfalls and their management. *J Laryngol Otol* 1995;109:583-9.

Brackmann DE, Shelton C, Arriaga MA. *Otologic Surgery.* Philadelphia: WB Saunders Company, 1994.

Caparosa R. *An Atlas of Surgical Anatomy and Techniques of the Temporal Bone.* Springfield: Thomas, 1972.

Caylan R, Titiz A, De Donato G, Falcioni M, Russo A, Taibah A, Mancini F, Sanna M. Meatoplasty technique in canal wall down procedures. *Proceedings of the Fifht International Conference on Cholesteatoma and Mastoid Surgery,* Alghero-Sardinia, Italy, 1-6 September 1996. CIC Edizioni Internazionali.

Celikkanat S, Saleh E, Khashaba A, Taibah A, Russo A, Mazzoni A, et al. Cerebrospinal fluid leak after translabyrinthine acoustic neuroma surgery. *Otolaryngol Head Neck Surg* 1995;112:654-58.

Charachon R. *La tympanoplastie.* Grenoble: Presses Universitaires, 1990.

Charachon R, Roulleau P, Bremond G et al. *Les ossiculoplasties: état actuel.* Paris: Arnette, 1987.

Chole RA. Petrous apicitis: surgical anatomy. *Ann Otol Rhinol Laryngol* 1985;94:251-57.

Cody DTR, Taylor W. Mastoidectomy for acquired cholesteatoma: long-term results. In: McCabe BF, Sadè J, Abramson M, eds. *Cholesteatoma: First International Conference.* Birmingham, AL: Aesculapius, 1977;337-51.

Cohen D. Location of primary cholesteatoma. *Am J Otol* 1987;8:61-5

Coker NJ, Jenkins HA, Fisch U. Obliteration of the middle ear and mastoid cleft in subtotal petrosectomy: indications, technique and results. *Ann Otol Rhinol Laryngol* 1986;95:5-11.

Cokkeser Y, Naguib M, Aristegui M, Saleh E, Lanfolfi M, Russo A, Sanna M. Revision stapes surgery: a critical evaluation. *Otolaryngol Head Neck Surg* 1994;111:473-7.

Cokkeser Y, Aristegui M, Naguib M, Saleh E, Sanna M. Surgical anatomy of the vertebral artery at the craniovertebral junction. In: Mazzoni A, Sanna M, eds. *Skull Base Surgery* Update, vol. 1. Amsterdam: Kugler, 1995;43-8.

De Donato G, Caylan R, Falcioni M, Landolfi M, Titiz A, Russo A, Taibah A, Sanna M. Facial nerve management and results in petrous bone cholesteatoma surgery. *Proceedings of the Fifth International Conference on Cholesteatoma and Mastoid Surgery.* Alghero-Sardinia, Italy, 1-6 September 1996. CIC Edizioni Internazionali.

De Donato G, Taibah A, Falcioni M, Mancini F, Russo A, Sanna M. Management of tympano-jugularis chemodectomas. *Skull Base* 2001;11(Suppl 2):48ff.

Deguine C. Long-term results in cholesteatoma surgery. *Clin Otolaryngol* 1978;3:301-10.

De la Cruz A. The transcochlear approach to meningiomas and cholesteatoma of the cerebellopontine angle. In: Brackmann DE, ed. *Neurological Surgery of the Ear and Skull Base.* New York: Raven Press, 1982;353-60.

Derlacki EL, Clemis JD. Congenital cholesteatoma of the middle ear and mastoid. *Ann Otol Rhinol Laryngol* 1965;74:706-27.

Di Chiro G, Fisher RL, Nelson KB. The jugular foramen. *J Neurosurg* 1964;21:447-60.

Donaldson A, Duckert LG, Lambert PM, Rubel EW. *Anson and Donaldson Surgical Anatomy of the Temporal Bone.* New York: Raven Press, 1992.

Dort JC, Fish U. Facial nerve schwannomas. *Skull Base Surgery* 1991;1:51-6.

Falcioni M, De Donato G, Landolfi M, Ferrara S, Caylan R, Taibah A, Russo A, Sanna M. The modified Bondy technique in the treatment of epitympanic cholesteatoma. *Proceedings of the Fifth International Conference on Cholesteatoma and Mastoid Surgery.* Alghero-Sardinia, Italy, 1-6 September 1996. CIC Edizioni Internazionali.

Falcioni M, Sanna M. Usefulness of preoperative imaging in chronic ear surgery. *Proceedings of the Sixth International Conference on Cholesteatoma and Ear Surgery.* Cannes, France, 29 June-2 July 2000. Label Production.

Falcioni M, Frisina A, Taibah A, Piccirillo E, De Donato G, Mancini F. Surgical treatment of labyrinthine fistula in chronic ear surgery. *Proceedings of the Sixth International Conference on Cholesteatoma and Ear Surgery.* Cannes, France, 29 June-2 July 2000. Label Production.

Falcioni M, Caruso A, Avanzini P, Piccioni L, Russo A. Facial nerve iatrogenic palsy in chronic ear surgery. *Proceedings of the Sixth International Conference on Cholesteatoma and Ear Surgery.* Cannes, France, 29 June-2 July 2000. Label Production.

Farrior JB. Anterior facial nerve decompression. *Otolaryngol Head Neck Surg* 1985;93:765-68.

Farrior JB. The canal wall in tympanoplasty and mastoidectomy. *Arch Otolaryngol* 1969;90:706-14.

Farrior JB. Systematized approach to surgery for cholesteatoma. *Arch Otolaryngol* 1973;97:188-90.

Fisch U. Infratemporal fossa approach to tumors of the temporal bone and base of the skull. *J Laryngol Otol* 1978;92:949-67.

Fisch U. Infratemporal fossa approach for glomus tumors of the temporal bone. *Ann Otol Rhinol Laryngol* 1982;91:474-79.

Fisch U. The infratemporal fossa approach for nasopharyngeal tumors. *Laryngoscope* 1983;93:36-44.

Fisch U. *Tympanoplasty, Mastoidectomy, and Stapes Surgery.* Stuttgart: Thieme, 1994.

Fisch U, Esslen E. Total intratemporal exposure of the facial nerve. *Arch Otolaryngol* 1972;95:335-41.

Fisch U, Mattox D. *Microsurgery of the Skull Base.* New York: Thieme, 1988.

Fisch U, Fagan P, Valavanis A. The infratemporal fossa approach for the lateral skull base. *Otolaryngol Clin North Am* 1984;17:513-22.

Flood LM, Kemink JL. Surgery in lesions of the petrous apex. *Otolaryngol Clin North Am* 1984;7:565-75.

Friedberg J. Congenital cholesteatoma. *Laryngoscope* 1994;104 (Suppl):1-24.

Gamoletti R, Bellomi A, Sanna M, Zini C, Scandellari R. Histology of extruded Plasti-Pore ossicular prostheses. *Otolatyngol Head Neck Surg* 1984;92:342-5.

Gacek R. Surgical landmarks for the facial nerve in the epitympanum. *Ann Otol Rhinol Laryngol* 1980;89:249-50.

Gantz B, Fisch U. Modified transotic approach to the cerebellopontine angle. *Arch Otolaryngol* 1983;109:252-56.

Glasscock ME. Surgical technique for open mastoid procedures: how I did it. *Laryngoscope* 1982;92:1140-42.

Glasscock ME, Harris FH. Glomus tumors: diagnosis and treatment. *Laryngoscope* 1974;84:2006-32.

Glasscock ME, Miller GW. Intract canal wall tympanoplasty in the management of cholesteatoma. *Laryngoscope* 1976;86:1639-57.

Glasscock ME, Shambaugh GE. *Surgery of the Ear*, 4th ed. Philadelphia: Saunders, 1990.

Goodhill V. Tragal perichondrium and cartilage in tympano-plasty. *Arch Otolaryngol* 1967;85:480-91.

Guild SR. A hitherto unrecognized structure, the glomus jugularis, in man. *Anat Rec* (Suppl) 1941;79:28.

Guild SR. The glomus jugulare, a nonchromaffin paraganglion, in man. *Ann Otol Rhinol Laryngol* 1953;62:1045-71.

Hakuba A, Nishimura S, Jang BJ. A combined retro-auricolar and preauricolar transpetrosal-transtentorial approach to clivus meningiomas. *Surg Neurol* 1988;30:108-16.

Hoffman RA. Cerebrospinal fluid leak following acoustic neuroma removal. *Laryngoscope* 1994;104:40-58.

House WF. Surgical exposure of the internal auditory canal and its contents through the middle cranial fossa. *Laryngoscope* 1961;71:1363-65.

House WF. Middle cranial fossa approach to the petrous pyramid: report of 50 cases. *Arch Otolaryngol* 1963;78:460-68.

House WF. Transtemporal bone microsurgical removal of acoustic neuromas. *Arch Otolaryngol* 1964;80:599-756.

House WF, Sheehy JL. Functional restoration in tympanoplasty. *Arch Otolaryngol* 1963;78:304-9.

House WF, Glasscock ME III. Glomus tympanicum tumors. *Arch Otolaryngol* 1968;87:124-28.

House WF, Hitselberger WE. The transcochlear approach to the skull base. *Arch Otolaryngol* 1976;102:334-42.

House JL, Hitselberger WE, House WF. Wound closure and cerebrospinal fluid leak after translabyrinthine surgery. *Am J Otol* 1982;4:126-28.

House JW, Brackmann DE. Facial nerve grading system. *Otolaryngol Head Neck Surg* 1985;93:146-47.

Jackler RK. Overview of surgical neuro-otology. In: Jackler RK, Brackmann DE, eds. *Neuro-otology*. Baltimore: Mosby, 1993;651-84.

Jackson CG. *Surgery of Skull Base Tumors*. New York: Churchill Livingstone, 1991.

Jackson CG, Glasscock ME, McKennan KX, et al. The surgical treatment of skull base tumors with intracranial extension. *Otolaryngol Head Neck Surg* 1987;96:175.

Jackson CG, Cueva RA, Thedinger BA, Glasscok ME. Conservation surgery for glomus jugulare tumors: the value of early diagnosis. *Laryngoscope* 1990;100:10.

Jansen C. The combined approach for tympanoplasty. *J Laryngol Otol* 1968;82:771-93.

Jansen C. Posterior tympanotomy: experiences and surgical details. *Otolaryngol Clin North Am* 1972;5:79-96.

Jansen C. Intact canal wall tympanoplasty. In: Shambaugh G, Shea J, eds. *Fifth International Workshop on Middle Ear Microsurgery*. Huntsville: Strode, 1977:370-75.

Jenkins HA, Fisch U. Glomus tumors of the temporal region: technique of surgical resection. *Arch Otolaryngol* 1981;107:209-13.

Karmarkar S, Bhatia S, Saleh E, De Donato G, Taibah A, Russo A et al. Cholesteatoma surgery: the individualized technique. *Ann Otol Rhinol Laryngol* 1995;104:591-95.

Karmarkar S, Bhatia S, Khashaba A, Saleh E, Russo A, Sanna M. Congenital cholesteatomas of the middle ear: A different experience. *Am J Otol* 1996;17:288-292.

Krmpotic-Nemanic J, Draf W, Helms J. *Surgical Anatomy of the Head and Neck*. Berlin: Springer, 1985.

Kveton JF, Cooper MH. Microsurgical anatomy of the jugular foramen region. *Am J Otol* 1988;9:109-12.

Landolfi M, Taibah A, Russo A, Szymanski M, Shaan M, Sanna M. Revalidation of the Bondy technique. In: Nakano Y, ed. *Cholesteatoma and Mastoid Surgery*. Amsterdam: Kugler, 1993;719-21.

Lang J. Topographical anatomy of the skull base and adjacent tissues. In: Scheunemann H, Schurmann K, Helms J, eds. *Tumors of the Skull Base*. Berlin: de Gruyter, 1986;3-28.

Lau T, Tos M. Treatment of sinus cholesteatoma: long-term results and recurrence rate. *Arch Otolaryngol* 1988a;9:456-64.

Lau T, Tos M. Sinus cholesteatomas: recurrences and observation time. *Acta Otolaryngol* 1988b;449(suppl):191-93.

Lau T, Tos M. Tensa retraction cholesteatoma: treatment and long-term results. *J Laryngol Otol* 1989;103:149-57.

Lempert J. Radical subcortical mastoidectomy. *Ann Mal Oreille* 1929;48:111-37.

Levenson JM, Michaels L, Parisier SC. Congenital choleste-atomas of the middle ear in children: origin and management. *Otolaryngol Clin North Am* 1989;22:941-54.

Liden-Jerger. Tympanoplasty—procedures, interpretation and variables (pp. 103-155). In: Feldman AS, Wilber LA, eds. *Acoustic impedance and admittance—the measurement of middle ear function*. Baltimore: Williams and Wilkins, 1976.

Magnan J, Bremond C. Les conditions de guérison de l'otite chronique cholesteatomateuse. *Ann Otolaryngol Chir Cervicofac* 1985;102:565-73.

Magnan J, Chays A, Gignac D, Bremond G. Reconstruction of posterior canal wall: long-term results. In: Charachon R, Garcia-Ibanez E, eds. *Long-Term Results and Indications in Otology and Otoneurosurgery*. Amsterdam: Kugler, 1991;57-61.

Magnan J, Sanna M. *Endoscopy in neuro-otology*. Stuttgart: Thieme, 1999.

Mancini F, Russo A, Sanna M. Grafting technique for tympanoplasty. *Operative Techniques in Otolaryngol-Head and neck Surgery* 1996;7:34-7.

Mancini F, Taibah A, Falcioni M. Complications and their management in tympanomastoid surgery. *Otolaryngol Clin North Am* 1999;32:567-83.

Marquet J. Eradication of cholesteatoma. In: Tos M, Thomsen J, Peitersen E, eds. *Cholesteatoma and Mastoid Surgery*. Amsterdam: Kugler, 1989;811-16.

Martin CH, Prades JM. Removal of selected infralabyrinthine lesions without facial nerve mobilization. *Skull Base Surg* 1992;2:220-26.

May M. Total facial nerve exploration: transmastoid, extra-labyrinthine, and subtemporal indications and results. *Laryngoscope* 1979;89:906-17.

Mazzoni A. Internal auditory canal: arterial relations at the porus acusticus. *Ann Otol Rhinol Laryngol* 1969;78:794-814.

Mazzoni A. Internal auditory artery supply to the petrous bone. *Ann Otol Rhinol Laryngol* 1972;81:13-21.

Mazzoni A. Jugulo-petrosectomy. *Arch Ital Otyol Rhinol Laring* 1974;2:20-35.

Mazzoni A, Sanna M. The petro-occipital trans-sigmoid approach to the posterolateral skull base: results and indications [paper presented at the Third Annual Meeting of the North American Skull Base Society, Acapulco, Mexico, 15-20 February 1992].

Michaels L. An epidermoid formation in the developing middle ear: possible source of cholesteatoma. *J Otolaryngol* 1986; 15:169-74.

Morimitsu T, Nagai T, Nagai M, et al. Pathogenesis of cholesteatoma based on clinical results of anterior tympanotomy. *Auris Nasus Larynx* 1989;16(suppl):9-14.

Nadol JB. Causes of failure of mastoidectomy for chronic otitis media. *Laryngoscope* 1985;95:410-13.

Nager GT. *Pathology of the Ear and Temporal Bone*. Baltimore: Williams and Wilkins, 1993.

Naguib M, Aristegui M, Saleh E, Cokkeser Y, Landolfi M, Sanna M. Surgical anatomy of the petrous apex as it relates to the enlarged middle cranial fossa approaches. *Otolaryngol Head Neck Surg* 1994;111:488-93.

Naguib M, Saleh E, Aristegui M, Cokkeser Y. Management of epitympanic cholesteatoma with intact ossicular chain: the modified Bondy technique. *Otolaryngol Head Neck Surg* 1994;111:545-49.

Nakano Y. Cholesteatoma surgery and mastoid obliteration. In: Nakano Y, ed. *Cholesteatoma and Mastoid Surgery*. Amsterdam: Kugler, 1993;769-73.

Neely GJ, Alford BR. Facial nerve neuromas. *Arch Otolaryngol* 1974;100:298-301.

Palva T. Reconstruction of ear canal and middle ear in chronic otitis. *Acta Otolaryngol* 1963;188(suppl):228-33.

Palva T, Mäkinen J. The meatally based musculoperiosteal flap in cavity obliteration. *Arch Otolaryngol* 1979;105:377-80.

Palva T, Palva A, Kärjä J. Cavity obliteration and ear canal size. *Arch Otolaryngol* 1970;92:366-71.

Paparella MM, Jung TTK. Intact bridge tympanomastoidectomy (IBM): combined essential features of open vs. closed procedures. *J Laryngol Otol* 1983;97:575-85.

Paparella MM, Jung TTK. Intact bridge tympanomastoidectomy. *Otolaryngol Head Neck Surg* 1984;92:334-38.

Paparella MM, Shumrick DA. *Otolaryngology*, 3 vols. Philadelphia: Saunders, 1988.

Pellet W, Cannoni M, Pech A. A widened transchoclear approach to jugular foramen tumors. *J Neurosurg* 1988;69:887-94.

Piccioni L, Piccirillo E, Falcioni M, De Donato G, Russo A, Taibah AK. Middle ear cholesteatoma in children. *Proceedings of the Sixth International Conference on Cholesteatoma and Ear Surgery*. Cannes, France, 29 June-2 July 2000. Label Production.

Plester D. Tympanic membrane homografts in ear surgery. *Acta Otolaryngol* 1970;24:34-7.

Portmann M. *The Ear and Temporal Bone*. New York: Masson, 1979.

Proctor B. Surgical anatomy of the posterior tympanum. *Ann Otol Rhinol Laryngol* 1969;78:1026-41.

Proctor B. *Surgical Anatomy of the Ear and Temporal Bone*. Stuttgart: Thieme, 1989.

Rambo JHT. A new obliteration to restore hearing in conductive deafness of chronic suppurative otitis. *Arch Otolaryngol* 1957;66:525-32.

Rambo JHT. Musculoplasty for restoration of hearing in chronic suppurative ears. *Arch Otolaryngol* 1969;89:184-90.

Rhoton AL, Buza R. Microsurgical anatomy of the jugular foramen. *J Neurosurg* 1975;42:541-50.

Rhoton AL, Pulec JL, Hall GM, Boyd A. Absence of bone over the geniculate ganglion. *J Neurosurg* 1968;28:48-53.

Russo A, Taibah A, Landolfi M, Shaan M, Pasanasi E, Scandellari R, Sanna M. Congenital cholesteatoma. *Proceedings of the Fourth International Conference on Cholesteatoma and Mastoid Surgery*. Niigata, Japan 8-12 September 1992. Kugler Publications.

Russo A, Taibah AK, De Donato G, Falcioni M, Sanna M. Congenital cholesteatomas: A different experience. *Proceedings of the Fifth International Conference on Cholesteatoma and Mastoid Surgery*. Alghero-Sardinia, Italy, 1-6 September 1996. CIC Edizioni Internazionali.

Sadè J. Postoperative cholesteatoma recurrence. In: McCabe BF, Sadè J, Abramson M, eds. *Cholesteatoma: First International Conference*. Birmingham, AL: Aesculapius, 1977;284-89.

Sadè J. *Secretory Otitis Media and its Sequelae*. New York: Churchill Livingstone, 1979.

Saleh E, Miguel M, Taibah A, Mazzoni A, Sanna M. Management of the high jugular bulb in the translabyrinthine approach. *Otolaryngol Head Neck Surg* 1994a;110:397-99.

Saleh E, Taibah A, Achilli V, Aristegui M, Mazzoni A, Sanna M. Posterior fossa meningioma: surgical strategy. *Skull Base Surg* 1994b;4:209-19.

Saleh E, Achilli V, Naguib M, Taibah A, Russo A, Sanna M, et al. Facial nerve neuromas: diagnosis and management. *Am J Otol* 1995a;16:521-26.

Saleh E, Nagiub M, Aristegui M, Cokkeser Y, Sanna M. The lower skull base: anatomical study with surgical implications. *Ann Otol Rhinol Laryngol* 1995b;104:57-61.

Saleh E, Naguib M, Aristegui M, Cokkeser Y, Russo A, Sanna M. Surgical anatomy of the jugular foramen area. In: Mazzoni A, Sanna M, eds. *Skull Base Surgery* Update, vol. 1. Amsterdam: Kugler, 1995c;3-8.

Samii M, Draf W. *Surgery of the Skull Base*. Berlin: Springer, 1989.

Sanna M. Anatomy of the posterior mesotympanum. In: Zini C, Sheehy JL, Sanna M, eds. *Microsurgery of Cholesteatoma of the Middle Ear*. Milan: Ghedini, 1980;69-73.

Sanna M. Ossicular chain reconstruction in closed tympanoplasties. In: Zini C, Sheehy JL, Sanna M, eds. *Microsurgery of Cholesteatoma of the Middle Ear*. Milan: Ghedini, 1980;91-96.

Sanna M. Congenital cholesteatoma of the middle ear. In: Zini C, Sheehy JL, Sanna M, eds. *Microsurgery of Cholesteatoma of the Middle Ear*. Milan: Ghedini, 1980;149-156.

Sanna M. Cholesteatoma in children (Experience of 2nd ENT clinic of Parma). In: Zini C, Sheehy JL, Sanna M, eds. *Microsurgery of Cholesteatoma of the Middle Ear*. Milan: Ghedini, 1980;157-160.

Sanna M. Proceedings of the Fifth International Conference on Cholesteatoma and Mastoid Surgery, Alghero-Sardinia, Italy, 1-6 September 1996. CIC Edizioni Internazionali.

Sanna M, Magnani M, Gamoletti R. Ossicular chain reconstruction with plastipore prostheses. *Am J Otol* 1981;2:225-9.

Sanna M, Mazzoni A. The modified transcochlear approach to the tumors of the petroclival area and prepontine cistern [paper presented at the Third Annual Meeting of the North American Skull Base Society, Acapulco, Mexico, 15-20 February 1992].

Sanna M, Zini C, Scandellari R, Jemmi G. Residual and recurrent cholesteatoma in closed tympanoplasty. *Am J Otol* 1984;5:277-82.

Sanna M, Zini C. Congenital cholesteatoma of the middle ear: A report of 11 cases. *Am J Otol* 1984;5:368-78.

Sanna M, Gamoletti R, Magnani M, Bacciu S, Zini C. Failures with Plasti-Pore ossicular replacement prostheses. *Otolaryngol Head Neck Surg* 1984;92:339-41.

Sanna M. Management of labyrinthine fistulae. In: Marquet J, ed. *Surgery and pathology of the middle ear*. Boston: Martinus Niihoff; 1985.

Sanna M, Gamoletti R, Scandellari R, Delogu P, Magnani M, Zini C. Autologous fitted incus versus PlastiporeTM PORP in ossicular chain reconstruction. *J Laryngol Otol* 1985;99:137-41.

Sanna M, Gamoletti R, Bortesi G, Jemmi G, Zini C. Posterior canal wall atrophy after intact canal wall tympanoplasty. *Am J Otol* 1986;7:74-5.

Sanna M, Zini C, Gamoletti R, et al. Prevention of recurrent cholesteatoma in closed tympanoplasty. *Ann Otol Rhinol Laryngol* 1987a;96:273-75.

Sanna M, Zini C, Gamoletti R, et al. The surgical management of childhood cholesteatoma. *J Laryngol Otol* 1987b;101:1221-6.

Sanna M, Zini C, Gamoletti R, Delogu P, Russo A, Scandellari R, et al. Surgical treatment of cholesteatoma in children. *Adv Otorhinolaryngol* 1987c;37:110-16.

Sanna M, Zini C, Bacciu S, Gamoletti R, Russo A, Scandellari R, Taibah A, Jemmi G. Surgery for cholesteatoma in children. *Proceedings of the Third International Conference on Cholesteatoma and Mastoid Surgery*, Copenhagen, Denmark, 5-9 June 1988. Kugler & Ghedini Publications.

Sanna M, Zini C, Gamoletti R, Taibah A, Russo A, Scandellari R. Closed versus open technique in the management of labyrinthine fistulae. *Am J Otol* 1988;9:470-475.

Sanna M, Zini C, Gamoletti R, Pasanisi E. Primary intratemporal tumors in the facial nerve: diagnosis and treatment. *J Laringol Otol* 1990;104:765-71.

Sanna M, Shea C, Gamoletti R, Russo A. Surgery of the "only hearing ear" with chronic ear disease. *J Laryngol Otol* 1992;106:793-98.

Sanna M, Zini C, Bacciu S, Scandellari R, Russo A, Shaan M, Taibah A, Szymanski M. Management of labyrinthine fistula. *Proceedings of the Fourth International Conference on Cholesteatoma and Mastoid Surgery*, Niigata, Japan, 8-12 September 1993. Kugler Publications.

Sanna M, Zini C, Gamoletti R, Frau N, Taibah A, Russo A, et al. Petrous bone cholesteatoma. *Skull Base Surg* 1993;3:201-13.

Sanna M, Mazzoni A, Saleh E, Taibah A, Russo A. Lateral approaches to the median skull base through the petrous bone: the system of the modified transcochlear approach. *J Laryngol Otol* 1994;108:1035-43.

Sanna M, Mazzoni A, Taibah A, Saleh E, Russo A, Khashaba A. The modified transcochlear approaches to the skull base: results and indications. In: Mazzoni A, Sanna M, eds. *Skull Base Surgery* Update, vol. 1. Amsterdam: Kugler, 1995a;315-23.

Sanna M et al. Atlas of Temporal Bone and Lateral *Skull Base Surgery*. Stuttgart: Thieme, 1995b.

Sanna M et al. *Atlas of Acoustic Neurinoma Microsurgery*. Stuttgart: Thieme, 1998.

Sanna M et al. *Color Atlas of Otoscopy*. Stuttgart: Thieme, 1999.

Saunders WH, Paparella MM. *Atlas of Ear Surgery*. St. Louis: Mosby, 1971.

Schuknecht HF. *Pathology of the Ear*, 2nd ed. Malvern: Lea & Febiger, 1993.

Schuknecht HF, Gylya JA. *Anatomy of the Temporal Bone with Surgical Implications*. Philadelphia: Lea and Febiger, 1986.

Shambaugh GE, Glasscock ME III. *Surgery of the Ear*, 3rd ed. Philadelphia: Saunders, 1980.

Shaan M, Landolfi M, Taibah A, Russo A, Szymanski M, Sanna M. Modified Bondy technique. *Am J Otol* 1995;16:695-7.

Shea JJ, Homsy CA. The use of Proplast in *otologic surgery*. *Laryngoscope* 1974;84:1835-45.

Shea MC, Gardner G Jr. Mastoid obliteration using homograft bone: preliminary report. *Arch Otolaryngol* 1970;92:358-65.

Sheehy JL. Surgery of chronic otitis media. In: Coates BM, Schenk HD, Miller MV, eds. *Otolaryngology.* Hagerstown: Prior, 1965.

Sheehy JL. Intact canal wall technique in management of aural cholesteatoma. *Laryngoscope* 1970a;84:1-31.

Sheehy JL. Tympanoplasty with mastoidectomy: a reevaluation. *Laryngoscope* 1970b;80:1212-30.

Sheehy JL. Surgery of chronic otitis media: In: English GM, ed. *Otolaryngology,* vol. 2. Hagerstown: Harper and Row, 1972;1-86.

Sheehy JL. Cholesteatoma surgery: canal wall down procedures. *Ann Otol Rhinol Laryngol* 1988;97:30-5.

Sheehy JL. Surgery for chronic otitis media. In: English GM, ed. *Otolaryngology,* 2d ed., vol. 1. Philadelphia: Lippincott, 1990;1-86.

Sheehy JL, Patterson MF. Intact canal wall tympanoplasty with mastoidectomy: a review of eight year's experience. *Laryngoscope* 1967;77:1502-42.

Sheehy JL, Brackmann D, Graham M. Cholesteatoma surgery: residual and recurrent disease. A review of 1024 cases. *Ann Otol Rhino Laryngol* 1977;86:451-62.

Smyth GDL. Preliminary report of the technique in tympanoplasty designed to eliminate the cavity problems. *Laryngoscope* 1962;76:460-63.

Smyth GDL. Combined approach tympanoplasty. *Arch Otolaryngol* 1969;89:250-51.

Smyth GD, Dowe AC. Cartilage canalplasty. *Laringoscope* 1971;81:786-92.

Taibah A, Russo A, Landolfi M, Shaan M, Sanna M. Open technique in cholesteatoma. *Proceedings of the Fourth International Conference on Cholesteatoma and Mastoid Surgery,* Niigata, Japan, 8-12 September 1993. Kugler Publications.

Taibah A, Russo A, Caylan R, Landolfi M, Mancini F, Sanna M. Canal wall down procedures: Causes of failure and pitfalls. *Proceedings of the Fifth International Conference on Cholesteatoma and Mastoid Surgery,* Alghero-Sardinia, Italy, 1-6 September 1996. CIC Edizioni Internazionali.

Takahashi S, Nakano Y. Tympanoplasty with mastoid obliteration using hydroxyapatite granules. In: Yanagihara N, Suzucki Y, eds. *Transplants and Implants in Otology.* Amsterdam: Kugler, 1992;159-63.

Tos M. Obliteration of the cavity in mastoidectomy. *Acta Otolaryngol* 1969;67:516-20.

Tos M. Pathogenesis and pathology of chronic secretory otitis. *Ann Otol* 1980;89:91-7.

Tos M. Modification of combined approach tympanoplasty in attic cholesteatoma. *Arch Otolaryngol* 1982;108:772-78.

Tos M. *Manual of Middle Ear Surgery,* vol. 1: *Approaches. Myringoplasty. Ossiculoplasty. Tympanoplasty.* Stuttgart: Thieme, 1993.

Tos M. *Manual of Middle Ear Surgery,* vol. 2: *Mastoid Surgery and Reconstructive Procedures.* Stuttgart: Thieme, 1995.

Tos M. *Manual of Middle Ear Surgery,* vol. 3: *Surgery of the External Auditory Canal.* Stuttgart: Thieme, 1997.

Tos M, Lau T. Attic cholesteatoma: recurrence rate related to observation time. *Am J Otol* 1988;9:456-64.

Tos M, Stangerup SE. The causes of asymmetry of the mastoid air cell system. *Acta Otolaryngol* 1985;99:564-70.

Tos M, Stangerup SE, Andreassen UK. Size of the mastoid air cells and otitis media. *Ann Otol Rhinol Laryngol* 1985;94:386-92.

Wigand ME, Trillsch K. Surgical anatomy of the sinus epitympani. *Ann Otol Rhinol Laryngol* 1973;82:378-84.

Wullstein H. The restoration of the function of the middle ear in chronic otitis media. *Ann Otol* 1956;65:1020-41.

Wullstein HL, Wullstein SR. *Tympanoplasty: Osteoplastic Epitympanotomy.* Stuttgart: Thieme, 1990.

Wullstein SR. Osteoplastic epitympanotomy. *Ann Otol Rhinol Laryngol* 1974;83:663-69.

Yanagihara N, Gyo K, Sasaki Y, Hinohira Y. Prevention of recurrence of cholesteatoma in intact canal wall tympanoplasty. *Am J Otol* 1993;14:590-94.

Zini C. Homotransplantation de dent en tympanoplastie. *Rev Laryngol* 1970; 91:258-61

Zini C, Sanna M, Jemmi G, Gandolfi A. Transmastoid extralabyrinthine approach in traumatic facial palsy. *Am J Otol* 1985;6:216-22.

Zini C, Sanna M, Bacciu S, Delogu P, Gamoletti R, Scandellari R. Molded tympanic heterograft: an eight-year experience. *Am J Otol* 1985;6:253-56.

Zini C, Sheehy JL, Sanna M. *Microsurgery of Cholesteatoma of the Middle Ear.* Milan: Ghedini, 1993.

Zöllner C, Büsing CM. How useful is tricalcium phosphate ceramic in middle ear surgery? *Am J Otol* 1986;7:289-93.

Zöllner F. Tympanoplasty. In: Coates G, Schenck HP, Miller MV, eds. *Otolaryngology,* vol. 1. Hagerstown: Prior, 1959.

Index